Medical Conditions in the Physically Active

FOURTH EDITION

T0314262

Medical Conditions in the Physically Active

FOURTH EDITION

Katie Walsh Flanagan, EdD, LAT, ATC
East Carolina University

Micki Cuppett, EdD, LAT, ATC, FNAP

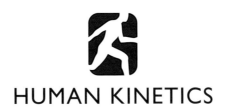

HUMAN KINETICS

Library of Congress Cataloging-in-Publication Data

Names: Cuppett, Micki, author. | Flanagan, Katie Walsh, author.
Title: Medical conditions in the physically active / Katie Walsh Flanagan,
  Micki Cuppett.
Other titles: Medical conditions in the athlete
Description: Fourth edition. | Champaign, IL : Human Kinetics, [2025] |
  Preceded by Medical conditions in the athlete / Katie Walsh Flanagan,
  Micki Cuppett. Third edition. [2017]. | Includes bibliographical
  references and index.
Identifiers: LCCN 2023029017 (print) | LCCN 2023029018 (ebook) | ISBN
  9781718215405 (paperback) | ISBN 9781718215412 (epub) | ISBN
  9781718215429 (pdf)
Subjects: MESH: Athletic Injuries | Sports Medicine--methods | Primary
  Health Care
Classification: LCC RC1210 (print) | LCC RC1210 (ebook) | NLM QT 261 |
  DDC 617.1/027--dc23/eng/20231201
LC record available at https://lccn.loc.gov/2023029017
LC ebook record available at https://lccn.loc.gov/2023029018

ISBN: 978-1-7182-1540-5 (print)

Acquisitions Editors: Jolynn Gower and Diana Vincer; **Managing Editor:** Amanda S. Ewing; **Copyeditor:** Christina West; **Proofreader:** Leigh Keylock; **Indexer:** Dan Connolly; **Permissions Manager:** Laurel Mitchell; **Senior Graphic Designer:** Joe Buck; **Cover Designer:** Keri Evans; **Cover Design Specialist:** Susan Rothermel Allen; **Photographs (cover):** Adamkaz/E+/Getty Images, Athletic Trainers Association of Florida, © Human Kinetics, © Human Kinetics; **Photographs (interior):** © Human Kinetics, unless otherwise noted; **Photo Asset Manager:** Laura Fitch; **Photo Production Manager:** Jason Allen; **Senior Art Manager:** Kelly Hendren; **Illustrations:** © Human Kinetics, unless otherwise noted; **Printer:** Premier Print Group

Printed in the United States of America

10 9 8 7 6 5 4 3 2 1

Human Kinetics
1607 N. Market Street
Champaign, IL 61820
USA

United States and International
Website: **US.HumanKinetics.com**
Email: info@hkusa.com
Phone: 1-800-747-4457

Canada
Website: **Canada.HumanKinetics.com**
Email: info@hkcanada.com

E8775

This book is dedicated to the memory of my brother, Kevin Brendan Walsh Jr., who lived life large and was taken too soon, and to my ever-patient husband, Sean, who believes wholly in me and keeps me laughing. Everyone should have a fantastic person like Sean in their lives.

—Katie Walsh Flanagan

This book is dedicated to the thousands of students whom I've had the privilege of teaching throughout my career. May you strive to provide the best patient care possible and continue to advance the athletic training profession. It is also dedicated to my loving husband, Michael, who supports me and believes in me in both my professional and personal life.

—Micki Cuppett

CONTENTS

CONDITION FINDER

PREFACE

This textbook is designed for the health care provider who works with a physically active population. Providers are referred to variously throughout the text as *athletic trainers*, *health care providers*, *examiners*, and *clinicians*. We use these multiple titles to help readers better understand the role they play in identifying and treating the conditions described in this text.

Although this text is not exclusively for athletic trainers, health care providers working in the collegiate and secondary school settings facilitate the primary care for their athletes and patients and are often the first to detect their potential medical issues. The athletic trainer continues to assume a greater role in the health care of patients, and this places more emphasis on the clinical diagnosis and the coordinated plan of care for patients' medical problems. In part, this is a result of advances in medical science that now enable athletes with certain medical conditions to compete at the highest levels. It also is the result of expanding employment opportunities for athletic trainers. They are employed in industries, inpatient hospitals, outpatient clinics, military, performing arts, fire and police, and other nontraditional workplaces as well as in the traditional realms of interscholastic, intercollegiate, and professional sport. Athletic trainers work carefully with and under the direction of physicians and see a more diverse population, including pediatric athletes, patients who are physically active, mature and older adults, and those with physical impairments. Athletic trainers establish a rapport with their patients and are familiar with their medical histories, their normal performance levels, as well as the demands of their sport, activity, or workplace on their bodies. This relationship may enable the athletic trainer to detect a condition that otherwise might go unnoticed. Although many athletic issues are orthopedic in nature, the conditions an athletic trainer encounters can also include infections, colds, and other maladies that need to be identified quickly and treated properly or referred in order for the patient to perform at optimal levels.

This book is a comprehensive resource that covers medical conditions by body system, their mechanism of acquisition, signs, symptoms, differential diagnoses, referral, treatment, and return-to-participation criteria. The text also includes associated chapters on diagnostic imaging and tests, pharmacology, psychological and substance abuse disorders, and special populations.

The purpose of this text is not only to provide information but also to help readers develop a framework for decision-making. We assume that readers are versed in basic human anatomy and physiology and basic health care such as bloodborne pathogens, communication, and patient-centered care.

Updates

Updates have been made throughout the text to showcase new content and references. In particular, the following updates were made to the fourth edition:

- Information about the prevention of disease transmission, bloodborne pathogens, and barriers to disease transmission is now included in the infectious diseases chapter.
- The systemic disorders chapter discusses new conditions, such as gout, pseudogout, rheumatoid arthritis, osteoarthritis, osteomyelitis, and polymyositis and dermatomyositis.
- Endocrine disorders, specifically pancreatitis, diabetes, and hyper- and hypothyroidism, are discussed in a standalone chapter.
- Updated photos show dermatological conditions on a greater variety of skin tones.

Organization

This textbook is separated into three parts. Part I, Introduction to Medical Conditions, begins with an overview of the medical examination, including communication skills, review of systems, and effective use of evaluation tools. These introductory chapters also include diagnostic imaging and testing that are mentioned throughout the textbook.

Part II, Pharmacology and Interventions, contains three chapters relating to pharmacology, therapeutic drug categories, and common invasive procedures seen in the athletic training clinic. It is important for on-site health care providers to know how to maintain a sterile field and the procedures for wound closure, injections, and intravenous administrations. Readers are reminded that practice acts in some states do not allow athletic trainers to perform some of the procedures included in chapter 5.

Part III, Medical Conditions by System, follows a systematic approach as the chapters address common conditions and diseases by body system. Most chapters follow a simple template. They begin with an overview of the relevant anatomy and physiology as they relate to the body system; identify specific conditions; explain signs and symptoms, including potential differential diagnoses; describe referral and diagnostic tests; discuss treatment and return to participation; and finally, discuss prognoses and prevention, if applicable. If a condition has related age- or sex-specific considerations, those issues are also discussed. Implications for pediatric and mature athletes are also included when relevant. Chapters relating to systemic conditions detail signs and symptoms that cross body systems, and the infectious diseases chapter begins with infection control and mitigation before discussing common childhood infectious diseases and other transmittable conditions. This section concludes with chapters on psychological and substance use disorders and working with active special populations.

Textbook Features

When applicable, we include current National Athletic Trainers' Association (NATA), National Collegiate Athletics Association (NCAA), and National Federation of State High School Associations (NFHS) position statements and references. Content is expanded and reinforced by clinical tips, red flags, and condition highlight elements.

- **Clinical Tips** present key points to help reinforce student understanding.
- **Red Flags** present warnings to readers.
- **Condition Highlight** spotlights a condition specific to the chapter that is either common or warrants additional emphasis.

More than 370 photos and illustrations enhance the reader's comprehension of anatomy, physiology, and pathophysiology. Pharmacological tables provide easy access to a full range of drug categories with generic and trade names, therapeutic uses, adult dosage information, and possible adverse effects. Important terminology is highlighted throughout the chapters, and a glossary appears at the end of the book.

Student Resources in HK*Propel*

Perhaps the most unique feature of this text is HK*Propel*, which contains three case studies per chapter. Each case study allows students to apply strategies taught in the text to the scenario presented in the case study.

Instructor Resources in HK*Propel*

Instructors have access to a full array of ancillary materials within the instructor pack in HK*Propel*:

- **Presentation package.** The presentation package includes more than 900 slides that provide detailed lecture notes and select art, photos, and tables from the text. Instructors can modify these slides as needed to best fit their classes and lecture format.
- **Image bank.** The image bank contains most of the art, photos, and tables from the text, which can be used to create custom presentations, student handouts, and other materials.
- **Instructor guide.** The instructor guide contains a file for each chapter that provides a chapter summary, a robust chapter outline, suggested activities, and suggested topics.
- **Test package.** The test package includes 540 questions in true-false, multiple-choice, fill-in-the-blank, short-answer, matching, and multiple response formats. These questions are available in multiple formats for a variety of instructor uses and can be used to create tests and quizzes to measure student understanding.
- **Chapter quizzes.** These LMS-compatible, ready-made quizzes can be used to measure student learning of the most important concepts for each chapter. Ten questions per chapter are included in true-false, multiple-choice, matching, and multiple response formats.

Adopting instructors receive free instructor ancillaries, including an ebook version of the text that allows instructors to add highlights, annotations, and bookmarks. Please contact your sales manager for details about how to access instructor resources in HK*Propel*.

Final Thoughts

We are athletic training educators and practitioners who have pooled our experience and worked with our colleagues in athletic training and medicine to design this textbook and the ancillary resources. We present it to you as an informative and easy-to-use instructional tool for beginning and advanced students as well as an indispensable reference guide for practitioners in the field. We look forward to your feedback and suggestions for future editions.

ACKNOWLEDGMENTS

We wish to thank the many people who made this project possible. First, we thank the current and past chapter contributors for providing their knowledge of the subject matter and expertise in their fields. They took time away from their busy practices and lives to ensure the text's accuracy and currency. We appreciate their spectacular responses to a tight timeline and their ongoing support of the project.

We are forever grateful to the Human Kinetics team that has made publication of this fourth edition an enjoyable process. It was a pleasure working with Jolynn Gower, our acquisitions editor, who shepherded us through the initial revisions for this edition. We had the great fortune to work once again with Amanda Ewing, our managing editor, who reviewed our work and provided excellent suggestions and edits. Her continuous communications, dedication, and patience kept us on task and focused. A thank-you will never truly convey our appreciation for her work. Diana Vincer who worked patiently with us as we strived to convey to her our vision for the cover of this edition. We appreciate her enduring stamina while we worked together to get it right.

Finally, we recognize and appreciate the tenacity of our friendship, which began more than two decades ago at a professional meeting and evolved into "Hey, let's do this project!" It has remained strong throughout the pursuit of our vision of improving the educational experience in the field of medicine for the athletic trainer. We have learned that with vision, drive, and determination, anything is possible if good friends keep pulling and pushing each other in the same direction with a common goal.

PART I

Introduction to Medical Conditions

This textbook begins with an overview of the basic information presented in subsequent chapters. (It is expected that this book is used later in the curriculum, so the roles of the athletic trainer and other rudimentary information are not covered.)

Chapter 1, Medical Examination, is the most critical chapter in this text. It discusses the basic evaluation tools that will assist the reader throughout the remainder of the book. Health history, observation and inspection, palpation, and diagnostic tests are explained thoroughly. Photographs and carefully detailed procedures instruct the reader on the use of special equipment and techniques for the medical examination. Topics covered include assessing blood pressure, pulse, respiration, and temperature; using evaluation tools, such as stethoscopes, ophthalmo-scopes, and otoscopes; and performing various diagnostic procedures, such as neurological testing (dermatomes, deep tendon reflex arc, and cranial nerve assessment), palpation, percussion, and auscultation.

Chapter 2, Diagnostic Imaging and Testing, describes various diagnostic imaging procedures (X-ray, radionuclide bone scan, fluoroscopy, computed tomography, positron omission tomography, and magnetic resonance imaging), their associated risks and side effects, and many diagnostic testing procedures (electrocardiography, Holter monitoring, stress tests, and laparoscopy). Many laboratory tests, such as urinalysis, complete blood count, and lumbar punctures, are described so that readers can tell their patients what to expect.

Medical
Examination

1

OBJECTIVES

At the completion of this chapter the reader should be able to do the following:

1. Perform a thorough patient history, including history of the current problem, past medical history, family history, and social history.

2. Perform a basic general medical examination, including a cephalocaudal review of systems.

3. Contrast the differences between orthopedic and medical assessment.

4. Differentiate between a focal orthopedic examination and a medical examination of conditions that may affect many organ systems.

5. Demonstrate the proper use of evaluation tools and techniques for the assessment of general health.

6. Apply the basics of palpation, percussion, and auscultation in a general medical examination.

The initial medical examination requires listening intently to patients as they provide a thorough history of the current problem. In addition, the clinician must complete a thorough medical history of past conditions, including family and social history. This chapter outlines the examination process and focuses on the evaluation techniques and equipment used in a medical examination. It introduces the use of the otoscope, ophthalmoscope, and stethoscope; presents basic techniques in palpation, percussion, and auscultation; and discusses general information about normal vital signs. The chapters that follow present a more detailed explanation of both normal and abnormal examination results as well as detailed signs and symptoms for common disorders for each body system. Later chapters assume that readers have reviewed and understood this chapter and are familiar with the equipment and techniques used in a general medical examination.

Examination of the Patient With a Medical Condition

Examination of the patient with a nonorthopedic condition may present the health care provider with a challenge. Often there is no identifiable onset, and there may be few signs that anything is wrong. Each evaluation begins with a thorough history, followed by an overall systemic review, and, finally, an examination specific to the condition. The clinician must rely heavily on the patient's history to guide the examination.

Comprehensive Medical History

A medical health history taken to ascertain the extent of a medical condition or illness is vastly different from an orthopedic history. In an athletic injury, the condition is

Clinical Tips

Effective Communication With Patients

- Ask open-ended questions.
- Maintain eye contact, if culturally respectful.
- Display an open, relaxed posture.
- Repeat key words spoken by the patient.
- Use simple phrases for encouragement, such as "go on" or "mm-hmm."

typically contained within one joint, muscle, or bone, and it usually involves only the musculoskeletal system. In contrast, a medical condition may involve many body systems, may be difficult to describe, and may not be at all obvious. The clinician must understand **comorbid** conditions that may exist with a medical condition. In addition, the clinician must understand how the questions asked when taking a health history for a medical condition differ from those for an orthopedic injury. Typical orthopedic questions inquire about the mechanism of injury, sounds associated with the onset (e.g., snap, crunch, or pop), and immediate disability associated with the injury, such as swelling, inability to bear weight, deformity, and radiculopathy. Questions in a medical health history review the patient's body systems as relevant. Questions about symptoms are critical because symptoms cannot be measured objectively, yet they may offer clues about the patient's condition. Consider the following questions when taking a patient's history for a medical condition.

- Describe your symptoms.
- How long have you had these symptoms?
- Do your symptoms interfere with activities of daily living?
- Are you currently taking any medications, vitamins, or supplements?
- Do your symptoms tend to occur at a specific time (e.g., after eating, when exercising, after exposure to an allergen, or at night)?
- Do your symptoms come and go, or are they constant?
- Are you sleeping well, according to your normal habits?
- Do you feel more fatigued than usual?
- Have you recently changed your diet, medication, activity level, or personal habits?
- Are you under more stress than usual?

- Are you having normal bowel and bladder function? (This may help to determine whether the condition is gastrointestinal.)
- Is there anything else going on that you would like to discuss?

Other aspects of a medical history include the duration of signs and symptoms, onset (e.g., rapid, insidious, or gradual), and resulting disability. Some medical situations may be life-threatening and may require complex information to make a correct but timely decision on treatment and patient referral. For example, a mild upper respiratory infection may be treated with over-the-counter medications, whereas a long-term respiratory tract infection or asthma requires physician intervention and medication.

Usually, the examiner begins to take a comprehensive medical history by identifying and recording a patient's age and biological sex. If race, ethnicity, marital status, occupation, and religion are important to the diagnosis or treatment, they may be documented as well.[1] Next, the patient's chief complaint is identified, including present illness, onset, and setting when symptoms were first apparent. Helpful information for the examiner may include the following descriptions of the chief complaint: location of discomfort, the quality or quantity of symptoms (including their frequency, onset, and duration), and any associated factors that aggravate or alleviate symptoms. Patients should be asked whether they are currently using medications, supplements, vitamins, home remedies, or poultices. Also, the examiner needs to know whether the patient has shared or borrowed prescription medications from someone else.

For patients with a medical condition, the next sections of a comprehensive history include past medical history, current health status, family history, and social history. Past medical history incorporates illnesses, as well as

Clinical Tips

Knowing the Difference Between a Sign and a Symptom

Although the terms *signs* and *symptoms* are generally used together during the assessment of a medical condition, they are not synonymous.

- A *sign* refers to something that the athletic trainer sees or feels, such as a temperature, respiration, heartbeat, or blood pressure. A sign can be objectively measured or assessed.
- A *symptom* refers to something the patient feels or tells the examiner about, such as headache, nausea, dizziness, or pain.

Chief Complaints

Descriptions important to evaluation are the following:

- Locations of discomfort
- Quality or quantity of symptoms
- Frequency
- Onset
- Duration
- Any associated factors that aggravate or alleviate the symptoms

accidents and injuries, in childhood and adulthood. Keep in mind that illnesses in adulthood also may include psychiatric, obstetrical, or gynecological conditions and surgery. Typically, the patient's current health status covers exercise, diet, immunizations, medications, and use of alcohol, illicit substances, or tobacco. The examiner asks questions about any history of allergies and specific reactions to antigens and ensures that the patient is up to date with routine screening tests (e.g., Papanicolaou or Pap smear, breast and testicular self-examinations), if relevant to the complaint, and with current vaccinations. It may also be appropriate to explore the environmental safety of the home and workplace.

A look into the patient's family history may be useful in identifying susceptibility to a given illness or disease and may prove helpful in the examination and care of the patient. Diabetes, heart disease, hypertension, kidney disease, cardiovascular disorders (e.g., deep vein thrombosis or stroke), allergies, asthma, mental illness, and addiction are all examples of conditions and diseases with a genetic tendency. Age, current health, cause of death, and age at death of immediate family members are also important in a family health history.

The personal and social history includes information to help clinicians better understand their patients. This category covers a patient's education, occupation, significant others, home life, daily activities, hobbies, and important beliefs. Although this information is not critical to diagnosing specific conditions, it profoundly affects the patients' overall health and attitude toward wellness.[2]

Review of Body Systems

The review of body systems is the health care provider's primary focus in the evaluation of medical conditions. Indeed, most health care professionals use the comprehensive medical history and review of body systems to assess medical issues. Traditionally, all body systems are reviewed, in contrast with an orthopedic assessment that focuses on the anatomical area or system believed to be affected. A medical review differs from an orthopedic evaluation in that the examiner may stop after crepitus is determined rather than continue to look for ligamentous injury. For example, if the patient has a clearly displaced fractured femur, the examiner does not continue the initial evaluation to determine whether the anterior cruciate ligament is intact.

The goal of the review of body systems during an examination for a general medical condition is to enable the clinician to gather enough information to provide treatment, make an intelligent decision about patient referral, and, if necessary, refer the patient to a specific type of practitioner.

The review of body systems always begins with a general assessment of the patient's condition, including weight and associated changes, fatigue, fever, and any reported sleep disturbances. Then the review continues system by system, starting with the skin and descending from head to toe. When assessing the skin, the examiner looks for obvious rashes, sores, dryness, color change, lumps, or swelling and asks the patient about itching or skin dryness.

A good mnemonic to help remember the order of the first part of the review of systems is HEENT:

Head
Eyes
Ears
Nose
Throat

Family Health History

Conditions and diseases that have a genetic tendency include the following:

- Diabetes
- Heart disease
- Hypertension
- Kidney disease
- Cardiovascular disorders (deep vein thrombosis, myocardial infarction, or stroke)
- Allergies
- Asthma
- Mental illness
- Addiction

Head

Beginning with signs and symptoms associated with the head, the examiner asks about the following:

- Headaches
- Seizures
- Syncope
- Tremors
- Paralysis
- History of a head injury

Eyes

Essential questions to ask about the eyes concern the following:

- Visual acuity
- Need to wear corrective lenses
- Surgical history that may include procedures that correct vision
- Date and results of last eye examination
- Any history of redness, tearing, diplopia, floaters, pain, dryness, or disease of the eye

Ears

Questions linked to the ears relate to symptoms of the following:

- Tinnitus
- Vertigo
- Earaches
- Signs of ear dysfunction, such as discharge

Nose

Patients with nasal problems or conditions of the accompanying sinuses can present with the following:

- Discharge
- Sinus pain
- Itching
- Sneezing
- Stuffiness

Throat

Mouth and throat problems are manifested by the following:

- Hoarseness
- Sores
- Caries
- Halitosis
- Bleeding gums

Pain or stiffness in the neck can indicate an infectious disease, and enlarged glands are palpable signs of a response to changes in the body.

Questions about breast discomfort, lumps, or nipple discharge may be relevant if the examiner is given information that points to pathology of the breast tissue. These questions may be pertinent to both sexes.

The review of systems continues with the respiratory, cardiovascular, gastrointestinal, urinary, and gynecological systems and follows the same **cephalocaudal** order.[1]

- *Respiratory.* Signs associated with respiratory problems include the presence of excessive sputum, altered respiratory sounds, and hemoptysis.
- *Cardiovascular.* The cardiovascular system encompasses the heart and blood vessels, including blood pressure. Symptoms of cardiovascular anomalies include murmurs, dyspnea, chest pain, vasovagal responses, hypertension, and syncope.
- *Gastrointestinal.* Gastrointestinal problems may manifest with symptoms such as heartburn, nausea, constipation, and food intolerance. Signs include vomiting, stool changes (e.g., in frequency, consistency, and/or color), rectal bleeding, diarrhea, gas, and jaundice.
- *Urinary.* Incontinence, pain, discolored urine, or any change in frequency of urination may indicate genitourinary system pathology, and referral is warranted. A male patient who complains of penile sores, discharge, or hesitancy in voiding should be referred to a physician.
- *Gynecological.* Gynecological disorders include delayed onset of menses, oligomenorrhea, dysmenorrhea, polymenorrhea, severe cramping, late menstrual period, abnormal pain, discharge, and vaginal sores. The examiner questions the patient about these symptoms if gynecological issues are raised when discussing the patient's current health history.

After the cephalocaudal systems review, the evaluation continues to other prevalent body systems: peripheral vascular, musculoskeletal, neurological, hematological, endocrine, and psychiatric. Important areas to explore include complaints of loss of sensation in the extremities, pitting edema, soreness and swelling in multiple joints, and abnormal fatigue.[2] Specific questions about these systems are discussed later in the appropriate chapters. After the review of all systems, the examiner begins a physical examination of the patient.

Physical Examination

Again, the examiner follows the universally accepted cephalocaudal sequence for the physical examination (see the Sequence of Symptom Review and Physical Examination sidebar). The general survey includes observation of the patient's apparent state of health, level of consciousness, signs of distress, height and weight, skin color, obvious lesions, and hygiene.[3] These are noted as the patient enters the examination area. The practitioner continues the physical assessment in the same order as the previously described review of systems, beginning with the vital signs and skin and advancing from the head down the body. The proper evaluation tools should be ready to expedite the examination.

Vital Signs

Assessment of all vital signs includes height and weight, blood pressure, heart and respiratory rate and rhythm, and body temperature.

Height and Weight

Recording a patient's height and weight is essential because it provides a baseline for future reference. Height is often critical to athletes but is typically of only mild

Sequence of Symptom Review and Physical Examination

General
Fatigue and energy
Desired weight
Fever

Diet
Appetite
Supplements
Restrictions

Skin, Hair, and Nails
Appearance
Color

Head and Neck
Supple neck
Headache
LOC
Dizziness

Eyes
Visual acuity
Corrective lenses
Visual disturbances

Ears
Vertigo
Tinnitus
Hearing acuity
Discharge

Nose
Functional
Congestion
History of bleeding

Mouth and Throat
Hoarseness
Sore throat
Dental issues
Chewing tobacco

Gastrointestinal System
Heartburn
Vomiting
Diarrhea
Constipation

Lymphatic System
Swelling
Pitting edema
Tenderness

Endocrine System
Heat or cold intolerance
Weight or energy change

Female
FMP/LMP
Regularity
Symptoms

Male
Testicular pain or swelling

Breasts
Swelling
Lumps
Pain

Chest and Lungs
SOB
Dyspnea
Night sweats
Cough
Sputum

Cardiovascular System
Chest pain
Exercise history
Exertional SOB

Hematology
Bruising history

Genitourinary System
Urine frequency, volume, or color
Dysuria

Musculoskeletal System
Joint or muscle pain or swelling
Neurological symptoms

Mental Status
Eating, sleeping, or social habits
Mood
Concentration

Note: FMP = first menstrual period; LMP = last menstrual period; LOC = level of consciousness; SOB = shortness of breath.

interest to the health care practitioner. Weight is more critical because a drastic change, whether gain or loss, can indicate a health problem and should be followed up in a timely fashion.

Height is typically measured with a stadiometer or, particularly with extremely tall patients, a tape measure fastened to the wall. The patient removes shoes and stands with the back to the stadiometer or wall, placing all weight on the heels. When using a stadiometer, the clinician stands to the side of the patient and raises the stadiometer to the patient's height. The horizontal arm rests at the crown of the patient's head. The height measurement is read on the instrument's vertical scale (figure 1.1). If not using a stadiometer, the athletic trainer must accurately mark increments on the wall or fasten a tape measure to the wall. The athletic trainer stands to the side of the patient (on a stool if necessary) and uses a flat surface on a sagittal plane along the crown of the patient's head to evenly mark the height measurement on the wall. Height may be recorded in either centimeters or inches and should be indicated as such in the medical record (1 in. = 2.54 cm).

Normal body weight is measured without shoes or excessive clothing. Weight is a confidential measurement, so the health care practitioner should ensure privacy

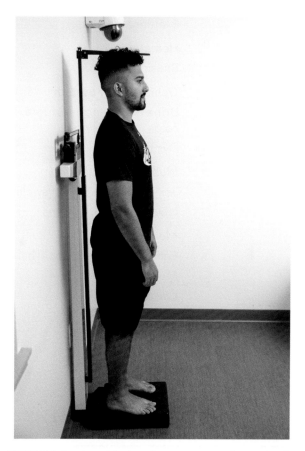

FIGURE 1.1   An athletic trainer measures the patient's height with a stadiometer.

for the patient during weighing when possible. Weight is typically recorded in medical records in kilograms but may also be recorded in pounds (1 kg = 2.2 lb). During preseason or excessively warm days, take weight measurements several times each day (preexercise and postexercise) to monitor proper hydration levels in an attempt to identify patients losing excessive amounts of fluid during exercise.[4] Standardization of measurements can be improved by following the same procedures each time height and weight are measured—for example, measuring both height and weight in the morning and having patients wear standard attire of gym shorts and a T-shirt. More accurate assessments of body composition exclusive of height and weight charts include hydrostatic weighing, skinfold calipers, bioimpedance, and body mass index.

Blood Pressure

A stethoscope and sphygmomanometer of the correct size will measure blood pressure properly. This is especially important for the athletic trainer, who often must evaluate extremely muscular or large patients for whom a regular-size blood pressure cuff is too small. Using a cuff that is too small results in a reading that is incorrect, indicating abnormally high blood pressure. Normal resting blood pressure is measured after the patient has been resting quietly for a period of time, never immediately after any physical exertion.[2,5]

The patient is positioned (e.g., seated in a chair) in a quiet area. The selected arm is free of clothing and positioned so the brachial artery is roughly at heart level; for example, the patient can rest the arm on a table next to the chair. The patient must not have their legs or arms crossed for this examination. The sphygmomanometer is placed around the upper arm, with the lower edge of the cuff about 2.5 cm above the antecubital crease (figure 1.2). The cuff is snugly secured around the arm with the Velcro fasteners, and the aneroid dial is positioned with its face toward the examiner. The diaphragm of the stethoscope is placed lightly over the brachial artery in the antecubital crease, under the sphygmomanometer, touching the skin.

The cuff is inflated first to greater than 200 mmHg and then gradually deflated at a rate of 2 to 3 mmHg/s. While deflating the cuff, the examiner listens for two consecutive beats, which will indicate the systolic pressure, and notes the numerical value on the aneroid dial when this occurs. The examiner continues to deflate the blood pressure cuff slowly until the sound becomes muffled and finally disappears. The level at which the sound disappears is the diastolic pressure; this is often referred to as the fifth **Korotkoff sound** (the last in a series of sounds produced by distention of an artery by the cuff). Systolic pressure is related to contraction of the heart ventricles, whereas diastolic pressure represents relaxation of the ventricles. The effect of the cuff on arterial blood flow is related to the auscultatory findings. Table 1.1 lists the phase and quality of each sound. Chapter 7 provides more details on cardiac output and blood pressure, and

Clinical Tips

Use of a Blood Pressure Cuff

- Blood pressure cuffs come in various sizes.
- A cuff that is too small gives an abnormally high blood pressure reading.

table 1.2 presents normal and abnormal blood pressure readings for adults.

Pulse Rate and Rhythm

The examiner determines the heart rate by feeling the radial pulse at the wrist with the pads of the index and middle fingers (figure 1.3). Once the pulse is found, the number of beats in 15 s is counted and then multiplied by 4 to estimate the heart rate (a normal, resting heart rate is 60-72 beats/min). The pulse is described by its rate, rhythm, and force.

Rate

Bradycardia: <60 beats/min

Tachycardia: >100 beats/min

Rhythm

Sinus arrhythmia: Heart rate speeds up at peak of inspiration and slows to normal with expiration

Force

4+	Bounding
3+	Increased
2+	Normal
1+	Weak, thready
Absent	

The examiner notes any irregular rhythms and further evaluates by auscultating with the stethoscope at the cardiac apex,[6] keeping in mind that it is normal for physically fit patients to have bradycardia—that is, a pulse rate of 60 beats/min or less. The pulse is also easily palpable at the carotid artery, the posterior tibial artery, and other pulse points (figure 1.4). Pulse characteristics at the distal extremities give the examiner information about the status of blood flow to those extremities.

Respiratory Rate and Rhythm

Evaluation of respiration includes the rate, effort, and depth of inspiration as well as the ratio of the depth of inspiration to expiration. The rate is quantified by counting the number of respirations in 1 min. The normal respiration rate for an adult is 12 to 20 breaths/min.[6] When assessing the rate, the examiner evaluates the patient's effort by watching for symmetry and the use of accessory muscles (sternocleidomastoid, trapezius, intercostals) to assist in breathing.

Temperature

Assessment of temperature can be omitted if there is no reason to suspect fever or heat-related illness. It may be wise, however, to record the temperature of any patient presenting with a nonorthopedic complaint, because temperature sometimes provides a defining clue to the severity of the condition. Normal temperature fluctuates considerably from the commonly reported oral temperature of 37 °C (98.6 °F); it may be as low as 35.8 °C (96.4 °F) in the early morning hours and as high as 37.3 °C (99.1 °F) in the evening. Rectal temperatures are higher than oral temperatures by 0.4 to 0.5 °C,[7] but this difference is also variable. In addition, athletes who have just finished a workout, recently experienced a heat modality (e.g., a warm whirlpool or Hydrocollator), or

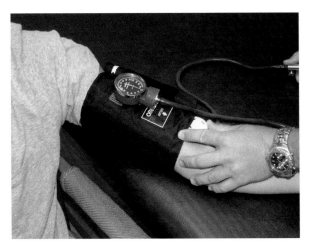

FIGURE 1.2 The sphygmomanometer is used to assess blood pressure.

© Micki Cuppett

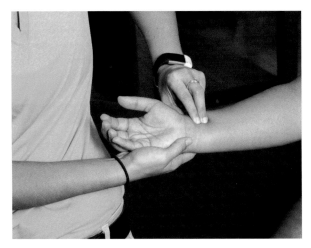

FIGURE 1.3 A pulse can be taken at the radial artery in the wrist.

TABLE 1.1   **Understanding Korotkoff Sounds When Assessing Blood Pressure**

Phase	Quality	Description	Rationale
Cuff inflated to occlude brachial artery	No sound		The brachial artery is compressed by exceeding the heart's systolic pressure with the cuff inflation; therefore, no blood is flowing under the stethoscope.
I	Tapping	Tapping sound, starting soft and increasing in intensity	As the pressure lessens, an audible sound is created as the blood flows into the brachial artery at a high velocity.
Auscultatory gap (abnormal sound)	No sound	Silence for up to 30-40 mmHg	In a person with hypertension, the sounds may temporarily disappear toward the end of phase I and then reappear in phase II. If undetected, this results in a falsely low systolic reading or a falsely high diastolic reading.
II	Swooshing	Softer murmur follows tapping	Because the artery is still partially occluded, the turbulent blood flow is audible as a swooshing sound.
III	Knocking	Crisp, high-pitched sounds	Sound is created with the less turbulent flow of blood through the artery. The artery closes momentarily during the latter part of diastole.
IV	Abrupt muffling	Sound mutes to a low-pitched, cushioned murmur; blowing quality	Once the artery is no longer occluded, the blood flow changes to a low-pitched murmur.
V	Silence		The disappearance of the last audible sound is called the fifth Korotkoff sound and defines diastolic blood pressure. Silence occurs when blood flow returns to normal velocity.

TABLE 1.2   **Understanding Blood Pressure Readings**

Blood pressure	Systolic (mmHg)	Diastolic (mmHg)
Normal	<120	<80
Elevated	120-129	<80
Hypertension		
Stage 1	130-139	80-89
Stage 2	≥140	≥90
Hypertensive crisis	>180	>120

A physician should evaluate low or high readings.

Adapted from "The Facts About High Blood Pressure," American Heart Association, last modified May 25, 2023, https://www.heart.org/en/health-topics/high-blood-pressure/the-facts-about-high-blood-pressure.

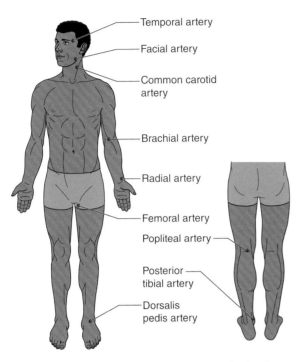

Temporal artery

Facial artery

Common carotid artery

Brachial artery

Radial artery

Femoral artery

Popliteal artery

Posterior tibial artery

Dorsalis pedis artery

FIGURE 1.4 Common pulse points on the body surface where arterial pulses can be assessed.

consumed a hot beverage can present with a slightly elevated temperature. It is important to note that temperature accuracy varies by thermometer type and anatomical site. Although some thermometers (e.g., contactless) may be fine for general screening purposes, the gold standard for evaluating conditions such as exertional heat illness is rectal temperature.[8,9]

It is important to maintain thermometer sanitation. Electronic thermometers must be covered with single-use plastic covers to ensure sanitation, and tympanic and temporal thermometers likewise must have single-use protective covers. Contactless thermometers must be cleaned frequently, but they require less sanitation because they have no skin contact. Figure 1.5 presents several types of thermometers:

- Figures 1.5*a* and 1.5*b* show both oral and tympanic thermometers.
- Figure 1.5*c* shows a contactless temporal thermometer. (Some clinics will use a temporal thermometer that actually touches the skin.) These thermometers are increasingly common, are safe, and measure temperature very quickly. However, they are not reliable for assessing heat-related illnesses.

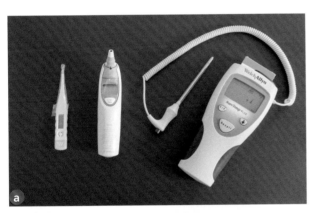

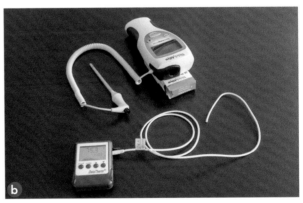

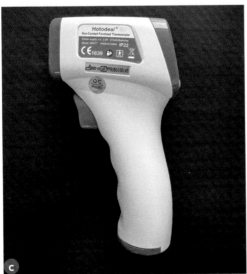

FIGURE 1.5 *(a)* Oral and tympanic thermometers. Note the blue coloring on the digital oral thermometer. *(b)* Both of these digital thermometers measure rectal (core) temperature. The Welch Allyn unit is interchangeable with the blue oral thermometer. The DataTherm unit is designed to have the sensor remain in the anus while cooling measures are administered to the body. *(c)* Contactless temporal thermometer.

(c) © Micki Cuppett.

Clinical Tips

Core Temperature

- When assessing conditions of suspected heat-related illness, one should use a rectal thermometer.

- A rectal temperature is the only temperature measurement proven to be a reliable measure of core body temperature.

If the patient is unconscious or suspected to have a heat-related illness, the examiner measures the rectal temperature to provide a better indicator of core temperature. The examiner places the patient in a side-lying position with the hip flexed. A probe cover is used with an electronic rectal thermometer. The examiner lubricates the thermometer tip with petroleum jelly or K-Y jelly before inserting it into the anal canal to 2.5 cm (1 in.). The cheeks of the patient's buttocks must be spread slightly to allow for proper insertion of the probe. If a digital thermistor is used, lubricate the thermistor tip before inserting it into the rectum. The thermistor is to be inserted 6 to 10 cm (2-3 in.).

Infrared wave sensors are most commonly used in tympanic thermometers. Tympanic thermometers are increasingly common, are safe, and measure temperature very quickly. However, their reliability has been questioned, especially in the athletic setting or in the assessment of heat-related illness. In suspected heat-related conditions, rectal temperature determination is the only method currently shown to reliably measure core temperature. A rectal probe with a remote display will allow monitoring of core body temperature even while the patient is being cooled in an ice bath.[8,10,11]

To use a tympanic thermometer, the examiner places the covered probe of the thermometer so that the beam has a direct route to the tympanic membrane. The auditory canal needs to be free of excessive cerumen. Within 2 to 3 s, the tympanic temperature registers on the thermometer. Temperatures taken with the tympanic thermometer are generally 0.8 °C (1.4 °F) higher than normal oral temperatures.

A temporal thermometer uses infrared waves to measure the temperature of the temporal artery in the forehead and is used more frequently than the tympanic thermometer.

Contactless thermometers do not touch the patient's skin. These thermometers were used extensively during the COVID-19 pandemic from 2020 to 2022 for regular temperature screening of large groups of people. It is important not to interchange measurements from peripheral thermometers (contactless) to digital or rectal as there is variability between them.[8,12]

The axillary method, in which a thermometer is placed in the axilla for 10 min, is sometimes used to measure temperature. This method was most often used with infants but is no longer as popular now that tympanic and temporal thermometers are readily available.

Evaluation Tools

In addition to hands for palpation, the examiner may use several tools during an examination. This section describes each tool and its proper use. Some tools require more practice than others.

Stethoscope

A good-quality acoustic stethoscope is sufficient for most examinations by athletic trainers. More sophisticated stethoscopes (magnetic, digital, stereophonic, or Doppler) are used to auscultate less obvious sounds. An acoustic stethoscope contains a diaphragm and a bell that are heavy enough to lay firmly on the body surface and thick, heavy tubing to conduct the sound (figure 1.6).[2] Earpieces fit snugly and comfortably.

To correctly use a stethoscope, the examiner first ensures that the tubing is "open" to the desired head (bell or diaphragm), depending on which side is against

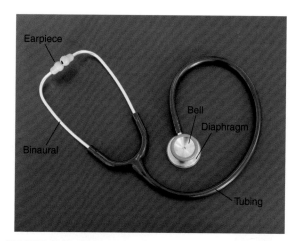

FIGURE 1.6 The parts of an acoustic stethoscope.

Clinical Tips

Using a Stethoscope

- The bell is used to hear low-pitched sounds.

- The diaphragm is used to hear high-pitched sounds.

- For best results, place the diaphragm or bell directly on the skin.

- Be sure the valve is open to the appropriate side of the stethoscope (bell or diaphragm).

the skin. The opening can be changed to the other head by twisting the stem. The examiner holds the end piece between the fingers, pressing the diaphragm (used for high-pitched sounds) firmly against the bare skin. When using the bell (for low-pitched sounds), the examiner holds it lightly on the skin to ensure that the entire bell is in contact with the skin. The tubing should not rub against itself or any other surface because extraneous noises will occur. Similarly, the environment must be noise free. The examiner listens not only for the presence or absence of sound but also for intensity, pitch, duration, and quality.[2] Listening to heart, lung, and bowel sounds through the stethoscope is called *auscultation*. Normal and abnormal sounds, as well as the order of auscultation points, are discussed at length in the respective chapters.

Ophthalmoscope

The ophthalmoscope is used to view the internal structures of the eye (figure 1.7). The head of the instrument contains a light source, which allows the examiner to visualize the inner eye through an aperture and lenses to allow for near or far focusing. The most commonly used aperture projects a large, round beam.

The ophthalmoscope also has other apertures. These include the small aperture; the slit-lamp aperture to examine the anterior eye; the red-free filter aperture,

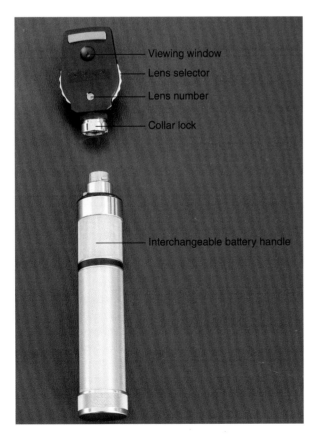

FIGURE 1.7   The parts of an ophthalmoscope.

Labels on figure:
- Viewing window
- Lens selector
- Lens number
- Collar lock
- Interchangeable battery handle

Using an Ophthalmoscope

- Viewing the interior of the eye is difficult without dilation.
- The room must be dark.
- Think of viewing a "field" through a "hole in a fence." Look through a small hole at a large object beyond the hole, and move the eye and the ophthalmoscope to adequately see the retina.
- Follow the vessels on the retina back to the optic disk for orientation to the anatomy of the retina (more on this in chapter 11).

which shines a green beam to check the optic disk; and the grid aperture used to estimate the size of fundal lesions.[2]

The diopter (magnification power of the lens) of the ophthalmoscope may be changed by turning the lens selector or disk to the corresponding magnification.[2] The black numbers and red numbers indicate positive and negative magnification power, respectively. Turning the wheel clockwise selects positive lenses, and rotating it counterclockwise selects negative lenses. Lens numbers range from ±20 to ±140 magnification power. The range of plus and minus lenses can compensate for myopia or hyperopia in both the examiner and the patient.[2]

The heads of both the ophthalmoscope and the otoscope (used to view the ears and nose) typically share a common handle containing a rechargeable battery. The heads are interchangeable and can easily be converted from one instrument to the other. To change from an otoscope head to an ophthalmoscope head, the examiner pushes down on the head currently on the handle while turning it to unlock the attachment, inserts the other head, and fastens it to the handle in the same manner.

Both instruments are turned in the same way—namely, by pushing the on/off switch while turning the black rheostat clockwise to the desired light intensity.

Otoscope

The examiner visualizes the external auditory canal and tympanic membrane with an otoscope (figure 1.8). The otoscope consists of a lamp to direct the light for illumination and disposable speculums that protect it from contamination. The disposable speculums come in various sizes, and each is attached to the otoscope by placing it and then twisting clockwise approximately one-half turn to secure it on the instrument. The instrument also has a viewing window that magnifies the area being visualized. Some otoscopes also contain a pneumatic attachment used to test tympanic membrane integrity. In addition, the instrument can be used as a nasal speculum.

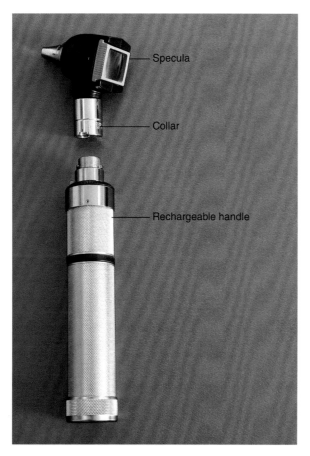

FIGURE 1.8   The otoscope uses various sizes of speculums and may have a pneumatic attachment. The chargeable base often enables the otoscope to be interchangeable with the ophthalmoscope.

Clinical Tips

Using an Otoscope

- Be sure to use a disposable speculum of the correct size.
- Pull up on the pinna of the patient's ear to straighten out the ear canal.
- Insert the speculum into the patient's ear canal before putting the otoscope to the eye.

Tuning Fork

A tuning fork (figure 1.9) is used as a diagnostic tool for many conditions. The most common uses are to check vibratory sensation or auditory sensitivity. A tuning fork with a frequency of 500 to 1,000 Hz mimics the range of normal speech and is used for auditory evaluation.[3] The examiner squeezes the fork or taps the prongs against the opposite hand to activate it while holding the tuning fork at its base.

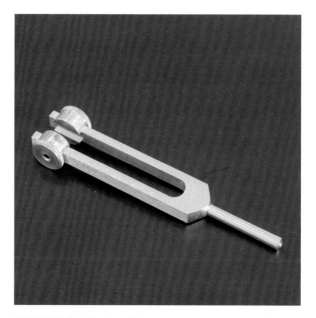

FIGURE 1.9   Tuning forks are used to assess vibratory sensations and to screen for auditory perception.

Snellen Chart

The Snellen chart is a quick and easy-to-use screening tool for distance vision and is used most often during preparticipation examinations to screen a patient's vision. The chart contains graduated sizes of letters with standardized acuity numbers at the end of each line (figure 1.10).

The patient is asked to read the lines on the chart while standing 20 ft away and covering one eye. The number corresponding to the row of the smallest letters the patient can read measures visual acuity. Although the patient is allowed to err in calling out a particular number or letter, two wrong answers on a line indicate the inability to correctly read at that distance. Visual acuity is recorded as a fraction, with the numerator of 20 indicating the distance away from the chart and the denominator being the distance at which a person with normal vision should be able to read the lettering.[13] A measurement of 20/20 is considered normal vision, with denominators greater than 20 indicating poorer vision. A person with a measurement of 20/200 is considered legally blind. Remember that this screening tool is for far visual acuity only and does not measure near vision or dynamic visual acuity. Referral to an optometrist or ophthalmologist for a complete visual assessment may be warranted. A patient who normally wears corrective lenses is screened without them, and the results of the examination are noted as being without corrective lenses. Near vision is assessed with the Rosenbaum or Jaeger chart or with a newspaper.[5]

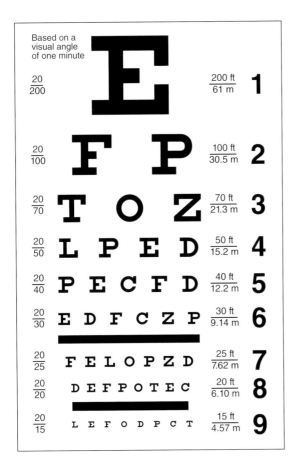

FIGURE 1.10 The Snellen chart is used to measure visual acuity.

Diagnostic Tests

Many common diagnostic tests are used to confirm specific conditions. The health care provider must be familiar with these tests, what they are used for, and what the results indicate. Common diagnostic testing and imaging is discussed in detail in chapter 2.

Neurological Testing

Neurological tests provide information about sensory, motor, and deep tendon reflexes, which may indicate pathology associated with the central nervous system or peripheral nerve trauma. The examiner performs neurological testing whenever a patient complains of paresthesia, heightened sensations, or muscular weakness.

A dermatome is a specific area of skin innervated by a dorsal or sensory nerve root. These areas tend to make a circular pattern over the body and are associated with very specific nerve roots (figure 1.11). Myotomes are single muscles or groups of muscles innervated by a single ventral or motor nerve.[6] A detailed description of dermatome and myotome evaluation is found in chapter 10.

A deep tendon reflex (DTR) is an involuntary motor reaction to a stimulus. This reflex depends on several conditions, beginning with the hammer stimulus. The dorsal fibers of sensory nerves transmit impulses from the hammer tap on the stretched tendon to sensory receptors in the muscle and along to the spinal cord. In the gray matter of the spinal cord, a flex reaction can occur if the dorsal fibers synapse with the ventral or motor fibers, which in turn travel back to stimulate the muscle to contract (figure 1.12).

This reflex will not occur if the patient's synapses are not functioning correctly or if there is damage to or disease involving either dorsal or ventral nerve fibers. The instruments used to test these pathological conditions are the reflex hammer and the neurological hammer. When conducting a neurological assessment, test bilaterally to note any differences between sides.

Reflex and Neurological Hammers

The reflex hammer is commonly used to test DTRs. The examiner holds it loosely between the thumb and index finger (figure 1.13a). The wrist is snapped rapidly downward when striking the tendon to elicit the best reflex response. Common locations for DTRs are the insertion of the biceps brachii, distal triceps tendon, distal brachioradialis tendon, patellar tendon, and Achilles tendon. The ulnar aspect of the hand or the fingertips can provide the same effect and may be used in place of the hammer when necessary. DTRs have a common rating scale for responses (table 1.3). When using the reflex hammer, the examiner places the patient in a relaxed position (sitting is best) and provides slight tension on the tendon to be tested. The examiner should palpate the tendon first to ensure they strike it correctly rather than striking the muscle.

A neurological hammer is a reflex hammer that also includes a brush and a sharp implement (stored within its handle) to use when eliciting the sensations a patient can feel, thereby assessing the integrity of dermatomes (figure 1.13b). Patients close their eyes during the test. This ensures a nondiscriminatory assessment because patients cannot witness the application of the tool. The pointed end of the tool is used to lightly depress the skin over a given dermatome, and the patient is asked if they perceive any sensation; the same dermatome on the contralateral side is then tested. Care must be taken when using the sharp implement (e.g., a toothpick lightly touched to the skin) to avoid puncturing the skin. Likewise, the brush is used to lightly brush a specific area and then test for the same sensation on the opposite limb. Other instruments that can provide a sharp, dull, and brushing effect can be used to conduct these sensory tests.

When assessing myotomes, the examiner asks the patient to actively move and then resist a given muscle group. The examiner then compares bilaterally. Tests of dermatomes and myotomes are common in orthopedic assessment and are used in many neurological assessments as well.

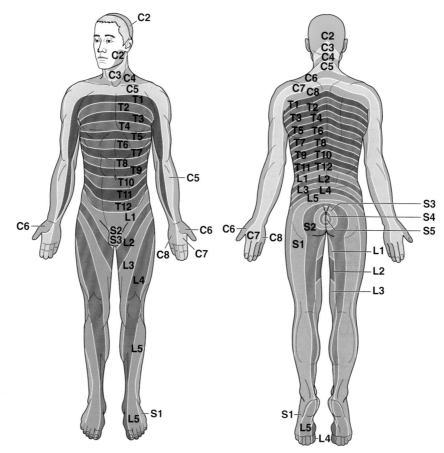

FIGURE 1.11 Dermatomes are areas of the skin supplied by a single nerve or nerve root. Shown here is the distribution of dermatomes throughout the body.

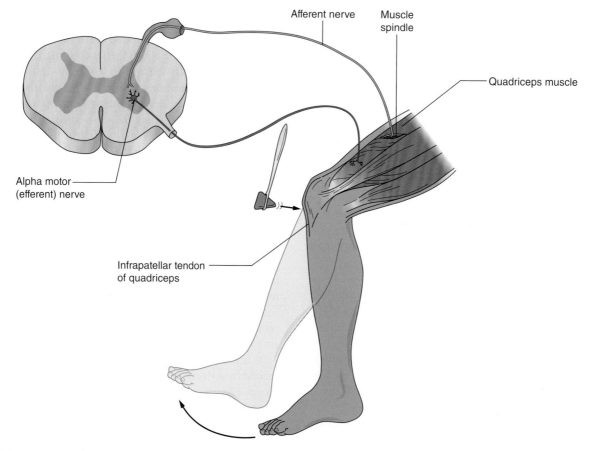

FIGURE 1.12 The deep tendon reflex arc.

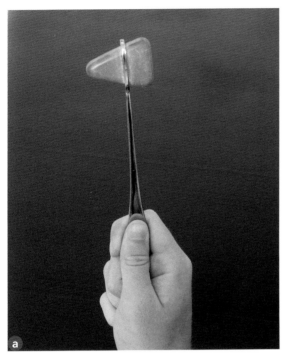 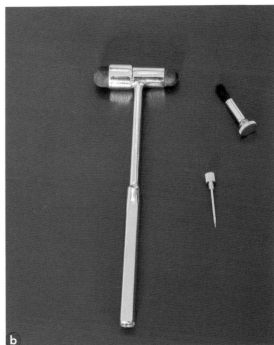

FIGURE 1.13   *(a)* Reflex hammer. *(b)* Neurological hammer.

TABLE 1.3   **Deep Tendon Reflex Grades**

Grade	Interpretation	Indication
0	Absent reflex	Complete loss of neuromuscular integrity (injury to nerve root or peripheral nerve)
+1	Diminished reflex	Reduced neurological function (incomplete injury to a nerve route or peripheral nerve)
+2	Normal reflex	Normal neurological integrity and function
+3	Exaggerated reflex	Upper motor neuron lesion (brain or spinal cord injury); hypersensitivity may also occur following brief, intense bouts of activity
+4	Clonus	Upper motor neuron lesion

Reprinted by permission from S. Shultz, P. Houglum, and D. Perrin, *Examination of Musculoskeletal Injuries*, 4th ed. (Champaign, IL: Human Kinetics, 2016), 118.

Cranial Nerve Assessment

Cranial nerve assessment is another valuable area of testing. When a patient has a suspected head injury, evaluation of these nerves is critical. Familiarity with their source and function is also important in evaluating many other neurological conditions. Table 1.4 provides an overview of these critical nerves, and chapter 10 covers the neurological system in depth.

Palpation

Palpation involves the use of the hands and fingers to gain information about a patient's condition through the sense of touch. The athletic trainer typically is profi-

cient in palpation of orthopedic conditions and can gain valuable information about general medical conditions by using systematic palpation. The clinician uses the fingertips for palpation during the medical examination to feel for skin texture and quality as well as temperature, underlying masses, rigidity, fluid, or crepitus. The ulnar surface of the hand should be used to palpate vibrations during inspiration or expiration because it is more sensitive, whereas the dorsal surface of the hand is best for estimating temperature.

Palpation may be done with one or both hands. The examiner uses palpation with or after visual inspection, except when assessing the abdomen, where palpation is completed after auscultation. Light palpation is per-

TABLE 1.4   **Cranial Nerve Function**

Source	Nerve	Sense	System
CN I	Olfactory nerve	Smell	Sensory
CN II	Optic nerve	Vision	Sensory
CN III	Oculomotor nerve	Extraocular muscle movement Pupillary light reflex	Motor
CN IV	Trochlear nerve	Extraocular (upward) muscle movement	Motor
CN V	Trigeminal nerve	Muscles of mastication	Sensory/motor
CN VI	Abducens nerve	Extraocular (lateral) muscle movement	Motor
CN VII	Facial nerve	Muscles of facial expression Taste Tears and saliva	Sensory/motor
CN VIII	Vestibulocochlear nerve	Balance Hearing	Sensory
CN IX	Glossopharyngeal nerve	Taste sensation of the mouth	Sensory/motor
CN X	Vagus nerve	Swallowing Gag reflex	Motor Sensory
CN XI	Spinal accessory nerve	Sternocleidomastoid, trapezius movement	Motor
CN XII	Hypoglossal nerve	Tongue movement	Motor

Note: CN = cranial nerve.

formed at a depth of approximately 1 cm and is useful for feeling skin and underlying tissue. Light palpation is always done before deep palpation. It helps the examiner to gain the patient's trust, identify areas of tenderness, and establish a systematic method of palpation from superficial to deep tissues. Deep palpation may approach 4 cm and must be done carefully because it may elicit tenderness or disrupt underlying tissue (figure 1.14). The patient should be relaxed during palpation because muscle guarding, especially of the abdominal region, will prevent the clinician from obtaining significant information from the examination. The patient is draped with consideration given to privacy and modesty, and only the area being palpated is exposed.

Percussion

Percussion is the process of assessing sounds transmitted through body organs and cavities and is generated by tapping. It involves striking one object (fingers or hand) against another to produce vibrations and subsequent sound waves. The techniques of percussion are the same regardless of the structure being percussed and include either direct or indirect percussion.

Direct percussion involves lightly striking the chest or abdominal wall with the ulnar aspect of the fist. Indirect percussion involves the finger of one hand acting as the hammer, striking the finger of the other hand that is resting on the body part being percussed (figure 1.15). The striking action creates a vibration or resonance that

with training and practice can be identified and quantified.

Practice is necessary to become proficient with percussion technique. The downward snap of the striking finger originates from the wrist and not the forearm or shoulder. The tap is sharp and rapid with the tip of the finger, not the pad. The ulnar surface of the fist may also be used for light percussion and is generally used to elicit tenderness over solid organs, such as the liver or kidneys.

Percussion-generated sounds may be recognized based on various characteristics, including intensity, pitch, and location. The general percussion tone over air is loud, over fluid it is less loud, and over solid areas it is soft.[2,13] It is often difficult to quantify percussion tones, especially for the novice examiner. The examiner should practice identifying tones from various parts of the body to learn how to quantify them, specifically noting the change from one tone to another when moving from percussing a known air-filled body part, such as the lungs, to the abdomen or a muscle.

Auscultation

Auscultation is the skilled listening by a trained ear for sounds produced by the body. Most body sounds, including the heart, lung, and bowel, are rarely audible without the use of a stethoscope. Auscultation takes practice so that the sounds can be identified and isolated from each other. It is strongly suggested that the learner practice listening to both normal and abnormal heart and lung sounds to train the ear. Just as health care professionals

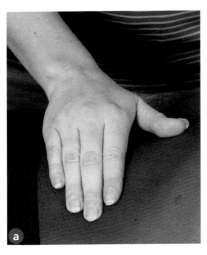 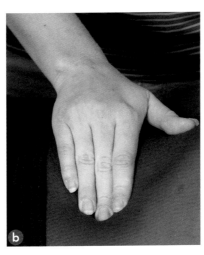 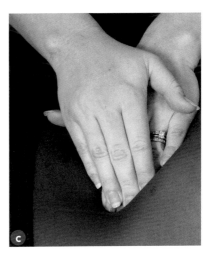

FIGURE 1.14 *(a)* Light palpation. *(b)* Deep palpation. *(c)* Bimanual palpation.

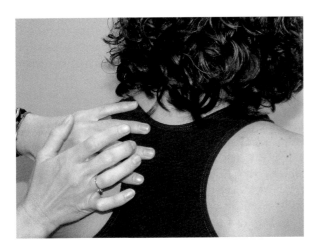

FIGURE 1.15 Indirect percussion.
© Micki Cuppett

train their fingers and touch with palpation, considerable practice is necessary to discriminate the subtle differences in sound during auscultation.

Certain basic principles apply to auscultation regardless of the system being examined:

- Perform auscultation after history, observation, and palpation (except for the abdomen) in order to gather as much information as possible from other sources first.
- Perform auscultation in a quiet environment. Ideally, the stethoscope should be placed directly on the skin and not through clothing.
- Point the earpieces of the stethoscope toward the face.
- Make sure the earpieces of the stethoscope fit comfortably, following the angles of the ear canal.

- Listen for the presence or absence of sounds as well as their frequency, loudness, quality, and duration.

As mentioned previously, auscultation of the abdomen is done before palpation. The examiner uses the part of the stethoscope that best relays the pitch of the sound sought. The diaphragm is used for high-pitched sounds, such as bowel, lung, and normal heart sounds, whereas the bell is used for low-pitched sounds.[6] Abnormal heart and vascular sounds have a lower pitch and may be heard better with the bell.[13] Table 1.5 describes common characteristics of sounds heard during auscultation. Specific placement of the stethoscope for auscultation of lung, heart, and bowel sounds and what the sound characteristics may indicate are discussed in the chapters covering respiratory, cardiac, and gastrointestinal disorders.

Preparticipation Examination

The medical examination is used for several purposes. For the athletic trainer, one of the more common uses is the preparticipation examination (PPE). The purpose of a PPE is not only to determine readiness for a specific sport but also to identify any potential or correctable conditions that may impair the patient's ability to fully perform. In general, the PPE is the first interaction a health care provider has with an athlete. The PPE is not a true physical examination; rather, it is a screening procedure that sheds light on potential problems associated with activity. The American Academy of Pediatrics (AAP), the American College of Sports Medicine, the American Medical Society for Sports Medicine, the American Orthopaedic Society for Sports Medicine, the American Osteopathic Academy of Sports Medicine, and the American Academy of Family Physicians have created

TABLE 1.5   **Characteristics of Sound**

Characteristic	Description
Pitch	Number of sound wave cycles generated per second by a vibrating object. The higher the frequency, the higher the pitch of a sound and vice versa.
Loudness	Amplitude of a sound wave. Auscultated sounds are described as *loud* or *soft*.
Quality	Sounds of similar frequency and loudness from different sources. Terms such as *gurgling*, *blowing*, *musical*, *sharp*, or *dull* describe quality of sound.
Shape	Heart sounds can be thought of in music vocabulary and include words like *crescendo* (sound that increases in intensity), *decrescendo* (sound that decreases in intensity), and *crescendo–decrescendo* (sound that increases then immediately decreases in intensity).
Duration	Length of time from when the sound is first heard to when the sound stops. The duration of sound is *short*, *medium*, or *long*.

a *Preparticipation Physical Evaluation* monograph that provides recommendations for PPE frequency, screenings, and participation.[14] This document recommends that all athletes have a PPE for the primary purpose of identifying any medical problems or conditions that could affect participation in sports. Without this examination, an athlete with systemic illnesses or a family history of cardiovascular disease may not be diagnosed or treated appropriately.[15] The AAP, along with other medical societies, requires the PPE to be signed by either a doctor of medicine (MD) or a doctor of osteopathic medicine (DO), although some states or school districts allow a health care provider other than a DO or MD to perform a PPE.

Student-athletes are required to have a comprehensive PPE upon entry into middle or high school or transfer to a new school, although each state is responsible for determining PPE frequency. The AAP recommends these comprehensive evaluations at 2 to 3 yr intervals for older students, with annual updates on a comprehensive health history, problem-focused areas, and vital signs.[14] Although some in the medical community still contend that PPEs are not thorough enough, especially in the realm of conditions related to sudden death, these evaluations have come a long way from the mass gymnasium physicals of the early 2000s.

According to the National Collegiate Athletics Association (NCAA) *Sports Medicine Handbook*,[16] a PPE is required for a student's entrance into the intercollegiate athletics program, and an updated cardiovascular screening, as well as interim history and blood pressure measurement, is required every 2 yr. Although many institutions use this examination largely as a medical history that focuses on orthopedic issues, it is also a venue to address medical problems as well as questions on mental health, physical abuse, and substance abuse, among other topics.[14] The PPE monograph from the AAP is available online and includes up-to-date medical history questions, interim COVID-19 forms, physical examination forms, and clearance forms for the sports PPE.

Proper administration of the PPE requires good communication skills, which are also critical to the assessment of medical conditions. Health care providers must be aware of their tone, body positioning, and language when talking with patients.

The NCAA and the National Federation of State High School Associations are constantly reviewing and updating the PPE process and regulations. The failure of personnel to recognize a sickle cell trait medical emergency contributed to the 2010 NCAA ruling that all athletes who are not certain of their status must be tested for the sickle cell trait as part of the medical examination with the university.[16] Changes like this are intended to provide better care to the student-athlete and to help health care providers obtain a thorough medical history that can contribute to safer participation.

An overview of the process of establishing and conducting PPEs is provided next. It is best that the PPE be conducted at least 6 wk before onset of the sport season, so physicians have time to order additional screening tests if needed and to analyze the results. There are two basic types of PPEs: office visit and station based. Both have advantages and disadvantages.

Office Visit

- The office visit is more private and is typically performed by a physician who has a working relationship with the patient.
- It is potentially expensive and rarely covered by insurance.
- The examining physician may not be as familiar with the requirements of the sport as would the team physician.

Station Based

- Patients move from station to station (medical history, orthopedic evaluation, visual screening, and lung and cardiac auscultation).

- Station-based PPEs often occur as a courtesy or community service from a group of physicians. Although they are cost-effective (nominal fee or free) and feature physicians with different specialties, they are not as private as office visits and can be loud or confusing to patients.[14]

- The traditional station-based PPE ends with a thorough review of the patient's medical history and a final checkout by the team physician. In this scenario, patients are all seen by the team physician, who has a better appreciation for the rigors of a particular sport than might the patient's personal physician.

Determining Sport Qualification

There are certain medical conditions (e.g., loss of one paired organ) that may disqualify a patient from certain sports or from competitive activity altogether. Chapter 7 provides extensive information about the 36th Bethesda Conference eligibility recommendations for competitive athletes with cardiovascular abnormalities. These recommendations identify safe competitive areas for patients with specific cardiovascular ailments. Pulmonary insufficiency, certain dermatological conditions, and organ mutations all must be addressed on an individual basis with the patient, parent or caregiver (if the patient is age <18 yr), medical specialist, and team physician. Ultimately, it is the physician's responsibility to determine the level of risk inherent in a given sport for a patient with a medical condition. If a patient is not cleared to participate, the physician should provide recommendations to correct any medical condition that can be modified with medication, treatment, or rehabilitation. If the medical situation preventing activity is acute and temporary, a follow-up appointment should be made.

Summary

The health care provider must be comfortable with general examination techniques in order to differentiate among the many disorders discussed in this text and to provide the best possible care for patients. The athletic trainer is often the first person the athlete approaches with a medical complaint and often serves as the gatekeeper to the medical community for the athlete. The clinician should appreciate the differences between a focal orthopedic examination and the examination of a medical condition that may affect multiple organ systems. Many techniques discussed in this chapter, such as palpation, percussion, and auscultation, are important skills for the health professional to master but take considerable practice. Practice these techniques on a variety of people of varying ages and health statuses to appreciate the range of normal and abnormal findings.

Apply It! Go to HK*Propel* to complete the case studies for this chapter.

HK*Propel* also provides access to online resources to help you practice auscultations and the use of an otoscope and ophthalmoscope.

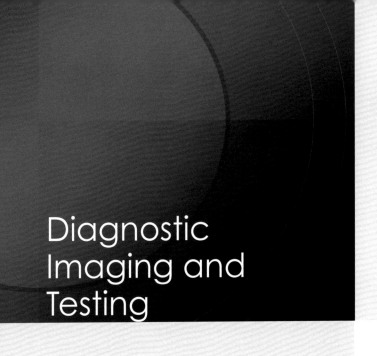

Diagnostic Imaging and Testing

At the completion of this chapter the reader should be able to do the following:

1. Choose the appropriate diagnostic imaging and laboratory tests for a given medical condition.

2. Explain test preparation and procedures to patients undergoing diagnostic evaluation.

3. Affirm patient consent after describing the benefits and possible adverse effects of imaging or testing.

4. Describe the risks and side effects of specific procedures.

5. Explain which medical conditions can be diagnosed with diagnostic imaging or laboratory testing.

6. Ask patients appropriate pre-MRI testing health questions.

7. Interpret normal values for urine and blood.

8. Identify the radiation levels of assorted diagnostic tests.

Diagnostic imaging refers to special impressions usually produced by radiologists and radiology technicians to determine specific medical conditions. Imaging captures impressions of internal structures so clinicians can distinguish normal from abnormal anatomy and view structures not seen with the naked eye. Not all diagnostic imaging involves radiation; for example, an ultrasound uses sound waves and magnetic resonance imaging (MRI) uses magnets to create images of internal structures. The specific imaging type is typically ordered by a physician and is based on patient signs and symptoms and their location. The images ensure that an accurate diagnosis and treatment plan can be implemented. Radiologists are medical doctors who have completed residency training in radiology (often in a specific area). Radiologists read and interpret the images and provide the treating physician with a report of any abnormal findings.

Diagnostic testing refers to medical tests performed primarily in a laboratory setting, such as blood, urine, and cardiovascular tests. A medical technologist analyzes the blood and/or tissue sample and then sends a report to the provider. A cardiac technician or nurse administers special cardiac tests, which are read and interpreted by the physician or a cardiologist.

Diagnostic Imaging

Radiography: X-Rays

An **X-ray** is a form of electromagnetic radiation that, when passed through a patient, allows viewing of the internal structures. The X-ray beam is absorbed to different extents by the various body tissues. Less dense tissue appears darker because the radiation is not absorbed in these structures. For example, the lungs appear dark

Informed Consent

Before clinicians perform any evaluation, diagnostic testing, imaging, or specimen collection, they must inform the patient of the reasons for the testing, describe possible associated risks, and obtain patient consent to the treatment or procedure. Obtaining consent is paramount and the clinician's legal responsibility. Consent can be assured verbally or in writing (signature) or via assent from a legal guardian if the patient is younger than age 18 yr, incapacitated, or unable to make medical decisions. In the era of patient-centered care, it is critical to fully explain side effects, describe possible outcomes, and allow the patient time to ask questions and decide independently whether to proceed with the plan.

because air does not absorb radiation. Fat is gray, and bone and calcium are light or white (figure 2.1). Most of the X-ray beam is absorbed by the tissues or is scattered, while a small amount passes through the body part to the receptor, creating the image. The image may be developed on film or, in the case of digital radiographs, may be saved and viewed on a computer.

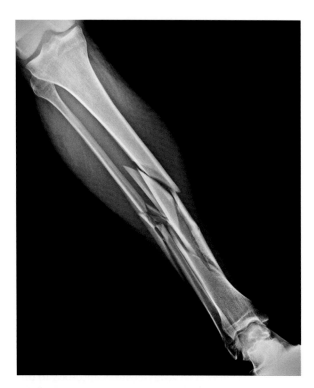

FIGURE 2.1   An anterior–posterior (AP) X-ray demonstrating multiple fractures to the tibia and fibula.

thesleepless1/iStockphoto/Getty Images

Because a radiograph is a two-dimensional picture of a three-dimensional body part, X-rays from several different angles may be administered in succession. Views are often named for the direction in which the X-ray beam passes through the body. For example, an image taken with the X-ray beam passing from the patient's anterior to posterior aspects is called an **AP view**, whereas an image taken from back to front is called a posterior–anterior view (**PA view**). A view shot from the side is called a **lateral view**. Other views may be named for the person who first produced them or perhaps for the place where they were first used.

Before the procedure, the patient may be asked to disrobe and wear a gown over the part to be X-rayed. Metal absorbs X-rays and shows up as white on the image, obscuring the content behind it. Therefore, patients need to remove jewelry and some clothing (especially with metal zippers, clasps, or buckles) in or near the X-ray–exposed area to achieve a clear image. During the procedure, the patient is asked to stand, sit, or lie still and to not move until the image has been taken. Depending on the radiograph type, patients may be asked to hold their breath so the image is not blurred by rib cage movement. The test is painless and lasts only a few seconds, although an entire series of X-rays may last 10 min. More than one view of an area may be taken.

Radiographs are ordered when there is a possibility of a fracture, dislocation, bony abnormality or deformity, tumor, arthritis, bone cancer, foreign object, infection, or dental caries. For structures that cannot normally be imaged (e.g., blood vessels or hollow organs), a contrast medium (e.g., barium or iodine) may be introduced either by mouth or intravenously. Contrast agents appear white inside the hollow organ or blood vessel to allow visualization of these structures.[1] Because the image is two-dimensional, anything in the path of the X-ray beam, including items not necessarily in the patient's body, shows up on the image.

Risks or Side Effects

For pregnant females, radiographs should not be taken because radiation may affect the fetus. Pregnancy status must be determined with a blood or urine test before radiography is allowed. For all patients, a protective barrier is placed over the reproductive organs if the pelvis is not the

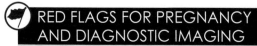

RED FLAGS FOR PREGNANCY AND DIAGNOSTIC IMAGING

Any female who has begun menses must have her pregnancy status determined before being subjected to diagnostic imaging. A simple blood or urine test can verify pregnancy status and prevent possible harm to a fetus.

focus of the test. Any time that radiation is used, there is a slight chance of developing certain types of cancer, such as leukemia and melanoma. Physicians try to minimize X-ray exposure by using the lowest amount of radiation necessary and by screening patients based on criteria such as the Ottawa ankle or knee rules, which are used to determine whether radiographs should be taken after an ankle or knee injury. Criteria for the ankle and foot are based on the location of bone pain, tenderness, and weight-bearing ability. Criteria for the knee are slightly different, with consideration of age (>55 yr), patella or fibular head tenderness, ability to flex the knee, and weight-bearing ability. Table 2.1 illustrates the amount of radiation introduced into the body for common diagnostic tests, including radiographs.

Radionuclide Bone Scan

A **radionuclide bone scan** is a nuclear imaging test involving the injection of a short-lived radionuclide to assess bone abnormalities. Patients are asked to remove their clothing and wear a gown for the procedure. A radio-nuclide tracer, which emits gamma rays, is injected into the brachial vein in the cubital fossa of the elbow. The tracer is attracted to increased metabolic activity. The patient may feel a warm sensation as the tracer circulates throughout the body. The technician administering the injection typically wears a radiation-protective lead vest and gloves. Time is allowed for the isotope to circulate in the body (30 min to 2 h), then the patient is moved to the examination room and placed supine on a table. The patient lies still as a special camera moves around them. The camera identifies gamma radiation, high levels of which indicate increased metabolic activity in bone, and the images are viewed on a computer or radiograph. Images are taken at various time intervals, revealing the rate at which the tracer is absorbed into the bone. The actual procedure is painless, save for any discomfort during the injection.

Areas of inflammation or injury appear dark on a bone scan; these are called **hot spots**. Lighter areas on the bone scan show normal tissue and bone (figure 2.2).[2]

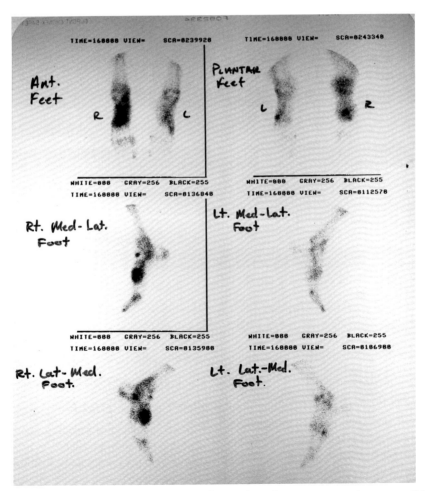

FIGURE 2.2 A bone scan showing uptake in the tarsal cuneiform bones, suggesting a possible stress reaction.
© Katie Walsh Flanagan

TABLE 2.1 **Comparison of Radiation From Imaging Versus Natural Radiation Exposure**

Examination	Radiation dose (mSv)	Time to accumulate comparable natural background dose
Computed tomography		
Abdomen and pelvis	10.0	3 yr
Abdomen and pelvis, with and without repeated contrast	20.0	7 yr
Chest	7.0	2 yr
Chest (pulmonary embolism)	10.0	3 yr
Colonography	6.0	2 yr
Head	2.0	8 mo
Multiphase abdomen and pelvis	31.0	10 yr
Sinuses	0.6	2 mo
Fluoroscopy		
Barium swallow	1.5	6 mo
Coronary angiography	5.0-15.0	20 mo to 5 yr
Nuclear medicine		
Bone scan	4.2	1 yr, 4 mo
Brain (PET)	1.0	4 mo
Cardiac perfusion (sestamibi)	12.5	4 yr
Lung ventilation/perfusion	2.0	8 mo
Tumor/infection	18.5	6 yr
Other		
Bone density (DEXA)	0.001	<1 d
Mammography	0.7	3 mo
Radiography		
Abdomen	1.2	5 mo
Chest	0.1	10 d
Extremity	0.001	<1 d
Lumbar spine	0.7	3 mo
X-rays, single exposure		
Dental (lateral)	0.02	<10 d
Dental (panoramic)	0.09	10 d
Hand or foot	0.005	<1 d
Hip	0.8	3 mo

Note: DEXA = dual-energy X-ray absorptiometry; PET = positron emission tomography.

Bone scans are used to identify stress fractures, bone infections, bone cancer, and arthritis. The same nuclear technology may be applied to other structures, such as the thyroid and heart, and may be used to identify abscesses or tumors. Nuclear medicine may also be combined with computed tomography (CT) to allow visualization of structures in *slices*, or sections.

Risks or Side Effects

Before radionuclide injection, the clinician should ask the patient if they are allergic to red dye. If the patient is female, her pregnancy status should be determined before the test; patients who may be pregnant should not have a bone scan. Once the test is completed, the patient should drink plenty of water to flush out the radionuclide tracer.

Most materials used in the test are not detectable even a day later, as most have a half-life of only a few hours.

Fluoroscopy

Fluoroscopy is performed when the clinician wants to see a "live" image to determine the size, shape, and movement of tissue. This test is not as detailed as an X-ray–based radiograph. Fluoroscopes are commonly found on-site at professional and large university athletic venues; they are a quick and noninvasive means of determining whether a fracture has occurred or a joint is disarticulated, thereby warranting further studies. Fluoroscopic evaluation also assists in return-to-play decisions, because the image can be taken with the patient in a weight-bearing position, thus allowing the diagnosis to be made immediately. Clothing should be removed from the area to be examined. Female patients should notify the technician if they might be pregnant, and they may be asked to undergo urinalysis or a blood test before fluoroscopy to rule out pregnancy.

The patient stands or sits next to the machine and the technician lines up the machine and the structure to be evaluated (figure 2.3). Radiation is allowed to pass through the skin, creating light and shadows that are viewed on a computer screen and can be printed. Dense areas, such as bone, will appear white on the film, and less dense areas, such as the lungs, will appear darker.

The fluoroscope can also be used to look at blood flow, tumors, fractures, organs, foreign bodies, and some soft tissue. It can also be used to assist with biopsy, injections, catheter insertion, and even pacemaker insertion.

Risks or Side Effects

Any time that radiation is used, there is a slight chance of developing certain types of cancer, such as leukemia or skin cancer.

Computed Tomography Scan

A **computed tomography (CT) scan** (also a *computerized axial tomography scan*) combines specialized high-resolution radiographs with computers to give better visualization of internal structures in cross sections or three dimensions (3D). It works by passing rotating beams of X-rays through the patient and measuring the transmission at thousands of points. The images may be seen individually as a series of cross sectional slices, but 3D images can be produced by a computer. The CT scan exposes a patient to much greater levels of radiation than do X-rays (see table 2.1), and the risks of additional radiation exposure must outweigh the benefits of the definitive

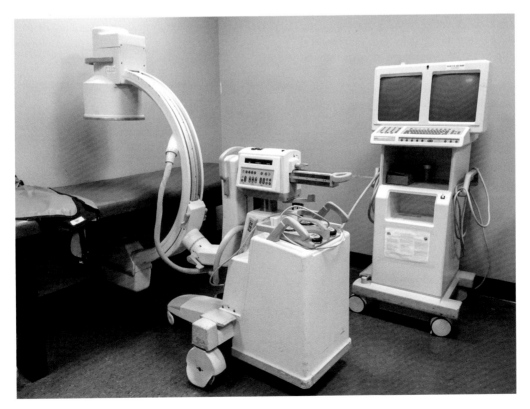

FIGURE 2.3   A mobile fluoroscope.

© Katie Walsh Flanagan

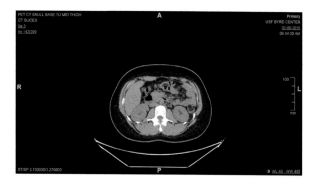

FIGURE 2.4 Computed tomography (CT) demonstrates the shoulders of a patient lying supine. The scapula, spine, and sternum are all visible in white.

© Lawrence Collins, PA-C, ATC

diagnosis. Depending on the structures to be examined, the patient may receive a contrast dye injection or be asked to consume a barium or other contrast solution at various intervals before or during the CT scan. Contrast agents are usually the same iodinated agents used in other imaging studies. Patients may feel a warm or cool sensation if the contrast dye is administered intravenously.[3]

The patient must lie very still on a table that moves in and out of an open tube. At times, the patient must hold the breath so that the images produced are clear. There is a whirring sound when the machine is operating, and it can sometimes be very noisy. The test is painless and lasts from 15 min to 1 h, depending on the structures to be examined.

CT scans are performed to look at cross sections of internal organs, bone, soft tissue, and blood vessels (figure 2.4).

Risks or Side Effects

As with any radiation, there is a slight risk of developing certain types of cancer such as leukemia or melanoma. On occasion, a patient will have an allergic reaction to the contrast dye. Every precaution is taken to avoid allergic reactions by taking an appropriate medical history, including allergies to food, medications, or dyes. Before a CT scan is performed, physicians typically require proof via a serum blood test that a female patient of childbearing age is not pregnant.

Positron Emission Tomography Scan

A **positron emission tomography (PET) scan** is ordered to examine the cell metabolism and biochemistry of tissue and organs. PET scans can identify abnormal metabolic activity before it becomes apparent on a CT scan or by MRI. The patient receives a glucose-based radionuclide

injection intravenously or tablets by mouth, depending on the suspected condition. These radioactive materials (radiotracers) identify tissue changes at the cellular level and can indicate disease before more specific signs or symptoms appear.[4]

Patients are asked a series of questions, including history of any allergic reactions to dyes or certain medications. After the patient has changed into a dressing gown, and voided, they are placed on a table and the imaging unit takes pictures of specific areas of the body. The patient must remain still and may be asked not to breathe for brief periods so that the image produced is clear. The table moves the patient in and out of the machine, similar to a CT scan. At times, the machine may move around the patient. The scanning process can take up to 2 h. The glucose-based radionuclide is absorbed by the area of abnormal metabolic activity and will appear dark on the body image view, similar to a bone scan, or as bright colors on 3D images (figure 2.5). This imaging mode is used to identify certain types of cancer, thyroid conditions, infection, and bleeding and to evaluate kidney function.

Risks or Side Effects

PET scans expose patients to a low dose of radiation, but the benefits outweigh the risks. Before the injection or ingestion of radionuclide, patients are asked if they are allergic to dyes. They are also asked to drink plenty of water after the scan to flush the radionuclide from their

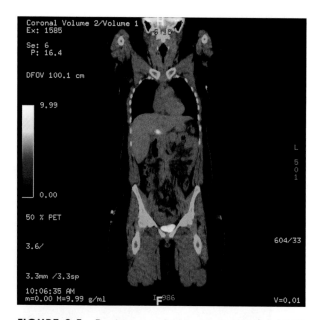

FIGURE 2.5 Positron emission tomography (PET) image demonstrating a healthy pelvis. The patient is in the supine position. The bright color at the bottom of the image is the bladder.

© Lawrence Collins, PA-C, ATC

system. As with other imaging, women who could be pregnant should undergo a urinalysis or blood test; if the patient is pregnant or nursing, the PET scan should not be performed.

Magnetic Resonance Imaging

A **MRI scan** is a test that applies a magnetic field to the body. The magnetic field aligns the body's atoms and nuclei (protons, actually) in such a way that when acted upon by external radio energy, they temporarily realign. A computer analyzes the data and creates an image. This image provides detailed information about organs, soft tissue, bones, tumors, bleeding, or infection. MRI scans are used to identify tumors, musculoskeletal injuries, soft-tissue conditions, fractures, and bleeding (figure 2.6).

The two most common imaging parameters are T1- and T2-weighted images, typically referred to as **T1** and **T2** images. On a T1 image, fat shows up as a white or light signal, whereas water appears dark. Conversely, on a T2 image, fat appears dark, whereas blood, edema, and cerebrospinal fluid (CSF) appear white (table 2.2). Calcium and bone do not show up well on MRI scans; however, the normal fat within bone marrow makes long bones appear white. At times, a contrast MRI scan is used to view structures such as the brain or cartilage more vividly. A contrast agent (gadolinium) can be introduced into the patient's body to better view structures and to delineate a solid structure from a fluid one. Knowing the image type (T1 or T2) assists the radiologist in determining which structures are typical and which are abnormal.

Patients who need an MRI scan will be asked a series of yes-or-no questions before scheduling. The results of this screening will be reviewed before the test is performed to determine whether patients are at risk of injury

if they undergo an MRI scan. Possible contraindications for MRI testing include the following:

- Cochlear implant
- Pacemaker
- Implantable cardio-verter defibrillator (ICD)
- Heart or valve surgery
- Shunt, stent, filter, or intravascular coil
- Aneurysm clips
- Insulin pump (implanted)
- Pregnant
- Gunshot wounds or shrapnel
- History of working with metal (e.g., welding)
- History of ocular injury involving metal or metal slivers
- Claustrophobia
- Allergies to dye
- Tattoos or permanent makeup
- Orthopedic clips, staples, plates, screws, and so on
- Implanted stimulator device (bone, neurological)
- Prosthesis

On arrival for the MRI, patients will be asked to wear a gown and to remove all metal jewelry, watches, body piercings, removable dental appliances, hearing aids, TENS (transcutaneous electrical nerve stimulator) units, glasses, hair accessories, and writing utensils. Metal items can interfere with the magnetic field of the MRI and alter the images. No metal or electronic devices are allowed in the room. The patient should also inform the technician of any metal implants before the test. MRI is safe for most patients with metal implants, screws, and pins, but there are a few exceptions.[5] Patients will need to remain still throughout the entire test to avoid blurring of the image.

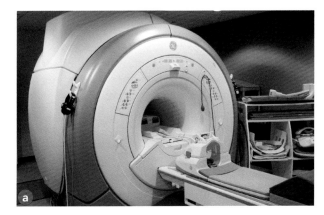 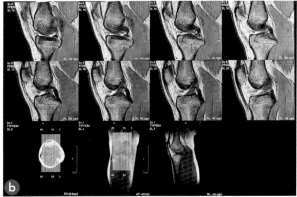

FIGURE 2.6   (a) A magnetic resonance imaging (MRI) machine. (b) An MRI scan of the knee, clearly showing the posterior cruciate ligament (PCL) on the posterior aspect of the knee. Note the lower-left aspect of the image, which displays the levels of slices this image portrays.

(a) © Micki Cuppett; (b) © Katie Walsh Flanagan

TABLE 2.2　**Differences Between T1 and T2 Images**

Image type	Fat	Water/fluid
T1	Bright/white	Dark
T2	Dark	Bright/white

There will be whirring, clicking, and knocking noises during the test, and the technician may provide earplugs or a headset for listening to music to eliminate some of the noise. If the patient receives a headset, the technician may use it to communicate with the patient during the test. The MRI scan may last 30 min to 1 h.

The patient must lie still on a movable table that slides into the magnetic area. The patient areas in older MRI machines are very small tunnels that could be uncomfortable for a patient who is claustrophobic; however, newer models are more open, and the magnetic cylinder is much larger and thus more tolerable for patients. A series of images is taken while the patient is moved into the magnetic area. The signals are processed by a computer to show detailed slices, or sections of tissue, or the data can be rendered as a 3D image.

Risks or Side Effects

MRI operates via magnets and has no documented side effects so long as the patient is honest and forthright in answering the preexamination questions. Patients who are claustrophobic should request an open MRI. If one is not available and a closed MRI will be used, patients may request a sedative so they can be more comfortable. Females should notify the technician if they might be pregnant and should undergo a urinalysis or blood test before imaging. The effects of magnetic imaging on the fetus have not been widely researched.

Diagnostic Ultrasound

Ultrasound consists of high-frequency sound waves that penetrate the body to produce images of internal structures in real time (figure 2.7). Images are produced by the magnitude and timing of returning echoes, which are the result of interfaces or changes in tissue density. An ultrasound examination is often thought of in the context of a pregnant female undergoing a sonogram to determine the developmental status (and sex) of the fetus. Gel is applied to the skin and a transducer is moved over the area to be examined. Sound waves are released through the transducer and transmitted into the tissue. Once the sound waves come in contact with internal organs, fluid, or tissue, they bounce back, creating an image on the computer.

To prepare for an ultrasound, patients remove their clothing and jewelry from the area to be examined so as

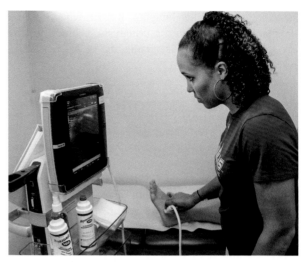

FIGURE 2.7　Diagnostic ultrasound of the ankle.
© Micki Cuppett

not to distort the images, and they lie still during the test. The patient rarely feels anything except the transducer moving on the skin. The examination usually takes about 30 min. When used to examine the heart, this test is called an echocardiogram (ECHO) and is performed in conjunction with an electrocardiogram (ECG).

Ultrasound is used to identify tumors, enlarged lymph nodes, heart abnormalities, soft-tissue injury, bleeding, and fetal development. It is useful in the diagnosis of tissue tears, blood clots, and deep vein thrombosis. In addition, a Doppler analysis can be performed, allowing the identification of moving blood. Diagnostic ultrasound is becoming more widely used to diagnose soft-tissue (musculoskeletal) injuries to athletes, thus improving the promptness and safety of return-to-play decisions. Recent uses for nontherapeutic ultrasound in athletics include diagnosis of muscular strains, tendon strains, and inflammatory pathologies as well as guided intraarticular injections.

Risks or Side Effects

Because ultrasound uses sound waves, there are no documented side effects. Ultrasound is safe for pregnant women and is used to assess fetal development and sex.

Laparoscopy

Laparoscopy is an invasive procedure in which small incisions are made in the abdomen and a scope is inserted into the incision to view the inside of the abdomen. Because the abdomen is distended with a gas before the scope is introduced, the abdominal organs are separated from the abdominal wall to allow for easier viewing. There is a camera on the scope, which allows the physician to see the internal structures of the abdomen and to determine any abnormalities. Other instruments may be introduced through another portal to facilitate moving the viscera for better viewing or to perform surgery.

Laparoscopy can be used to diagnose conditions of the abdomen, to perform biopsies, and to provide a venue for surgical procedures for the gallbladder, appendix, uterus, ovaries, and colon. Before a laparoscopic procedure, patients will fast for several hours, possibly use an enema or complete a colon preparation, and shower with antibacterial soap. As with any surgery, patients will also be cautioned to stop using any anticoagulant medications (including over-the-counter aspirin, naproxen [Naprosyn], ibuprofen [Motrin], and supplements that can promote bleeding) for at least 5 d before laparoscopy.

Risks and Side Effects

General anesthesia is used for laparoscopy. As such, patients are warned of possible side effects of anesthesia, including headache, nausea, vomiting, dizziness, and constipation. The patient may be slightly sore for a few days, depending on the procedure performed. Gas is introduced into the abdomen before the procedure; therefore, it is possible that not all gas was released before wound closure. Gas-like abdominal discomfort is common but dissipates rapidly. If surgery was performed, the patient may have limited physical activity for a period of time. With advances in technology, many major surgeries can be carried out via laparoscopy. Therefore, patients should be cautioned that the size of the scar (2-5 cm) is not necessarily indicative of the full scope of the surgery. Each patient should be informed about signs of infection. If any symptoms of infection occur, the patient should call the physician immediately.

Colonoscopy

Colonoscopy is an invasive procedure in which the colon and rectum are examined for abnormalities. A scope with a camera on the end, inserted through the rectum and into the colon, displays an image of these structures, allowing the physician to identify any abnormalities. The American Cancer Society recommends that adults undergo a colonoscopy at age 45 yr to detect and prevent colorectal cancer or earlier if there is a history of colon cancer in the patient's immediate family. Colonoscopy is used to examine the patient for any early indication of colon cancer or polyps and to help explain bleeding or changes in normal bowel habits. Those without a trace of colon cancer are advised to undergo a colonoscopy every 10 yr following the initial one at age 45.

Preparation for the Test

The patient must eliminate all solid waste from the gastrointestinal tract. A liquid diet will be required, beginning 1 to 3 d before the procedure. The patient will be asked to take a laxative, to drink a special liquid and/or take tablets, and to consume only clear liquids. Clear liquids include bouillon or broth, flavored gelatin, water, coffee, tea, electrolyte drinks, or clear soft drinks. Patients taking any medication should inform the physician in advance of the procedure. On the day of the procedure, patients are given a sedative to increase their comfort. Air is introduced into the colon to make visualization clearer. The procedure usually takes 30 to 60 min.

Risks and Side Effects

Colonoscopy involves sedation and thus has associated risks. Typically, a person trained in anesthesiology is present to provide and supervise light medical sedation, but not intubation as with general anesthesia. Biopsies can be obtained during colonoscopy, so bleeding and colon tears or perforation are risks of this procedure.

Side effects of a routine colonoscopy include temporary cramping or bloating after the procedure. Because of the sedative, patients should not drive for 24 h. At times, the patient may experience dizziness, weakness, and some blood in bowel movements after the procedure.

Endoscopy

Endoscopy is an invasive procedure used to examine cavities within the body, most often the upper digestive tract, stomach, and proximal small intestine. The physician inserts a flexible tube with a lighted camera into the mouth to view the esophagus, stomach, and duodenum. During this process, the physician can view the lining of the aforementioned structures, examine the integrity of the associated valves, and extract biopsies, if warranted.

Preparation for the Test

Preparation for an endoscopy is easier than that for a colonoscopy. The patient must fast for a period of time (usually nothing by mouth after a specific time the night before the procedure). The physician will determine whether any prescribed medicine should be delayed until after the procedure or taken as usual. Patients usually receive some level of intravenous sedation before endoscopy. Both colonoscopies and endoscopies are typically considered nonsurgical procedures. The endoscopy usually takes less than 30 min.

Risks and Side Effects

There are minimal risks or side effects of a routine endoscopy. The type of sedative used may affect patients differently, and the physician will determine the restrictions for that day, if any.

Diagnostic Testing

Electromyography and Nerve Conduction Studies

Electromyography is done to measure electrical activity in muscle. The result is recorded on an **electromyogram (EMG)**, which involves inserting a needle into a muscle and recording its electrical activity. A normal muscle will have no electrical activity at rest. A **nerve conduction study (NCS)** is typically performed in conjunction with electromyography. The NCS measures the electrical signals of a nerve associated with a specific muscle. An NCS involves stimulating a nerve (via an electrical impulse delivered via a small needle inserted into the muscle) and recording the strength of the neurological reaction and the amount of time taken to contract the muscle being tested (figure 2.8). Results are displayed on an oscilloscope, as an audio signal, or both. Abnormal electrical activity will elicit an abnormal waveform (time of contraction) or sound.

EMGs are used to determine the cause of muscle weakness and abnormal nerve conduction, which may be attributable to medical conditions such as muscular dystrophy, myasthenia gravis, or amyotrophic lateral sclerosis. Nerve irritation or injury to the carpal tunnel, cubital tunnel, brachial plexus, or lumbar plexus or other neuropathies may also cause abnormal electrical activity.

Preparation for electromyography involves cleaning the area to be evaluated and inserting a needle into the muscle to be tested. The patient may experience some discomfort at the insertion site, similar to receiving an injection. During the test, the patient may be asked to contract the muscle. Typically, groups of muscles are assessed and compared with muscles on the contralateral side. The only side effect associated with electromyography is the possibility of slight soreness in the tested muscle.

Electrocardiography

Electrocardiography is done to determine whether the electrical activity of the heart is normal. Electrodes are placed on the chest and extremities (if 10- to 12-lead electrocardiography is being done) to detect the electrical activity of the heart (figure 2.9). The number of leads used (range, 3-12) depends on the information the physician needs from different areas and structures of the heart. For 10- to 12-lead electrodes, placement is as follows:

Six Precordial Leads (Chest Leads)

- V1—Fourth intercostal space on the right lateral border of the sternum
- V2—Fourth intercostal space on the left lateral border of the sternum
- V3—Midway between the V1 and V2 electrodes
- V4—Fifth left intercostal space, at the midclavicular line
- V5—Anterior axillary line, horizontally equal to V4
- V6—Mid-axillary line, horizontally equal to V4 and V5

Standard Limb Leads (Four)

- Right arm (anywhere between the right shoulder and elbow)

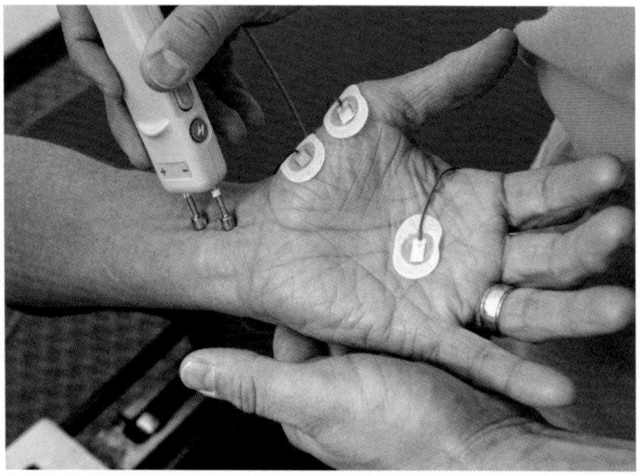

FIGURE 2.8 Electromyography and nerve conduction studies are traditionally evaluated at the same time by recording the electrical impulses in the muscle and the speed at which they travel when stimulated.

BanksPhotos/Getty Images

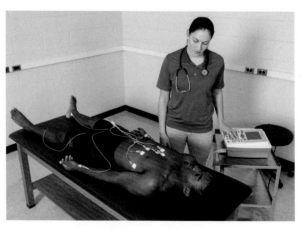

FIGURE 2.9 Some athletes undergo 12-lead electrocardiography as a baseline test in their preparticipation physical.

- Right lower leg
- Left arm (anywhere between the left shoulder and elbow)
- Left lower leg

The electrical activity is charted on a graph (an **electrocardiogram**, or **ECG**) as waveforms. An ECG records electrical activity as two phenomena: depolarization (the spread of electricity through the cardiac muscle) and repolarization (the return of the stimulated heart to rest) (figure 2.10).[6] The basic components of the ECG represent important aspects of cardiac function:

- P wave—Electrical stimulus through the atria (atrial depolarization)
- PR interval—Time between stimuli of atria and ventricles
- QRS complex—Stimuli traveling through ventricles (ventricular depolarization)
- ST segment and T wave—Ventricular repolarization (relaxing)
- U wave—Final stage of ventricular repolarization

An ECG is used to identify ischemia, heart attack, pericarditis, valvular disorders, electrolyte imbalances, palpitations, angina, and other related heart problems.

The patient removes all jewelry and clothing in the chest area. The chest is cleaned and may be shaved. If the test uses 12-lead electrodes, the patient's wrists and ankles are also bared and cleaned. A gel is applied between the skin and the electrode. The patient should not feel anything during the test and may be asked to lie very still because movement may affect the results. The examiner should be informed if the patient is taking any medication or has a pacemaker. There are no known risks associated with electrocardiography.

Cardiac Event Monitor

A **cardiac event monitor** (or event monitor, formerly called a *Holter monitor*) is a device worn by a patient to monitor the heart's electrical activity. It is used to identify arrhythmias, ischemia, cardiomyopathies, and premature ventricular contractions and to monitor pacemakers. A cardiac event monitor works in the same manner as electrocardiography. It traces the electrical activity of the heart, identifying any arrhythmias. Generally, three to eight electrodes are applied to the patient's skin with a glue backing, and the leads are attached to a monitoring device (figure 2.11). The monitor is worn for between 24 h and 1 mo, depending on the suspected condition, and it records the heart rhythm. Patients must keep a diary of their activity and record any symptoms (skipped or racing heartbeat, or angina) they experience while wearing the monitor. Patients can also push a button on certain models to indicate that they are feeling an irregular heartbeat or chest pain; in essence, they mark an event to be reviewed by technicians. Those wearing the device longer than 24 h are given extra electrodes and taught how to apply them correctly. The electrodes may be removed daily for bathing. The typical cardiac event monitor is smaller than a deck of cards, with some about the size of a matchbook.

Individuals who are prescribed cardiac event monitoring undergo the same preparation as for an ECG. They should perform their normal activities, but they will not be able to bathe while wearing the monitor.

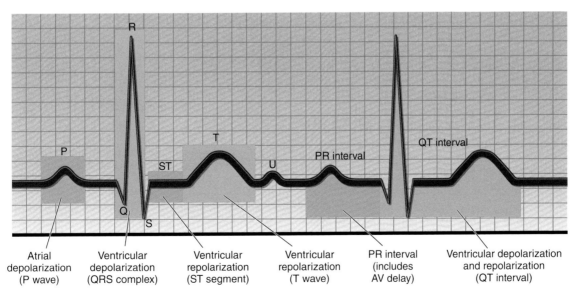

FIGURE 2.10 Graphic illustration of phases of the resting electrocardiogram. Waveforms are analyzed to determine whether there are any abnormalities.

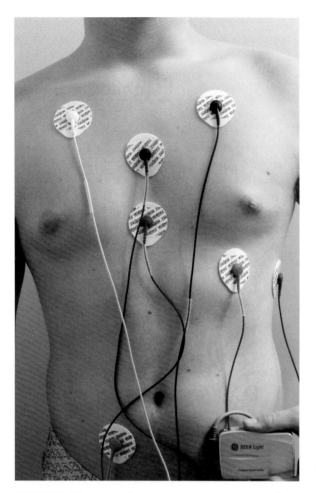

FIGURE 2.11 A cardiac event monitor is an excellent tool with which to evaluate a person's cardiac activity while performing activities of daily living.

Photo courtesy of Kathleen Knott / Johns Hopkins University.

Female athletes can wear the monitor in their sports bra. Patients are asked to provide a comprehensive history of prescribed medications, vitamins, supplements, and herbs taken routinely. For the most part, patients may continue their normal activities without interruption. As with electrocardiography, there are no known risks associated with cardiac event monitor testing.

Interpretation of Results

The physician reviews the information from the cardiac event monitor. Some units have a call-in number or indicator that patients should use if they feel pain or cardiac arrhythmia. The cardiac event monitor then communicates with a computer or telephone to deliver live cardiac readings. Otherwise, the data are downloaded on completion of the test and analyzed by a cardiologist or cardiovascular technician.

Cardiac Stress Test

A **cardiac stress test** is used to examine patients' heart rhythm during exercise in a controlled environment. This test is often used with patients who have several risk factors or are at moderate risk of coronary heart disease. The patient is connected to an electrocardiography machine, with a blood pressure cuff on the arm and a pulse oximeter on one finger to measure oxygen levels. A baseline ECG is taken for comparison. The cardiac stress test is done while the patient walks on a treadmill or pedals on a stationary bicycle (e.g., an Exercycle) (figure 2.12). At three-minute intervals, the grade or intensity of the exercise increases. For a maximal stress test, the patient is asked to continue exercise until fatigued. In a submaximal stress test, the patient continues exercise to a predetermined level. During the cardiac stress test, heart rhythm, blood pressure, pulse, and oxygen levels are recorded.

A cardiac stress test is used to identify coronary artery disease, ischemia, and angina and to monitor the functional capacity of patients with heart disease. If radioactive nuclides are used in conjunction with the stress test, it is then called a **nuclear stress test**. This allows the cardiologist to detect regional areas of decreased blood flow. The risks are the same for a cardiac stress test as they are for exercise.

RED FLAGS FOR ENDING A CARDIAC STRESS TEST

Parameters for ending a cardiac stress test before submaximal effort include the following: patient desire to stop, signs of cyanosis or pallor, sustained ventricular tachycardia, patient dizziness, near syncope, moderate to severe angina, and hypertensive response (systolic blood pressure >250 mmHg and diastolic blood pressure >115 mmHg), among other criteria.[7]

Laboratory Tests

Many common diagnostic tests are performed to confirm specific conditions. An athletic trainer should be familiar with these tests, what they are used for, and what the results indicate. Two of the most common laboratory examinations, urinalysis and complete blood count (CBC), and the lumbar puncture are discussed next. Athletic trainers rarely perform laboratory tests, with the possible exception of urine test strips (e.g., Chemstrips),

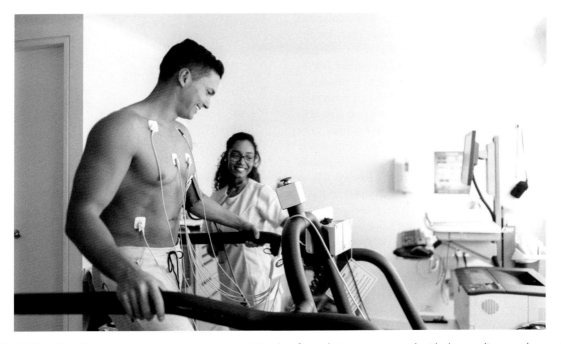

FIGURE 2.12   Cardiac stress tests can uncover a multitude of conditions associated with the cardiovascular system.

andresr/Getty Images/Getty Images

but they need to appreciate the normal values of these examinations. Elsewhere in this text, results of these common tests related to a specific condition or disease are discussed; here, emphasis is on the common normal values found in urinalysis and CBC.

Urinalysis

Urinalysis is a urine test to determine pH, protein, glucose, ketone, bilirubin, hemoglobin, nitrite, leukocytes, urobilinogen, and specific gravity levels. The patient is asked to urinate into a clean plastic cup.

Urinalysis may be ordered for various reasons. The results can indicate urinary tract infection, diabetes, starvation (including anorexia nervosa), liver problems, intravascular hemolysis, kidney injury or bleeding, and renal or glomerular damage. Illicit drugs, anabolic steroids, and alcohol can also be screened for in a urinalysis. A specific urinalysis can also confirm pregnancy.

If a *clean-catch* specimen is ordered, then the patient cleans the external area of the urethra with a disposable cloth before voiding into a cup. Collected urine should be refrigerated if it will not be assessed within 1 h.

In the athletic environment, the urinalysis may consist of a simple dipstick placed in a container of urine. This is often used to determine the presence of hematuria to rule out trauma to the renal system. These dipsticks, or Chemstrips, are flexible, coated paper with multiple test

Clinical Tips

Conditions a Urinalysis May Reveal

- Blood in the urine (hematuria) can indicate a kidney injury or can occur benignly after an intense workout.

- The color of urine can reveal dehydration or may be the by-product of certain medications.

- Glucose is not normally present in urine unless high levels exist in the body; therefore, glucose in the urine might indicate diabetes.

- Ketones also can reveal diabetes or fasting.

- pH is the acidity or alkalinity of the urine. A higher acid reading can be found with diabetes or dehydration, whereas an alkaline reading indicates kidney infection or urinary tract infection.

- Specific gravity of urine indicates its ion concentration and attests to hydration level and the ability of the kidney to process fluids.

- Urine tests can also indicate medication and illicit drug use, electrolyte levels, and the presence of infection.

components on each stick; they are dipped into collected urine and subsequently compared with a chart on the bottle label to determine whether the color reaction matches a given component of urine. Common assessments include pH, red blood cells (RBCs; if present, a sign of injury), white blood cells (WBCs; if present, a sign of infection), glucose, specific gravity, and protein values. The dipstick bottle is dark to prevent light from penetrating and altering reliability of the sticks; the bottle must be tightly sealed to preserve the reactive chemicals on each stick. The side of the bottle is labeled with a chart for various parameters (e.g., blood or pH) and with associated color squares that indicate the presence or concentration of each (figure 2.13). Each value has a specific time frame for correct reaction response, typically from immediately to 2 min, and the stick must be read within the allotted time frame to obtain accurate results. Normal values and possible conditions from abnormal results for urine are found in table 2.3.

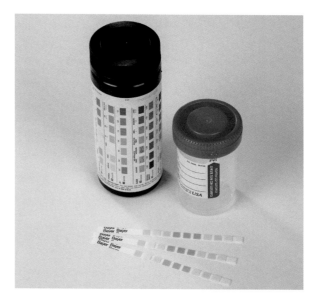

FIGURE 2.13 The label on a Chemstrip bottle can be used to assess strips for results of urinalysis.

TABLE 2.3 **Normal Values for Urine**

Aspect measured	Normal value	Low range may indicate*	High range may indicate*
Color	Pale yellow to amber	High hydration status	Dehydration (colored urine may be related to specific foods or drugs)
pH	Tends to be acidic (4.6-8.0)	Acidic—kidney health, stones, some medications, drug overdose	Alkaline—UTI, rhabdomyolysis, certain kidney stones, some medications, drug overdose
Specific gravity	1.003-1.030	Kidney dysfunction (diabetes insipidus, sickle cell nephropathy)	High protein or ketoacids
Red blood cells	<5/HPF		Kidney injury, liver condition, menstruation
White blood cells	<5/HPF		Pyuria (pus in urine), STI
Protein†	Negative		Strenuous exercise, stress, fever, seizure disorder, congestive heart failure
Glucose	Negative		Diabetes, pregnancy
Ketones	Negative		Skipped meals, uncontrolled diabetes, vomiting, pregnancy
Nitrites	Negative		Bacteria in urine, UTI
Crystals	None		Acute kidney injury, gout, UTI
Volume	800-2,500 mL/24 h	Dehydration	Euhydration or hyperhydration

Note: HPF = high-power field; STI = sexually transmitted infection; UTI = urinary tract infection.

*This list is not exhaustive.

†Can have false-positive results.

Complete Blood Count

A **complete blood count (CBC)** presents a microscopic review of a blood sample. It is used to examine specific components of whole blood and expresses those components in designated units (per volume of blood). Physicians often order a CBC as a basic screening test of overall health and to provide information about the ratios of cells per volume of blood. A CBC does not typically furnish information about cell shape or blood type.

The CBC determines the number and types of WBCs and RBCs, hematocrit (volume of RBCs in whole blood), and hemoglobin level. The number of platelets per unit is also estimated. Abnormal blood values can indicate a variety of conditions, described in subsequent chapters. Common disorders, such as anemia, can be present when the hemoglobin level or hematocrit is low. High WBC counts can indicate infections ranging from a skin infection to mononucleosis to leukemia; low RBCs and platelets can be caused by internal bleeding. Table 2.4 shows normal CBC values for adults.

For some blood tests, the patient will be asked to fast overnight, but this is not typical for the common CBC. The cubital fossa of the arm is cleaned, and a compression tourniquet is placed around the upper arm. The technician inserts a needle into a vein in the cleaned area of the patient's arm to draw blood into a tube or syringe. The needle is removed, and gauze is taped over the needle puncture site. The amount of blood removed depends on the type of blood test ordered, and the procedure is called a **venous puncture**. If multiple vials of blood are needed, the technician will collect them via the one venous puncture.

There are no risks or side effects when a CBC is performed under sterile conditions. There might be slight bleeding or bruising over the puncture site. The test results can be affected by stress, dehydration, or overhydration.

In addition to basic screening, a CBC is used to diagnose viral and bacterial infections, such as upper respiratory infection, mononucleosis, anemia, and leukemia. It is also typically ordered to determine cholesterol levels, identify vitamin and mineral deficiencies, and screen for drugs and substances.

Lumbar Puncture

A lumbar puncture can be used to withdraw CSF for examination. It can also be used to give injections to assist in radiographic imaging or to relieve the pain of a herniated disc. The CSF is tested when meningitis is suspected or when there is a need to measure CSF pressure. In the case of diagnostic imaging, a radiopaque substance is injected into the subarachnoid space for clarification of structures in the radiographic image.

Lumbar puncture is performed by placing the patient in a side-lying position with the knees pulled up to the chest and the head fully flexed. This position helps to open the spaces between the vertebrae in the lumbar column. Lumbar puncture is performed under strict sterile conditions. A sterile hollow needle is inserted between two lumbar vertebrae (typically L3 and L4) and enters the subarachnoid space to draw out CSF for assessment (figure 2.14).

The CSF is assessed for pressure and color before it is sent to the laboratory for evaluation of WBCs, glucose, and protein. The lumbar puncture is a good diagnostic tool for meningitis, Lyme disease, Guillain-Barré syndrome, multiple sclerosis, tumors, and other neurological disorders. A physician will sometimes use this procedure to inject medication or anesthetic for other medical procedures. After the puncture, the patient is typically kept prone for 4 to 6 h to reduce the risk of headache.

Pulse Oximeter

A pulse oximeter is a noninvasive device that quickly measures the amount of oxygen saturation in a person's blood. It is used to determine whether a patient may

---

Clinical Tips

Components of Human Blood

- *Human blood* is composed of 52% to 62% plasma and 38% to 48% cells. A typical adult has about 5 L of blood, which is typed A, B, AB, or O, and has a positive or negative rhesus factor.

- *Blood plasma* is largely water; the three chief cell components are erythrocytes (red blood cells [RBCs]), leukocytes (white blood cells [WBCs]), and thrombocytes (platelets). Leukocytes are further divided into five subtypes: neutrophils, basophils, lymphocytes, monocytes, and eosinophils. The function of RBCs is to carry oxygen to working tissues, whereas the WBCs primarily fight the invasion of unrecognized or foreign elements in the body.

TABLE 2.4   **Normal Adult Values for Complete Blood Count**

Parameter measured	Normal range	Low range may indicate*	High range may indicate*
WBC count	$3.8\text{-}10.8 \times 10^3$ cells/μL	Autoimmune disease, viral infection	Infection, inflammation, stress, leukemia
WBC differential			
Absolute neutrophils	1,500-7,800 cells/μL	Immunosuppression, bone marrow issue	Infection, inflammation, leukemia
Absolute eosinophils	50-550 cells/μL	Not typically a concern	Parasitic infection
Absolute basophils	0-200 cells/μL	Not typically a concern	Acute allergic response
Absolute lymphocytes	850-4,100 cells/μL	Immunosuppression, chemotherapy	Viral infections, leukemia
Absolute monocytes	200-1,100 cells/μL	Immunosuppression, chemotherapy	Autoimmune disease, chronic infection
RBC count	Males: $4.4\text{-}5.8 \times 10^6$ cells/μL Females: $3.9\text{-}5.2 \times 10^6$ cells/μL	Acute or chronic blood loss; vitamin B_{12}, iron, or folate deficiency	Dehydration, renal system issue, pulmonary or cardiac issue
Mean corpuscular volume (average size of RBCs)	78-102 fL	Iron deficiency	Vitamin B_{12} or folate deficiency
Mean corpuscular Hb	27-33 pg/RBC	Iron deficiency	Sickle cell disease
Mean corpuscular Hb concentration (Hb/RBC)	32-36 g/dL	Iron deficiency	Sickle cell disease
Distribution width (variation of RBC size)	11%-15%	Not a concern typically	Vitamin B_{12} or folate deficiency, recent blood loss
Hb	Males: 13.8-17.2 g/dL Females: 12.0-15.6 g/dL	Vitamin B_{12}, iron, or folate deficiency; acute or chronic blood loss	Dehydration, renal system issue, pulmonary or cardiac issue
Hct (percentage of RBCs)	Males: 41%-50% Females: 35%-46%	Vitamin B_{12}, iron, or folate deficiency; acute or chronic blood loss	Dehydration, renal system issue, pulmonary or cardiac issue
Platelet count	150,000-450,000/μL	Viral infections, bone marrow failure, lupus, leukemia, lymphoma	Leukemia, inflammatory disorders

Note: Hb = hemoglobin; Hct = hematocrit; RBC = red blood cell; WBC = white blood cell.

*This list is not exhaustive.

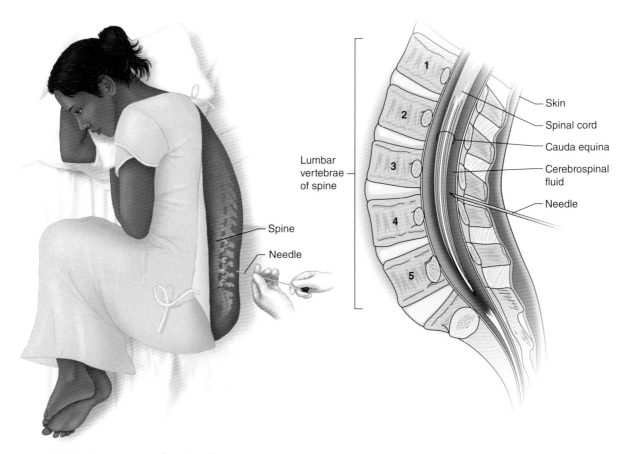

Lumbar
vertebrae
of spine

Spine

Needle

Skin

Spinal cord

Cauda equina

Cerebrospinal
fluid

Needle

FIGURE 2.14   Proper setup for a lumbar puncture.

benefit from supplemental oxygen. Most of these units operate via a pair of light-emitting diodes (LEDs) within a selected wavelength. The light passes through a translucent area, such as an earlobe or fingertip (figure 2.15), and is used to determine the amount of oxygen bound to hemoglobin. The signal vacillates with each heartbeat to display LED absorption in arterial blood. The instrument provides the saturation of peripheral oxygen (SpO_2). Normal SpO_2 values are 95% to 100%. Values below 95% saturation identify hypoxia, and those below 85% are critical.

Limitations that may lead to inaccurate readings in oxygen saturation include external interference (motion, bright light), hypotension, hypothermia, carbon monoxide poisoning, and dark nail polish.

When recording results in a patient's chart, include the date, time, reading, patient position, and activity level. Also include the probe placement site and whether the reading was accompanied by supplemental oxygen.

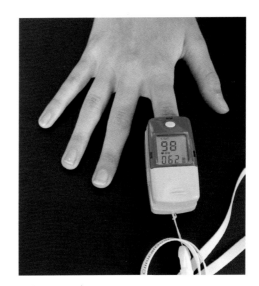

FIGURE 2.15   Pulse oximeter.

Summary

Health care providers must understand common diagnostic imaging and laboratory tests administered to active people. Being able to explain procedures and their expected results is important to help assuage patient anxiety. Knowing how much radiation these procedures emit (see table 2.1) can help in determining which type of evaluation may be best for a given condition and patient. Health care providers can also explain the risks and side effects of tests so patients can be informed and prepared.

Apply It!

Go to HK*Propel* to complete the case studies for this chapter.

PART II
Pharmacology and Interventions

Part II covers issues related to pharmacology, therapeutic drugs, and common procedures in athletic training. Chapter 3, Basic Principles of Pharmacology, describes pharmacokinetics and pharmacodynamics and provides an overview of generalized pharmacologic science. It discusses the regulation of pharmaceuticals, including the roles of the Drug Enforcement Administration and the Food and Drug Administration, and the differences between administering a drug and dispensing a drug. This information is important to athletic trainers because it offers guidance on which drugs may be permissible in sport and describes the legal issues involved in working with medications.

Chapter 4, Drug Categories, discusses the categories of medications and their effects on the body. Mechanism of action and delivery, side effects, and adverse effects are discussed within each drug category. The therapeutic categories of drugs covered include anti-inflammatory agents, analgesics, antibiotics, antivirals, antifungals, bronchodilators, antihistamines, decongestants, and antidiabetic agents. Their individual indications and contraindications and their effects on athletic participation are reviewed. Red Flags features in this chapter include drugs that can have an adverse effect on participation. Also covered are medications that are banned by national and international organizations because they are considered dangerous or because they create unfair advantages for athletes.

Chapter 5, Common Procedures in the Athletic Training Clinic, starts with a brief discussion on informed consent, infection prevention, and the importance of maintaining a sterile field. The chapter provides step-by-step photographic instructions for opening and donning sterile gloves, opening a sterile pack, and opening wrapped supplies. It also describes the use of adhesive skin tape, liquid skin adhesive, and sutures (including photographic demonstrations of various types of knot tying). Step-by-step photographic demonstrations (on pig skin) show simple interrupted sutures, vertical mattress sutures, and horizontal mattress sutures and present the removal of sutures and staples used for wound closure. Joint aspiration and injections are also discussed, and step-by-step intravenous procedures are described and illustrated. The reader is reminded, once again, that practice acts in some states do not allow athletic trainers to perform some of the procedures included in this chapter; however, all of these skills are included in the required educational content for accredited athletic training programs.

Basic Principles
of Pharmacology

3

At the completion of this chapter the reader should be able to do the following:

1. Describe the basics of pharmacokinetics, including routes of drug administration, distribution throughout the body, metabolism, and elimination.

2. Explain the basics of pharmacodynamics, including mechanisms of action, drug interactions, side effects, adverse effects, and allergic reactions.

3. Administer medications via the appropriate route upon the order of a medical provider with appropriate prescribing authority.

4. Explain the regulation of over-the-counter and prescription medications and abide by laws governing their development, use, administration, distribution, and storage.

5. Recommend the safe and appropriate use of supplements, including educating patients that supplements are not regulated and may contain banned substances.

This chapter introduces the regulatory, pharmacological, and pharmaceutical information that athletic trainers must be familiar with and understand. The role of the athletic trainer or other health care professional will invariably involve pharmaceutical agents and their use by their patients. Important U.S. regulatory agencies discussed in relation to athletic trainers include the Food and Drug Administration (FDA), the Drug Enforcement Administration (DEA), and the National Collegiate Athletics Association (NCAA). The basic principles of pharmacology cover pharmacokinetics, routes of administration, drug storage and resources, pharmacodynamics, indications and contraindications, and special considerations for athletes or other physically active people. Content about pharmaceuticals is organized by drug categories and identifies available drug forms and dosages, routes of administration, correct methods for storage of specific drugs, and side effects. This chapter also reviews some popular supplements and cautions the reader that although they are widely used, supplements are not regulated by the FDA or any other agency and may contain ingredients that are banned or that may interfere with other medications. Drug information resources also are reviewed. This chapter is designed as an overview and lists additional sources for continued reading and expanded content.

Regulation of Pharmaceuticals

Athletic trainers must understand the legal regulations that apply to the use of medications. Two entities of the U.S. federal government are charged with controlling the use of pharmaceutical products: the FDA and the DEA. Health Canada is the FDA-equivalent agency in Canada. Health Canada's various subdivisions are responsible for regulating food and health products, including pharmaceuticals, biological agents, and genetic therapies.[1]

Drug Enforcement Administration

The DEA is situated within the Department of Justice. Its function is to ensure compliance with the Controlled Substances Act of 1970 and to implement the regulations found in Title 21, Code of Federal Regulations, Part 1300 to the end. The DEA registers health care practitioners who prescribe or dispense drugs that are considered controlled substances and advises them on how to comply with controlled substance regulations.

Controlled substances are drugs that have a high potential for abuse (e.g., morphine, codeine). The DEA has established five categories or *schedules* of controlled substances (Schedules I-V). Table 3.1 provides examples of controlled substances in these five categories based on their likelihood for abuse.

Food and Drug Administration

The FDA is an agency of the Department of Health and Human Services. This agency has three main responsibilities:

1. The FDA is responsible for protecting the public health.
2. The FDA is also responsible for advancing the public health.
3. The FDA plays a significant role in the nation's counterterrorism capability.

The mission of the FDA is to "protect the public health by ensuring the safety, efficacy, and security of human and veterinary drugs, biological products, and medical

TABLE 3.1   Drug Enforcement Administration Schedules of Controlled Substances

Schedule	Description	Examples of drugs*
I	Drugs with no accepted medical use in the United States High abuse potential	Hallucinogens (heroin, LSD, mescaline) Methylenedioxymethamphetamine (ecstasy) Marijuana (cannabis)†
II	Drugs with high abuse potential Severe psychic or physical dependence liability Tightly controlled prescribing requirements, including written prescription (*no* verbal orders) from physician No refills without additional prescription from physician	Methadone Meperidine (Demerol) Fentanyl Morphine Oxycodone (OxyContin, Percocet) Amphetamine (Dexedrine, Adderall) Methylphenidate (Ritalin) Methamphetamine (Desoxyn)
III	Drugs with less abuse potential than those in Schedule I or II	Products with <90 mg of codeine (Tylenol with codeine) Benzphetamine (Didrex) Ketamine Depressants Anabolic steroids
IV	Drugs with less abuse potential than those in Schedule III	Alprazolam (Xanax) Carisoprodol (Soma) Clonazepam (Klonopin) Diazepam (Valium) Lorazepam (Ativan) Midazolam (Versed)
V	Drugs with less abuse potential than those in Schedule IV Class consists of preparations containing limited quantities of certain narcotic ingredients generally for antitussive and antidiarrheal purposes	Cough preparations containing <200 mg of codeine or opium per 100 g (Robitussin AC)

Note: LSD = lysergic acid diethylamide.

*Examples of drugs in each schedule do not represent an all-inclusive list.

†As of December 2023, marijuana was still a Schedule I controlled substance, according to the Drug Enforcement Administration; however, many states have legalized marijuana for both medical and recreational use and a federal task force has been established to explore the appropriate location for marijuana within the controlled substance table.[2]

devices; and by ensuring the safety of our nation's food supply, cosmetics and products that emit radiation."[3] Through oversight of science-based information, the FDA seeks to speed innovations that make medicines more effective, safer, and more affordable for the public. In its role in promoting the nation's counterterrorism capability, the FDA fulfills this responsibility by ensuring the security of the food supply and by fostering the development of medical products to respond to deliberate and naturally emerging public health threats.[3]

The FDA is responsible for approving and overseeing manufacturers who may produce medications for consumption, the approval of new chemical formulations for marketing and sale via either prescription or nonprescription (e.g., over-the-counter [OTC] products), and the approval of generic drug products that must exhibit the bioequivalence of a trade-name product.

The FDA is also charged with determining how drugs may be marketed and sold in the United States, including the drug's indications, information contained in the product's package insert, and how the drug is manufactured. Pharmaceutical product manufacturers must meet very stringent manufacturing guidelines and pass FDA inspections. The drug products that they produce must consistently pass dissolution and bioequivalence tests. The FDA does not oversee the marketing or sale of food supplements and herbal products, and neither does any other government agency, even though these supplements are used by the general population and especially by athletes.

Administration Versus Dispensing

Most states regulate both administration and dispensing of drugs. The athletic trainer must understand the differences between these two actions. **Dispensing** is generally defined as the act of delivering a medication to an ultimate user pursuant to a medical order issued by a practitioner authorized to prescribe (however, this can vary by state).[4] This includes the packaging, labeling, or compounding necessary to prepare the medication for such delivery. A facility that dispenses prescription medication must have a separate DEA certification.[5] **Administration** is the act of applying a medication by injection, inhalation, ingestion, or any other means to the body of a patient in a single dose.[4]

Both dispensing and administration of prescription medications require a written prescription from a physician. Current state laws prohibit physicians from delegating the duty of prescription drug dispensing to providers not licensed to do so, including athletic trainers.[4] The athletic training facility (whether the main facility or ancillary facilities such as a sideline, bus, or hotel) must comply with both state and federal regulations governing prescription medications. Most states require that an athletic training facility have a DEA certificate and a signed agreement with a physician in cases in which medical staff serve as an "agency" in the care of the physician's patients. In these situations, the athletic trainer is acting as an agent assigned by the DEA and is not acting under the scope of the state practice act for athletic trainers; at no time does the agent make any discretionary decisions about the administration or dosage of a medication.

Sports medicine teams must ensure that medication is properly stored, packaged, and labeled. Athletic training facilities may want to consider a pharmacy service, which is a system to provide and inventory individually packaged and labeled medications (including both prescription and OTC agents). These services provide unit dosing so that medication is not repackaged from larger quantities to individual doses for a patient or for a medical kit. All medication should be stored in a dry, environmentally controlled space, with all prescription medications stored in a locked space accessible only by

---

Clinical Tips

Bioequivalence

Bioequivalence is the quality of having the same drug strength and providing an equivalent amount of drug to the target tissue in the same dosage form as another sample of a given drug substance. For example, for two drugs to be considered bioequivalent, they must meet the following criteria:

- Have the same dosage form (e.g., tablet, suspension)
- Have the same drug strength
- Provide equivalent blood levels or tissue levels of the drug

---

Clinical Tips

Administration Versus Dispensing

- Administration is the direct application of a single dose of a drug.
- Dispensing includes packaging and labeling prescription medication (multiple doses).
- Facilities that dispense medications must have a Drug Enforcement Administration (DEA) certificate on file. Individuals do not hold DEA certificates; only facilities apply for and obtain DEA certificates.

appropriate personnel.[6] Most states do not allow athletic trainers to dispense prescription medications even with standing orders; however, the administration of certain drugs, especially lifesaving medications such as epinephrine or naloxone, is allowed by many state statutes.[7] The appropriate administration of these medications is taught in all athletic trainer educational programs, as required by the standards set forth by the Commission on Accreditation of Athletic Training Education.[8]

Pharmacology

Pharmacology is the science of drugs and includes pharmacokinetics and pharmacodynamics.

- **Pharmacokinetics** is the study of how the body acts on the drug. Pharmacokinetics includes the absorption, distribution, metabolism, and elimination of the drug in the body.
- **Pharmacodynamics** is the study of the actions of a drug on the body, including the mechanism of action and medicinal effects (i.e., the biochemical and physiological effects of the drug). This may involve a stimulatory or inhibitory reaction at the receptor.

To better understand how drugs work within the body, it is important to understand the process by which a drug gets into the body, is distributed, is metabolized, and, finally, is eliminated (figure 3.1). The methods of absorption, distribution, metabolism, and elimination are discussed here.

Absorption (also called *administration*) is the process of getting the drug into the body. Drugs may be absorbed through various routes, including the rectal, intestinal, and dermal tissues. Which route is used depends on many different patient-related and drug-related factors. Patient-related considerations include age, level of consciousness, and disease being treated; drug-related factors include solubility and stability. The desired route of absorption will determine the formulation used. For example, rectal absorption generally indicates the use of a suppository, but tablets, capsules, liquids, and suspensions may also be absorbed rectally.

Absorption has a major influence on the bioavailability of a drug. *Bioavailability* describes how much of the drug is available to the tissues after its administration. Bioavailability is an important concept in drug development, especially as it pertains to generic drugs. For any generic drug to be considered equivalent to a trade-name preparation, it must be shown to have bioavailability that is equal to the trade-name product.

Distribution refers to the process of moving the drug throughout the body. Most drugs are distributed throughout most or all body tissues, but this distribution is not necessarily even. For example, many drugs do not cross the blood–brain barrier to enter the central nervous system (CNS). Factors such as the drug's pH, **hydrophilicity** (water solubility), and **lipophilicity** (fat

Clinical Tips

Pharmacokinetics

- absorption—Process of getting the drug into the body through a variety of routes, including oral, rectal, vaginal, intravenous, intramuscular, inhalation, and topical application to the skin; also called *administration*
- distribution—Process of moving the drug throughout the body tissues and fluids; whether a drug is fat or water soluble is a factor, and the medication's ability to cross the blood–brain barrier also affects distribution
- metabolism—Process by which the drug is changed into chemical entities in the body different from the drug itself
- elimination—Process of getting the drug out of the body

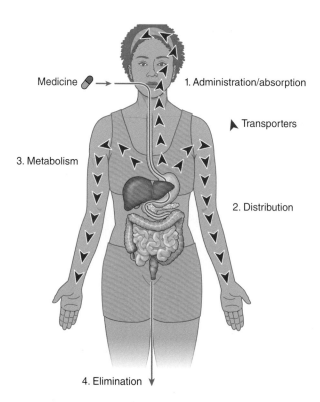

Medicine → 1. Administration/absorption

Transporters

3. Metabolism

2. Distribution

4. Elimination

FIGURE 3.1 Pharmacokinetics.

solubility) affect its distribution throughout the body.[9] The concept of *volume of distribution* is used to describe the effective space in the body available to contain a drug. This is the ratio of the total amount of drug in the body to the plasma concentration of drug. Drugs with a high volume of distribution have lower plasma concentrations and are more greatly distributed into extravascular tissues. Drugs with a lower volume of distribution have higher plasma concentrations and less distribution into extravascular tissues.

Metabolism is the complex process by which a drug is changed into one or more chemical entities that differ from the parent drug. These entities may be active metabolites that have a pharmacological effect or inactive metabolites with no pharmacological effect.[10] Drug metabolism occurs primarily in the liver through the action of various hepatic enzymes, although some metabolism occurs in a few other tissues in the body, such as the lungs.

Elimination is the process of getting the drug out of the body. A drug and its metabolites are eliminated through some combination of renal or fecal excretion. Although some drugs are completely eliminated either through renal or fecal excretion, most drugs and their metabolites undergo elimination through a combination of these two mechanisms. Additional means of excretion, although to a much lesser extent, are by the lungs, through sweat, or by salivary and mammary glands. The kidney is the most important excretion channel for most drugs. In persons with renal or hepatic impairment, the rate of drug elimination is slowed to a degree dependent on the level of impairment. This means that the dose of a drug or the frequency of administration often needs to be adjusted in patients with renal or hepatic dysfunction.

Clearance and *half-life* are two concepts used to describe the elimination of a drug from the body. **Clearance** is the measure of the body's ability to eliminate a drug. It describes the volume of blood that is cleared of a drug over a given period, usually expressed in milliliters per minute. Drugs with a higher clearance rate are removed from the body more quickly. Creatinine clearance is the rate of removal of creatinine from the serum into the urine and is used as a measure of renal function. Normal creatinine clearance is 100 mL/min for men and 80 mL/min for women.[10] In patients with impaired renal function, it is important to determine creatinine clearance. In pharmaceutical reference books, dosage adjustments for renal impairment are given based on creatinine clearance.

Half-life is the length of time that it takes for blood levels or tissue levels of a drug to decrease by one-half. The clearance rate of a drug and the drug's volume of distribution both determine the drug half-life. The half-life is directly proportional to the volume of distribution and inversely proportional to the clearance. This means that a drug with a high clearance rate and a small volume of distribution has a short half-life and is eliminated from the body rapidly. A drug with a large volume of distribution and a low clearance rate has a long half-life.[9]

Half-life is one of the major determining factors in how often a drug will be given. As a rule, a drug with a long half-life has a long dosage interval. A drug with a short half-life has a short dosage interval. If the clearance rate of a drug is decreased by renal or hepatic dysfunction, this increases the half-life of the drug and necessitates an increase in the dosage interval.[9] Patients with an altered volume of distribution attributable to disease (e.g., ascites) also will have an altered drug half-life. It is important to know the effects of disease on drug half-life so that changes in the dosage regimen may be made.

Routes of Administration

Drugs can enter the body through a variety of routes, and these paths of administration promote the drug's absorption. Following are the routes of administration:

Oral	Intraarterial
Ophthalmic	Sublingual
Otic	Rectal
Intravenous	Topical
Intramuscular	Intravaginal
Subcutaneous	Intranasal
Inhalation	Subarachnoid

The oral route of administration is the most common, but often it is more appropriate to use a parenteral (nonoral) route. The preferred route is determined by many factors, including ease of administration, patient adherence, desired onset of action, local versus systemic distribution, and properties of the drug itself. An example is the destruction of insulin in the gastrointestinal tract, which necessitates its administration through a nonoral route.

Oral

The oral route is a convenient, noninvasive way to deliver drugs that are distributed systemically. Tablets, capsules, solutions, and suspensions are dosage forms used to deliver drugs orally. Tablets contain the drug compressed or embedded along with inert ingredients into a compact unit, and they may be either uncoated or coated. Enteric coatings are used to ensure that a tablet does not dissolve in the low pH of gastric acid but instead passes into the small intestine, where the tablet is dissolved and the drug absorbed. Drugs that are destroyed by gastric acid or that may cause local irritation in the stomach, such as aspirin, are delivered in an enteric coating. Other tablet coatings provide controlled release of drug over an extended period, allowing for less frequent dosing. *Delayed release*, *extended release*, and *controlled release* are all terms used to refer to dosage forms that are constructed to prolong the release of drug from the tablet or capsule so that the drug may be given at extended dosage intervals.

Other mechanisms allow for controlled release of the drug from a tablet, such as an osmotic delivery system used to deliver the antihypertensive drug nifedipine (Procardia XL). In such systems, the drug is contained in an osmotically active core surrounded by a semipermeable membrane. When the tablet is exposed to water in the gastrointestinal tract, water is drawn into the core at a controlled rate, resulting in a suspension of the drug that is pushed out through an orifice in the tablet.

Capsules are solid oral dosage forms that contain powdered, beaded, or liquid drug inside a gelatin shell. Some shells are formulated to dissolve in the stomach; others dissolve in the intestines. Some capsule shells are designed to release the drug in a controlled fashion over an extended period.

Oral solutions, elixirs, and syrups contain drug completely dissolved in a liquid medium. Elixirs typically contain alcohol to aid in drug dissolution. Syrups contain high concentrations of sugar to make them more palatable. Oral suspensions are also liquids, but they contain undissolved drug dispersed or suspended throughout the liquid. All suspensions must be shaken before administration to ensure that the drug is dispersed evenly throughout the liquid. Antibiotic suspensions often require refrigeration and may have a short expiration date, after which they must be discarded.

Clinical Tips

Dissolution

Dissolution is the process of dissolving a substance. In the context of pharmaceuticals, it is the process of a solid, oral dosage form (e.g., tablet or capsule) being dissolved in the gastrointestinal tract so that it can be absorbed. Poorly manufactured products may not dissolve at all and may be passed through the gastrointestinal tract and into the stool without allowing the expected dose of medication to be absorbed.

Inhaled

Inhaled drugs are most often used for their local effect on the bronchial passages. Bronchodilators and corticosteroids are the drugs most often given via this route to treat bronchoconstriction from asthma and sinusitis. These drugs may be administered via metered-dose inhalers (MDIs), dry-powder inhalers, or **nebulizers** (figure 3.2). MDIs and dry-powder inhalers deliver a set dose of drug with each inhalation. Nebulizer machines use compressed air to cause aerosolization of a liquid drug, which is then inhaled through a mask or mouthpiece. Intranasal sprays and inhalers are used for a local effect on the intranasal passages. Corticosteroids and decongestants are the most common drugs delivered intranasally to treat allergic rhinitis symptoms. Naloxone may also be administered intranasally for emergency opioid overdose.

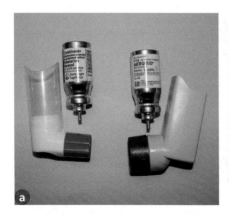 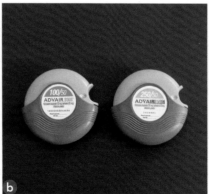 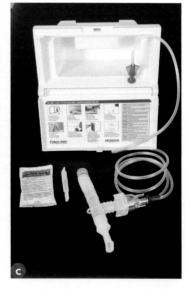

FIGURE 3.2   *(a)* Metered-dose inhalers, *(b)* dry-powder inhalers, and *(c)* nebulizers are commonly used to administer inhaled medications.

(a) © Micki Cuppett

Ophthalmic

Ophthalmic administration of drugs may be used to treat eye infections, allergies, dryness, glaucoma, and other eye disorders. Droppers used to administer drugs into the eye must be kept sterile and must never touch the eye. Administration of drops into the lateral area of the eye also increases comfort, because the medial area, pupil, and iris are much more sensitive. Applying the drops laterally also helps bathe the eye, because tears are produced laterally and flow medially to the nasolacrimal duct (figure 3.3).

Otic

Otic administration of drugs is used primarily to treat otitis, decrease pain from otitis, and prevent recurrence of otitis in patients whose ear canals are often exposed to moisture, such as swimmers. Droppers used to administer drugs into the ear canal do not need to be sterile, but every attempt must be made to avoid touching the dropper to the ear during administration. Administration of ear drops requires the patient to be in a sitting or side-lying position. The ear canal is straightened by pulling up and back on the pinna. The dropper is held approximately 1/2 in. above the ear canal (figure 3.4). After the drops are administered, gently massage the tragus of the ear and have the patient remain quiet for a few minutes so all the medication can work into the ear. Although it is not uncommon for ophthalmic drops to be prescribed for use in the ear, otic drops are never used in the eye.

Topical

Topical administration refers to application of a drug to the outer areas of the body for a local effect rather than a systemic effect. Creams, ointments, gels, and solutions are the most common dosage forms used for topical administration. Topical drugs may be used for several

Clinical Tips

Administration of Ophthalmic and Otic Drops

Individuals who administer ophthalmic or otic drops must wash their hands thoroughly before and after administration. Warming the drops to body temperature by rolling the dropper bottle rapidly between the hands may increase patient comfort during administration.

purposes, such as treatment of infection, inflammatory skin disorders (e.g., dermatitis), or acne. The drug and its intended use determine the frequency of application, whether it should be applied in a thick layer or sparingly, and if a dressing or bandage should be used after application. The area where the drug is to be applied should be as clean and dry as possible. Individuals who apply topical preparations must wash their hands before and after application of the drug; some drugs necessitate the wearing of gloves.

Transdermal

Transdermal administration is the application of a drug to the skin, usually in the form of a patch. Once the drug is absorbed, it produces a systemic effect. Nitroglycerin, estrogen, testosterone, and fentanyl (a pain medication) are all available in patch form for transdermal administration. The frequency with which old patches are removed and replaced with new ones varies depending on the drug. Patches should be applied to hairless areas on the trunk, with the exception that estrogen patches should not be applied to the breasts. When an old patch is removed and a new one applied, the new patch is put in a different area

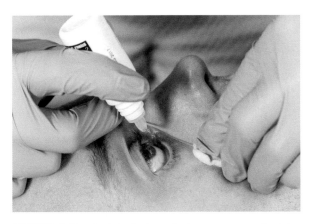

FIGURE 3.3 Ophthalmic solutions are applied by holding the eyedropper above the conjunctival sac laterally to allow the drops to flow toward the nasolacrimal duct.

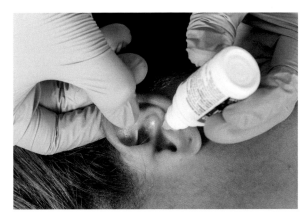

FIGURE 3.4 Administration of otic drops.

to minimize irritation. The old patch is then folded in on itself (sticky side in) and discarded in the trash so that it cannot be reapplied.

Intravenous

Intravenous (IV) injection of a drug directly into a vein (figure 3.5) is used in situations in which immediate onset of drug action is required or where the use of other routes is not possible because of the patient's condition or the drug's characteristics. The athletic trainer will see the IV route most often in situations in which IV fluids (typically without medication added) are administered to achieve rapid hydration of a patient experiencing heat-related illness. Athletic trainers must be aware of state practice laws to understand the limits of their role in administering IV fluids. Many states allow athletic trainers with formal training to administer IV fluids under the supervision of a physician.

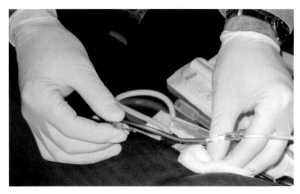

FIGURE 3.5   Intravenous injection.
© Micki Cuppett

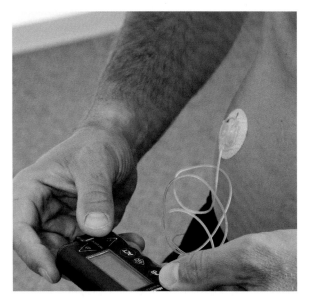

FIGURE 3.6   Insulin pump.

Intramuscular

The intramuscular (IM) route may be used for various reasons. In situations where a rapid, reliable onset of drug action is required but IV access is impractical, the IM route is the best alternative. Typically, IM injections are given in large muscle groups such as the deltoid or gluteus muscles. Meperidine (Demerol) can be administered via IM injection for migraine. The IM route is also used for injection of suspensions that will be slowly absorbed to deliver a drug over prolonged periods. Medroxyprogesterone (Depo-Provera), a birth control injection lasting for 3 mo, is given via the IM route. The IM route is used to administer nearly all vaccinations.

Subcutaneous, Intrasynovial, and Intraarticular Injections

The subcutaneous route is used for injection of a drug into subcutaneous fat and for rapid, reliable onset of drug action when IV access is impractical. This route is also preferred for self-injected medications (e.g., insulin, epinephrine in pen form [EpiPen], and some pain medications such as morphine). Pumps are available that provide a continuous infusion of drug into a subcutaneous catheter.[11] Patients with diabetes who use subcutaneous insulin pumps adjust the insulin infusion rate based on their current blood glucose level, activity level, and food intake to achieve much better control of blood glucose than with conventional subcutaneous injections (figure 3.6). Epinephrine is often self-administered through an autoinjector or EpiPen for treatment of emergency anaphylaxis (figure 3.7).

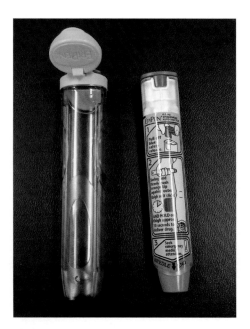

FIGURE 3.7   EpiPen.
© Katie Walsh Flanagan

Using an EpiPen

1. Take the EpiPen out of the protective tube.
2. Remove the blue protective safety cap.
3. Quickly jab the orange tip into the thigh. (The autoinjector is designed to go through clothing.) The EpiPen will click so the user knows that it worked.
4. Hold the EpiPen against the thigh for 3 s and then remove.

Intrasynovial injection is used to place a drug, usually an anti-inflammatory corticosteroid suspension, into the synovial cavity of a joint. The drug will not be absorbed systemically but will act locally to decrease inflammation.

Intraarticular injection refers to injection of the drug into the joint. As with intrasynovial injection, the drug will not be absorbed systemically but will act locally to decrease inflammation.

Iontophoresis and Phonophoresis

Drugs may also be introduced into the body through use of electricity (iontophoresis) or ultrasound (phonophoresis). Both delivery methods drive ionized medication into the subcutaneous tissues. Iontophoresis uses low-voltage, high-amperage direct current and requires the use of customized electrodes (figure 3.8). Transdermal introduction has advantages over oral ingestion because it bypasses the liver, reducing metabolic breakdown of the medication, and can be concentrated in a local area. It provides advantages over injected medications because it is less painful and does not result in high concentrations in the soft tissue, which have been associated with tendon rupture.[12]

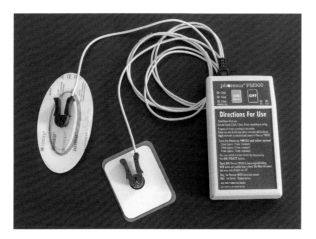

FIGURE 3.8 Iontophoresis delivers ionized medication using low-voltage, high-amperage direct current (DC).

Iontophoresis also has disadvantages. It cannot reach deep tissue structures or areas of thick skin. Many medications may be used with iontophoresis, and they are usually dissolved in a carrier. Typical medications include acetic acid, dexamethasone, lidocaine, and epinephrine in varying combinations.

Phonophoresis does not actually drive the ions of the medication through the skin; rather, it opens pathways that allow the medication to diffuse through the skin and pass deeper into the tissue. Some medications have been shown to be delivered up to 6 cm into the tissue with phonophoresis.[13] Medications typically administered this way include corticosteroids, such as hydrocortisone and dexamethasone, salicylates, and anesthetics.

Additional research has produced significant breakthroughs for the delivery of topical medications.[12,14] Athletic trainers will be expected to master new techniques as they are developed, because they are the ones who provide most topical medications for their patients.

Drug Storage

The proper storage of drugs is essential to maintain drug potency. Temperature, humidity, and exposure to light must all be considered. Most drugs are best stored in a cool, dry, dark place. This means room temperatures of 65 to 80 °F, with low humidity (<50%) and limited exposure to sunlight.[9] Drugs requiring refrigeration are typically oral antibiotic suspensions, immunizations, insulin, and injected drugs that have been reconstituted from powders.

Some refrigerated drugs may be kept for limited time at room temperature, whereas others lose potency rapidly if left unrefrigerated. Many emergency drugs (e.g., epinephrine, phenylephrine) degrade rapidly on exposure to sunlight or high temperatures. Other drugs cannot tolerate freezing.

It is particularly important to consider the storage needs of all drugs during transportation. Medical kits for use at outdoor athletic events must be inspected regularly to ensure integrity of the stocked drug products. Security of the drugs must also be ensured. All prescription medications must be stored in a locked cabinet or a locked portable medical treatment kit. Protocols must be followed that do not violate state practice acts or federal DEA guidelines for dispensing prescription medication. Dispensing prescription medications is not within the scope of practice for athletic trainers in most states. However, some states may allow the athletic trainer to be licensed as an agent for the physician. The athletic trainer must only be assigned duties that are allowed by applicable state law.[4]

Pharmacodynamics

Pharmacodynamics is the study of how medications work in the body, including the mechanisms of action, drug interactions, side effects, adverse reactions, and allergic reactions. Some concepts necessary for later discussion are reviewed here.

A drug's mechanism of action may be very simple. An example is the action of magnesium hydroxide in the stomach, where it neutralizes stomach acid through a simple acid–base reaction. Another simple mechanism of action is exhibited by bulk-forming laxatives, in which insoluble fibers cause increased stool volume in the large intestine.

Other drugs act through more complicated mechanisms. **Agonists** are drugs that exert their effect by attaching to cellular receptors in the body, causing stimulation of the receptors (figure 3.9). Agonists mimic the effects of endogenous chemicals, which normally target cellular receptors.[9] Morphine, an opiate agonist, stimulates opiate receptors in the body that are normally targeted by the body's own endorphins. Endorphins cause decreased sensitivity to pain and impart a sense of well-being or euphoria. Intense exercise causes the release of endorphins in the body, which explains the euphoria and pain tolerance that occur in many athletes during endurance events. Morphine is used for its therapeutic effect of decreasing sensitivity to pain. The euphoria produced by morphine is the reason for its high abuse potential.

Antagonists also act by binding to cellular receptors, but they do not cause stimulation of the receptor. An antagonist binds to the receptor and blocks other chemicals or agonists from binding to it. Antihistamines bind to histamine receptors in the body but do not cause stimulation of the receptors. Rather, antihistamines block the binding of histamine to histamine receptors, thereby preventing the itching, rhinitis, and edema that histamine causes when it is released by immune system cells in response to an allergen.[9]

Inhibition of enzyme action is another important mechanism of action for several of the drugs discussed later in this chapter. Enzymes are proteins that act as biochemical catalysts for chemical reactions that occur in the body. Some drugs exert their effect by breaking down enzymes or blocking the effect of enzymes, thereby preventing or slowing down the reactions for which these enzymes are responsible. The cyclooxygenase (COX)-1 and COX-2 enzymes are involved in the biochemical transformation of arachidonic acid into prostaglandins. Prostaglandins are chemicals that cause pain and inflammation.

Anti-inflammatory drugs are COX inhibitors that prevent COX-1 or COX-2 from facilitating the prostaglandin production. A drug's mechanism of action often

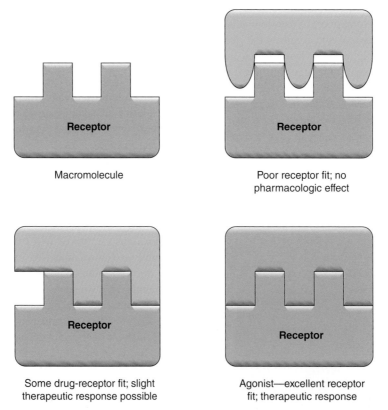

Macromolecule

Poor receptor fit; no pharmacologic effect

Some drug-receptor fit; slight therapeutic response possible

Agonist—excellent receptor fit; therapeutic response

FIGURE 3.9 Drug–receptor interaction can take place when agonists with shapes that match an endogenous chemical fit exactly into a cell receptor or when an antagonist binds to a receptor, thereby blocking the agonist and preventing it from stimulating the receptor.

is directly related to its side effects and drug interactions. For example, β-adrenergic agonists, which stimulate β-adrenergic receptors, cause bronchodilation and are used to treat asthmatic attacks. People who take β-blockers to treat hypertension may have a decreased response to β-agonists.[9,10]

Indications

Indications outline conditions for which a drug shows a therapeutic effect. The indications are FDA approved, meaning that (1) the drug manufacturer has provided a body of research to the FDA supporting the use of the drug for a particular indication and (2) the FDA has approved the use of the drug for that indication. FDA-approved indications are found on the drug package insert.

Contraindications

Contraindications are situations in which a drug must be avoided. Disease states, other medications, pregnancy, age, and sex may all be reasons for a particular drug to be contraindicated. For example, tetracycline antibiotics are contraindicated in children younger than age 7 yr because their use stains permanent teeth. Decongestants, which can cause profound, transient elevations in blood pressure, are contraindicated in people with uncontrolled hypertension.[10] Although athletic trainers do not prescribe or dispense medications, they must be aware of contraindications to medications commonly used by their patients. It is important for athletic trainers to be aware of

---

Clinical Tips

Indications and Contraindications

- indications—Conditions for which the drug has been found to have a therapeutic effect
- contraindications—Situations in which a drug should be absolutely avoided

---

RED FLAGS FOR HYPERTENSION AND DECONGESTANTS

Patients with uncontrolled hypertension should avoid pseudoephedrine as a decongestant because it may cause profound, transient elevations in blood pressure. Many multisymptom cold medications contain these decongestants, and it may not be obvious that their use is not safe for individuals with high blood pressure. OTC decongestants are available that are marked safe for people with high blood pressure.

---

their patients' medication history. Working closely with the physician and pharmacist will ensure the best health care for the patient.

Warnings and precautions are statements that alert health care professionals to the serious adverse events associated with the use of a drug. Black box warnings are strong precautions that the FDA mandates be printed inside a black box at the very top of a product's package insert (figure 3.10). As with contraindications, the athletic trainer must be familiar with the warnings and precautions for all drugs prescribed for their patients.

The term *drug interaction* most commonly refers to the interaction of one drug with another drug, but it may also refer to interactions between drugs and foods and drugs with disease states. Drug interactions with foods occur most commonly when the minerals in a particular food inhibit drug absorption (table 3.2). For example, administration of fluoroquinolone antibiotics with calcium-containing foods decreases absorption of the antibiotic because the calcium binds to the antibiotic and forms an insoluble complex.

Drug–disease interactions may occur for a variety of reasons. For example, the administration of drugs that block β-adrenergic receptors, or β-blockers, is not recommended for people with diabetes because these drugs

---

WARNING
Cardiovascular Risk
May increase risk of serious and potentially fatal cardiovascular thrombotic events, MI (heart attack), and stroke; risk may increase with duration of use; possible increased risk with cardiovascular disease or cardiovascular disease risk factors; contraindicated for CABG peri-operative pain.

GI Risk
Increased risk of serious GI adverse events include bleeding, ulcer, and stomach or intestine perforation, which can be fatal; may occur at any time during use and without warning symptoms; elderly patients at greater risk for serious GI events.

FIGURE 3.10 Sample black box warnings from the FDA.

TABLE 3.2 **Selected Drug–Food Interactions**

Drug	Food	Interaction
Analgesics and antipyretics	Alcohol	Increased risk of liver damage
Antihistamines	Alcohol	Can increase drowsiness caused by these medications
Benzodiazepines	Caffeine	Antagonism of antianxiety action
Bronchodilators	Caffeine Alcohol	Can cause increased excitability, nervousness, and rapid heartbeat Increased chance of nausea, vomiting, headache, and irritability
Griseofulvin	Fatty foods	Increased blood levels of griseofulvin
Fluoroquinolones (ciprofloxacin, moxifloxacin)	Dairy products Caffeine	Dairy products can interfere with absorption May increase the effects of caffeine
MAO inhibitors	Coffee, tea, chocolate (caffeine-containing)	Excessive consumption can lead to hypertensive crises or dangerous cardiac arrhythmias
Statins	Grapefruit juice	Increased bioavailability, inhibition of first-pass metabolism, increased toxicity
Tetracyclines	Dairy products high in calcium, ferrous sulfate, antacids	Impaired absorption of tetracycline
Thiamine	Blueberries, fish, alcohol	Decreased intake, absorption, and utilization, owing to thiaminase-containing foods
Timed-release drug preparations	Alcoholic beverages	Increased rate of release for some

Note: MAO = monoamine oxidase.

mask symptoms of hypoglycemia that are mediated by the sympathetic nervous system, such as tremors.

Drug–drug interactions occur when one drug affects the absorption, metabolism, distribution, receptor binding, or elimination of another drug. For example, many antibiotics, such as penicillin, change the bacterial composition of the intestine, which in turn alters the metabolism of oral contraceptives. As a result, the effectiveness of oral contraceptives may be decreased in females taking certain antibiotics. Although many drug interactions are undesirable, some interactions can be used for a beneficial therapeutic effect. Histamine$_2$ (H$_2$) receptor blockers, such as famotidine (Pepcid), interact with orally administered pancreatic enzymes (Pancreaze) in a beneficial way.[10] Pancreatic enzymes are susceptible to acid–peptic enzyme degradation. Administration of an H$_2$ blocker increases gastric pH and decreases acid–peptic degradation of pancreatic enzymes, thereby decreasing the dose of pancreatic enzymes required.

Drug allergies occur when the medicine produces a response different from what is expected. Symptoms may include severe itching and hives, which are signs of an allergic response. Some allergic reactions may be anaphylactic and may include bronchospasm and shock.

It is important to distinguish drug allergies from drug side effects. Drug side effects are conditions reported by the majority of people who take a particular medication, whereas a drug allergy is an unusual presentation seen in approximately 6% to 10% of patients who take that medication.[15] Because of the potential severity of drug allergy reactions, it is important to know whether the patient is allergic to any medications. Allergy to a medication is obviously a contraindication for taking that medication.

The side effects of or adverse reactions to a drug are the drug's nontherapeutic actions. Usually, drugs of the same class have similar side-effect profiles. For exam-

RED FLAGS FOR DRUG ALLERGIES

- Severe itching
- Hives or other signs of allergic response
- Bronchospasm
- Dysphagia (difficulty swallowing)
- Dysarthria (difficulty speaking)
- Shock

ple, the nonsteroidal anti-inflammatory drugs ibuprofen (Advil, Motrin) and naproxen (Naprosyn, Aleve) have nearly identical side effects.[16] Serious adverse effects of a drug should be reported to the FDA MedWatch program. These include any adverse effect that results in death, disability, hospitalization, life-threatening condition, or congenital anomaly. Adverse drug effects that require medical or surgical intervention to prevent permanent impairment should also be reported. The pharmacy that dispensed the medication or the office of the prescribing physician may assist in producing the report. Reporting of adverse reactions is extremely important, especially in the case of newly approved drugs, because it is used to identify potentially serious adverse effects of a drug that may lead to changes in the product's labeling or even withdrawal of the drug from the market.

Many drugs are being given expedited, fast-tracked FDA approval. Compared with other drugs that are not fast tracked, fewer people will have used these drugs before they are approved. Serious adverse reactions or serious drug interactions may not be discovered until after the drug has received FDA approval. The FDA and the drug manufacturers rely on postmarketing surveillance, including the MedWatch program, for reports of these adverse incidents.

Dosages

Drug dosages take many factors into consideration. The first consideration is age. Children older than age 12 yr may generally be given dosages using guidelines for adults. For children younger than age 12 yr, many dosages are simply based on age. This approach presumes that a child is of normal weight. For premature infants and underweight or overweight children, determining doses by age range is not optimal.

On the opposite end of the age spectrum, older adults may require decreased drug dosages. The two main reasons for this are as follows:

1. advanced age causes increased sensitivity to many drugs, such as CNS depressants, and

2. aging also is associated with diminished hepatic and renal function, which decreases the rate at which drugs are eliminated from the body and necessitates the use of smaller doses.

Dosages based on weight or body surface area are preferable for prescribing medications for children. Numerous resources are available to calculate pediatric dosages based on known weight, including electronic references such as Epocrates, Lexicomp, and Micromedex and desk references such as *The Harriet Lane Handbook* and *The Pediatric and Neonatal Dosage Handbook*. In addition, dosages for some medications administered to adults, such as cancer chemotherapy drugs or certain antibiotics, are based on weight or body surface area. In children and adults with obesity, the prescriber may need to use an ideal body weight or adjusted body weight to calculate an appropriate drug dose.

For some drugs given by weight, the dose is expressed in terms of milligrams, grams, or units per kilogram per dose (e.g., acetaminophen, 10 mg/kg/dose given every 4-6 h). For other drugs, the dosage is published as milligrams, grams, or units per kilogram per day,[19] followed by the recommended number of divided doses per day (e.g., amoxicillin, 40 mg/kg/d divided every 8 h, or in three divided doses). It is important to make the distinction between whether the dose is being expressed as the total daily dose or as the quantity to be given in a single dose. Physicians typically express dosages on prescription pads or orders as abbreviations. Therefore, the athletic trainer must be familiar with common medical abbreviations used in prescribing.

Special Considerations for Athletes

Sometimes the drug of choice for an athlete with a particular condition is not viable because it may be banned during competition or is ergolytic and negatively affects athletic performance. Therefore, a particular agent may not be the drug of choice but rather the most viable one. Athletes, athletic trainers, coaches, and compliance officers are expected to know the most current list of prohibited agents. The list is published by the World Anti-Doping Agency (WADA), with the U.S. Anti-Doping Agency (USADA) being a signatory of the WADA

🚩 RED FLAGS FOR COX-2 ANTI-INFLAMMATORY AGENTS

In 2004, the manufacturer of a COX-2 anti-inflammatory medication, rofecoxib (Vioxx), voluntarily pulled it from the market amid concerns that it increased the risk of cardiovascular problems.[17] Interestingly, almost two decades later, rofecoxib has received an *orphan drug designation* and there is a proposal to return it to the market.[18] Although cardiovascular concerns with the drug are still present, the risks must be taken in context and must consider the potential benefits of the drug and patient quality of life. As with any medication, potential benefits must be weighed against the drug's adverse side effects. The athletic trainer must remain current on drug cautions and recalls.

published list.[20,21] The NCAA maintains a similar list of banned and monitored substances.[22] The WADA specifies which medicinal agents are permanently banned, as opposed to specific cases when an agent may be banned. There may be instances when an athlete has a medically diagnosed illness or condition that requires the use of a medication listed on the WADA prohibited list. In these cases, the athlete may apply for a therapeutic use exemption from the WADA. Adequate documentation will be required, and the athlete must comply with all testing requirements. NCAA athletes have a similar process for requesting medical exceptions.[22] Because the WADA, USADA, and NCAA lists are subject to change, consult the agency websites when questions arise.

Potential Drug Misuse

It is often thought that if some of a thing is good, more is better. This is extremely problematic when dealing with medication. Patients may self-medicate with OTC drugs using prescription-strength dosages. Lang and colleagues[23] found that almost a third of female high school volleyball athletes reported using OTC pain medications in the past week during the study. Those with a history of injury were more likely to use OTC medications.[23] Similarly, Omeragic and colleagues[24] found that 36% of the athletes surveyed used OTC medications during the season, with 95% of those surveyed indicating they used OTC analgesic drugs and 40% of the athletes used two or more OTC drugs concomitantly without medical supervision.[24] The athletic trainer must help to educate patients about the dangers of self-medicating or taking medications in dosages other than indicated on the label for prescription and OTC medications.

Athletes and physically active individuals may also be tempted to use medications in ways other than intended or indicated, in hopes of improving their performance. Educating individuals about the dangers of using drugs for purposes other than those prescribed is paramount for their continued safety. Although drug testing may be a deterrent for some athletes, the technology used to circumvent drug tests is typically years ahead of the technology for detecting the drugs.

Supplements

No U.S. federal agency, not even the FDA, regulates the content of food supplements and herbal products. It is assumed that these products contain the ingredients or the quantities of each ingredient listed on the label and that the ingredients listed are safe. This puts the person using these products at risk because there has been no regulatory follow-up to make sure the products provide what is listed and, further, are safe for human consumption.

In Canada, however, the Natural and Non-prescription Health Products Directorate enforces the natural health products regulations, ensuring all Canadians ready access to natural products that are safe, effective, and of high quality.

Ephedra (*ma huang*) and ephedrine, substances closely related to pseudoephedrine, are used in weight-loss products, thermogenics, and other products sold for their energy-producing properties. Many products sold as nutritional supplements and herbal products for weight loss or energy may contain ephedra or ephedrine. These two substances are also stimulants on the USADA and NCAA banned drug lists.[20,22]

Both ephedra and ephedrine can cause hypertension, increased cardiac workload, and arrhythmias, especially in high doses (>150 mg/24 h). Use of these agents has been associated with hemorrhagic stroke.[25] Other problems associated with the use of food supplements or herbal products containing ephedra or ephedrine include the lack of both consistency and reliability of active ingredient content in these products.[26]

Caffeine is another CNS stimulant that is banned in high doses from international competition. Caffeine concentrations greater than 12 mg/mL in the urine are banned. Athletes who drink a couple of cups of coffee before competition will not be at risk of such high urinary concentrations. However, those who take a supplement containing guarana or a caffeine pill may be over the limit, because these supplements do not metabolize at the same rate and they produce higher urine concentrations of caffeine than coffee or soft drinks.

Other supplements, such as anabolic steroids, are typically not used therapeutically and are not covered in this chapter. The NCAA and USADA are good sources of information on additional banned substances for athletes.

Resources

The number of pharmaceutical products on the market, among generic, trade-name, and biologic medications, continues to grow steadily each year. With the continued emphasis on biomedical research and the vast volume of research being published, it is essential that individuals involved in health care have up-to-date resources available. The best options are electronic references that are updated frequently, such as Epocrates, Lexicomp, or Micromedex, but full subscriptions to these services can be costly. Those who work at universities may have access to online drug information resources through their library's subscription. There are also free services online that are sufficient for many practitioners.

Drug information programs are also available for use with mobile applications on smartphones or tablets. Both desktop and mobile app versions are available for many online drug information programs. The advantages of electronic drug references over printed references are that the medical professional may easily select two or more drugs and access comparative information, including drug interactions. In addition, the electronic drug references are updated on a regular basis and do not rely on publication schedules to be updated.

Popular printed drug information references are now available electronically. These references include Facts and Comparisons, which receives timely updates and is designed for retail pharmacists; American Hospital Formulary Service Clinical Drug Information, which is published by the American Society of Health-System Pharmacists; and the U.S. Pharmacopoeia, which contains information for the patient in nontechnical language. Information for pediatric patients is available in *The Harriet Lane Handbook*, which is still available in print and updated every 3 yr. When foreign medications are needed, the health professional may refer to the *Martindale's Health Science Guide*, which provides information in print and online. The ability to synthesize the drug information available and apply it to real-world situations requires advanced level training.

Summary

The athletic trainer is responsible for monitoring for and preventing allergic reactions when possible, recognizing and reporting adverse drug reactions, and recognizing situations in which drug interactions may occur. The athletic trainer is often asked by patients to recommend OTC or herbal supplements. In complex situations in which multiple medications or supplements are involved, it is advisable to seek an opinion from either a physician or pharmacist.

Apply It!

Go to HK*Propel* to complete the case studies for this chapter.

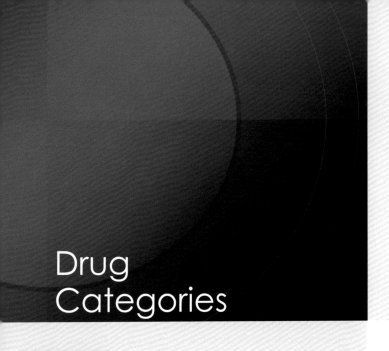

Drug Categories

OBJECTIVES

At the completion of this chapter the reader should be able to do the following:

1. List the basic drug categories in which drugs are classified, including mechanism of action, side effects, and adverse effects.

2. Describe the inflammatory process and discuss appropriate pharmacological management of inflammation.

3. List common narcotic analgesics and understand federal restrictions for administration of these drugs and their potential for addiction.

4. Appreciate the risks to individuals who participate in athletics while using local anesthetics.

5. Understand the actions, including bactericidal and bacteriostatic, of antibiotics.

6. List the common antivirals and antifungals, along with their indications, contraindications, dosage, and side effects.

7. Describe the indications, contraindications, dosage, and side effects of antihistamines and decongestants and their implications for athletic participation.

8. Describe the key points for using a metered-dose inhaler (MDI) and the medications commonly administered with a MDI.

9. Educate patients on the types and use of gastrointestinal medications, their indications, and side effects.

10. Describe the various antidiabetic agents commonly used with physically active individuals.

11. Describe the basic use of anticoagulants in athletics, their mechanism of action, and precautions for this drug class.

This chapter discusses the various categories in which drugs are classified. Within each category, the mechanism of action in the body for various drugs is discussed. Side effects and adverse effects of drugs are also discussed. For information about pharmacodynamics and pharmacokinetics, please see chapter 3.

Anti-Inflammatory Agents

One of the most common conditions that athletic trainers encounter is inflammation. Following injury, irritation, or overuse, inflammation occurs to limit the spread of the damage to adjacent tissue. Inflammation is both a chemical and a vascular response at the site of injury or exposure to the injurious agent. The process is nonspecific and is the same regardless of whether the injury or irritation is mechanical or is caused by a noxious foreign substance.

Initially, a vasoconstriction occurs to prevent blood loss, which is followed by release of chemical mediators such as prostaglandins, histamine, leukotrienes, and bradykinins. These mediators cause vasodilation and increase cell wall permeability, which results in the escape of fluid from the cells into the interstitial spaces in a quickly progressing inflammatory cascade. Inflammation results in pain, redness, warmth, swelling, and loss of function. The inflammatory process is covered in detail in many therapeutic modality texts for athletic trainers.

The physician may prescribe anti-inflammatory medication to limit the extent of the inflammatory process or cascade. Anti-inflammatory medications are classified as steroidal anti-inflammatory agents or nonsteroidal anti-inflammatory drugs (NSAIDs).

Steroidal Anti-Inflammatory Agents: Corticosteroids

Corticosteroids are defined as hormones secreted by the adrenal cortex or synthetic analogs of these hormones. Although corticosteroids and anabolic steroids, which are analogs of testosterone, both contain a steroid ring, corticosteroids have very different pharmacological actions from anabolic steroids. The actions of corticosteroids can be classified as either mineralocorticoid or glucocorticoid. Mineralocorticoid actions are those that affect electrolytes, fluid balance (with the net effect being sodium and fluid retention), and potassium and hydrogen excretion. Glucocorticoid actions decrease inflammation, cause immune system suppression, and stimulate gluconeogenesis. They also promote protein catabolism, redistribute peripheral fat to central areas, decrease intestinal absorption of calcium, and increase renal excretion of calcium. The pharmacological effects of corticosteroids are most likely caused by their complex influence on various enzyme systems. For the athletic trainer, the most important effects of corticosteroids are their anti-inflammatory properties, which are beneficial in the treatment of inflammatory joint disorders and environmental allergies (table 4.1).

Most corticosteroids used to treat joint disorders are administered in one of three ways:

1. Intrasynovial injection
2. Intraarticular injection
3. Iontophoresis

It is not unusual for these injections to be accompanied by a short-acting anesthetic such as lidocaine (Xylocaine).[1] Injectable corticosteroids are typically used after more conservative treatments have failed and the inflammatory process can be localized to a small area.

TABLE 4.1 Corticosteroids

Trade name	Generic name	Route	Usual dose or dosage
Cortef, Solu-Cortef	Hydrocortisone	Intraarticular or intralesional IM or IV PO Rectal	5-75 mg 15-240 mg/d 20-240 mg/d 100 mg/d
Various	Prednisone	PO	5-60 mg/d
Various	Prednisolone	IM IV Intraarticular or soft tissue PO	4-60 mg 5-60 mg/d
Medrol, Solu-Medrol, Depo-Medrol	Methylprednisolone	IM Intraarticular or soft tissue Topical IV PO	80-120 mg 4-80 mg 40-120 mg/wk 10-40 mg 4-48 mg/d
Kenalog, Kenacort	Triamcinolone	IM IA or intrabursal Topical Intralesional or sublesional PO	25-60 mg/d 2.5-40 mg/d 1 mg/site 5-48 mg 8-16 mg/d
Dexamethasone Intensol, Hemady	Dexamethasone	IM IA or soft tissue PO	4-8 mg 4-16 mg 0.75-9 mg/d
Flonase	Fluticasone propionate	Nasal inhalation Oral inhalation	55-250 µg/actuation
Rhinocort	Budesonide	Nasal inhalation	1-2 actuations in each nostril
Celestone	Betamethasone	IM IA Topical	0.25-9 mg/d

Note: IA = interarticular; IM = intramuscular; IV = intravenous; PO = oral (per os).

Data from Clinical Pharmacology (2022); Anderson (2023); Epocrates (2022).

The immunosuppressive properties of corticosteroids make them invaluable in the treatment of allergies and inflammatory joint conditions. Prednisone (Deltasone) and methylprednisolone (Medrol) are the oral agents used most often in the treatment of allergic reactions and acute joint inflammation. Typically, a large dose, equivalent to 30 mg of prednisone, is given on the first day of treatment and then the dose is reduced by 5 mg/d until the drug is completely tapered off. The initial dose and subsequent doses may be given as a single daily dose or in divided doses. The very popular Medrol Dosepak contains 4 mg methylprednisolone tablets in a six-row blister pack with complete instructions for how the drug is to be started and tapered off over the course of 6 d. For inflammatory conditions of a joint, the steroid taper is followed by a course of an NSAID, such as ibuprofen or a cyclooxygenase (COX)-2 inhibitor. If the condition being treated is exacerbated during the taper, then the dose of steroid is increased and maintained for a short time before the taper is restarted.

Inhaled Corticosteroids

Intranasal steroids are also used in the treatment of allergic rhinitis or allergies. These include fluticasone propionate (Flonase, Flovent HFA) and mometasone furoate (Nasonex). These steroids are manufactured as intranasal metered-dose sprays, which provide a local anti-inflammatory effect and reduce the effects of environmental allergens through immunosuppressive mechanisms.

Inhaled corticosteroids are used in the treatment of asthma. Beclomethasone dipropionate (QVAR Redi-Haler), fluticasone (Flovent), and budesonide (Pulmicort) are dispensed from metered-dose inhalers (MDIs); the dry-powder inhaler ADVAIR DISKUS dispenses a combination of two drugs: fluticasone propionate and salmeterol. Inhaled corticosteroids provide a local anti-inflammatory effect in the airways. They should never be used for acute exacerbations of asthma because they do not cause immediate bronchodilation.

Side Effects

The side effects of corticosteroids depend on the dose and the route of administration. They are minimal with intrasynovial injection, intraarticular injection, intranasal application, inhalation, or short-term therapy. However, tendon ruptures have occurred in patients receiving

Clinical Tips

Inhaled Corticosteroids

The anti-inflammatory benefits of inhaled corticosteroids are not realized until after 1 to 4 wk of therapy.

corticosteroid injections.[2] The Achilles tendon and the rotator cuff are especially susceptible to this effect.[1] In a previous study, the incidence of rotator cuff tear after corticosteroid injection was almost 3%; without the injection, rotator cuff tear occurred in approximately 1% of the population studied.[2]

For orally administered short-course tapers, the most common side effects are increased appetite, restlessness, insomnia, fluid retention, gastrointestinal disturbances, and decreased glucose tolerance. Gastrointestinal effects are diminished if doses are taken along with food. Less common but serious effects of corticosteroids are the development of and the impaired healing of peptic ulcers.

In addition, high doses or prolonged use of corticosteroids to treat systemic inflammatory or autoimmune diseases, such as lupus, multiple sclerosis, or inflammatory bowel syndromes (e.g., Crohn's disease), may produce devastating side effects. These may include changes in physical appearance caused by changes in fat deposition, adrenal suppression, cataracts, or peptic ulcers. Long-term corticosteroid use decreases bone density and contributes to osteoporosis.[3]

In individuals with diabetes, corticosteroids (even in short courses) must be used with caution because of their effects on glucose tolerance. Changes in insulin doses or diet may be required for these patients during treatment with corticosteroids.

Intranasal corticosteroids are generally very well tolerated. The most common side effects are nasal irritation, pharyngeal irritation, and dryness. Use of intranasal corticosteroids is shown to be safe in the adult population and does not increase intraocular pressure as once feared.[4] Second-generation intranasal corticosteroids result in minimal systematic adverse effects, such as hypothalamic–pituitary–adrenal axis suppression, growth retardation, and glaucoma, but these effects rarely occur in childhood.[5] Similarly, the most common side effects of inhaled corticosteroids are hoarseness, dry mouth, sore throat, and oropharyngeal fungal infections, such as *Candida albicans* or *Aspergillus niger*. After an inhaled corticosteroid is used, the mouth should always be rinsed to prevent oral fungal infections.

Repeated intrasynovial or intraarticular injection does not result in any systemic effects but causes damage to the joint. Intraarticular injections in major weight-bearing joints are not recommended because of the potential softening of joint cartilage. Even after a single injection, damage may occur if the joint is not allowed proper time to heal. Iontophoresis is a much less invasive way to administer corticosteroids superficially, because it uses direct electrical current to introduce ions into the body. Often, ionized medications can be introduced through iontophoresis; however, the most common are corticosteroids in combination with a topical anesthetic, such as lidocaine.[6] Research has suggested that iontophoresis may be beneficial for both pain and function, but it is more effective for superficial conditions rather than deeper conditions or larger joints.[7]

Nonsteroidal Anti-Inflammatory Agents

Among the most common medications used in the athletic setting are the NSAIDs (table 4.2). NSAIDs decrease pain, inflammation, and fever (i.e., they have an **antipyretic** effect). Many of these drugs are available over the counter (OTC), so their use is common.

Drugs in the NSAID class exert their pharmacological effects through inhibition of prostaglandin synthesis. NSAIDs inactivate the COX-1 and COX-2 enzymes and the prostaglandin G/H synthase 1 and 2 enzymes that catalyze the formation of prostaglandins from arachidonic acid (figure 4.1). COX-2 inhibitors, such as celecoxib (Celebrex), are selective for the COX-2 enzyme. NSAIDs are given primarily by the oral route (PO), although ketorolac (Toradol) may be given via the PO, IM, or IV route. Lower doses are adequate for treating pain and fever (200-400 mg of ibuprofen or 5-10 mg/kg/dose for children age 6 mo to 12 yr), whereas higher doses are required for anti-inflammatory effects.[8] The best results in inflammatory conditions are obtained when scheduled doses of 600 to 800 mg every 6 to 8 h around the clock are given for several weeks.[9]

Side Effects

The major side effects of NSAIDs are gastrointestinal and include dyspepsia, heartburn, nausea, vomiting, abdominal pain, peptic ulcer, and gastrointestinal bleeding. Prostaglandins stimulate the secretion of a protective mucosal layer in the gastrointestinal tract.

Prostaglandin inhibition leads to a breakdown in the protective mucosal layer, which leads to ulceration. Aspirin administered without an enteric coating, buffers, or antacids causes increased entry of acid into the gastric mucosa, leading to cellular damage at the dissolution site. As mentioned previously, enteric-coated aspirin undergoes dissolution in the small intestine, and thus avoids direct effects on the gastric lining. Administration

TABLE 4.2 Nonsteroidal Anti-Inflammatory Drugs

Trade name	Generic name	Usual dose	Maximum dose per day
Propionic acids			
Advil, Motrin	Ibuprofen	400 mg every 4-6 h	3,200 mg
Aleve, Anaprox, Naprosyn	Naproxen	250 mg every 6-8 h	1,250 mg
Orudis, Orudis KT	Ketoprofen	25-50 mg every 6-8 h	300 mg
Daypro	Oxaprozin	1,200 mg/d	1,800 mg
Salicylates, acetylated			
Bayer, Asatab, Arthritis Pain Formula	Aspirin	325-650 mg PO every 4 h	325-500 mg
Acetic acids			
Cataflam, Voltaren	Diclofenac	50 mg PO 3 times daily	200 mg
Lodine	Etodolac	200-400 mg every 6-8 h	1,200 mg
Indocin	Indomethacin	25-50 mg PO or rectally 2 or 3 times daily	200 mg
Toradol	Ketorolac	IV: 30 mg × 1 dose or 30 mg every 6 h IM: 60 mg × 1 dose or 60 mg every 6 h PO: 20 mg initially, then 10 mg every 4-6 h	120 mg 120 mg 40 mg
Oxicams			
Mobic	Meloxicam	7.5 mg/d	15 mg
Feldene	Piroxicam	20 mg/d or twice daily	40 mg
COX-2 inhibitors			
Celebrex	Celecoxib	100-200 mg twice daily	400 mg

Note: COX-2 = cyclooxygenase-2; IM = intramuscular; IV = intravenous; N/A = not applicable; PO = oral (per os).

Data from Lexicomp Online (2022); Epocrates (2022).

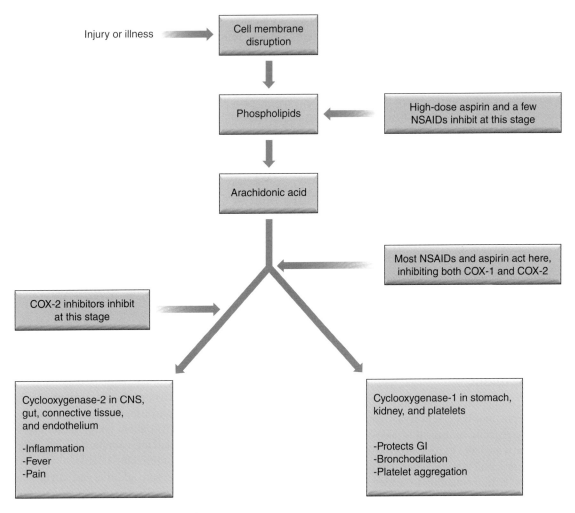

FIGURE 4.1   The inflammatory cascade.

of NSAIDs with food or milk minimizes gastrointestinal adverse effects.[10] Coadministration of aspirin and other NSAIDs along with corticosteroids increases the risk of gastrointestinal lesions. People who drink alcohol or individuals with alcohol use disorder who take aspirin or NSAIDs have higher risk of upper gastrointestinal bleeding, and this risk is elevated by increased alcohol consumption.[10]

Aspirin, salicylates, and NSAIDs, although to a much lesser extent, have hematological effects that must be considered in physically active individuals. Aspirin inhibits platelet aggregation and decreases hepatic synthesis of blood coagulation factors. At normal dosages of up to 6 g/d, aspirin rarely increases **prothrombin time (PT)**, the time it takes blood to clot, by more than 2 to 3 s. Higher doses, fever, and increased metabolic rate may cause larger increases in PT.[11] For individuals in contact sports, especially those with a high likelihood of head trauma, aspirin may not be a good therapeutic choice. The risk or extent of intracranial bleeding may increase in an individual who experiences head trauma in an anti-

coagulated state. Research is mixed on whether aspirin causes increased intracranial bleeding following head trauma for the patient receiving low-dose aspirin therapy.

Other NSAIDs, such as ibuprofen, inhibit platelet aggregation but to a lesser extent than aspirin. This has raised some concern that NSAIDs not be used by athletes in sports that may put them at risk of head trauma. Physicians have varying views on this subject, and athletic trainers must know and uphold these views.

The renal effects of NSAIDs are also of concern. Prostaglandins play a role in maintaining renal perfusion in people with certain renal conditions (e.g., decreased

Clinical Tips

Anti-Inflammatory Agents

It typically takes 2 wk for the maximum anti-inflammatory response to occur, although some decrease in inflammation occurs after 2 to 7 d.

extracellular fluid depletion). A patient receiving long-term NSAID therapy who becomes dehydrated may be at risk of renal impairment and needs to be monitored for symptoms of azotemia, such as malaise, fatigue, or loss of appetite. Other adverse effects of NSAIDs include rash, dermatitis, photosensitivity (sun block use is recommended), dizziness, headache, nervousness, fatigue, drowsiness, fluid retention, anaphylaxis, bronchospasm, tinnitus, and visual disturbances.

The safety of COX-2 NSAIDs has been questioned, with the voluntary recall of rofecoxib (Vioxx) after increased risk of cardiovascular events was reported. Studies involving celecoxib, a COX-2 inhibitor, have reported conflicting results. Many clinical reviews have determined that at least a moderately increased risk of cardiovascular events is associated with COX-2 inhibitors.[12,13] Athletic trainers and patients must remember that along with its benefits, potential adverse effects occur with any drug. Individual patient needs and risk factors must be considered to make the best drug therapy choices. The lowest possible effective dose of a drug should always be used to minimize the chance of adverse events.

Contraindications

NSAIDs are contraindicated for individuals who have experienced a previous hypersensitivity reaction or other severe allergic reaction to aspirin or any other NSAID and for those who have experienced bronchospasm, angioedema, or nasal polyps when taking aspirin or other NSAIDs. Extreme caution is needed when giving aspirin or other NSAIDs to individuals with a history of gastrointestinal lesions (e.g., peptic ulcer), those with sickle cell anemia, and those taking blood thinners such as enoxaparin (Lovenox) or warfarin (Coumadin).[10]

Interactions

Because many OTC NSAIDs are readily available, individuals may be tempted to take them with acetaminophen.[14] These two drugs have different mechanisms of action; therefore, it is safe to combine them if the maximum dosage of OTC NSAIDs is not providing enough analgesia. However, better prescription medications are likely available; if the patient's discomfort is not relieved with OTC medications, a physician should be consulted about the condition. The athletic trainer must also teach patients that many products contain the same active ingredients and, therefore, care must be taken when combining OTC medications of any kind.[15]

Narcotic Analgesics

Narcotic analgesics affect pain by stimulating the opiate receptors (table 4.3). Some of these agents, such as morphine, codeine, and oxycodone, are derived from opium. Others, including meperidine (Demerol), sufentanil, and fentanyl, are synthetic opiate agonists that share structural similarities. A third group of related opiate agonists includes methadone. Many previous trade-name narcotic analgesics have been taken off the market in favor of their generic equivalents.

Narcotic analgesics stimulate opiate receptors, causing analgesia, sedation, and euphoria. The analgesia is produced not by an actual decrease in the level of pain but rather by altering the way that pain is perceived. Opiate agonists cause dissociation from the pain. A person who takes an opiate agonist still has pain but does not care about it. Because these drugs also cause a feeling of euphoria, there is significant potential for addiction.

Opiates are found in combination with aspirin, ibuprofen, or, most commonly, acetaminophen. Their combination is very effective because aspirin and ibuprofen decrease the production of pain mediators (e.g., prostaglandins), and the opiate agonist minimizes the perception of pain.

Side Effects

The side effects of opiate agonists are constipation, physical dependence or addiction, sedation, drowsiness, dry mouth, blurred vision, urinary retention, nausea, vomiting, histamine release, respiratory depression, and allergic reactions. The patient taking these medications must avoid alcohol and use caution if taking other drugs that cause sedation of the central nervous system (CNS). These sedating effects are additive and can be very dangerous. Patients taking opiate agonists also should avoid operating any machinery that could be dangerous, such as an automobile.[8] Obviously, the individual who is in enough pain to warrant narcotic analgesics should not participate in sports. The use of patient-controlled infusion pumps allows the hospitalized individual to self-administer the narcotic analgesic as needed to control pain.

To minimize the constipating effects of opiate agonists, fluid and fiber intake can be increased. A stool softener, such as docusate sodium (Colace), may be needed to alleviate constipation. To minimize nausea and vomiting, opiate agonists are taken with food rather than on an empty stomach.

 RED FLAGS FOR NARCOTIC ANALGESICS

- Alcohol and other sedating drugs must be avoided when taking narcotic analgesics because their additive effects may be dangerous.
- Athletes should not operate motor vehicles or other heavy or dangerous machinery while taking narcotic analgesics.

TABLE 4.3   **Narcotic Analgesics**

Trade name (opioid, ASA, or APAP)	Combination	Dosage
Generic	Oxycodone with ASA	1 every 6 h
Endocet (5/325, 7.5/325, 7.5/500, 10/325, or 10/650 mg)	Oxycodone with APAP	1 every 6 h*
Percocet (2.5/325, 5/325, 7.5/325, 7.5/500, 10/325, or 10/650 mg)	Oxycodone with APAP	1 every 6 h*
Norco (5/325, 7.5/325, or 10/325 mg)	Hydrocodone with APAP	1-2 tablets every 4-6 h*†
Contin, Avinza, or Kadian	Morphine sulfate	200 mg 30 mg/24 h (maximum, 1,600 mg) SC/IM: 10 mg every 4 h IV: 2-10 mg/70 kg over 4-5 min
Generic	Codeine with APAP	1 or 2-4 every 4 h*
Dolophine, Methadose	Methadone	2.5-10 mg IM, SC, or PO every 3-4 h
Demerol	Meperidine	50-150 mg IM, SC, or PO every 3-4 h
Actiq, Lazanda, Fentora, or Subsys	Fentanyl	Nasal spray, IM, patches, sublingual sprays, tablets

Note: APAP = acetaminophen; ASA = aspirin; IM = intramuscular; IV = intravenous; PO = oral (per os); SC = subcutaneous.

*Daily dose of APAP should not exceed 4,000 mg.

†Daily dose of hydrocodone should not exceed 60 mg.

Data from Lexicomp Online (2022); Epocrates (2022); Anderson (2023).

Opiate agonists can also cause the release of histamine, which may result in mild to severe itching, especially in the facial area. This itching can be alleviated by antihistamines, such as diphenhydramine (Benadryl); again, caution is needed because of the additional sedative effects. The itching is sometimes confused with an allergic reaction, but itching alone in the absence of a rash or hives is an irritating but harmless side effect. An allergic reaction to opiate agonists manifests through hives, difficulty breathing, and facial or tongue swelling. Allergic reactions to opiates are a contraindication to prescribing these medications. Cross-allergenicity occurs between agents that share structural similarities (e.g., codeine and morphine or methadone and propoxyphene). If a patient reports an allergy to opiates, the athletic trainer must determine whether the reaction is simply itching caused by histamine release.

Narcotic analgesics have very high potential for misuse, and their nonmedical and recreational use is increasing among young students and athletes. See chapter 17 for more information on substance use and abuse. Tramadol use by individuals with a history of opioid use disorder may cause this dependence to reemerge. Although the athletic trainer must be alert for signs of dependence, such as drug-seeking behavior, the majority of individuals who take opioids for legitimate pain never experience a physical dependence.

Clinical Tips

Narcotic Analgesics

Almost all narcotic analgesics are banned by the U.S. Anti-Doping Agency and the National Collegiate Athletics Association. See www.usada.org for the latest information.[16-18]

Local Anesthetics

Local anesthetics produce their effects by reversibly blocking nerve conduction near the site of administration (table 4.4). Blocked nerve conduction is caused by a decrease in the permeability of the nerve cell membrane to sodium ions. Small nerve fibers (e.g., C- and A-δ) are affected more than large fibers (e.g., A-α and A-β). Autonomic activity is affected first, then loss of sensory functions, and, finally, loss of motor activity. The anesthetic effects regress in the reverse order.

Although allergic reactions to local anesthetics occur rarely, there is cross-allergenicity between agents with the same type of linkage but not with agents with different linkages. Therefore, a person who is allergic to procaine (Novocain) will also be allergic to benzocaine but not to lidocaine.

TABLE 4.4 **Local Anesthetics**

Type	Trade name	Generic name	Route of administration	Duration of action
Ester	Lanacane, Orajel Nesacaine Novocain Pontocaine Septocaine	Benzocaine Chloroprocaine Procaine Tetracaine Articaine	Topical Parenteral Parenteral Parenteral, topical Topical	Short Short Short Long Long
Amide	Marcaine Nupercainal Duranest Chirocaine Xylocaine	Bupivacaine Dibucaine Etidocaine Levobupivacaine Lidocaine	Parenteral Topical Parenteral Parenteral Parenteral and topical	Long Long Long Long Intermediate

Data from Clinical Pharmacology (2022); Lexicomp Online (2022); Epocrates (2022).

As their name implies, local anesthetics are used to produce a temporary, localized loss of sensory function. In some cases, these drugs may be used for a therapeutic effect in treating pain. In other cases, the anesthetic effect is desired for dental and surgical procedures or sutures. Local anesthetics may be administered in several ways. Topical administration, ophthalmic administration, infiltration, and nerve block are the most common methods seen by the athletic trainer.

Infiltration anesthesia involves the injection of the local anesthetic intradermally, subcutaneously, or submucosally across the nerves that supply the area being anesthetized. Nerve block is the injection of the anesthetic agent into or around the nerve trunks or ganglia that supply the area being anesthetized. Local anesthetics for injection are often combined with vasoconstrictors, usually epinephrine, to decrease systemic absorption of the anesthetic and to decrease bleeding. Epinephrine is especially useful when a patient needs sutures because it helps control bleeding, but it is contraindicated in areas that have poor blood supply, such as the tips of the fingers or nose.[19]

Topically administered agents, such as lidocaine or lidocaine-prilocaine cream (EMLA), may be used to numb the skin before certain procedures. Benzocaine and dibucaine are used in topical preparations for the relief of sunburn pain. Benzocaine is also found in otic preparations for the relief of ear pain associated with otitis. Other topical anesthetics, such as benzocaine-containing oral gels or throat lozenges, are formulated for application to the oral mucosa to relieve minor irritations of the mouth or throat. These agents are for short-term use only. Any persistent pain in the ears, mouth, or throat should be evaluated by a physician.

Proparacaine and tetracaine are examples of topical ophthalmic anesthetic agents. Topical anesthetics should be used in the eye only to desensitize or anesthetize the eye before ophthalmic procedures, such as corneal scraping or foreign body removal. They should never be used for pain control because prolonged use of topical ophthalmic anesthetics has been associated with severe keratitis and permanent corneal opacity and scarring.

Side Effects

Adverse effects associated with local anesthetics vary with the site of application. The most common adverse effect is a burning or stinging sensation associated with an application or injection. For the injected agents, adverse reactions usually result from high concentrations of the local anesthetic in the blood, either from inadvertent IV injection or from high doses.[20] These adverse reactions affect the CNS and cardiovascular system. When anesthetic agents are combined with epinephrine, adverse effects of the epinephrine must be considered. Table 4.5 lists side effects of local anesthetics. Anxiety, palpitation, dizziness, headache, restlessness, tremor, tachycardia, and hypertension may result from high blood levels of epinephrine.

The use of local anesthetics by athletes often presents difficult decisions for the team physician. Athletes may want to receive anesthetics so they can participate; however, such use must be strictly monitored to prevent further harm to athletes. In a 2016 survey of National Football League physicians, 100% of responding physicians used local anesthetic injections on players to facilitate play.[21] The literature suggests that the use of

Clinical Tips

Local Anesthetics

Local anesthetics are restricted by the U.S. Anti-Doping Agency and the National Collegiate Athletics Association. See www.usada.org for the latest information.

TABLE 4.5 **Side Effects of Local Anesthetics**

System	Effect
Central nervous system (initial)	Anxiety Restlessness Confusion Tremors Seizures
Central nervous system (delayed)	Drowsiness Respiratory arrest
Cardiovascular	Bradycardia Cardiac arrhythmias Hypotension Cardiovascular collapse Cardiac arrest
Integumentary	Vasoconstriction occurs when coupled with epinephrine; problematic when used as local anesthetic in fingers, toes, ears, and tip of nose

local anesthetics seems to be safe, but there is a lack of long-term follow-up and evaluation of functional and satisfaction outcomes with these athletes.[22] Local anesthetics should only be administered when medically justifiable. The risks of participation must be fully explained to the athlete and only allowed when there is no increased chance for injury in the anesthetized body part.

Antibiotics

Antibiotics are drugs used to treat bacterial infections. The discussion of antibiotic medications or antimicrobial therapy is very broad and complex. Although the coverage in this text is neither comprehensive nor exhaustive, it includes the most commonly used agents encountered by the athletic trainer.

Antibiotics may be classified in many ways based on their chemical structure, mechanism of action, or the spectrum of bacteria for which they are used. The four primary mechanisms of action are disruption of the cell wall, disruption of cytoplasmic metabolism, disruption of deoxyribonucleic acid replication, and disruption of protein synthesis. Tables for each class of antibiotic, along with common indications, dosages, and adverse reactions, are listed within each section that follows.

Antibiotics that disrupt cell wall synthesis are **bactericidal**. They bind to enzymes in the cytoplasmic membrane that are essential to cell wall synthesis. β-lactam antibiotics (cephalosporins, penicillins, carbapenems, vancomycin) act through this mechanism. Polymyxin B, which is found in many topical antibiotic creams and ointments, exerts its bactericidal effect through cell wall disruption.

A few antibiotics exert their effect by interfering with cellular metabolism. Sulfonamides, such as sulfamethox-

azole, a component of co-trimoxazole (Bactrim, Septra), interfere with the early stages of folic acid production in organisms that synthesize their own folic acid.

Antibiotics that disrupt protein synthesis do so by binding irreversibly to ribosomal subunits. Aminoglycosides, macrolides, clindamycin, and tetracyclines fall into this category. Aminoglycosides are bactericidal. Macrolides and tetracyclines are **bacteriostatic**.

The physician determines which antibiotic is appropriate to use in a particular situation, ideally based on a culture of body fluids or tissues from the infected area. For practical reasons, culture is reserved for those situations when the infection is serious or resistant to empirical therapy. In most cases, choosing an antibiotic empirically will suffice.

Patient age, history of allergic reactions, and adverse reactions to previous antibiotic therapy must be considered. Broad-spectrum antibiotics are reserved for infections that may be caused by resistant or multiple organisms. Antibiotics must be used appropriately to achieve complete eradication of the infecting organisms.

Clinical Tips

Antibiotic Actions

- Bactericidal antibiotics cause bacterial cell death.
- Bacteriostatic antibiotics inhibit further replication of the bacteria but do not cause cell death.
- Bacteriostatic antibiotics may be bactericidal at high concentrations or against highly susceptible organisms.

Incomplete courses of antibiotic therapy, inappropriate use of broad-spectrum antibiotics, and the use of antibiotics to treat viral infections all contribute to bacterial resistance.

If antibiotic therapy is discontinued prematurely, then not only is the chance of infection reoccurrence increased but the infecting organisms are also likely to show resistance to the antibiotic used. This resistance arises because the bacteria most susceptible to the antibiotic will be eradicated first, while the bacteria with some resistance to the antibiotic will linger; the latter organisms will be those that cause a recurrence of the infection.

When antibiotic therapy is initiated unnecessarily (e.g., to treat viral infections), then bacteria in the body are exposed to antibiotics unnecessarily. Exposure of bacteria to any antibiotic gives the organism an opportunity to develop adaptive resistance mechanisms to the agent. The more often that bacteria are exposed to an antimicrobial agent, the greater the likelihood that resistance will develop. Each year, more than 2.8 million people acquire an antibiotic-resistant infection. The two most common antibiotic-resistant bacteria are methicillin-resistant *Staphylococcus aureus* and drug-resistant *Streptococcus pneumoniae*.[23] Antibiotic use must be minimized to prevent the development of resistant bacteria.

The use of broad-spectrum antibiotics is reserved for situations in which the infecting bacteria have exhibited resistance to other antimicrobials, either through culture results or treatment failure. Broad-spectrum antibiotics are the most powerful tools in the antimicrobial arsenal. They should be used only when no other agents will work.

Side Effects

Adverse reactions associated with antibiotics include nausea, vomiting, diarrhea, and abdominal pain (table 4.6). Specific side effects for various antibiotics, along with common uses and dosages, are also discussed individually next. A more serious gastrointestinal adverse effect associated with the use of certain antibiotics is antibiotic-associated pseudomembranous colitis and diarrhea. The seriousness of this infection ranges from mild to life-threatening.[24] Pseudomembranous colitis may respond to discontinuation of the antibiotic or may require additional antibiotic therapy and supportive treatment to resolve.

Clinical Tips

Viral Infections

Viruses are not susceptible to antibiotic therapy; therefore, antibiotics are not used to treat a viral infection, such as the common cold.

Clinical Tips

Broad-Spectrum Antibiotics

Broad-spectrum antibiotics exhibit activity against a wide variety of organisms, including drug-resistant strains.

Antibiotic therapy commonly contributes to the overgrowth of nonsusceptible bacteria or fungi, often described as a *superinfection*. It is common for females taking antibiotics to develop vaginal fungal infections because of the disruption of normal vaginal flora. The physician may choose to prescribe an antifungal agent for use as needed whenever antibiotic therapy is prescribed to female patients who commonly experience such infections.

Rash, pruritus, urticaria, and other dermatological reactions are also common with various antibiotics. The rash may or may not be associated with a hypersensitivity or allergic reaction. Amoxicillin often causes rash in the presence of certain viral infections, but the rash is not attributable to an allergic reaction to the drug. **Stevens-Johnson syndrome** is a very serious, sometimes fatal, dermatological reaction to antibiotics. This syndrome is a severe form of erythema multiforme that involves the oronasal mucosa, eyes, and viscera and results in malaise, headache, fever, and arthralgia.[24]

Aminoglycosides

Aminoglycoside antibiotics are administered primarily via the IV, topical, and ophthalmic routes (table 4.7). They are active against aerobic gram-negative and aerobic gram-positive bacteria. The athletic trainer will see these drugs used most often for the treatment of eye infections and sometimes for skin infections. When used for eye infections, the most common adverse effects are transient burning or stinging.

Macrolides

Macrolide antibiotics are administered primarily via the PO, IV, and topical routes. Athletic trainers will see these drugs used most often as oral preparations for the treatment of infection. Some athletes may use erythromycin topical preparations (A/T/S, Benzamycin) to treat acne.

Erythromycin is used in the treatment of several sexually transmitted diseases, Lyme disease, diphtheria, pertussis, and Legionnaires' disease and of penicillin-sensitive infections in individuals with penicillin allergy. Clarithromycin (Biaxin) is used in the treatment of upper and lower respiratory tract infections, pharyngitis, tonsillitis, otitis media, Lyme disease, skin and skin structure infections, and *Helicobacter pylori* infections associated

TABLE 4.6   **Common Adverse Effects of Antibiotics**

Gastrointestinal	Dermatological	Central nervous system	Systemic	Gynecological	Cardiovascular	Metabolic
Nausea Vomiting Diarrhea Abdominal pain Cramping Heartburn Anorexia	Rash Pruritus Urticaria	Headache Behavioral changes Hallucinations Insomnia Tremor Vertigo Tinnitus	Fever Chills Arthralgia Lymphadenopathy	Vaginal candidiasis Decreased effectiveness of birth control pills	Tachycardia Hypotension	Hepatic dysfunction

Data from Clinical Pharmacology (2022); Lexicomp Online (2022); Epocrates (2022).

TABLE 4.7   **Aminoglycosides**

Medication	Common indications	Usual adult dosage	Adverse reactions
Gentamicin (Garamycin) 0.3% ophthalmic ointment 0.3% ophthalmic solution 0.1% topical cream 0.1% topical ointment	Ocular bacterial infection Dermatological infection	Ointment: 1/2 in. to affected eye, 2-3 times daily Solution: 1-2 drops into affected eye every 4 h Topical cream and ointment should be applied 3-4 times daily to affected area	Ointment: stinging, blurred vision Solution: stinging
Tobramycin (Nebcin, Tobrex) 0.3% ophthalmic ointment 0.3% ophthalmic solution	Ocular bacterial infection Dermatological infection	Ointment: 1/2 in. to affected eye, 2-3 times daily Solution: 1-2 drops into affected eye every 4 h	Ointment: stinging, blurred vision, hypersensitivity (tearing, itching, edema, conjunctival erythema) Solution: stinging, hypersensitivity (tearing, itching, edema, conjunctival erythema)

Data from Clinical Pharmacology (2022); Lexicomp Online (2022); Epocrates (2022).

with peptic ulcer disease.[8] Azithromycin (Zithromax) is used in the treatment of mild to moderate upper and lower respiratory tract infections, uncomplicated skin and skin structure infections, sexually transmitted diseases, acute otitis media, pharyngitis, tonsillitis, and pelvic inflammatory disease. The major advantage of azithromycin over other antibiotics is its once-daily dosage frequency and five-day duration of therapy. Several sexually transmitted diseases may be treated with a single 1 g dose of azithromycin.[19]

Table 4.8 lists the most common adverse effects of macrolides. Less common are heartburn, anorexia, melena, pruritus ani, and reversible mild acute pancreatitis. Prolonged or repeated erythromycin therapy has been associated with pseudomembranous colitis. These adverse gastrointestinal effects occur less often

with clarithromycin and azithromycin than with erythromycin. Azithromycin interacts with aluminum- and magnesium-containing antacids, which decrease the rate of absorption of azithromycin.

Erythromycin and clarithromycin also have a significant interaction with warfarin (similar to heparin). Patients stabilized with warfarin experience prolonged PT and bleeding when erythromycin or clarithromycin therapy is initiated. PT needs to be monitored closely in patients receiving warfarin and one of these macrolides simultaneously. Hepatic dysfunction may occur in patients receiving erythromycin. Erythromycin estolate can cause hepatotoxicity or reversible cholestatic hepatitis in adults who have received the drug for 10 d or longer. The estolate salt of erythromycin should not be used in adults.

TABLE 4.8 **Macrolides**

Medication	Common indications	Usual adult dosage	Adverse reactions
Erythromycin (E-mycin, Erythrocin)	Sexually transmitted diseases Lyme disease Diphtheria, pertussis Legionnaires' disease Penicillin-sensitive infections in individuals with penicillin allergy	250 mg PO 4 times daily 333 mg PO 3 times daily 500 mg PO 2 times daily	Nausea, vomiting, diarrhea, abdominal pain, cramping, stomatitis, heartburn, anorexia, melena, pruritus ani, reversible mild acute pancreatitis, pseudomembranous colitis Hepatic dysfunction, reversible cholestatic hepatitis (estolate) Mild allergic reaction: rash, urticaria
Clarithromycin (Biaxin)	Upper and lower respiratory tract infections Skin and skin structure infections Otitis media *Helicobacter pylori* infections (peptic ulcer) Pharyngitis, tonsillitis Lyme disease	250-500 mg PO 2 times daily	Nausea, vomiting, diarrhea, abdominal pain, cramping, stomatitis, heartburn, anorexia, melena, pruritus ani, reversible mild acute pancreatitis, pseudomembranous colitis Mild allergic reaction: rash, urticaria Abnormal taste, headache, behavioral changes, hallucinations, insomnia, tinnitus, tremor, vertigo
Azithromycin (Zithromax)	Mild to moderate upper and lower respiratory tract infections Uncomplicated skin and skin structure infections Sexually transmitted diseases Acute otitis media Pharyngitis, tonsillitis Pelvic inflammatory disease	500 mg on the first day of treatment, followed by 250 mg daily for 4 d A single 1 g dose may be used in the treatment of sexually transmitted diseases	Nausea, vomiting, diarrhea, abdominal pain, cramping, stomatitis, heartburn, anorexia, melena, pruritus ani, reversible mild acute pancreatitis, pseudomembranous colitis

Note: PO = oral (per os).

Data from Clinical Pharmacology (2022); Lexicomp Online (2022); Epocrates (2022).

Penicillins

Penicillins may be administered by the PO, IM, or IV route (table 4.9). These drugs were the "magic bullet" against bacterial infection in the early 20th century but can be rendered ineffective by some enzymes. The athletic trainer most often will see these agents being given via the PO route. The orally administered penicillins are addressed here, including penicillin V, dicloxacillin, ampicillin, and amoxicillin. Penicillin V is classified as a natural penicillin exhibiting activity against *S. pneumoniae*, streptococci (groups A, B, C, G, H, K, L, and M and nonenterococcal group D), and many other bacteria as well.

Penicillin V is used principally for the treatment of upper and lower respiratory tract infections and skin and skin structure infections caused by susceptible organisms (e.g., group A β-hemolytic streptococci) and Lyme disease. This antibiotic may also be used for the treatment of upper and lower respiratory tract infections caused by susceptible strains of *S. pneumoniae*. The prevalence of *S. pneumoniae* resistance to penicillin ranges between 24% and 28%.[23] For this reason, the prevalence and pattern of penicillin resistance of *S. pneumoniae* in the local community must be considered before using penicillin for empirical therapy. Penicillin G or some other form of IM penicillin may be used in the treatment of sexually transmitted diseases caused by susceptible organisms, such as syphilis.

The most common adverse reaction to penicillins is an allergic reaction ranging from mild to severe (see table 4.9). The most serious reaction to penicillins, occurring in

TABLE 4.9 **Penicillins**

Medication	Common indications	Usual adult dosage	Adverse reactions
Natural penicillins (penicillin VK)	Upper and lower respiratory tract infections	250-500 mg every 6 h for 7-14 d	Mild to severe allergic reactions: rash, urticaria, pruritus, Stevens-Johnson syndrome, fever, chills, malaise, arthralgia, myalgia, lymphadenopathy, splenomegaly, angioedema, anaphylaxis Gastrointestinal disturbances: nausea, vomiting, diarrhea
Aminopenicillins (ampicillin)	Upper and lower respiratory tract infections Gastrointestinal tract infections Skin and skin structure infections, genitourinary tract infections Otitis media	250-500 mg PO every 6 h	Same as for the natural penicillins Mild, nonallergic maculopapular rash (especially in viral infection) Candidal or bacterial superinfections
Aminopenicillins (amoxicillin)	Upper and lower respiratory tract infections Gastrointestinal tract infections Skin and skin structure infections, genitourinary tract infections Otitis media	250-500 mg PO every 8 h	Same as for the natural penicillins Mild, nonallergic maculopapular rash (especially in viral infection) Candidal or bacterial superinfections
Penicillinase-resistant penicillins (dicloxacillin, oxacillin, nafcillin)	Skin and skin structure infections Acute or chronic osteomyelitis	250-500 mg PO every 6 h for at least 14 d Osteomyelitis may require up to 2 mo of oral therapy after initial course of therapy with an IV penicillinase-resistant penicillin	Same as for the natural penicillins Prolonged therapy: hematological, renal, and hepatic adverse events

Note: IV = intravenous; PO = oral (per os).

Data from Clinical Pharmacology (2022); Lexicomp Online (2022); Epocrates (2022).

0.05% of people receiving the drug, is anaphylaxis, which is fatal in 5% to 10% of cases. Anaphylactic reactions usually occur within 30 min of the drug administration.[19]

Oral contraceptives have a highly significant drug interaction with penicillins and many other antibiotics. The use of penicillins and many other antibiotics concomitantly with estrogen-containing oral contraceptives may decrease contraceptive efficacy and increase the incidence of breakthrough bleeding.

Dicloxacillin is classified as penicillinase-resistant penicillin. It is used mainly in the treatment of skin and skin structure infections, such as cellulitis, that are caused by staphylococci. Dicloxacillin may also be used in the treatment of acute or chronic osteomyelitis after an

initial course of IV therapy with penicillinase-resistant penicillin (e.g., nafcillin).

The adverse reactions associated with the use of dicloxacillin are the same as for the natural penicillins.

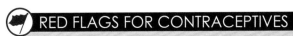 **RED FLAGS FOR CONTRACEPTIVES**

Many antibiotics interact with and decrease the efficacy of oral contraceptives. This can increase the incidence of breakthrough bleeding. The female athlete taking oral contraceptives and receiving antibiotic therapy should use a second form of birth control during sexual intercourse to prevent pregnancy.

Prolonged therapy with penicillinase-resistant penicillins, such as therapy for osteomyelitis, has been associated with adverse hematological, renal, and hepatic events.

Amoxicillin and ampicillin are classified as aminopenicillins. Aminopenicillins have the same spectrum of antimicrobial activity as the natural penicillins with enhanced activity against gram-negative bacteria. Aminopenicillins are used in the treatment of upper and lower respiratory tract infections, gastrointestinal tract infections, skin and skin structure infections, genitourinary tract infections, and otitis media caused by susceptible organisms.

The aminopenicillins exhibit the same adverse reactions as the natural penicillins (see table 4.9). In addition to hypersensitivity reactions, ampicillin and amoxicillin often cause a mild maculopapular rash that resolves in 1 to 2 wk even if drug therapy continues. This rash, which is not an allergic reaction, is more intense at pressure areas (e.g., knees, elbows). It occurs more often when aminopenicillins are used by patients with viral disease and will resolve in 1 to 7 d if the drug is discontinued. This amoxicillin rash must be differentiated from a true allergic reaction, and those experiencing it must not be labeled as penicillin allergic. Prolonged therapy with aminopenicillins needs to be accompanied by periodic monitoring of renal, hepatic, and hematological function. The drug interactions of the aminopenicillins are the same as those for the natural penicillins.

Cephalosporins

Cephalosporin antibiotics may be administered by the PO, IV, or IM routes. The agents in this class that will be discussed are cephalexin (Keflex), cefadroxil (Duricef), cefuroxime (Ceftin), cefdinir (Omnicef), and cefixime (Suprax) (table 4.10).

Cefadroxil and cephalexin are classified as first-generation cephalosporins. First-generation cephalosporins are active against gram-positive cocci, including *S. aureus*, *Staphylococcus epidermidis*, group A β-hemolytic streptococci, group B streptococci, and *S. pneumoniae*. Cefadroxil and cephalexin are used in the treatment of mild to moderate respiratory tract infections, skin and skin structure infections, acute bacterial otitis, pharyngitis, and tonsillitis caused by susceptible bacteria. They also are used in the treatment of mild to moderate urinary tract infections caused by susceptible gram-negative organisms.

Cefuroxime (Ceftin) is classified as a second-generation cephalosporin and is used in the treatment of mild to moderate respiratory tract infections caused by susceptible bacteria, acute otitis media, uncomplicated urinary tract infections, uncomplicated gonorrhea, and early Lyme disease.

Cephalosporins should be used with caution in patients with a history of penicillin hypersensitivity because there is a partial cross-allergenicity between penicillins and cephalosporins. Hypersensitivity reactions occurring with cephalosporins are rash, urticaria, pruritus, fever, chills, arthralgia, edema, hypotension, Stevens-Johnson syndrome, and, rarely, anaphylaxis. Other adverse reactions reported with cephalosporins include renal dysfunction, nephropathy, hepatic dysfunction, dizziness, headache, malaise, fatigue, cough, rhinitis, and superinfections. Cefixime causes adverse events in 50% of individuals, most commonly gastrointestinal (30%), headache (15%), and hypersensitivity reactions (≤7%). Cefuroxime use has been associated with decreased hemoglobin and hematocrit in 10% of patients.[19]

Fluoroquinolones

Ciprofloxacin (Cipro) is a broad-spectrum fluoroquinolone antibiotic active against most gram-negative aerobic bacteria and many gram-positive aerobic bacteria except for streptococci.

Ciprofloxacin is used orally in the treatment of urinary tract infections, acute sinusitis, lower respiratory tract infections, skin and skin structure infections, or bone and joint infections. Oral ciprofloxacin has also been used in the treatment of *Salmonella* infections, uncomplicated gonorrhea, and infectious diarrhea and in the prevention or empirical treatment of travelers' diarrhea. Ciprofloxacin and hydrocortisone otic drops (Cipro HC) are used in the treatment of otitis externa and chronic otitis media. Ciloxan, ophthalmic ciprofloxacin, is used in the treatment of bacterial conjunctivitis and corneal ulcers caused by susceptible bacteria.

Levofloxacin (Levaquin) is a fluoroquinolone with a similar antimicrobial spectrum to ciprofloxacin but with increased activity against gram-positive organisms, including *S. pneumoniae*. Levofloxacin is used in the treatment of acute sinusitis, lower respiratory tract infections (e.g., community-acquired pneumonia), skin and skin structure infections, and urinary tract infections. Oral levofloxacin has also been used in the treatment of traveler's diarrhea.

Adverse reactions for ciprofloxacin and levofloxacin are similar to those that occur with other antibiotics (see table 4.11). Tendon ruptures have been reported in patients receiving fluoroquinolones;[25] however, this is of particular concern in the athlete. Any athlete taking a fluoroquinolone who experiences pain or inflammation of a tendon must discontinue use of the drug immediately. The risk of rupture may increase in athletes taking fluoroquinolones and corticosteroids simultaneously.

The safe use of fluoroquinolones in children younger than age 18 yr has not been established. Although altered skeletal growth in children has not been reported, fluoroquinolones cause arthropathy in young animals. Therefore, fluoroquinolones are avoided in children and adolescents whose skeletal growth is incomplete.

TABLE 4.10 Cephalosporins

Medication	Common indications	Usual adult dosage	Adverse reactions
First generation			
Cephalexin (Keflex)	Mild to moderate respiratory tract infections Skin and skin structure infections Acute bacterial otitis Pharyngitis, tonsillitis Mild to moderate UTIs	250-500 mg every 6 h Uncomplicated UTIs: 500 mg every 12 h	Gastrointestinal reactions (including pseudomembranous colitis) Headache Hypersensitivity reactions: rash, urticaria, pruritus, fever, chills, arthralgia, edema, hypotension, Stevens-Johnson syndrome, and rarely anaphylaxis Renal dysfunction, nephropathy, increases in serum hepatic enzyme concentrations, increased serum bilirubin, hepatic dysfunction, dizziness, malaise, fatigue, cough, rhinitis, superinfections
Cefadroxil (Duricef)	Mild to moderate respiratory tract infections Skin and skin structure infections Acute bacterial colitis Pharyngitis, tonsillitis Mild to moderate UTIs	500 mg twice daily Uncomplicated UTIs: 1 or 2 g single dose Other UTIs: 1 g twice daily	Same as for cephalexin
Second generation			
Cefuroxime (Ceftin)	Mild to moderate respiratory tract infections Acute otitis media Uncomplicated UTIs Uncomplicated gonorrhea Early Lyme disease	250-500 mg every 12 h Uncomplicated UTIs: 125-250 mg every 12 h Uncomplicated urethral, endocervical, or rectal gonorrhea: single 1 g dose	Same as for cephalexin Decreased hemoglobin and hematocrit in 10% of individuals
Third generation			
Cefdinir (Omnicef)	Mild to moderate upper and lower respiratory tract infections Acute otitis media Streptococcal pharyngitis and tonsillitis Uncomplicated skin and skin structure infections	600 mg once daily *or* 300 mg twice daily	Gastrointestinal reactions (including pseudomembranous colitis) Headache Hypersensitivity reactions: rash, urticaria, pruritus, fever, chills, arthralgia, edema, hypotension, Stevens-Johnson syndrome, and rarely anaphylaxis Renal dysfunction, nephropathy, increases in serum hepatic enzyme concentrations, increased serum bilirubin, hepatic dysfunction, dizziness, malaise, fatigue, cough, rhinitis, superinfections
Cefixime (Suprax)	Uncomplicated UTIs Acute otitis media Streptococcal pharyngitis and tonsillitis Respiratory tract infections	400 mg once daily *or* 200 mg twice daily	Same as for cefdinir

Note: UTI = urinary tract infection.

Data from Clinical Pharmacology (2022); Lexicomp Online (2022); Epocrates (2022).

TABLE 4.11 **Fluoroquinolones**

Medication	Common indications	Usual adult dosage	Adverse reactions
Ciprofloxacin (oral, Cipro; ophthalmic, Ciloxan; otic, Cipro HC)	UTIs Acute sinusitis, lower respiratory tract infections Skin and skin structure infections Bone and joint infections *Salmonella* infection Uncomplicated gonorrhea Infectious diarrhea, traveler's diarrhea Otic: otitis externa, chronic otitis media Ophthalmic: bacterial conjunctivitis, corneal ulcers	Oral: 250-750 mg every 12 h Ophthalmic: 1-2 drops every 2-4 h Otic: 3-5 drops twice daily	Bone marrow depression, eosinophilia, hemolysis in individuals with G6PD deficiency, ECG changes, CNS disturbances, nausea, vomiting, diarrhea, taste disturbances, tendon rupture
Levofloxacin (oral, Levaquin; ophthalmic, Quixin)	Acute sinusitis, lower respiratory tract infections (e.g., community-acquired pneumonia) Skin and skin structure infections Urinary tract infections, acute pyelonephritis Traveler's diarrhea Ophthalmic: bacterial conjunctivitis, corneal ulcers	Oral: 250-500 mg once daily; single-dose therapy may be used for STIs Ophthalmic: 1-2 drops every 2-4 h	Bone marrow depression, eosinophilia, hemolysis in individuals with G6PD deficiency, ECG changes, CNS disturbances, blood glucose disturbances, nausea, diarrhea, taste disturbances, nephrotoxicity; rash, hypersensitivity reactions, Stevens-Johnson syndrome, arthralgias, tendon rupture Ophthalmic: ocular pain, burning, dryness, transient decreased vision
Ofloxacin (oral and otic, Floxin; ophthalmic, Ocuflox)		Oral: 300-400 mg twice daily; 400 mg single dose used for STIs Ophthalmic: 1-2 drops every 2-4 h Otic: 10 drops 1-2 times daily	Blood dyscrasias, hemolysis in individuals with G6PD deficiency, CNS disturbances, nausea, vomiting, diarrhea, taste disturbances, vaginitis, dysuria, skin eruptions, rash, eczema, photosensitivity, arthralgia, myalgia, tendon rupture, hypersensitivity Otic: dizziness or vertigo Ophthalmic: burning, redness, itching, blurred vision, dryness

Note: CNS = central nervous system; ECG = electrocardiogram; G6PD = glucose-6-phosphate dehydrogenase; STI = sexually transmitted infection; UTI = urinary tract infection.

Data from Clinical Pharmacology (2022); Lexicomp Online (2022); Epocrates (2022).

Aluminum, magnesium, calcium, iron, and zinc decrease the absorption of orally administered fluoroquinolones; therefore, antacids and multivitamin or mineral supplements containing these minerals should be avoided during fluoroquinolone therapy. If concomitant use is unavoidable, then the minerals or antacids should not be ingested within 2 to 4 h of the fluoroquinolone.

Fluoroquinolones cause blood glucose disturbances, both hypoglycemia and hyperglycemia, in individuals taking either oral antidiabetic agents or insulin. These agents must be used with caution in athletes receiving oral hypoglycemic agents or insulin to treat diabetes. Ciprofloxacin may cause adverse events, including nausea, vomiting, dizziness, headache, tremor, agitation, confusion, seizures, tachycardia, and respiratory failure. Levofloxacin occasionally causes anemia, leukopenia, thrombocytopenia, eosinophilia, fever, chills, rash, and itching. Levofloxacin, which has been associated with seizures, may lower the seizure threshold and must be used with caution in persons with a history of seizure. The risk of seizure is increased if NSAIDs and levofloxacin are used concomitantly.

Tetracyclines

Tetracyclines are antibiotics with activity against most *Rickettsia*, *Chlamydia*, *Mycoplasma*, and spirochetes bacteria. Many gram-negative bacteria are susceptible to tetracyclines. Most gram-positive bacteria are susceptible to the tetracyclines, although staphylococci and streptococci are becoming increasingly resistant. Tetracyclines are used in the treatment of the following: rickettsial infections (including Rocky Mountain spotted fever and Q fever), urogenital chlamydial infections, psittacosis,

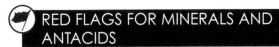

RED FLAGS FOR MINERALS AND ANTACIDS

Patients should avoid minerals and antacids when taking fluoroquinolones, if possible. These agents decrease absorption of orally administered fluoroquinolones. If minerals and antacids cannot be avoided, they should be taken 2 to 4 h after the antibiotic.

Mycoplasma pneumoniae, nongonococcal urethritis, gonorrhea, anthrax, acne, syphilis, Lyme disease, cholera, leprosy, *H. pylori* gastrointestinal infections, and infections caused by uncommon gram-negative bacteria (e.g., brucellosis).[19] Tetracyclines may also be used to prevent malaria. The athletic trainer most often will see the oral tetracyclines doxycycline (Vibramycin), minocycline (Minocin), and tetracycline (Sumycin) used for the treatment of acne.

Common adverse reactions associated with tetracyclines are similar to other antibiotics (see table 4.12). Dysphagia, sore throat, and black, hairy tongue have also been reported. Photosensitivity reactions can be striking; they can appear almost immediately or within a few hours after ingestion. Other dermatological reactions, such as rash and nail discoloration, may occur occasionally. A Jarisch-Herxheimer reaction occurred in some cases when tetracyclines were used to treat spirochetal infections, Lyme disease, or brucellosis. This reaction consists of headache, fever, malaise, myalgia, and arthralgia, and it typically occurs within 12 to 24 h after initiation of tetracycline therapy. Minocycline use is associated

TABLE 4.12 **Tetracyclines**

Medication	Therapeutic use	Usual adult dosage	Adverse effects
Doxycycline Minocycline Tetracycline	Rocky Mountain spotted fever Q fever Urogenital chlamydial infections Psittacosis *Mycoplasma pneumoniae* ("walking" pneumonia) Nongonococcal urethritis, gonorrhea, syphilis Anthrax Acne Lyme disease, *Helicobacter pylori* gastrointestinal infections, cholera, leprosy	100 mg twice daily 100 mg twice daily 250-500 mg orally 1 or 2 times daily	Gastrointestinal reactions: nausea, vomiting, diarrhea, anorexia, abdominal discomfort Rash, discoloration of the nails Jarisch-Herxheimer reaction: headache, fever, malaise, myalgia Tetracycline and doxycycline: photosensitivity Minocycline: lightheadedness, dizziness, vertigo, ataxia, drowsiness, headache, fatigue, nausea, vomiting

Data from Clinical Pharmacology (2022); Lexicomp Online (2022); Epocrates (2022).

RED FLAG FOR PHOTOSENSITIVITY

- Photosensitivity can occur with tetracycline antibiotics. This reaction appears as a severe sunburn that can develop a few minutes to a few hours after sun exposure and may last 1 to 2 d after discontinuing the offending antibiotic.
- Sunscreen is of little value in preventing a photosensitive reaction.
- Because minocycline is a tetracycline antibiotic that rarely causes this reaction, it may be the best choice in this case for sun-exposed individuals.

with a high incidence of vestibular symptoms (≤90%).[8] These symptoms include lightheadedness, dizziness, vertigo, ataxia, drowsiness, headache, fatigue, nausea, and vomiting.

Tetracyclines bind to orally administered aluminum, calcium, and magnesium ions, resulting in decreased gastrointestinal absorption of the antibiotic. Antacids containing these minerals should not be taken within 2 h of tetracycline. Iron more significantly decreases tetracycline absorption and should not be ingested within 3 h of tetracyclines. Antidiarrheals containing kaolin, pectin, or bismuth subsalicylate also impair tetracycline absorption and should not be used concurrently.

Oral tetracyclines can reduce the effectiveness of oral contraceptives. Concurrent use has resulted in pregnancy and breakthrough bleeding. Females taking oral contraceptives and tetracyclines should use a second form of birth control during sexual intercourse to avoid pregnancy.

Antivirals

The antiviral agents discussed here are used to treat herpes and influenza infections. Antivirals used in the treatment of human immunodeficiency virus are not covered. Acyclovir and valacyclovir (a prodrug of acyclovir) are used in the treatment of herpesvirus, which causes infection of the skin and mucous membranes. Genital herpes infections are contracted through sexual contact, but there are many ways in which herpesvirus may be spread through nonsexual contact. For example, wrestlers may experience herpes infection of the skin contracted through skin-to-skin contact with infected wrestlers (see chapter 16 for a discussion on viral skin infections).

Acyclovir (Zovirax) is most often administered as a topical agent applied five or six times per day directly on the herpes lesions. Before valacyclovir became available, acyclovir was the only oral drug that could treat herpes infections. Unfortunately, oral acyclovir must be administered five or six times per day, which makes it extremely inconvenient. Valacyclovir (Valtrex) oral tablets are administered only one to three times daily. For treatment of acute, localized herpes lesions, the dosage of valacyclovir is 1 g every 8 h for 7 d.[8,19]

Wrestlers are often given valacyclovir prophylaxis throughout the wrestling season to prevent the occurrence of cutaneous herpes infections. The dosage for prophylaxis is 500 mg twice daily.

For athletes with genital herpes, the treatment dosage of valacyclovir is 1 g twice daily for 10 d. For the treatment of cold sores, two doses (2 g each) are given separated by an interval of 12 h. Regardless of the condition, treatment is most effective if started within 48 h of symptom onset.

Side Effects

Oral acyclovir and valacyclovir are generally well tolerated. The most common adverse effects are gastrointestinal in nature and include nausea, vomiting, or diarrhea. Malaise and headache have also been reported. Occasionally, dermatological reactions such as rash, pruritus, or urticaria may be seen. It is extremely rare to see any adverse reaction from topical acyclovir, although patients using this agent to treat genital lesions may experience burning and pain on application.

Antifungals

Discussion of antifungal agents is limited to those used in the treatment of dermatological and vaginal fungal infections. The most common fungal conditions are tinea pedis, tinea corporis, and tinea cruris, which are generally caused by *Trichophyton* species or *Epidermophyton floccosum* (see chapter 16 for descriptions of these conditions).

Antifungal agents exert their fungicidal effects through a variety of mechanisms: alteration of fungal cell wall permeability, inhibition of transmembrane transport, interference with fungal cellular metabolism, and growth inhibition. Topical fungal infections are common, and patients can often safely self-medicate with OTC agents. These agents include miconazole products (Desenex, Micatin) or clotrimazole (Lotrimin) products. Terbinafine creams (Lamisil) and tolnaftate-containing products (Tinactin) are also popular. OTC antifungal medications are available in spray, powder, and cream forms. The typical rule of thumb is that sprays and powders are used prophylactically, and creams are used for active fungal infection. Topical antifungal agents are sometimes combined with corticosteroids (e.g., Lotrisone), which relieve the itching and burning that may be caused by the fungal infection. Caution is necessary when using these combination products because the corticosteroid may inhibit the activity of some antifungal agents against certain pathogens.

Oral antifungals may be prescribed by the physician if the infection has not resolved by the end of the recommended antifungal treatment duration, if the infection is recurring, or if a hastier recovery is needed, such as in returning a wrestler to competition.

Vaginal fungal infections are caused by *C. albicans* or other *Candida* species. Many females experience vaginal candidiasis during antibiotic therapy as a result of suppression of the normal vaginal flora, which allows for *Candida* overgrowth. These infections may be safely self-medicated in otherwise healthy individuals. Any athlete with diabetes or a compromised immune system should consult a physician rather than self-medicate. If vaginal candidiasis occurs during menstruation, the patient should either delay therapy until after the flow has stopped or begin treatment but avoid the use of tampons. Several products for the treatment of vaginal candidiasis have a petroleum base that may interact with the rubber or latex used in condoms or contraceptive diaphragms.[19] Condoms or diaphragms should not be used within 72 h of a dose of these products. As with topical fungal infections, if relief of vaginal candidiasis is not achieved by the end of the recommended duration of therapy, then the advice of a physician is needed.

Oral candidal infections, which may also occur during antibiotic therapy, should be treated using either clotrimazole or nystatin under the advice of a physician. Table 4.13 lists various antifungal agents, their uses, and the adverse effects associated with each. Two oral antifungal agents, griseofulvin and ketoconazole, are used in the prevention and treatment of topical fungal infections in wrestlers. These athletes are at risk of developing fungal infections from skin-to-skin contact with other wrestlers or contact with wrestling mats.[26] Griseofulvin (Fulvicin, Gris-PEG) comes in two forms: microsize and ultramicrosize. The difference between the two is the particle size in the drug, which affects absorption. The microsize drug has a particle size of 4 mm; anywhere from 25% to 70% of an oral dose is absorbed.[19] Absorption is increased by administering the drug with a high-fat meal. The ultramicrosize drug has a particle size of 1 mm and is almost completely absorbed. The griseofulvin microsize dosage is 500 to 1,000 mg once daily. The griseofulvin ultramicrosize dosage is 330 to 750 mg once daily.

The most common side effects of griseofulvin therapy are headache, which often resolves with continued therapy, as well as fatigue, dizziness, insomnia, gastrointestinal disturbances, rash, urticaria, and photosensitivity. Griseofulvin rarely causes proteinuria, hepatotoxicity, and leukopenia but because of the serious nature of these disorders, it is recommended that hepatic function, renal function, and white blood cell counts be monitored periodically throughout the course of therapy.

Griseofulvin may cause tachycardia and flushing when taken concurrently with alcoholic beverage consumption. Griseofulvin may also potentiate the effects of alcohol; therefore, it may be wise to advise patients to avoid ingestion of alcohol during treatment. Griseofulvin may also decrease the effectiveness of warfarin. In individuals taking warfarin and griseofulvin concurrently, PT and **international normalized ratio (INR)** should be monitored. The dose of warfarin also may need to be adjusted during therapy with griseofulvin.[27] Griseofulvin is known to decrease the effectiveness of oral contraceptives and cause amenorrhea or breakthrough bleeding. A form of contraception other than birth control pills must be used during therapy. Griseofulvin also has significant teratogenic potential, which makes the requirement for an alternative form of birth control even more urgent. Because griseofulvin has caused sperm abnormalities in mice studies, it is recommended that men wait at least 6 mo after the discontinuation of griseofulvin therapy before fathering a child.

Ketoconazole (Nizoral) is prescribed in a single daily dose of 200 to 400 mg. The most common side effect of ketoconazole is gastrointestinal disturbance, which may be lessened by administration with food. Gynecomastia with breast tenderness has also been reported in males taking ketoconazole.[28] This condition may resolve with continued therapy, but some cases may require discontinuation of the drug. Because of its unusual nature, all men receiving ketoconazole should be advised of this reaction and encouraged to continue therapy.

Rarely, ketoconazole can cause hepatotoxicity. More frequently, increases in liver function tests (LFTs) will be transient. The hepatotoxicity usually resolves on discontinuation of the drug and usually occurs very early during therapy. Individuals receiving ketoconazole should have LFTs performed before initiation of therapy, every 2 wk thereafter for the first 2 mo of therapy, and then every month until therapy is discontinued.

Ingestion of alcohol during treatment with ketoconazole may result in an Antabuse-like reaction consisting of flushing, rash, nausea, vomiting, and headache. Although this reaction is not dangerous, it is uncomfortable. Individuals receiving ketoconazole therapy are cautioned not to ingest alcohol within 48 h of a dose of ketoconazole.

The absorption of ketoconazole is significantly decreased by drugs that decrease gastric acidity. For this reason, ketoconazole should not be administered within 2 h of the following: antacids; H_2 antagonists, such as ranitidine (Zantac) or famotidine (Pepcid); or proton pump inhibitors, such as omeprazole (Prilosec) or lansoprazole (Prevacid).

TABLE 4.13   **Antifungal Agents**

Antifungal agent	Trade names	Uses	Duration of therapy	Adverse effects
Butenafine 1% cream	Mentax	Tinea pedis, tinea corporis, tinea cruris, tinea versicolor	Tinea pedis: 4 wk Tinea corporis, tinea cruris, tinea versicolor: 2 wk	Burning, stinging, local irritation
Butoconazole 2% vaginal cream*	Femstat-3, Myclex-3	Vulvovaginal candidiasis	3 d	Burning, itching
Ciclopirox 0.77% gel, cream, lotion	Loprox	Tinea pedis, tinea cruris, tinea corporis, tinea versicolor	Tinea versicolor: 2 wk All other conditions: 4 wk	Pruritus, transient burning
Clotrimazole 1% cream, solution, lotion, lozenges	Mycelex, Lotrimin, Gyne-Lotrimin, Lotrisone (with betamethasone)	Tinea pedis, tinea cruris, tinea corporis Vulvovaginal and oral candidiasis	Tinea cruris: 2 wk Tinea corporis and tinea pedis: 4 wk Vulvovaginal candidiasis: 7 d Oral candidiasis: 14 d	Erythema, pruritus, burning, stinging, peeling, contact dermatitis
Econazole 1% cream	Spectazole	Tinea corporis, tinea cruris, tinea pedis, tinea versicolor	Tinea cruris, tinea corporis, tinea versicolor: 2 wk Tinea pedis: 1 mo	Burning, stinging, pruritus, erythema
Ketoconazole 2% cream and shampoo	Nizoral	Tinea corporis, tinea cruris, tinea pedis, tinea versicolor	Tinea corporis, tinea cruris, tinea versicolor: 2 wk Tinea pedis: 6 wk	Irritation, pruritus, stinging, contact dermatitis
Miconazole 1% and 2% aerosol, cream, lotion, powder, solution, vaginal cream, vaginal suppositories (100 mg and 200 mg)*	Desenex, Lotrimin AF, Micatin, Ting, Monistat, Femizol-M, Nystat-Rx	Tinea pedis, tinea cruris, tinea corporis, tinea versicolor Vulvovaginal candidiasis	Tinea cruris, tinea corporis, tinea versicolor: 2 wk Tinea pedis: 1 mo Vulvovaginal candidiasis: 3-7 d	Irritation, burning, contact dermatitis
Nystatin oral suspension, tablets, lozenges, cream, ointment, powder	Mycostatin, Nystex, Nystop, Mycolog with triamcinolone, Mycogen with triamcinolone	Vulvovaginal and oral candidiasis	Vulvovaginal candidiasis: 14 d Oral candidiasis: 14 d	Irritation
Oxiconazole 1% cream and lotion	Oxistat	Tinea corporis, tinea cruris, tinea pedis, tinea versicolor	Tinea corporis, tinea cruris, tinea pedis: 2-4 wk Tinea versicolor: 2 wk	Pruritus, burning, contact dermatitis
Sulconazole 1% cream or solution	Exelderm	Tinea corporis, tinea cruris, tinea pedis, tinea versicolor	Tinea corporis, tinea cruris, tinea pedis: 2-4 wk Tinea versicolor: 2 wk	Pruritus, erythema, burning, irritation, stinging, tingling

Antifungal agent	Trade names	Uses	Duration of therapy	Adverse effects
Terbinafine 1% cream or solution	Lamisil	Tinea corporis, tinea cruris, tinea pedis, tinea versicolor	Tinea corporis, tinea cruris, tinea versicolor: 1 wk Tinea pedis: 2 wk	Burning, pruritus, erythema, skin discoloration
Terconazole 0.4% and 0.8% cream, suppositories (80 mg*)	Terazol	Vulvovaginal candidiasis	Vulvovaginal candidiasis: 3-7 d	Itching, burning, pruritus, irritation, abdominal pain, dysmenorrhea, fever, chills, headache
Tioconazole 6.5% ointment*	Monistat-1, Vagistat-1	Vulvovaginal candidiasis	Vulvovaginal candidiasis: single dose, improvement in 3 d	Burning, vaginitis, pruritus, headache, abdominal pain, dysuria, nocturia, pharyngitis, rhinitis
Tolnaftate 1% powder, cream, solution	Tinactin, Aftate, Zeasorb-AF	Tinea corporis, tinea cruris, tinea pedis, tinea versicolor	Tinea corporis, tinea cruris, tinea pedis, tinea versicolor: 4-6 wk	Slight local irritation

*These products contain a petroleum base that may interact with the latex or rubber of condoms or contraceptive diaphragms. Do not use condoms or a contraceptive diaphragm within 72 h following a dose of these products.

Data from Clinical Pharmacology (2022); Lexicomp Online (2022); Epocrates (2022).

Ketoconazole may increase the anticoagulant effect of warfarin. PT and INR should be monitored when the two drugs are used together, and the dose of warfarin adjusted accordingly. When ketoconazole is administered with phenytoin or theophylline, metabolism of the latter two drugs may be altered. Serum levels need to be monitored and doses adjusted accordingly.

Ketoconazole may cause increased plasma concentrations of systemically administered corticosteroids. In addition, ketoconazole may potentiate the adrenal suppression caused by corticosteroids. For these reasons, the dose of corticosteroids may need to be decreased when they are administered with ketoconazole.

Bronchodilators

Bronchodilators are β-adrenergic agonists (table 4.14). These agents stimulate the β-adrenergic receptors in the bronchi and bronchioles to cause widening of these airways and allow for improved airflow. In the athlete, exercise-induced bronchospasm is the most common cause of airway constriction requiring treatment with bronchodilators. Albuterol is the agent used to treat exercise-induced bronchospasm. Albuterol is available as a MDI, which offers the most convenient dosing, but proper technique must be used for the drug to be maximally effective (see figure 4.2).

Here are step-by-step instructions for using a MDI:

1. Remove the dust cap and shake the inhaler system before each use.

2. Inspect the mouthpiece for contamination or foreign objects.

3. Breathe out through the mouth, exhaling as completely as possible.

4. Hold the inhaler system upright with the mouthpiece in the mouth and the lips closed tightly around the mouthpiece.

5. Breathe in slowly while pressing down on the metal cartridge.

6. Hold the breath as long as possible.

TABLE 4.14   **Bronchodilators**

Drug	Administration
Albuterol (Ventolin, Proventil, ProAir RespiClick)	Metered-dose inhaler, oral tablets, oral solution, solution for nebulization
Levalbuterol (Xopenex)	Solution for nebulization
Racemic epinephrine (AsthmaNefrin, S2 inhalant)	Solution for nebulization

Data from Clinical Pharmacology (2022); Lexicomp Online (2022).

7. Release pressure while still holding the breath.

8. Remove the mouthpiece.

9. Wait for the container to repressurize, shake, and then repeat steps 3 through 8 when more than one inhalation is prescribed.

10. Rinse the mouth with water after the prescribed number of inhalations.

11. Clean the inhaler system every few days by removing metal cartridge and rinsing the plastic inhaler and cap with running warm water. Replace the cartridge and cap.

Another appropriate technique is described here:

1. With the inhaler properly positioned, have the patient hold the inhaler with the thumb at the mouthpiece and the index finger and middle finger at the top. This is a three-point or bilateral hand position.

2. Instruct the patient to tilt the head back slightly, inhale slowly and deeply through the mouth for 3 to 5 s, and then depress the medication canister fully.

3. Have the patient hold the breath for approximately 10 s.

4. Instruct the patient to remove the MDI from the mouth before exhaling, then exhale slowly through the nose or pursed lips.

A spacer that holds the puff of medicine between the inhaler device and the patient can increase the ease of use. When a spacer is used, the actuation of the inhaler does not have to be timed to the inhalation of the drug; the inhaler delivers the drug into the spacer (figure 4.3). The patient then inhales the drug slowly and often more completely through the spacer as a separate step.

Nebulizers are machines that use air pressure to aerosolize the drug and then deliver the quickest onset and maximized amount of drug. They are expensive and bulky to transport, but the drug can be delivered simply by placing a tube inside the mouth or wearing a mask over the mouth and nose (figure 4.4).

Side Effects

The main adverse effects of bronchodilators are tremor, nervousness, dizziness, headache, nausea, and tachycardia. A paradoxical bronchospasm also has been reported in 8% of individuals using bronchodilators. It is usually associated with the first use of a new MDI canister and

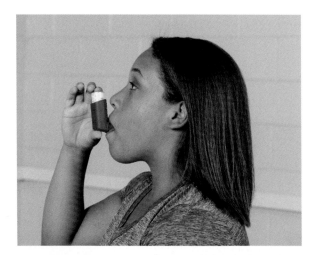

FIGURE 4.2   Proper technique for metered-dose inhaler use.

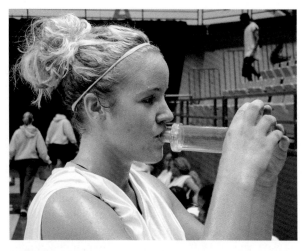

FIGURE 4.3   Proper use of a metered-dose inhaler with a spacer.

© Micki Cuppett

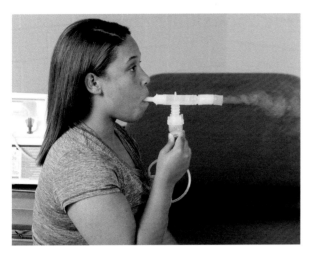

FIGURE 4.4 A nebulizer contains a pump and compressor that deliver a mist of medication through a face mask or tube.

may be related to exposure to the propellant. To avoid this reaction, a new MDI can be actuated into the air a few times before its first use. Nebulized albuterol caused coughing in 4% of individuals in various clinical trials. Side effects that occurred in less than 3% of individuals but that may be significant in the athlete include muscle cramping, muscle spasm, and dilated pupils.[29]

Levalbuterol (Xopenex) is the *R*-enantiomer of albuterol. It is only available as a solution for nebulization. Levalbuterol is considerably more expensive than albuterol, but it is associated with a lower rate of adverse effects. Albuterol, the less expensive alternative, is adequate for treating exercise-induced bronchospasm in the athlete.[30]

Antihistamines

Antihistamines are drugs used to treat allergies. When the body's immune system reacts to an allergen, histamine is released by the mast cells and basophils. Histamine binds to histamine receptors in the nose, eyes, respiratory tract, and skin, causing the classic allergic signs (e.g., rhinitis, sneezing, watery eyes, itching, dermatitis). Antihistamines are antagonists that block the histamine receptors and prevent histamine from binding to the cell's receptors.

The histamine antagonists are classified into two groups based on their likelihood of causing sedation. The first-generation, or sedating, antihistamines are older agents with a much higher incidence of anticholinergic adverse effects, including sedation (table 4.15). They are used in the treatment of seasonal allergies and some cold symptoms. The sedating properties associated with these drugs also make them useful in the short-term treatment of insomnia. In addition, some antihistamines, such as meclizine (Antivert) and hydroxyzine (Atarax, Vistaril), are used in the treatment of nausea, vertigo, motion sickness, and hives. Sedating antihistamines are commonly used to treat allergy symptoms associated with seasonal allergies and are usually formulated in combination with decongestants.

The second-generation, or nonsedating, antihistamines are used to treat and prevent seasonal allergies and to treat chronic idiopathic urticaria. These antihistamines are often the drug of choice for athletes and physically active individuals because of their nonsedating effects (table 4.16), and they typically are available without a prescription. Many are also formulated in combination with the decongestant pseudoephedrine (Zyrtec-D, Allegra-D).

TABLE 4.15 **Sedating Antihistamines**

Antihistamine	Trade name	Usual adult dosage
Azatadine	Optimine, 1 mg Rynatan and Trinalin, 1 mg	1-2 mg twice daily
Brompheniramine	Numerous	4 mg every 4 h *or* 6-12 mg every 12 h (extended release)
Carbinoxamine with pseudoephedrine	Rondec, Arbinoxa	4 mg 4 times daily *or* 8 mg every 12 h (extended release)
Chlorpheniramine	Chlor-Trimeton, Ahist, Aller-Chlor	4 mg every 4-6 h *or* 8-12 mg twice daily (extended release) *or* 16 mg once daily (extended release)
Clemastine	Tavist	1.34 mg every 12 h
Diphenhydramine*	Benadryl, Sominex, Unisom	25-50 mg every 4-6 h
Promethazine	Phenergan	6.25 mg every 4-6 h
Triprolidine	Actifed	2.5 mg every 4-6 h

*Available over the counter.
Data from Clinical Pharmacology (2022); Lexicomp Online (2022).

The adverse effects most often associated with the first-generation sedating antihistamines are those caused by CNS depression, such as drowsiness, muscular weakness, and dizziness. Therefore, antihistamines should be used with caution by athletes participating in events where coordination and alertness are needed to prevent injury. Even mild sedation may increase the incidence of injury and decrease performance. Anyone taking antihistamines should avoid alcohol intake because of the additive effect on CNS depression.

Additional adverse effects seen with first-generation antihistamines are gastrointestinal and include nausea, vomiting, diarrhea, or constipation. These antihistamines also cause anticholinergic side effects, such as dry mouth, blurred vision, urinary retention, impotence, nervousness, and irritability.

Antihistamines must be used with caution in people with hyperthyroidism and hypertension (see chapter 7). Although there is some controversy over the potential for antihistamines to induce asthma attacks by virtue of their drying effect on bronchial tissues, antihistamines are contraindicated in those who experience acute asthmatic attacks. The drug interactions of the sedating antihistamines are primarily with other CNS depressants, which will cause an additive CNS depressant effect.

Decongestants

Decongestants are drugs that primarily stimulate the α-adrenergic receptors and to a lesser extent the β-adrenergic receptors (table 4.17). The beneficial result of this α-adrenergic stimulation is vasoconstriction in the nasal mucosa that shrinks swollen nasal passages, thereby relieving nasal congestion. The decongestants are used orally either alone or in combination with other agents used to treat cold and allergy symptoms, such as antihistamines. Topical decongestants like Afrin can also be applied directly to the nasal mucosa to provide relief from congestion without systemic side effects. Ophthalmic decongestants like Visine are applied to the eyes to produce vasoconstriction of the conjunctival vasculature, reducing redness of the eyes.

Pseudoephedrine (Sudafed) is the oral decongestant most used alone or in combination products. Pseudoephedrine is a naturally occurring substance found in plants of the genus *Ephedra* and is an isomer of ephedrine. The usual adult dosage of pseudoephedrine is 30 to 60 mg every 4 to 6 h. Sustained-release products of pseudoephedrine are available as 120 mg tablets given every 12 h and 240 mg tablets given every 24 h. Side effects associated with the use of pseudoephedrine include mild

TABLE 4.16　**Nonsedating Antihistamines**

Antihistamine	Trade names	Usual adult dosage	Drug interactions	Adverse effects
Cetirizine*	Zyrtec	5-10 mg once daily		Somnolence, fatigue, dizziness, dry mouth
Desloratadine*	Clarinex, Clarinex RediTabs	5 mg daily		
Fexofenadine*	Allegra	60 mg twice daily *or* 180 mg once daily	Aluminum- and magnesium-containing antacids decrease absorption and peak plasma levels; do not take fexofenadine within 2 h of antacids	Headache, insomnia, dizziness, back pain
Loratadine*	Claritin, Alavert	10 mg once daily		Headache, sedation, insomnia, nervousness, dry mouth, abdominal pain

*Available over the counter.

Data from Clinical Pharmacology (2022); Lexicomp Online (2022).

TABLE 4.17 **Decongestant Sprays**

Generic name	Trade names	Usual adult dosage	Adverse effects
Naphazoline	Privine	2 drops every 3-6 h	Rebound congestion, burning, stinging, nasal dryness, sneezing, headache, hypertension, palpitations, tachycardia, reflex bradycardia, nervousness, nausea, dizziness, weakness, sweating
Oxymetazoline	Afrin Allerest Cheracol Dristan Genasal Neo-Synephrine	2-3 drops/sprays every 10-12 h for no more than 3 d	Rebound congestion, burning, stinging, rhinorrhea, nasal dryness, sneezing, hypertension, nervousness, nausea, dizziness, headache, insomnia, palpitations, tachycardia, reflex bradycardia
Phenylephrine	Neo-Synephrine Alconefrin Vicks Sinex	2-3 drops or 1-3 sprays every 4 h	Rebound congestion, burning, stinging, sneezing, rhinorrhea, nasal dryness, palpitation, tachycardia, PVCs, headache, pallor, tremors, sweating, hypertension, nausea, dizziness, nervousness
Propylhexedrine	Benzedrex	2 inhalations every 2 h	Rebound congestion, burning, stinging, nasal dryness, sneezing, headache, hypertension, nervousness, tachycardia
Tetrahydrozoline	Tyzine	2-4 drops/sprays every 4-6 h	Rebound congestion, burning, stinging, nasal dryness, sneezing, headache, hypertension, weakness, sweating, palpitations, tremor
Xylometazoline	Otrivin	2-3 drops/sprays every 8-10 h for no more than 3-5 d	Rebound congestion, burning, stinging, nasal dryness, sneezing, hypertension, nervousness, nausea, dizziness, headache, insomnia, palpitations, tachycardia, arrhythmias
Ophthalmic decongestants			
Naphazoline	Allerest Clear Eyes Naphcon VasoClear Comfort Vasocon	1-3 drops every 3-4 h	Blurred vision, mild stinging or irritation, pupil dilation, headache, hypertension, palpitations, tachycardia, reflex bradycardia, nervousness, nausea, dizziness, weakness, sweating
Oxymetazoline	OcuClear Visine LR	1-2 drops every 6 h	
Phenylephrine	Isopto Frin Ocu-Phrin Prefrin Relief Zincfrin Vasosulf	1-2 drops every 3-4 h	Headache, blurred vision, irritation, pupil dilation, palpitations, tachycardia, PVCs, headache, pallor, tremors, sweating, hypertension, nausea, dizziness, nervousness
Tetrahydrozoline	Collyrium Fresh Geneye Extra Murine Plus Visine	1-2 drops up to 4 times daily	Irritation, blurred vision, pupil dilation, rebound congestion, headache, hypertension, weakness, sweating, palpitations, tremor

Note: PVC = premature ventricular contraction.

Data from Clinical Pharmacology (2022); Lexicomp Online (2022).

CNS stimulation, such as nervousness, dizziness, weakness, insomnia, and headache. Because pseudoephedrine causes minimal blood pressure changes in patients with normal blood pressure, it should be used with caution by those with high blood pressure because α-adrenergic stimulation causes vasoconstriction and may raise blood pressure.

Pseudoephedrine can be used to make methamphetamine, a CNS stimulant with high addictive potential. For this reason, federal law limits the quantity of pseudoephedrine that can be sold by retail distributors. It is also vital that the athletic trainer be aware that as CNS stimulants, oral decongestants are listed by the National Collegiate Athletics Association (NCAA), U.S. Anti-Doping Agency, and World Anti-Doping Agency as banned drugs. For athletes subject to drug testing, the drug of choice for the treatment of allergic rhinitis within 24 h of competition or testing should not contain pseudoephedrine.[31]

Phenylephrine (Neo-Synephrine) is used as a topical decongestant in nasal drops and sprays. It is also listed on the NCAA list of banned drugs because of its stimulant properties. Phenylephrine nasal drops or sprays for adults are available as 0.25% or 0.5% solutions that are applied to the nasal mucosa every 4 to 6 h.[32] Adverse effects of phenylephrine nasal solutions include transient burning, stinging, sneezing, rhinitis, and nasal dryness. Prolonged use of phenylephrine nasal solutions should be avoided because it may result in chronic or rebound swelling of the nasal mucosa, which resolves within 1 wk of discontinuing the drug.

Oxymetazoline (Afrin, Dristan) and xylometazoline (Otrivin) are long-acting topical decongestants found in nasal sprays and drops. These long-acting agents should not be used for more than 3 d because significant rebound congestion often occurs and may promote their overuse.

Ophthalmic decongestants, such as tetrahydrozoline (Visine), provide relief of conjunctival redness and minor eye irritation. Prolonged use of ophthalmic decongestant solutions must be avoided, however, because rebound **hyperemia** may result and promote overuse of the products. It is also important that the use of ophthalmic decongestants not mask an underlying condition that may need medical attention. If ocular pain, redness, or irritation occurs or if visual changes are experienced during the use of these products, the patient must immediately stop using them and seek medical attention.[33]

Individuals with glaucoma should not use ophthalmic decongestants without consulting a physician or optometrist. Also, most manufacturers recommend that contact lenses be removed before using any ophthalmic decongestant product. Allergic reactions to the ophthalmic decongestants themselves are extremely rare, whereas allergic reactions to the preservatives used in these products are common.

Gastrointestinal Disorders

Medications to treat conditions such as heartburn, gastroesophageal reflux disorder (GERD), and peptic ulcer disease focus on several mechanisms. These mechanisms include neutralizing the acidity of gastric acid produced, inhibiting the secretion of acid, physically blocking the effect of acid on tissues, or increasing the protective effects of naturally occurring mucus in the digestive tract. (See chapter 8 for specific diagnosis and treatment of various gastrointestinal disorders.) For GERD, the goal is to prevent the disease from progressing, including first and foremost, lifestyle changes to suppress gastric acid. In addition to lifestyle modifications, such as elevating the head of the bed and eliminating offending foods, a simple change in the pH of the gastrointestinal system may allow the patient to start healing and decrease symptoms. There are several effective OTC antacids mostly consisting of calcium carbonate, sodium bicarbonate, magnesium hydroxide, or aluminum hydroxide.[19] Many products combine one or more of these ingredients for effectiveness in chemically neutralizing gastric acid. Examples of antacids include Maalox, Mylanta, Rolaids, Alka-Seltzer, and Tums or their generic counterparts.

The next line of treatment for gastrointestinal acid disorders includes histamine H_2-receptor agonists like cimetidine (Tagamet HB) and famotidine (Pepcid AC). These drugs compete with histamine for H_2 receptors in the stomach and therefore depress the production of gastric acid. They are absorbed in 1 to 3 h, with acid suppression lasting for several hours. These agents come in a variety of formulations, including capsules, pills, chewables, liquid, and effervescents, and they may be combined with antacids. If relief is not achieved after a few weeks of treatment with antacids and H_2 agonists, the patient may progress to a proton pump inhibitor taken 30 to 60 min before the first meal of the day. Common OTC proton pump inhibitors include omeprazole (Prilosec) and esomeprazole (Nexium). See table 4.18 for some common OTC drugs for gastrointestinal disorders.

Treatment of constipation includes the use of laxatives in four different categories: stool softeners, bulk-forming laxatives, osmotic laxatives, and stimulant laxatives. The category of laxative used is dependent on the patient and the circumstances that require treatment of constipation. Stool softeners lower the surface tension at the oil-water interface of the feces, helping to hydrate and soften the fecal material, facilitating movement through the colon. Docusate (Colace) is often used to prevent constipation, rather than as a specific treatment, and may be given with other medications known to cause constipation. Bulk-forming laxatives, such as methylcellulose (Citrucel) or psyllium (Metamucil), are generally made of nondigestible plant products and form a gel-like substance when combined with water. This gel

TABLE 4.18 **Common OTC Medications for GERD**

Generic name	Trade name	Dosage	Notes
Antacids			Quick onset of action Short duration of relief requiring frequent dosing
Aluminum hydroxide	Maalox* Mylanta*	200-400 mg	May cause constipation
Magnesium hydroxide	Maalox* Mylanta*	200-400 mg	May cause diarrhea
Calcium carbonate	Tums	500-1,000 mg	May cause belching and abdominal distention May cause constipation
Sodium bicarbonate	Alka-Seltzer	750-1,900 mg	May cause belching and abdominal distention Should not be used long term in sodium-sensitive patients
H$_2$ agonists			
Cimetidine	Tagamet	200 mg as needed, 1-2 times daily	
Famotidine	Pepcid	10-20 mg as needed, 1-2 times daily	
Proton pump inhibitors			
Esomeprazole	Nexium	20 mg/d	
Lansoprazole	Prevacid	15 mg/d	
Omeprazole	Prilosec	20 mg/d	

*Maalox and Mylanta use a combination of aluminum hydroxide and magnesium hydroxide, because aluminum hydroxide may cause constipation and magnesium hydroxide may cause diarrhea. Through combination of these ingredients, these symptoms are reduced.

Data from Clinical Pharmacology (2022); Lexicomp Online (2022); Epocrates (2022).

moves readily through the digestive tract and encourages peristalsis.[34] For specific information on treating various conditions of the gastrointestinal system, including both pharmacological and nonpharmacological treatment, please see chapter 8.

Antidiabetic Agents

With the increased prevalence of diabetes mellitus worldwide, athletic trainers will likely encounter patients with diabetes. There are also well-recognized genetic risk factors for the disease. There are two types of diabetes mellitus: Type 1 diabetes is associated with autoimmune-mediated destruction of B-cells of the pancreatic islets. This results in a total (or near-total) lack of insulin production by the pancreas. Type 2 diabetes is believed to be a combination of complex metabolic conditions that ultimately results in impaired insulin secretion and insulin action.[24] It is increasingly important for athletic trainers to understand diabetes, to be familiar with the pharmacological treatments that individuals may be using, and to understand the effects of these medications on training and rehabilitation.

There are many medications to treat diabetes. For patients with type 1 diabetes, the most prevalent treatment is insulin. Insulin is available in various forms and delivery methods, including insulin pens, pumps, and injectors, in addition to traditional needle injections.

Patients with type 2 diabetes have multiple pharmacological options, all designed to work on different organ systems. The coverage here is neither comprehensive nor exhaustive; this chapter simply focuses on the diabetes medications most likely to be encountered by the athletic trainer.

Insulin Secretagogues and Oral Hypoglycemic Agents

Several medications are designed to stimulate the secretion of insulin from the pancreas (table 4.19). Some are referred to as *hypoglycemic agents* because of their ability to induce low blood glucose levels in patients once introduced to the body. Other medications are called *insulin secretagogues* because they can promote insulin secretion without necessarily producing low glucose levels. These medications are for patients with type 2 diabetes.

Sulfonylureas and Meglitinides

Sulfonylureas and meglitinides are hypoglycemic agents that work by stimulating the sodium–potassium channels in pancreatic beta cells. The sulfonylureas are separated into first generation and second generation. The only first-generation sulfonylurea still in use today is chlorpropamide (Diabinese). Most of the second-generation sulfonylureas are used in smaller doses than chlorpropamide and generally are taken once or twice per day before meals. The meglitinides have a similar mechanism of action to the sulfonylureas, but their duration of activity is much less. Therefore, they must be taken more often, up to three times daily, usually before meals. Because these drug classes stimulate the release of insulin, it is important to monitor for signs and symptoms of hypoglycemia (sweating, shaking, chills, rapid heartbeat).

Dipeptidyl Peptidase-4 Inhibitors

The dipeptidyl peptidase-4 (DPP-IV) class of diabetes medications is commonly called the *gliptins*. They raise incretin levels in the body by preventing their degradation. This, in turn, results in increased insulin secretion when the secretion is stimulated by a meal. Gliptins have few adverse effects, but they do increase the risk of hypoglycemia. At present, all gliptins are administered orally.

Antihyperglycemic Medications

As their name implies, antihyperglycemic medications aim to prevent significant increases in glucose levels through means other than pancreatic insulin secretion. The most common medication in this category is metformin, which is classified as a biguanide. Metformin has multiple mechanisms of action to control glucose levels in patients. Its primary action is to decrease liver glucose production and increase peripheral glucose uptake

TABLE 4.19 Diabetes Medication Classes

Diabetes medication class	Glycemic action	Generic name	Trade name
α-glucosidase inhibitors	Antihyperglycemic*	Acarbose Miglitol	Precose Glyset
Biguanides	Antihyperglycemic	Metformin	Glucophage
Dopamine-2 agonists	Antihyperglycemic	Bromocriptine	Cycloset Parlodel
DPP-IV inhibitors	Antihyperglycemic	Alogliptin Sitagliptin Linagliptin Saxagliptin	Nesina Januvia Tradjenta Onglyza
Meglitinides	Hypoglycemic†	Repaglinide Nateglinide	Prandin Starlix
SGLT2 inhibitors	Antihyperglycemic	Dapagliflozin Empagliflozin Canagliflozin	Farxiga Jardiance Invokana
Sulfonylureas	Hypoglycemic	Glyburide Glipizide Glimepiride	DiaBeta Glucotrol Amaryl
Thiazolidinediones	Antihyperglycemic	Pioglitazone Rosiglitazone	Actos Avandia

Note: DDP-IV = dipeptidyl peptidase-4; SGLT2 = sodium-glucose cotransporter 2.

*Antihyperglycemic agents control elevations in blood glucose levels by decreasing the amount of glucose produced by the liver; they usually do not promote hypoglycemia.

†Hypoglycemic agents can produce hypoglycemia because of facilitated insulin secretion from the pancreas.

Data from Clinical Pharmacology (2022); Lexicomp Online (2022); "Oral and Other Injectable Diabetes Medications," American Diabetes Association, accessed May 2023, https://diabetes.org/healthy-living/medication-treatments/oral-other-injectable-diabetes-medications.

in target cells. Metformin has a very minimal effect on glucose levels in patients with normal levels, and it does not promote insulin secretion. This results in very rare instances of hypoglycemia being reported. Adverse effects for metformin include gastrointestinal effects (e.g., nausea, cramping, diarrhea) and a rare association with lactic acidosis. Because of the potential for lactic acidosis, renal function should be monitored periodically.[35] Other classes of antihyperglycemic medications include the thiazolidinediones, α-glucosidase inhibitors, and the newest class called sodium-glucose cotransporter 2 inhibitors.

Insulin

When oral medications have not succeeded in controlling a patient's glucose levels, insulin is the next level of medication to be used. There is wide variability in the prescribing and administration of insulin because of the need to individualize insulin therapy for each patient. Patients with type 1 diabetes require insulin as their primary source of glucose control, whereas patients with type 2 diabetes may be prescribed insulin after all other forms of treatment have failed to produce desired glucose control. The specific nature of the diabetes may also affect insulin therapy. Experienced clinicians should be in control of the type of insulin regimen recommended for each patient.

Insulin is primarily categorized according to its duration of action: short acting versus long acting (see table 4.20). Short-acting insulin is administered to quickly control and reduce glucose levels in patients. This rapid control may be used in response to meals to prevent postprandial glucose increases, in response to very significant elevations in glucose levels, or as a feature of insulin pumps that release very small amounts of insulin in a very controlled manner. Long-acting insulin is administered to provide continuous control of glucose levels over a span of 10 to 24 h in single or multiple administrations. Patients should be taught the proper administration techniques for insulin injections and how to monitor for both positive glucose control and possible adverse effects. Because insulin can cause hypoglycemia, patients should also know how to manage these episodes if they should occur. Athletic trainers may also benefit greatly from understanding how to manage hypoglycemic episodes should they occur in their presence.

Biologics

Biologics are medications developed from blood, proteins, viruses, or living organisms and are used to treat a variety of conditions from autoimmune disorders to cancers. Readers may be familiar with many biologics, such as onabotulinumtoxinA (Botox) and adalimumab (Humira), because pharmaceutical companies have heavily advertised these medications in recent years. Biologics go through a different approval process from most drugs approved by the Food and Drug Administration (FDA), because they are not made from chemicals like most drugs but instead are made from living sources.[32,36] They are typically administered as injections and infusions and there are no generics available. Recently, similar drugs have been synthetically developed and are called *biosimilars*, which may prove to be less expensive than the biologics.

A few common biologics are Botox, Humira, and etanercept (Enbrel). While these biologics are used to treat very different conditions, they are all derived from living cells. Botox is produced by using the bacterium *Clostridium botulinum* and has been used for cosmetic procedures for years. Recently, Botox has been used to treat numerous other conditions, such as muscle spasms, migraine, eyelid twitching, and overactive bladder, because it blocks the nerves and muscles from

TABLE 4.20 **Types of Insulin**

Insulin	Onset	Peak	Duration
Insulin lispro (Humalog), insulin aspart (Novolog)	<15 min	1-2 h	3 h
Regular	0.5-1 h	2-3 h	2-5 h
NPH and insulin zinc (lente)	2-4 h	6-10 h	10-12 h
70/30, 50/50	0.5-1 h	2-10 h	10-12 h
Humalog 75/25, Novolog 70/30	<15 min	1-8 h	10-12 h
Insulin glargine (Lantus, Semglee)	1-2 h	Flat	24 h
Insulin detemir (Levemir)	1-2 h	Flat	12-24 h
Insulin degludec (Tresiba)	1-2 h	Flat	24 h
Inhaled (Afrezza)	<15 min	1-2 h	3 h

Note: NPH = neutral protamine Hagedorn.

Data from Clinical Pharmacology (2022); Lexicomp Online (2022).

activating. Humira is a monoclonal antibody, which is an artificial protein used to target specific elements in the body. Humira is used to treat certain inflammatory conditions, like rheumatoid arthritis, by blocking the specific molecules in the body that would otherwise trigger inflammation.[32,36]

Supplements

No U.S. federal agency, not even the FDA, regulates the content of food supplements and herbal products. It is assumed that these products contain the ingredients or the quantities of each ingredient listed on the label and that the ingredients listed are safe. This puts the person using these products at risk because there has been no regulatory follow-up to make sure the products provide what is listed and, further, are safe for human consumption. Consumers should exercise caution when purchasing herbal and fitness supplements, as most of their packaging does not list adverse effects and drug interactions. Fortunately, many drug formularies now include supplements in their drug interaction search engines. See chapter 3 for a discussion of supplements.

Summary

This chapter describes several commonly used classes of medications prescribed to treat various medical conditions. Although medication dispensing is not within the scope of practice of certified athletic trainers, they must understand the range of common medications that patients may be using as well as potential interactions with other medications or foods and possible adverse reactions. It is also important for athletic trainers to be familiar with the basic drug classifications used in the athletic population, along with their indications, contraindications, drug and food interactions, and typical patterns of use. In addition, the athletic trainer must know how to access current drug information and should have a good working relationship with the physician and the pharmacist to ensure the best treatment for patients.

Apply It!

Go to HK*Propel* to complete the case studies for this chapter.

Common Procedures in the Athletic Training Clinic

5

At the completion of this chapter the reader should be able to do the following:

1. Demonstrate attainment of appropriate informed consent before performing any of the procedures described herein.

2. Employ fundamental aseptic procedures, including the use of sterile gloves and the creation of a sterile field.

3. Properly unpack a sterile package and prepare for a sterile procedure.

4. Compare the various types of sutures and suture needles and their specific applications.

5. Describe the differences among interrupted, running, and mattress sutures and the advantages and disadvantages of each.

6. Complete a simple interrupted suture.

7. Prepare the patient for injection and aspiration.

This chapter begins with a disclaimer about state practice acts. At present, 49 U.S. states regulate the practice of athletic training in some fashion, whether by certification, licensure, or other regulation.[1] It is important to remember that the practice acts for athletic trainers as well as other health care professionals vary widely by state. Clinicians must be familiar with the practice acts of their state. By recognizing the limitations of their own practice acts, athletic trainers can fully use their skills and knowledge base to provide appropriate health care to patients.

The techniques and procedures outlined in this chapter may be prohibited or not addressed in particular state rules and regulations. Despite this, learning new techniques allows practitioners to evolve with changes in the profession and revisions in state practice acts, or to practice to the full scope of the profession if they move to a state with a different set of guidelines. The skills in this chapter are required to be taught within all Commission on Accreditation of Athletic Training Education–accredited athletic training programs. With the growing number of athletic trainers working in physician offices and other health care settings, many are now performing the procedures described in this chapter in their daily practice. Even if they do not perform the procedures themselves, many athletic trainers are asked to help prepare patients and the environment for invasive procedures in the athletic training clinic.

Informed Consent

Informed consent ensures an individual's right to participate in decisions about their own health care. All individuals should receive enough information to make an informed decision about whether to consent to a treatment or procedure. Legally, it is the physician who must obtain informed consent, but the physician may delegate this responsibility to another health care provider. A health care provider who is substantially involved with the patient's care must obtain informed consent. Figure 5.1 provides an example of an informed consent form. Informed consent should include, at a minimum, a thorough discussion of the following:

- The patient's diagnosis
- The nature and purpose of a proposed treatment or procedure
- The risks and benefits of a proposed treatment or procedure
- Alternatives to the proposed treatment or procedure (regardless of the cost or the extent to which the treatment options are covered by health insurance)
- The risks and benefits of the alternative treatment or procedure
- The risks and benefits of not receiving or undergoing a treatment or procedure

Preventing Infection

The Centers for Disease Control and Prevention (CDC) defines *universal precautions* as a simple set of effective practices designed to protect health care workers and patients from infection by a range of pathogens, including bloodborne viruses. Specific instructions and details regarding universal precautions are detailed in chapter 14. These practices are used when caring for all patients regardless of diagnosis.[2]

Universal precautions apply to blood and to other body fluids that contain visible blood, semen, and vaginal secretions. Universal precautions also apply to tissues and to cerebrospinal, synovial, pleural, peritoneal, pericardial, and amniotic fluids. Universal precautions do not apply to feces, nasal secretions, sputum, sweat, tears, urine, and vomitus unless they contain visible blood. Universal precautions do not apply to saliva except when visibly contaminated with blood or in the dental setting where blood contamination of saliva is predictable.

Universal precautions provide for the use of protective barriers such as gloves, gowns, aprons, masks, and protective eyewear, which can reduce the risk of exposing the health care worker's skin or mucous membranes to potentially infective materials. It is also recommended that all health care workers take precautions to prevent injuries caused by needles, scalpels, and other sharp instruments or devices.[2]

Asepsis and Aseptic Technique

Preventing infection and maximizing healing should be the primary goals when performing any invasive proce-

---

Clinical Tips

Preventing Sharps Injuries

Use the following best practices for handling sharps in the medical clinic:

- Use standardized sterile field setups.
- Keep all sharps on instrument tables or trays with the points away from staff members.
- The hands-free or neutral zone method should be used for passing all sharps.
- Dedicate the neutral zone for sharps only (these include suture and hypodermic needles, scalpels, and other sharp instruments).
- Only one sharp at a time should be in the neutral zone.
- Use a needle holder or forceps to handle suture needles. Avoid manually handling needles. Do not hold a sharp and any other instrument simultaneously.
- Do not multitask when using sharps. Focus on making safe passes and exchanges and nothing else.
- Look before reaching.
- Confine and contain all sharps in a disposable, puncture-resistant needle container.

---

dure. The term **asepsis** means the absence of infectious organisms, and the goal of **aseptic technique** is to prevent the transfer of microorganisms into the wound.[3,4] Preventing site contamination requires all team members to use their knowledge and experience in aseptic practices.

Whenever an invasive procedure is performed, these aseptic practices *must* be followed:

- Assess the patient for any risk factors.
- Assess any environmental concerns.
- Ensure proper disinfection and sterilization of instruments.
- Observe the use of universal precautions.

Sterile Versus Nonsterile Individuals

Both sterile and nonsterile individuals must be aware of aseptic techniques. Once a person dons sterile equipment (gown, gloves, etc.), they must pay particular attention to maintaining sterility. Nonsterile personnel must be careful not to contaminate the sterile person or the sterile field. Before performing a sterile procedure, the clinician must don sterile gloves. This procedure is very different from the use of latex gloves under normal universal precautions.

ASSUMPTION OF RISK AND RELEASE: ASTHMA

State of _____

This release, executed by _____ , a resident of (city), (state) and a student at (university), is given to the (university), its Board of Governors, administrative staff, agents and employees, and to (university), (state), its Board of Trustees, administrative staff, physicians, including those physicians who provide services to the University pursuant to a contract, and all agents and employees of the University having any connection with the athletic program at (university), and particularly the _____ program.

Statement of Facts and Intent

The student is a _____ (freshman, sophomore, junior, senior) at (university), and is a member of the University's _____ team.

As a result of a preexisting asthmatic condition, the student has been determined to be at risk when involved in strenuous physical activities including conditioning exercises and playing and practicing college _____ .

Dr. XXXX, who is designated as the (university) team physician, has conferred with (student) and advised them as to the risk of participating in intercollegiate _____ and has further recommended that if (student) elects to participate in intercollegiate _____ despite these risks, they should take certain precautions.

Based on the foregoing statement of facts, and in consideration of (university) permitting (student) to participate in intercollegiate _____ , the (student) (and parents if student is a minor) execute the following assumption of risk and release:

Operative Provisions

1. (Student) acknowledges that they are fully aware that playing or practicing in any sport can be a dangerous activity involving many risks of injuries. Further, that the dangers and risks of playing or practicing in _____ _____ include, but are not limited to, death or serious injury resulting from an asthmatic attack or an exercise-induced asthma attack.

2. (Student) acknowledges that they have been fully advised by the team physician and (university) that because of their preexisting asthmatic condition, their participation in intercollegiate _____ could result in death or serious injury secondary to bronchospasm following an asthmatic attack or exercise induced asthmatic attack.

3. (Student) understands that if they elect to play _____ despite the risks noted herein, the team physician and (university) officials have advised them to use a short acting bronchodilator inhaler. Specifically, the team physician and these University officials have advised them to administer two puffs ten to fifteen minutes prior to any strenuous activity and two puffs every four hours as needed.

4. (Student) agrees to inform a member of the (university's) athletic training staff whenever they experience any symptoms related to their asthmatic condition including wheezing, cough, shortness of breath, and tightness in the chest during exercise.

5. By execution of this assumption of risk and release and in consideration of (university) permitting them to engage in intercollegiate _____ , (student) acknowledges and assumes the risk of serious injury or death that could result from an asthmatic attack or exercise induced asthmatic attack.

6. (Student) agrees that no representation has been made to them by (university) except as set forth in this assumption of risk and having had the risks explained to them, they wish to continue their participation in intercollegiate _____ despite these risks.

This is the _____ day of _____ 20 _____ .

_____
Signature of student-athlete

_____
Signature of parent (if student-athlete is a minor)

_____
Witness

_____
Witness

FIGURE 5.1 An informed consent form for asthma should outline the responsibilities of each party as well as the risks and benefits of athletic participation with the condition. This sample consent form is for an athlete on a university team.

Proper Technique for Opening and Donning Sterile Gloves

1. Peel away the packaging, exposing the sterile gloves *(a)*.
2. Hold the opened package horizontal to the table *(b)*.
3. Flip the contents onto the table without releasing either end of the packaging *(c)*.
4. While keeping the package flat on the table, pinch the bottom corners and open *(d)*.
5. Pinch the bottom corners inside the package and unfold *(e)*.
6. Pinch the top corners inside the package and unfold *(f)*.
7. Without touching the fingertips of the gloves, gently unfold the packaging, leaving it flat on the table *(g)*.
8. Pick up the right glove and gently slide the fingertips inside, using the left hand for guidance and assistance *(h, i)*. Make sure not to touch the fingertips of the glove.
9. Properly applied sterile glove *(j)*.
10. With the gloved right hand, place the fingertips inside the pocket of the left glove, while sliding the left hand into the glove *(k, l)*.
11. Properly applied sterile gloves *(m)*.

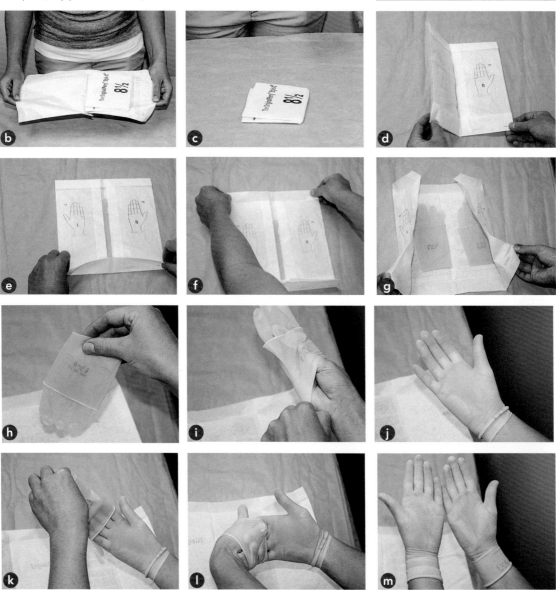

FIGURE 5.2

© Micki Cuppett

Before donning sterile gloves, the clinician must perform a thorough hand scrub with antibiotic soap. If close contact with body fluids or tissue is likely, or in the event of potential splash, a surgical mask and protective eyewear should also be worn.

Sterile Field

Sterile drapes are used to create a sterile field. The sterile field may be thought of as an imaginary "box" that also encompasses the space above the patient. Sterile drapes should be placed on the patient to leave only the procedural area exposed. Sterile drapes are used to establish an aseptic barrier between nonsterile and sterile areas.

All items placed within the sterile field must be sterile. Only sterile packages, instruments, and materials should be placed in the sterile field. Under no circumstances should sterile and nonsterile items be mixed. Nonsterile people (e.g., a student who is observing) should never reach across or into the sterile field. To ensure sterility, all sterile items should be inspected for package integrity. If a package has been compromised, it should be considered contaminated and should not be used. When a sterile packaged item is dropped on the floor, air can penetrate the sterile package. The force that is created when the package contacts the floor can cause the sterile barrier to be penetrated by forcing sterile air out and allowing contaminated air and particles into the package.[5,6] Nonsterile personnel must use good judgment when dispensing sterile items onto the sterile field either by presenting them directly to the sterile person or by placing them securely on the sterile field. Proper technique must be used when opening wrapped supplies.

Clinical Tips

Sterile Field

Keep in mind that after draping, only the top surface of the draped area is considered sterile.

Proper Technique for a Nonsterile Person Opening a Sterile Pack

1. Grasp the tip of the folded paper and open *away* from the pack *(a)*.
2. Unfold each flap individually *away* from the pack *(b, c)*.
3. *Do not* reach under the folds or flaps *(d)*.

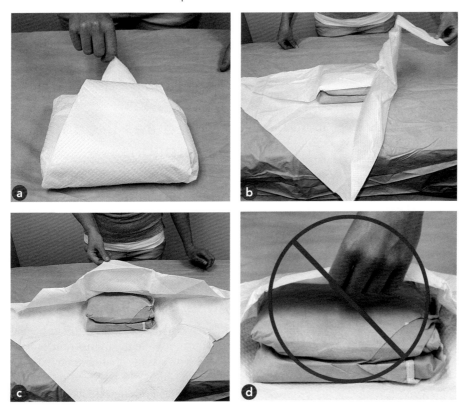

FIGURE 5.3
© Micki Cuppett

Proper Technique for Opening Wrapped Supplies

1. A nonsterile person opens sterile packs for a person wearing sterile gloves (a).
2. Peel packs are opened by peeling back the wrapping at the corner and holding the package open for a sterile person to reach in and remove sterile items (b, c).

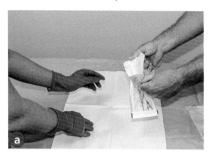 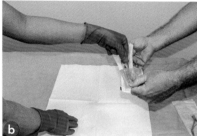 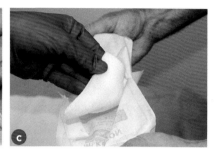

FIGURE 5.4
© Micki Cuppett

A sterile field should be maintained throughout the procedure and monitored constantly. Sterility can never be guaranteed, but every reasonable effort to reduce the likelihood of contamination should be taken, and personnel should be vigilant to avoid breaches in sterility.

When a breach of sterility occurs, medical team members must take immediate and appropriate action to correct the break in technique to reduce further risk of contamination. If there is doubt about an item's sterility, consider it not sterile. The sterile field should be prepared as close as possible to the time of use. Once set up, the sterile field needs to be monitored constantly.[4]

Everyone moving near or in a sterile field should do so in a manner that maintains the sterile field. Once gloved, personnel should remain in or close to the sterile field without wandering around the room. To avoid any accidental contact with nonsterile items or areas, gloved personnel should keep their arms and hands within the sterile field at all times. Just as the sterile person must maintain a safe distance from nonsterile areas and persons, nonsterile personnel must always be aware of and maintain a *margin of safety* when approaching sterile fields and scrubbed personnel. Finally, when delivering sterile supplies to the sterile field, nonsterile team members must always maintain a margin of safety between themselves and the sterile field, never contacting or reaching over any portion of the sterile area. This margin of safety is considered to be a minimum of 12 in. (30 cm).[6]

Policies and procedures for maintaining a sterile field should be written, reviewed annually, and readily available within the practice setting. These recommended practices for aseptic technique should be used as guidelines for developing policies and procedures within the practice setting. Training in aseptic technique requires experienced surgical team members to demonstrate these skills to new and inexperienced personnel. New personnel should be assigned an experienced mentor who will be a good role model and teacher in perioperative practice.

Maintaining Asepsis

All medical team members must practice aseptic technique to help prevent the transfer of microorganisms into the wound during the procedure. Team members must develop a strong conscience, adhering to the principles of asepsis and rectifying any improper technique they see during the procedure. In addition, proper surgical attire plays an important role in the reduction of site infections by reducing the amount of hair and skin contaminants reaching the sterile field.[4]

Procedures Used to Close Lacerations

Caring for a laceration is a common occurrence in the athletic training clinic. Often, simply cleaning the wound and applying an antibiotic ointment and an adhesive bandage are sufficient. Sometimes, however, more aggressive measures must be used to close the laceration to achieve good healing and cosmetic results. This section discusses common skin closure materials and techniques.

Adhesive Skin Tape

Adhesive skin tape is used to close small, superficial, low-tension wounds and to reinforce larger wounds closed with sutures or after removing sutures to protect the wound during the proliferation and early remodeling periods of healing (figure 5.5).

Adhesive skin tape is designed to facilitate quick, simple closure of minor wounds with minimal risk. The noninvasive application technique reduces tissue

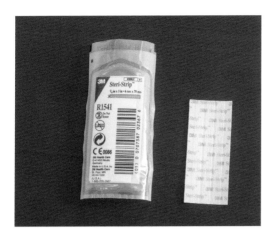

FIGURE 5.5 Adhesive closures can be used to close minor wounds, or they can be used after sutures have been removed.

trauma and is relatively pain free. In an athletic setting, it is also used to temporarily close wounds during competition before more definitive wound closure after the competition.

Topical Liquid Skin Adhesives

Tissue adhesives are polymers formulated to be used in place of nonabsorbable sutures for primary closure of skin wounds and have been used in the United States since 1998.[7] Tissue adhesive is used to approximate wounds that do not require deep-layer closure and do not have significant tension on the edges of the wound.

Commercially available tissue adhesives include butyl cyanoacrylate (Histoacryl, Indermil) and 2-octyl cyano-acrylate (Dermabond). These products are approved for closing skin wounds and forming barriers against certain bacterial infections. They have shown a lower incidence of wound infection and wound **dehiscence** than other wound closure techniques.[7]

Skin tissue adhesives may be used in place of non-absorbable sutures for primary closure of skin wounds. For wounds that are under tension, deep sutures are recommended. These products should not be used on the oral mucosa or across joints, where repetitive movement may cause the adhesives to slough prematurely. These adhesives do not replace the necessity for appropriate wound care. Wounds still need careful examination and exploration with irrigation and debridement when appropriate.[8] These tissue adhesives polymerize to form a firm, pliable film that bridges the edges of the wound and binds to the epithelium. The adhesives are water resistant enough to permit showering after 48 h, and the material typically sloughs off with keratinized epithelium about 5 to 10 d after application.[7,8]

If used appropriately, the adhesive will act as a strong bridge to hold well-apposed wound edges together. When necessary, deep dermal sutures (vertical mattress stitches) are used to bring the skin edges into everted apposition. Everted edges are extremely important to successful closure with tissue adhesives because they prevent scar broadening and improve the cosmetic result. Everted skin apposition should be maintained with forceps or fingers during the application of adhesive.

Application Technique for Adhesive Skin Tape

1. Clean the wound.
2. Inspect the wound.
3. Dry the edges and surrounding skin.
4. Consider application of an adhesive, such as a tincture of benzoin or Mastisol. Both may be applied to the skin with a cotton-tipped applicator before applying tape. They may offer some degree of protection from allergy to the adhesive in the skin tape, and they improve tape adherence. Mastisol appears to have superior adhesion and fewer adverse reactions. If significant swelling is anticipated, it is likely best not to apply an adhesive. Elastic tape may be used, but it should be used with caution if swelling is anticipated because it may also cause blistering of the skin.

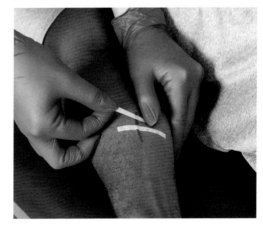

FIGURE 5.6

5. Ensure that the wound edges are nicely aligned. Starting at the center of the wound, apply strips in an evenly spaced manner opposing gravity until the edges of the wound are approximated.
6. Do not apply too much tension across a wound that may swell, or the tape may cause blisters.

Application Technique for Liquid Tissue Adhesive

1. Hold the wound together with forceps, gauze, or gloved fingers.
2. Expel droplets of the adhesive through the cotton-tipped applicator at the end of the container. Three to four thin layers should be applied along the length of the wound and extending slightly past each side of the wound.
3. Hold the edges of the wound together for at least 1 min while the adhesive dries.

Clinical Tips

Tissue Adhesives

Everted edges are extremely important to successful closure with tissue adhesives because they prevent scar broadening and improve the cosmetic result.

The adhesive should be applied to dry tissue that is under very little tension. For best results, a thin layer should be applied over the epidermis and allowed to dry for approximately 20 to 30 s.[7] This method prevents pooling and running of the tissue adhesive, and it also provides a layer of protection from the heat generated by the exothermic polymerization. Subsequent layers of the adhesive are then applied over this initial layer.

When applying tissue adhesives, it is important to ensure that the adhesive does not leak into the wound.[5] If leakage into the wound occurs, the adhesive acts as a barrier to epithelialization. The adhesive may also cause a foreign body reaction and potentially increase the risk of infection if it enters the wound. It is also important to remember to use proper sterile technique and to minimize tissue trauma while applying these products. Always reduce skin tension at the site of the laceration and ensure that no dead space is present before sealing with a tissue adhesive.

Sutures

It is essential to understand the principles of wound healing before learning and mastering suturing techniques. This chapter assumes that readers are well versed in these principles. Sutures are used to approximate wound edges in good apposition to facilitate the healing process, and they should be left in place long enough to allow healing to proceed to a sufficient degree that the natural properties of the skin can hold the wound together. Remove facial sutures after 3 to 5 d. (The physician may give instructions to remove every other suture on day 3 and the rest on day 5.) For the extremities and trunk, sutures should remain in place for 5 to 7 d. On the scalp, back, feet, hands, and over the joints, sutures may need to be left in place for 10 to 14 d. Leaving sutures in place for an extended period may increase the risk of leaving permanent marks in the skin. Although athletic trainers may not perform the actual suturing, depending on the state practice act or the direction of the physician, they may often be asked to assist in preparing the patient and materials to expedite the suturing process. Athletic trainers should be familiar with the materials and techniques used in suturing. Sutures are made of various materials with various tensile strengths and degradability. Suture materials can be categorized according to the following characteristics:

- Absorbable versus nonabsorbable
- Natural versus synthetic
- Monofilament versus multifilament

Absorbable Sutures

Absorbable sutures degrade and are eventually eliminated either by inflammatory reactions caused by enzymes in the body or by hydrolysis. Absorbable sutures include the following:

- Purified collagen (catgut, chromic; see their description in the Natural Sutures section)
- Polyglycolic acid (Vicryl, Monocryl)
- Polydioxanone (PDS II)

Nonabsorbable Sutures

Nonabsorbable sutures, although they do weaken, are permanent and do not dissolve in the body. Examples of nonabsorbable sutures include the following:

- Polyester (Ethibond)
- Polypropylene (Prolene)
- Nylon (Ethilon)
- Stainless steel
- Silk (not a truly permanent material; silk eventually degrades over a prolonged period, such as years)

Natural Sutures

Natural sutures are biological in origin and typically cause a more intense inflammatory reaction in tissue. Examples of natural sutures include the following:

- Catgut (purified collagen fibers from the intestines of healthy sheep or cows)
- Chromic (treated with chromium salts; resists enzymes, and prolongs time to degradation)
- Silk

Synthetic Sutures

Synthetic sutures are made from various polymers and do not cause as intense an inflammatory reaction as that seen with natural sutures. Examples include the following:

- Polyglycolic acid (Vicryl, Monocryl)
- Polydioxanone (PDS II)
- Polyester (Ethibond)
- Polypropylene (Prolene)
- Nylon (Ethilon)

Monofilament

Suture material may also be characterized as being *monofilament* (a single strand of suture material) or *multifilament* (multiple fibers twisted or braided together). Monofilament sutures generally cause less tissue trauma and have better resistance to microorganisms. Monofilament sutures do require more knots than multifilament sutures because there is more "memory" in these sutures.

- Polyglycolic acid (Monocryl)
- Polydioxanone (PDS II)
- Polypropylene (Prolene)
- Nylon (Ethilon)

Multifilament

Multifilament sutures may have greater resistance in tissue, although they do require fewer knots and may be significantly stronger. Examples are as follows:

- Polyglycolic acid (Vicryl, braided)
- Chromic (twisted)
- Silk (braided)
- Ultrahigh molecular weight polyethylene ("super") sutures (Orthocord, FiberWire)

Suture Sizes

Sutures are sized according to diameter, with 0 as the reference size. Numbers alone indicate progressively larger sutures (1, 2, 3, etc.), whereas numbers followed by a 0 indicate progressively smaller sutures (2-0, 4-0, 6-0, etc.). A human hair is roughly the size of a 6-0 suture.

Needles

Needles are classified according to shape (curved or straight), the type of point (taper point, cutting, reverse cutting, etc.), and the degree of curvature. Curved needles are designed to be held with a needle holder and are typically used for suturing. Straight needles are handheld and may be used to secure percutaneously placed devices, such as central lines and arterial lines. Cutting needles are typically used for tougher tissue, such as skin. Taper-point needles are used for easily perforated tissues, such as the gastrointestinal tract and muscle fascia, or may be used when tearing through tissue, such as a tendon, may be a risk.

Technique

The goal for suturing or closing any wound should be to optimize the potential for a good outcome by adhering to the principles of wound healing and by appropriately approximating the tissues. Proper wound preparation and assessment should include the evaluation and stabilization of deep tissues and copious irrigation to remove dirt, foreign bodies, and loose nonviable tissue. On occasion, debridement of wound edges may be needed to eliminate nonviable tissue.

Here are some tips to improve and facilitate the ease of suture placement:

- A proper grip on the needle with the needle holder should be ensured from the beginning. The needle may be inserted directly into the needle holder, or it may be loaded directly from the suture packet (figure 5.7).
- Introduce the needle perpendicular to the tissue surface (figure 5.8).
- Supinate the forearm—do not push the needle.
- If the needle is inserted inappropriately, then remove the needle from the wound and reinsert to ensure entrance into the skin.
- To help ensure everted edges, sutures should be placed deeper rather than wider.
- Use the rule of halves: Insert the first suture at the wound's midpoint, the next two sutures at the midpoints of the two halves created by the first suture, and so on.
- Bridge the gaps of the wound to avoid *dog ears*, or flaps of skin protruding from the wound.

Knot Tying Sutures need to be tied off to make them secure and to keep them from sliding through the skin during the healing process. The *two-hand square knot* is the easiest and most reliable and is used to tie most suture material.

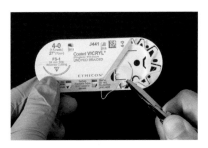

FIGURE 5.7 Load the needle holder: Clamp the needle holder approximately one-third the distance from the swage or eye to the point of the needle. Note that the clinician is not wearing a glove on the right hand at this time because it is easier to take the needle out of the holder without a glove. The glove would be put on prior to touching the patient, however.

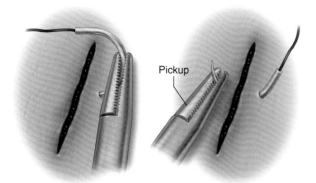

FIGURE 5.8 Correct way to introduce a suture needle into the skin.

The *instrument tie* is the most common technique used for laceration repair (see the Simple Interrupted Suture section that follows). It is useful when one or both ends of the suture material are short. Techniques for suturing should include closing the wound in layers if needed. Proceed from deep to superficial, while obtaining adequate hemostasis, to ensure good skin apposition with minimal tension and evert skin edges.

Basic Suturing Techniques There are several suturing techniques that may be used depending on the wound type, the area to be sutured, and the preference and experience of the person suturing (figure 5.9). This section describes some of the more common techniques and the advantages and disadvantages of each.

Simple Interrupted

- Quick, easy
- Single stitches, individually knotted
- Used for uncomplicated laceration repair and wound closure
- Often done poorly—may result in poor cosmetic outcome

Continuous (Running)

- Good for hemostasis

Vertical Mattress

- Better eversion with precise approximation of skin edges
- Two-step stitch:
  - Simple stitch made "far, far" relative to wound edge (large bite)
  - Needle reversed and second simple stitch made inside the first "near, near" (small bite)
- Increased "crosshatching": poor **cosmesis**

Horizontal Mattress

- Better for thicker tissues
- Provides added strength in fascial closure
- Useful in callused skin (e.g., palms and soles)
- Two-step stitch:
  - Simple stitch made
  - Needle reversed and second simple stitch made adjacent to first (same-size bite as first stitch)
- Increased ischemia possible if too tight

Subcuticular (Intradermal)

- Best cosmetic results
- Fast, easy
- Requires good approximation of underlying dermis
- Usually a running stitch but can be interrupted
- Intradermal horizontal bites
- Ability to allow the suture to remain in the tissue for a longer period without the development of crosshatch scarring

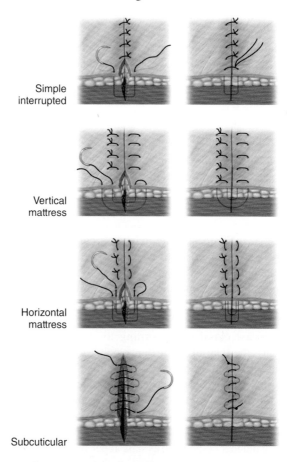

Simple interrupted

Vertical mattress

Horizontal mattress

Subcuticular

FIGURE 5.9 Types of sutures.

Note: A colored rope is used to clearly represent the two ends of the suture being tied.

1. Hold the purple strand in the left hand, with the index finger supporting the strand *(a)*.
2. Bring the white strand (held in the right hand) forward, crossing the purple strand on the index finger *(b)*.
3. Then loop the white strand over and under the purple strand *(c)*.
4. Use the right hand to pull the white strand away from the body, and use the left hand to pull the purple strand toward the body *(d)*.
5. Completed first *throw* (the term used to describe the first part of the knot.
6. With the purple strand held in the left hand, loop the purple strand *behind* the left thumb. Hold the white strand away *(e)*.
7. Use the right hand to pull the white strand toward the body, crossing the purple strand over the thumb *(f)*.
8. Then loop the white strand under the purple strand *(g)*.
9. Use the right hand to grasp the white strand *(h)*.
10. Use the right hand to pull the white strand toward the body, while the left hand pulls the purple strand away from the body *(i)*.
11. Finished square knot. Be sure the knot lies flat *(j)*.

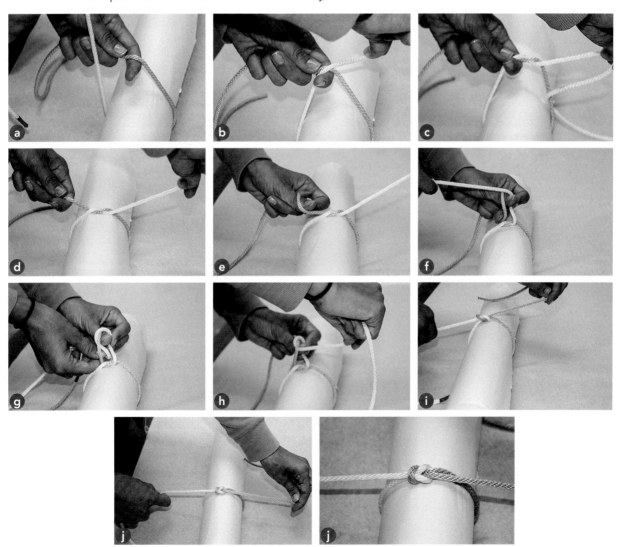

FIGURE 5.10

© Micki Cuppett

Simple Interrupted Suture

1. With Adson forceps everting the skin and with the needle perpendicular to the skin on the opposite side of the incision, supinate the wrist, allowing the needle to penetrate the skin (a).

2. With Adson forceps holding the skin, the needle should now be perpendicular to the subcutaneous tissue (b).

3. Supinate the wrist, allowing the needle to penetrate through the skin. Grasp the needle with Adson forceps (c).

4. Pull the suture through, leaving some excess with which to tie a knot (d).

5. With the hand holding the forceps, wrap the suture around the needle holder twice (e).

6. Once the suture is wrapped around twice, use the tip of the forceps to grasp the end left in excess (f).

7. Exert tension on both ends until the knot lies flat; this completes the first throw (g).

8. Wrap the suture around the needle holder once; be sure it is in the opposite direction from which the suture was initially wrapped around, and exert tension (h). The direction in which the needle holder is being pulled should not be the same direction pulled after the first throw (i).

9. Continue these alternating throws two more times.

10. Cut the suture, leaving approximately 1/2 in. for tails (j).

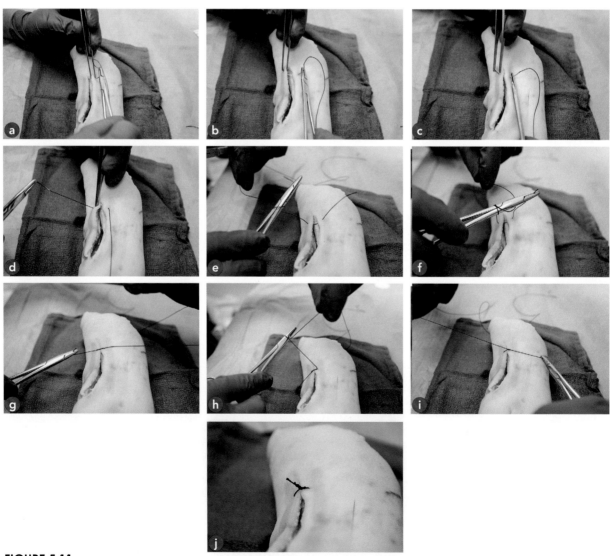

FIGURE 5.11

© Micki Cuppett

Vertical Mattress Suture

Here is an easy way to remember the vertical mattress suture: It is called a *far-far, near-near stitch*.

1. Holding the skin with forceps, insert the needle perpendicular to the skin at point A *(a)*.
2. Holding the other side of the incision with forceps, insert the needle through the subcutaneous tissue and skin at point B *(b)*.
3. Holding the same side of the incision with forceps, insert the needle perpendicular to the skin at point C *(c)*.
4. Holding the opposite side of the incision with forceps, insert the needle through the subcutaneous tissue and skin at point D *(d)*.
5. After pulling the excess suture through and leaving a small tail, wrap the suture around the needle holder twice *(e)*.
6. Exert tension on both ends of the suture, allowing the knot to lie flat *(f)*.
7. Wrap the suture around the needle holder once *(g)*. Exert tension on both ends of the suture, locking the knot. This completes one throw knot *(h)*.
8. Repeat single throws two more times, in opposite directions (for a total of four throws).
9. A completed vertical mattress suture *(i)*.

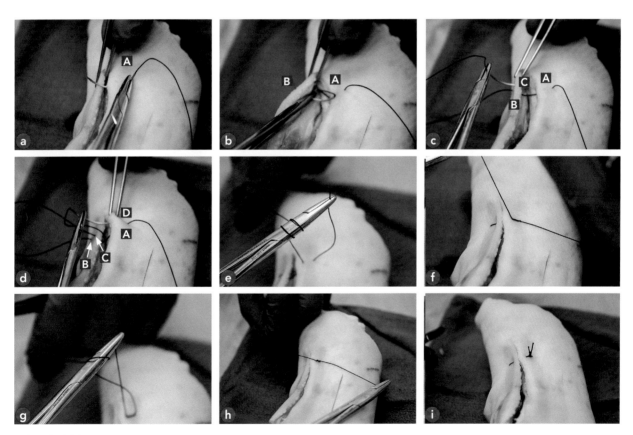

FIGURE 5.12
© Micki Cuppett

Suture Aftercare and Complications Wound infections can be minimized with meticulous attention to wound debridement and irrigation, strict aseptic technique, and antibiotics if indicated. The sutured area should be kept clean and dry for 24 to 48 h and should be inspected for signs of infection. The sutured wound is typically covered with a bandage. Wound tattooing or discoloration may occur if dyed sutures are used too close to the skin and if dirt or grit is left superficially in the wound. Wound scarring can be minimized by decreasing the tension across the closed wound and by ensuring that the tension is unidirectional and that the skin edges are

Horizontal Mattress Suture

1. With the needle perpendicular to the skin, supinate the wrist, allowing the needle to penetrate from the skin to the subcutaneous tissue at point A *(a)*.
2. The needle then penetrates from the subcutaneous tissue to the skin at point B *(b)*.
3. Either just distally to point A or just proximally to the previous suture at point B, to the point at which the needle exits the skin, reinsert the needle, penetrating the skin to subcutaneous tissue at point C *(c)*. Cross the wound and reinsert the needle, penetrating from subcutaneous tissue at point D.
4. Exert tension on the suture, keeping some excess suture for knot tying *(d)*.
5. Wrap the suture around the needle holder twice *(e)*.
6. Grasp the end of the suture with the tip of the needle holder and exert tension. The suture should lay flat *(f)*.
7. A completed horizontal mattress suture. Snip the ends, leaving approximately 1/2 in. for tails *(g)*.

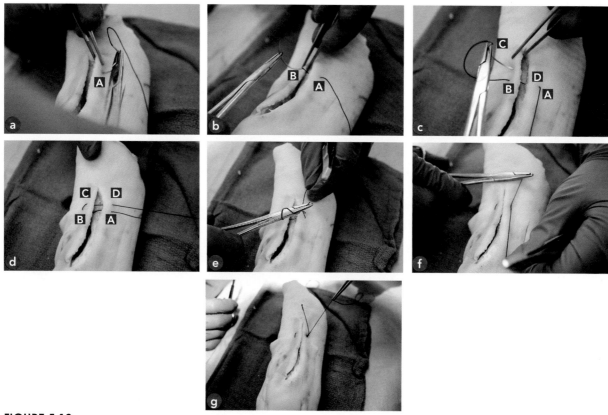

FIGURE 5.13

© Micki Cuppett

everted.[6] The risk of wound dehiscence can be reduced by using appropriate techniques and proper suture placement and knot tying.

Suture Removal   Many athletic trainers may not be in a position to suture, but most will have the opportunity to remove sutures. To remove sutures, open the sterile suture removal kit per previous instructions in this chapter. Put on gloves, and then remove and discard the dressing on the wound. Inspect the wound for healing and signs of infection. With forceps, lift the suture. Snip the suture as close to the skin as possible (figure 5.14a). Grasp the knotted end with forceps and slowly pull the suture through from the other side (figure 5.14b). Place the removed suture on gauze for disposal. Cover the healing wound with appropriate dressing or adhesive bandage.

RED FLAGS FOR SUTURES

- Excessive redness
- Inflammation or soreness
- Discoloration or discharge
- Fever

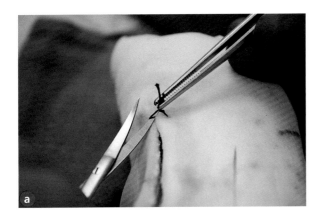

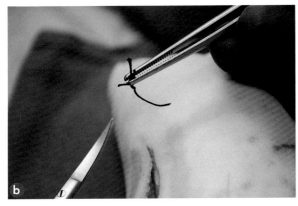

FIGURE 5.14 Removing sutures. *(a)* Seize the knot with needle holders and gently pull upward. With suture-cutting scissors, snip the suture. Make sure to leave the knot intact. *(b)* Complete suture removed.

© Micki Cuppett

Staples

Metal skin staples are commonly used to approximate skin after surgery or for wound closure. Staples have been shown to be similar to sutures in their mechanical and histological characteristics, and contaminated wounds often demonstrate lower infection rates when stapling is employed.[9,10] Staples also provide other advantages, including decreased inflammatory response, wound width, and wound closure times, as well as promotion of wound edge eversion, formation of an incomplete loop with decreased tissue strangulation, and a lack of residual cross-marks compared with sutures. Studies have also demonstrated that total costs and patient satisfaction can be improved with the use of skin staples compared with sutures.[10]

Using a Skin Stapler

To use a skin stapler, approximate and evert the skin edges with forceps. Hold the stapler at a 90° angle to the skin while applying gentle pressure (figure 5.15*a*). The staple is then ejected from the device, typically by gently squeezing the handle and then releasing it. Move the device to position the next staple and repeat the procedure. Staples are typically placed 1/4 to 1/2 in. (6-13 mm) apart. Each staple should hold the edges of the wound slightly everted with the edges nicely apposed (figure 5.15*b*).

Staple Removal

Staple removal requires a special staple extractor kit. As in suture removal, open the sterile staple removal kit and put on the sterile gloves provided. Inspect the wound and suture line for healing and signs of infection. Cleanse the suture line and staples with antiseptic swabs. Place the lower tip of the staple extractor under the first staple (figure 5.16*a*). Close the handle on the extractor to depress the center of the staple, causing the outer edges to bend upward simultaneously, away from the skin (figure 5.16*b*).[4] Apply appropriate dressing if necessary.

Joint Aspiration and Injection

Joint aspirations (**arthrocentesis**) and injections are performed for a variety of reasons, most commonly for diagnostic or therapeutic purposes. Aspirations are typically performed to evaluate joint fluids for the presence of crystals, white blood cells, or bacteria; to confirm an acute hemarthrosis; and to relieve pressure attributable to an abnormal amount of fluid. Joint injections are usually performed to provide pain relief for arthritic or painful inflammatory conditions. Contraindications to joint aspirations or injections include the following:

- Local osteomyelitis
- Bacteremia
- Infectious arthritis
- Periarticular cellulitis
- Poorly controlled diabetes mellitus
- Uncontrolled coagulopathy

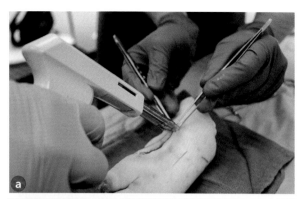

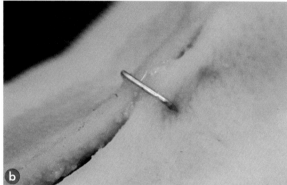

FIGURE 5.15   Using a skin stapler. *(a)* Have an assistant evert the skin edges while staples are applied. The stapler is held at a 90° angle to the skin with gentle pressure. *(b)* Once the staple is ejected from the stapler, it should hold the edges of the wound slightly everted with the edges nicely apposed.

© Micki Cuppett

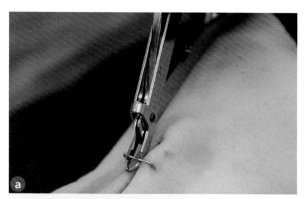

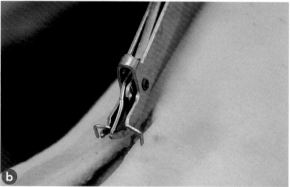

FIGURE 5.16   Staple removal. *(a)* Place the lower tip of the staple extractor under the first staple. *(b)* Close the handle of the extractor to depress the center of the staple, causing it to bend and be released from the skin.

© Micki Cuppett

The most commonly injected joints are the knees and the shoulder. Common medications used for joint injections include a combination of a local anesthetic and a corticosteroid or hyaluronic acid (e.g., Synvisc). Other substances are also occasionally used. See figure 5.17 for typical supplies and equipment necessary for joint injections and aspirations.

Corticosteroid injections are relatively safe and have few systemic side effects. Common side effects include allergic reactions, steroid flare, or temporary exacerbation of underlying diabetes. Hyaluronic acid injections also have proven to be safe with few side effects. As with suturing, some athletic trainers may not be able to perform injections or aspirations, but they may be asked to assist the physician in preparing the patient and supplies. Athletic trainers who are employed as physician extenders may be asked to perform these techniques on a regular basis.

After diagnostic arthrocentesis, interventions will be dictated by the results of the fluid analysis. Large effusions can recur and may require repeat aspiration. It is helpful to inform the patient that the immediate relief from the local anesthetic may wear off after 4 to 6 h and that the joint may be sore until the corticosteroid

effects begin, which may take a day or so. Applying ice several times for 20 to 30 min will help relieve some of the soreness. Resting the joint will also help.

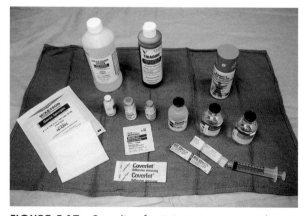

FIGURE 5.17   Supplies for joint injections and aspirations are alcohol, povidone–iodine solution, ethyl chloride spray, sterile gauze, alcohol wipe, bandage, and a 10 cm³ syringe. Also needed but not shown are an 18-gauge needle (to draw up an injection) and a 22-gauge needle (for injection).

© Micki Cuppett

Technique for Knee Aspiration and Injection

The lateral approach is the most functional and is outlined here. Sterile gloves should be worn for asepsis and universal precautions, but there is no consensus as to whether gloves are necessary.

1. The patient lies supine on the table with the knee extended.

2. The superior lateral aspect of the patella is palpated. The skin is marked with a pen, one fingerbreadth above and one fingerbreadth lateral to this site. This location provides the most direct access to the suprapatellar pouch. The most distal aspect of the vastus lateralis also is a good landmark in many patients.

3. The skin is washed with povidone–iodine (or alcohol) solution (a). An 18-gauge, 1 in., or 1 and 1/2 in. needle is attached to a 20 or 60 mL syringe, depending on the anticipated amount of fluid present for removal. The barrel of the syringe should be slid in and out once or twice before the procedure in order to remove air and reduce friction in the syringe.

4. Ethyl chloride spray may be applied topically to the skin after preparation and immediately before needle insertion. Stretching the skin with the opposite hand can also reduce needle insertion discomfort by stretching the pain fibers in the skin. The needle is directed at a 45° angle distally, with the needle held just below parallel to the table (b).

5. Pay particular attention as the needle is inserted, to sense when the needle penetrates the joint capsule—there is usually a subtle but palpable "pop." Maintain slight backpressure on the syringe while inserting the needle; once the needle has entered the joint, aspirate should begin filling the syringe (c). It is not necessary to fully insert the needle, although the entire needle (or occasionally a 3 in. spinal needle) may be needed in patients with obesity. Continue to draw back on the plunger with steady pressure, holding the syringe and needle still. Using the nondominant hand, or employing an assistant, to compress the opposite side of the joint and the patella may aid in arthrocentesis.

6. Once the aspirate is completely removed, a sterile hemostat may be placed on the hub of the needle and used to hold the needle steady while the syringe is removed (unscrewed) (d), and the injection syringe is attached to the needle or another syringe for aspirate is used (e).

7. Various mixtures are used for injection, based on the provider's experience. The author prefers 3 mL of betamethasone (6 mg/mL of Celestone) mixed with 7 mL of 0.25% bupivacaine for injection alone or 3 mL of betamethasone and 2 mL of bupivacaine after aspiration. After injection of the medication, the needle and syringe are withdrawn.

8. The skin is cleansed with alcohol and a bandage is applied over the puncture site. Apply compression wrap.

Note: If no aspiration is being performed (i.e., for an injection only), a 22-gauge, 1 and 1/2 in. needle may be used instead of an 18-gauge needle. The clinician may choose to have the patient sitting with the knee at a 90° angle.

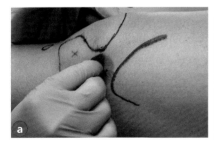
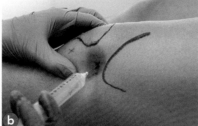
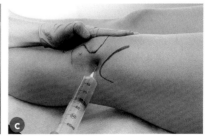
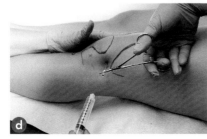
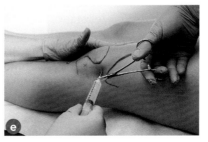

FIGURE 5.18

© Micki Cuppett

Technique for Knee Injection Only

If no aspiration is needed, the clinician can more easily administer a joint injection to the knee with the patient in a seated position.

1. Cleanse the injection area with povidone–iodine (Betadine) *(a)*.

2. Insert the needle into the anterolateral side of the joint, keeping it parallel to the ground *(b)*.

3. Keep one hand in contact with the skin surface while keeping the other hand on the syringe. This will help with proprioception of the syringe *(c)*.

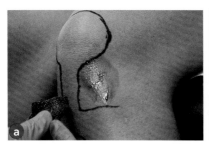 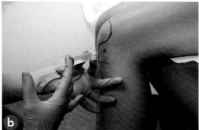 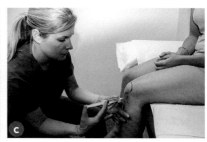

FIGURE 5.19

© Micki Cuppett

Subacromial Injection Technique

1. The patient should be seated in a chair with the affected shoulder exposed. The arm is resting in the lap or next to the body. The posterolateral approach is direct and avoids having the patient observe the procedure. After taking the appropriate medical history, performing a physical examination, and discussing with the patient the procedure and obtaining informed consent, complete the following steps.

2. The acromial border is palpated, and the posterolateral corner is marked with a pen, one fingerbreadth below the acromion on the posterior aspect of the shoulder. A soft area will be able to be palpated at that location.

3. The skin is washed with povidone–iodine (or alcohol) solution *(a)*. Sterile gloves should be worn for asepsis and universal precautions, but there is no consensus as to whether gloves are necessary.

4. A 22-gauge, 1 and 1/2 in. needle is attached to a 10 mL syringe. Slide the barrel of the syringe in and out once or twice before the procedure to remove air and to reduce friction in the syringe. Ethyl chloride spray may be used topically on the skin after the preparation and immediately before needle insertion. Stretching the skin with the opposite hand may also reduce needle insertion discomfort by stretching the pain fibers in the skin *(b)*.

5. The needle is directed at an angle corresponding to the slope of the acromion. The acromion may be palpated with the opposite hand, which is also useful for proprioception of the needle. There should be almost no resistance when injecting *(c)*. Pay attention as the needle is inserted; it is possible to sense when the needle penetrates the subacromial space. Maintain slight backpressure on the syringe while inserting the needle; once the needle has entered the space, begin injecting the solution. A common subacromial injection is 3 mL of betamethasone (6 mg/mL of Celestone) mixed with 7 mL of 0.25% bupivacaine. After injection of the medication, the needle and syringe are withdrawn.

6. The skin is cleansed with alcohol and a bandage is applied over the puncture site.

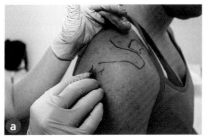
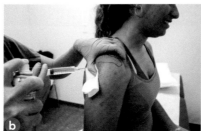
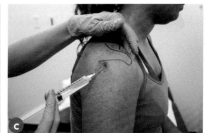

FIGURE 5.20
© Micki Cuppett

Intraarticular Injection Technique

1. Cleanse the injection area with povidone–iodine.
2. Insert the needle from the posterolateral aspect of the shoulder, below the acromion. The needle should be parallel to the floor. There should be almost no resistance when injecting.

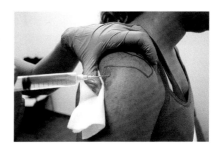

FIGURE 5.21
© Micki Cuppett

Acromioclavicular Injection Technique

1. Cleanse the injection area with povidone–iodine.
2. Palpate the distal end of the clavicle and the acromion. Insert the needle perpendicular to the joint. There should be almost no resistance when injecting.

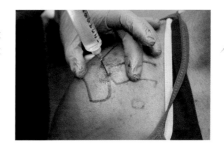

FIGURE 5.22
© Micki Cuppett

Subungual Hematoma Drilling and Drainage

Nail **trephination** usually can be performed up to 36 h after injury or recognition of hematoma. Before performing the procedure, appropriate physical examination should be performed and informed consent obtained.

There are several ways to drain the nail bed. Melting a small hole in the nail by means of a heated paper clip or a surgical electrocautery device is an effective and simple technique. There are also several commercially available devices specifically designed for this purpose. Another method is to use an 18-gauge needle as a handheld drill. This method is quick, inexpensive, and easy to learn.

Antibiotics are not usually necessary unless there is gross contamination of the wound. Instruct the patient to elevate the hand for several days to prevent swelling.

Soaking the digit in warm water with povidone–iodine solution for 15 min, three or four times a day, will help prevent infection. Make sure that the patient understands that the nail may be lost (although it will often regrow), and that there is a small risk of permanent nail deformity because of the initial injury to the nail bed.

Paronychial Incision and Drainage

A paronychia is a tender, inflamed infection of the hand (most commonly) or foot, where the nail and skin meet. It is usually caused by a bacterial infection, but it may also be fungal or viral. Paronychia is often associated with nail trimming. If the infection is noticed early, antibiotics and soaking in warm water and povidone–iodine solution may be effective. Incision and drainage are indicated to control pain, speed healing, and prevent the spread of infection.

Subungual Hematoma Drilling Technique

1. Cleanse the digit with povidone–iodine solution or alcohol. Local anesthesia is usually not necessary for isolated nail trephination.
2. Position an 18-gauge needle with the tip in the center of the hematoma.
3. Hold the hub of the needle between the thumb and index finger.
4. Roll the needle back and forth quickly and observe as it begins to bore into the nail.
5. Blood should soon begin to emerge from the hole—be careful, the blood may be under pressure and may spray from the hole.

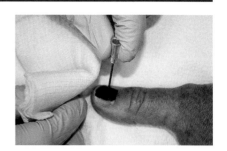

FIGURE 5.23
© Micki Cuppett

6. It will not be necessary to press any deeper, but slowly enlarge the hole by drilling. Be careful not to press too deeply or the nail bed will be violated, and this will be painful.
7. Cleanse the nail again and apply a sterile dressing.
8. If possible, allow a small portion of the gauze to enter the hole as a wick to keep it from clotting.

Paronychial Incision Technique

1. Cleanse the digit with povidone–iodine solution.
   - *Note:* A cutaneous nerve block is usually tolerated much better than local infiltration of anesthetic.
   - The digital cutaneous nerves run along the medial and lateral aspects of each finger.
   - These nerves can be blocked at any point above the distal phalanx.
2. Use a 25-gauge needle to raise a skin wheal by administering approximately 0.25 mL of lidocaine directly over the lateral and medial cutaneous nerve.

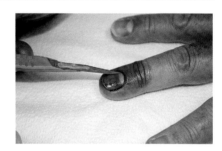

FIGURE 5.24
© Micki Cuppett

3. Advance the needle perpendicular to the digit (nerve) until the bone is reached.
4. Inject about 1 mL of lidocaine, sliding the needle up and down on the dorsal and volar sides of the finger.
5. Allow 5 to 10 min for the block to develop.
6. Cleanse the entire digit again with povidone–iodine solution.
7. Using a No. 11 scalpel, make an incision parallel to the axis of the finger.
   - *Note:* The incision should be an extension of the lateral and medial nail groove and deep enough to enter the abscess being treated.
   - Do not direct the scalpel toward the bone.
8. Using scissors, debride necrotic tissue if needed.
   - *Note:* If the infection has progressed under the nail, the proximal nail must be removed as well.
9. Use mosquito forceps to lever up and hold the nail.
10. Cut the nail off in a straight line, using the scissors.
11. Place gauze packing under the flap of overhanging tissue and the cuticle.
12. Culture the infected material removed from under the nail to determine the exact pathogen causing the infection.

Drainage is usually sufficient to clear up the infection. Topical antibiotics are typically used, and oral antibiotics may also be considered.

Instruct the patient to elevate the hand or foot for several days to prevent swelling. Follow-up should be performed within 2 to 3 d, at which time the packing should be removed. After the packing is removed, the digit should be soaked in warm water with povidone–iodine solution for 15 min, three or four times a day. After each soaking, a dry, nonstick dressing should be applied. Inform the patient that the nail must be protected from being torn away from the nail bed until it regrows completely. This process may take several months. After the healing process is complete, the nail and cuticle may be deformed.

Inserting an Intravenous Catheter

The intravenous (IV) route involves the injection of a drug directly into a vein. This route of administration is used when drug action must begin immediately or when other routes cannot be used because of patient condition or drug characteristics.[5] This is a common occurrence in the hospital or surgical center. The athletic trainer will see the IV route used most often when IV fluids (typically without medication added) are administered to achieve rapid rehydration of a patient who is experiencing heat-related illness. Athletic trainers must be aware of state practice laws that address their potential role in administering IV fluids. Some states allow athletic trainers who have gone through IV training and certification to administer IV fluids under the supervision of a physician. In other situations, the athletic trainer may be asked to assist the physician in preparing the patient and materials for IV administration. It is up to the athletic trainer to know the laws and to work only under the authorized scope of practice. In addition, before starting an IV, the practitioner must make certain that an order for the IV line has been given and is noted in the patient's chart.

Equipment

The following equipment is required for starting an IV line:

- Towel
- Alcohol wipes (povidone–iodine wipes may also be used)
- Tourniquet
- Angiocatheter
- IV tubing
- IV fluid
- Sterile transparent dressing or tape
- Gloves
- Gauze

Anatomy

There are many acceptable sites for starting an IV line. The antecubital fossa and the dorsal veins of the hand are probably the most common because of the presence and easy accessibility of several large veins (cephalic, basilic, and median cubital) (figure 5.25).

Preparing the IV Tubing

Remove the sterile cover from the IV bag and portal and open the IV tubing set. Maintain aseptic technique when opening sterile packages and IV solution. Clamp the tubing; then uncap the spike on the tubing and insert the spike into the entry portal on the IV bag (figure 5.26*a*). Squeeze the drip chamber on the tubing set (figure 5.26*b*) and allow it to fill at least halfway (figure 5.26*c*). Open the clamp and allow enough fluid to flow until all air bubbles have disappeared from the tubing (figure 5.26*d*). Reclamp the tubing and maintain sterility of setup.

Catheter Selection

Selecting an appropriate-sized catheter is very important. A catheter that is too large will make it more difficult to enter the vein, increase the likelihood of vein rupture, and likely increase discomfort. A catheter that is too small will limit the amount of fluid that can be given over a period. Sometimes it is necessary to use a smaller-than-desired catheter to begin an IV treatment; later, if needed, another IV line can be installed at a different site once the patient is better hydrated. An 18- or 20-gauge catheter is typically used; occasionally a larger 16-gauge or a smaller 22-gauge catheter may be needed (figure 5.27).

Failed Attempt

If the first attempt is unsuccessful in entering the vein (or there is no flashback or the flashback disappears), slowly withdraw the catheter without pulling all the way out. Watch for the flashback to occur. If the vein has still not been entered, advance the catheter again in another attempt to enter the vein. If several attempts at entering the vein fail, the tourniquet should be released, gauze placed over the puncture site, the catheter withdrawn, and tape placed to hold the gauze. Identify another site for another attempt.

Adjusting Flow

In an emergency with a patient experiencing heat illness, the roller clamp is opened completely to allow for rapid rehydration with the IV fluid, and the flow rate is not determined. There may be situations in which the physician will want to determine the rate of infusion, and the roller clamp can be adjusted to increase or decrease the flow rate. The flow rate is determined by counting drops in the drip chamber for 1 min. There are many conversion charts and calculators available either in print or electronic format to

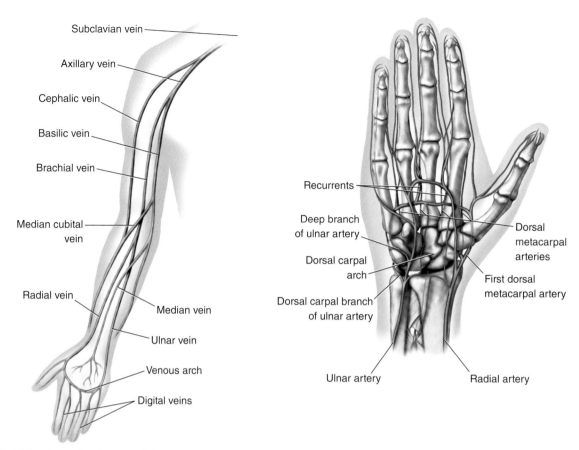

FIGURE 5.25 Superficial veins of the antecubital fossa typically are used for starting an IV line. The dorsal veins in the hand may also be used.

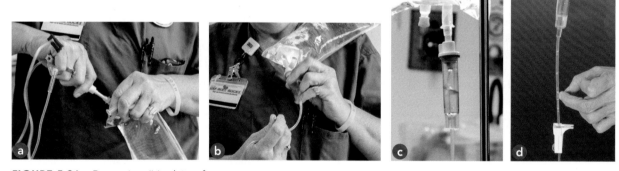

FIGURE 5.26 Preparing IV tubing for use.

Photos a-c © Micki Cuppett

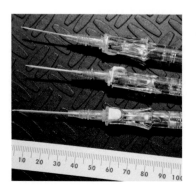

FIGURE 5.27 Typically an 18- or 20-gauge catheter is used to administer IV fluids; however, occasionally a large-bore (≥16-gauge) is used for rapid infusion. A smaller needle may be used for comfort when rapid infusion is not needed.

© Micki Cuppett

Technique for Inserting a Catheter

Preparing the Arm

1. Identify and palpate the selected site. For the antecubital area, apply a tourniquet high on the upper arm *(a)*. The tourniquet should be tight enough to restrict blood flow. One way to help increase venous engorgement is to ask the patient to squeeze their hand into a fist several times.
2. Reidentify the selected vein and palpate for patency *(b)*.
3. Clean the area by wiping several times with alcohol swabs. Some health care providers prefer to prep the area by wiping with povidone–iodine swabs and then a final wipe with alcohol.
4. Don gloves if not already wearing them.

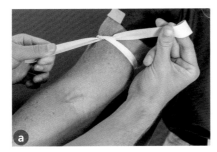 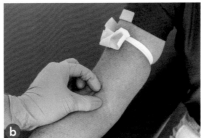

Inserting the Catheter

1. Remove the catheter from the sterile package. It may be helpful to slide the catheter in and out of the metal stylet once or twice to feel how much force is needed.
2. Use one hand to apply distal tension to the skin, toward the wrist in the opposite direction from that in which the needle will be advancing *(c)*. Be careful not to compress the vein and prevent flow, which may cause the vein to collapse.
3. Using a deliberate—but not too forceful—motion, advance the catheter through the skin and into the vein. Aim the catheter along the direction of the vein so as not to poke through the vein *(d)*. Slowly advance the catheter into the vein and look for the flashback of blood at the catheter hub *(e)*. This will indicate that the catheter is within the vein.
4. With the catheter positioned in the vein, slide the plastic catheter forward into the vein over the top of the metal stylet. The catheter should slide forward easily until the hub is all the way to the skin. Do not force it or the vein may rupture.
5. With the catheter advanced to the hub, release the tourniquet while simultaneously applying pressure over the vein to collapse it. This will prevent blood from flowing out of the catheter when the stylet is removed.[4]

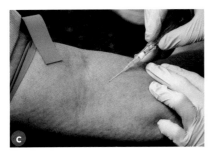 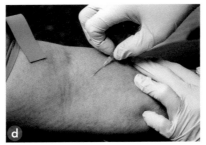 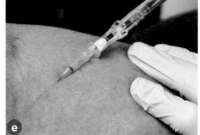

Attaching IV Tubing

1. Remove the stylet and set it aside to be disposed of in a sharps container, or drop it immediately into the sharps container.
2. Attach the IV tubing to the catheter *(f)*. This is usually done with a rotating *Luer-lock* mechanism, and successful locking is signaled by a click.
3. Release pressure from the vein; there should be a small amount of blood backflow into the tubing.
4. Open the clamp on the tubing and allow the IV fluid to flow into the catheter.

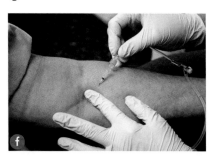

Securing the IV

1. Secure the catheter in place with the transparent sterile dressing and tape the IV in place using several strips of tape. This will prevent movement of the tubing. Another method is to place gauze over and under the tubing near the catheter to protect the skin and to soak up any blood droplets.
2. Place tape over the puncture site and over loops of tubing so there is less pressure on the tubing *(g, h)*.
3. Make sure the tubing is secure to prevent any accidental removal of the catheter.

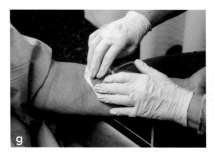 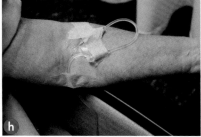

FIGURE 5.28

Photos c-h © Micki Cuppett

---

assist the health care professional in translating the drips for 1 min into milliliters per hour.

Summary

Many of the techniques outlined in this chapter may be new even to practicing athletic trainers or other health care professionals. It is crucial for athletic trainers to know which procedures are allowed under their state practice acts. Even if athletic trainers are not directly involved in the actual procedure, it is imperative that they understand asepsis and aseptic technique so as not to contaminate a procedure when near the patient and the sterile person performing it.

Many of these procedures take considerable practice to master. Simulators are available to allow clinicians to practice many of the techniques. There are injection models that realistically simulate the feeling of a correctly placed needle as it is inserted into the joint capsule. Similarly, models are available for suture practice.

Apply It!

Go to HK*Propel* to complete the case studies for this chapter.

PART III

Medical Conditions by System

Chapters 6 through 16 follow a systematic approach as they address common conditions and diseases by body system. Most chapters follow a simple template: They begin with an overview of the relevant anatomy and physiology as it relates to the body system; then identify specific conditions; explain signs and symptoms and differential diagnoses, referral, and diagnostic tests; and finally, discuss prognoses, treatment, and implications for sport participation. If a condition has conditions specific to age or biological sex, those issues are also discussed. If relevant, implications for pediatric and mature athletes are also included. The systems covered are as follows:

- Chapter 6, Respiratory System, covers conditions such as asthma, chronic obstructive pulmonary disease, upper respiratory infection, and pneumonia. All conditions discussed can occur in an otherwise healthy person. Knowing the early signs and symptoms of respiratory conditions and evaluation techniques unique to this system can help prevent a situation from becoming worse or, in cases of pneumothorax or hemothorax, can save a life.

- Chapter 7, Cardiovascular System, includes conditions such as causes of sudden cardiac death, Marfan syndrome, arrhythmia, and hypertension. Anemia and sickle cell trait are also discussed. Medical standards for safe athletic participation for athletes with cardiac conditions are discussed throughout the chapter.

- Chapter 8, Gastrointestinal System, covers the stomach, abdomen, and digestive system, including the appendix and gallbladder. In addition to common conditions such as nausea, vomiting, and diarrhea, this chapter covers food poisoning and parasitic infections. These conditions are especially critical to recognize in athletes, as they travel often and can be subjected to a variety of food that may cause these ailments. Gastroesophageal reflux disease and ulcers, irritable bowel syndrome, celiac disease, and inflammatory bowel conditions are all discussed, as are their implications for athletes who require proper nutrition to perform at optimal levels.

- Chapter 9, Genitourinary and Gynecological Systems, covers conditions found in both biological sexes, such as kidney stones, sports hematuria, urinary tract infection, and sexually transmitted infections. Specific to males, testicular torsion and testicular and prostate cancers are among the conditions discussed. Specific to females, vaginitis, pelvic inflammatory disease, conditions related to the menstrual cycle, ovarian and cervical cancers, and pregnancy are covered.

- Chapter 10, Neurological System, discusses concussions (traumatic brain injury), stroke, headaches, and chronic conditions such as seizure disorders, epilepsy, and vertigo. Also reviewed are amyotrophic lateral sclerosis, Bell's Palsy, rabies, and complex regional pain syndrome.

- Chapter 11, The Eye, covers infectious conditions, such as conjunctivitis, and acute traumatic injuries, such as hyphema, orbital fracture, and lacerations to the eyelid. Protective eyewear is also addressed, as there are national safety guidelines that govern eyewear in certain sports.

- Chapter 12, Ear, Nose, Mouth, and Throat, discusses conditions unique to the systems of hearing, smelling, and taste. It begins with a very common issue, especially in swimmers, otitis externa (swimmer's ear), but also addresses traumatic ruptured eardrum. Conditions that can be related to allergies, rhinitis, and sinusitis are covered, as is epistaxis (nosebleed). Mouth and throat ailments include tonsillitis, laryngitis, and lesions of the mouth, including oral cancers.

- Chapter 13, Systemic Disorders, describes conditions that cross body systems or present in more than one system, such as malignancies involving the lymphatic system and Lyme disease. Raynaud's Disease, systemic lupus erythematosus, fibromyalgia, chronic fatigue syndrome, multiple sclerosis, Guillain-Barré syndrome, and gout are also discussed. Medical conditions that affect the musculoskeletal system are also reviewed, including rheumatoid arthritis, osteoarthritis, osteomyelitis, polymyositis, and dermatomyositis.

- Chapter 14, Infectious Diseases, discusses conditions that are infectious and can be transmitted. Some of these infectious conditions are covered in chapter 16 on dermatological conditions. This chapter covers infection transmission and prevention. Conditions discussed include influenza, infectious mononucleosis, childhood conditions (e.g., mumps, measles, chicken pox), and hepatitis. Streptococcal and staphylococcal infections and the danger they present are reported. Life-changing or threatening infections, such as encephalitis, meningitis, and Zika virus, are discussed, as are the prevention of spread and treatment of these diseases.

- Chapter 15, Endocrine Disorders, describes conditions specific to that system. Type 1 and type 2 diabetes are discussed, including signs and symptoms, treatment options, implications for participation in athletic activities, and prevention techniques. The reader will be introduced to signs and symptoms of hyper- and hypoglycemia and diabetic ketoacidosis. Disorders of the pancreas, such pancreatitis and cholelithiasis, are presented. The functions of the thyroid gland and common disorders are also detailed in this chapter, including hyper- and hypothyroidism signs and symptoms, treatment, and return to participation.

- Chapter 16, Dermatological Conditions, discusses common viral, fungal, and bacterial skin disorders that can be found in the physically active population, including skin cancers and insect bites.

Chapter 17, Psychological and Substance Use Disorders, addresses these important topics because many active people have these conditions and it is critical to recognize them. Mood, anxiety, eating, and attention-deficit/hyperactivity disorders are discussed. Drug and alcohol abuse are also discussed.

Chapter 18, Working With Special Populations, specifically examines the medical concerns for specific pathological conditions. Issues concerning paraplegia, including boosting, hyperthermia, pressure sores, and spasms, are discussed. Other conditions covered are cerebral palsy, amputations, and sensory and intellectual disabilities. These topics are important because of the increasing number of athletes who have genetic disabilities or who compete after sustaining traumatic injuries. These athletes participate in local events, national trials, the Paralympics, and the Special Olympics. They should have appropriate medical care that may be outside the realm of the primary physicians who treat them.

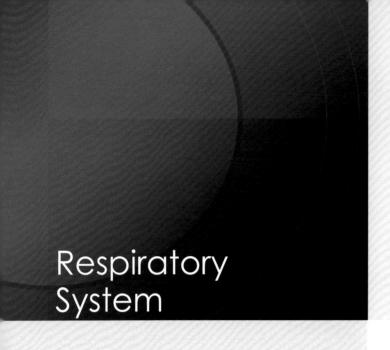

Respiratory System

At the completion of this chapter the reader should be able to do the following:

1. Describe the basic anatomy and physiology of the respiratory system.

2. Recognize common, normal, and abnormal respiratory patterns.

3. Perform a basic evaluation of the respiratory system, including auscultation and percussion.

4. Identify characteristics of normal and abnormal breath sounds.

5. Recognize common pathological conditions, including signs and symptoms, differential assessment, referral, standard medical treatment, and implications for participation in athletics.

Respiratory disorders can be very alarming to both the patient and the medical professional. Respiratory conditions not only affect performance, but acute respiratory distress can also be life-threatening. Great strides have been made in the recognition and treatment of common airway disease. Advances in the management of respiratory disorders have allowed patients to participate in the activities they love, even at competitive levels. Because so many more people with respiratory disorders are participating in physical activity, the athletic trainer must be able to recognize, evaluate, and refer patients with these conditions.

This chapter describes the techniques, including percussion and auscultation, used to evaluate individuals who exhibit a respiratory condition. Normal and abnormal breathing patterns are reviewed to identify potential respiratory system problems. Common respiratory disorders, such as asthma, influenza, pneumonia, bronchitis, and other viral upper respiratory infections (URIs), are discussed. Signs and symptoms of these conditions, as well as problems requiring medical attention, are presented. Respiratory health is integral to physical activity and must be assessed properly, with referral of the patient to a physician if warranted.

Overview of Anatomy and Physiology

The pulmonary system is primarily involved in the exchange of oxygen and carbon dioxide, and both are vital in producing the energy needed for cellular metabolism. This process, known as *respiration*, can be divided into two distinct but simultaneous steps: ventilation and oxygenation. During **ventilation**, air moves through the respiratory tract. **Oxygenation** describes the actual exchange of gases in the alveolar–capillary beds.

The organs of respiration are divided into the upper and lower respiratory tracts. The upper respiratory tract consists of the following:

- Nasal passages
- Paranasal sinuses
- Pharynx, including nasopharynx and oropharynx
- Larynx or voice box

The upper respiratory tract is mainly responsible for warming, humidifying, and filtering air as it reaches the lower respiratory tract.[1] As air is pulled from the external environment into the nasal passages, secretions from the paranasal sinuses add moisture. Cilia, which are tiny hairlike projections that line the upper airway, filter out fine particles of debris as air moves into the lower respiratory tract. The lower respiratory tract is composed of the following:

- Trachea
- Right and left bronchi
- Lung parenchyma

In the lungs, each mainstem bronchus is further divided into bronchioles and terminal alveoli (figure 6.1).

The tracheobronchial tree is a tubular system supported by cartilaginous rings that divide from the trachea into the right and left bronchi at approximately T4 or T5. These main bronchi then divide further into three branches on the right and two on the left. This tubular system serves as a passageway for air as it reaches the bronchioles and, finally, the terminal alveoli, where the exchange of oxygen and carbon dioxide from the surrounding capillary beds takes place. The right lung is divided into three separate lobes: upper, middle, and lower. The left lung has only an upper lobe and a lower lobe.

Evaluation of the Respiratory System

Considerable information can be gleaned from a physical examination of the respiratory system. The patient's history can provide telltale signs about the frequency, intensity, and triggers of respiratory issues. General observations of the patient's demeanor will provide the clinician with clues if there is any respiratory distress or discomfort with breathing. Breath sounds themselves provide clues as to the nature of the condition.

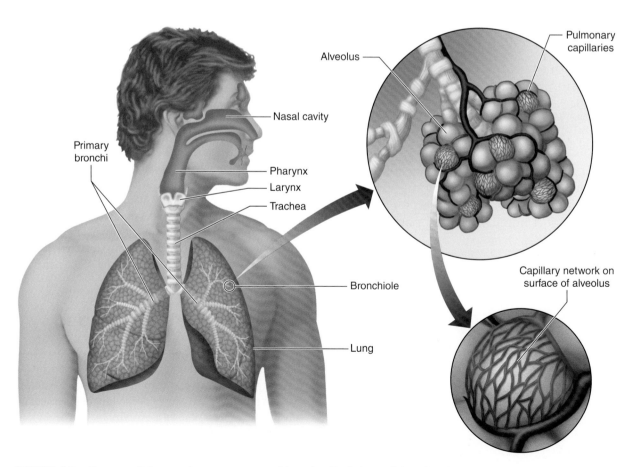

FIGURE 6.1   Organs of the respiratory system, with a detailed view of the alveolar sac.

History and Inspection

The patient may present with an acute or chronic respiratory condition while complaining of shortness of breath, an abnormal breathing pattern, or cough. Respiratory pathologies often present with nonspecific symptoms that can make initial diagnosis difficult. The first step in evaluation is to take a thorough history, which includes asking the patient about the length of the problem, exacerbating factors, and symptom severity. For a patient experiencing an acute respiratory attack, the history is abbreviated to only those questions needed to determine the immediate course of action. A more thorough history is taken once the immediate emergency is under control. If the patient complains of a cough, the examiner asks for a description of its characteristics: Is the cough "dry" or "barking," or does it produce sputum? Attention should also be paid to any discolored sputum with the cough. Timing of the cough is also important: Is the cough worse at night, as is often the case with asthma or gastroesophageal reflux disease (see chapter 8)? Or does the cough occur shortly after exertion, as in exercise-induced bronchospasm (EIB)? If the patient complains of shortness of breath or dyspnea, the examiner should determine the severity (e.g., how long the patient has felt short of breath, which activity precipitated it, and whether it occurs at rest or only with activity): Does the patient struggle with inhalation, exhalation, or both? Was there any trauma to the chest or abdomen? Associated chest pain is another important symptom to ascertain in considering cardiac causes for dyspnea. Is the patient's chest or throat tight? Throat tightness may indicate exercise-induced laryngeal obstruction (EILO).[2,3] Also, the examiner should ask the patient about any history of respiratory infections, smoking, and environmental exposure to potential allergens.

The chest is inspected after the history is taken. In the athletic training clinic, a chest examination is usually performed on a male athlete who has removed his shirt and on a female athlete dressed in a sports bra and shorts. The examiner inspects the chest for shape and configuration, including any skeletal deformities. Congenital deformities, such as scoliosis or kyphosis, and other chest deformities may be present and may affect not only the chest shape but also respiration efficiency. There are four common chest shapes:

- In adults with a normal chest, the thorax is elliptical in shape and is narrower anterior to posterior than it is across the transverse axis (figure 6.2*a*).
- A barrel chest presents as a rounded shape that is the same diameter from anterior to posterior as it is transversely (figure 6.2*b*). The barrel chest shape is associated with chronic emphysema and asthma but may also be present in the healthy, older adult.
- Pectus excavatum, a congenital shape, is usually not symptomatic but presents as a depression at the junction of the xiphoid with the sternum (figure 6.2*c*).
- Pectus carinatum presents as a forward protrusion of the sternum (figure 6.2*d*). It is less common than pectus excavatum, and minor conditions require no treatment.

The clinician also inspects the chest for potential bruising of the ribs or chest wall, while paying special attention to the patient's effort and posture while breathing and noting the respiration rate and rhythm.[4] Symmetry of chest wall movement with breathing is also important (symmetry can be measured as part of palpation, later in the examination).

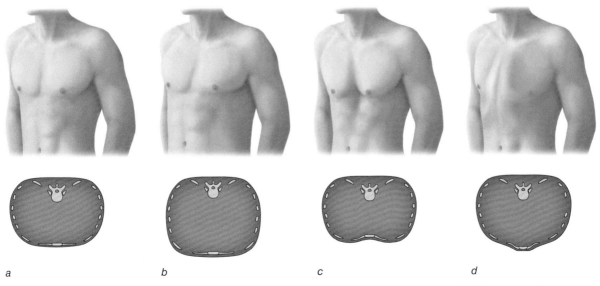

a *b* *c* *d*

FIGURE 6.2 Common chest shapes: (*a*) normal, (*b*) barrel, (*c*) pectus excavatum, and (*d*) pectus carinatum.

Respiratory Patterns

Breathing involves several simultaneous processes. Chemoreceptors in the medulla oblongata of the brain sense changes in pH and carbon dioxide levels. Decreases in pH, as well as corresponding increases in carbon dioxide, result from normal cellular metabolism and stimulate an increase in ventilation to remove these by-products. Neural control of breathing comes from the phrenic nerve, which arises from cervical nerve roots C3, C4, and C5 and innervates the diaphragm, and from the nerves that innervate the intercostal muscles. As the diaphragm and intercostal muscles contract, the thoracic cavity expands. This generates negative pressure, which causes air to move into the lungs during inspiration. When alveolar pressure equalizes with atmospheric pressure, intercostal stretch receptors fire and inspiration ceases. The elastic recoil of the thoracic cage results in the passive process of expiration. Accessory muscles of breathing, which include the abdominal, sternocleidomastoid, and scalene muscles, are relatively quiet during normal breathing but become active as the work of normal breathing increases.

Normal respiration is unlabored, with 12 to 20 breaths/min. When breathing becomes disordered, several patterns can emerge. The term **dyspnea** refers to the subjective sensation of breathing difficulty or shortness of breath. When patients have dyspnea, it is important to determine its severity. For example, does the difficulty occur at rest or only with exertion? Certain situations may produce dyspnea, such as eating, being exposed to cold **ambient temperatures**, or lying down at night. Patients with underlying congestive heart failure may experience **paroxysmal nocturnal dyspnea**, which causes shortness of breath when lying down at night. Dyspnea may accompany other symptoms in various disease processes, such as fever with lung infection, wheezing with asthma, or chest pain with acute myocardial infarction.

Tachypnea refers to breathing that is more rapid than 24 breaths/min. Tachypnea can be seen in several respiratory conditions that require the body to increase ventilation. For example, pulmonary embolism causes tachypnea. Conditions that limit diaphragmatic excursion, such as an enlarged liver or spleen, also cause tachypnea. **Hyperpnea** is a type of tachypnea in which breaths are

Clinical Tips

Neural Control of Breathing

Neural control of breathing comes from the phrenic nerve, which arises from cervical nerve roots C3, C4, and C5 and innervates the diaphragm, and from the nerves that innervate the intercostal muscles.

Clinical Tips

Classification of Breathing Terms

- tachypnea—Rapid breathing: >24 breaths/min
- hyperpnea—Tachypnea with very large breaths
- bradypnea—Slow breathing: <12 breaths/min
- hypopnea—Shallow, slow breaths
- orthopnea—Shortness of breath when lying down

unusually large and deep, resulting in hyperventilation. For some patients and individuals with anxiety, hyperpnea can be observed after normal exercise. Hyperpnea is also associated with certain central nervous system and metabolic disorders, such as **Kussmaul breathing** that occurs in patients with **diabetic ketoacidosis (DKA)**.

Breathing that slows to fewer than 12 breaths/min is called **bradypnea**. Electrolyte and acid–base disturbances can produce this slowed pattern, but well-conditioned individuals with higher levels of cardiorespiratory fitness can also develop it. Breathing that becomes slow and shallow is called **hypopnea** and is seen as an adaptive response to pleuritic pain situations, such as rib fracture. The absence of spontaneous respiration is known as **apnea**. *Obstructive sleep apnea* occurs primarily in patients with obesity during rapid-eye-movement sleep. Periods of apnea can also be found in **Cheyne-Stokes respiration**, or periodic breathing. The Cheyne-Stokes breathing pattern can be normal in children and infants during sleep, but it also occurs pathologically in individuals with brain damage. Figure 6.3 is a visual representation of the respiratory patterns.

As mentioned earlier, disordered breathing may have a cardiac origin. **Orthopnea**, which describes a type of dyspnea that begins or increases as the patient lies down, results from pulmonary edema caused by congestive heart failure. Orthopnea severity is often gauged by the number of pillows a patient needs to sleep. Dyspnea that reliably occurs with exertion may be attributed to cardiac **angina** rather than to a respiratory condition. The athletic trainer should consider the possibility of cardiac involvement when abnormal breathing or chest pain occurs.

Palpation and Percussion of the Chest

The next step in evaluation is to palpate the chest for any painful areas, masses, and symmetrical chest expansion.

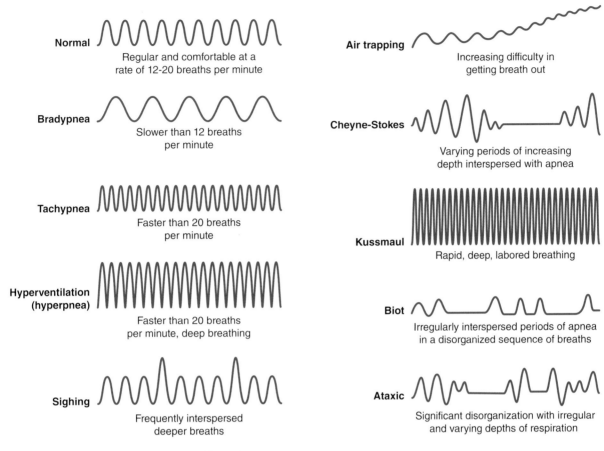

FIGURE 6.3 Normal and disordered breathing patterns.

To palpate for chest expansion, the examiner places the hands on the posterior chest wall with the thumbs placed on either side of the spine at thoracic vertebra 9 (T9) or T10 (figure 6.4a). The examiner asks the patient to inhale deeply and then watches the thumbs diverge away from the spine. The hands should move apart symmetrically with the chest wall.

Next, the examiner feels for **tactile fremitus**, which is a palpable vibration generated from the larynx and transmitted through the patient's bronchi and lungs to the chest wall. The examiner can use the palmar or ulnar surface of the hand to feel the vibrations over the posterior chest wall while the patient says "ninety-nine" (figure 6.4b). The intensity of the fremitus is not as important as the symmetry between lungs. Fremitus will decrease over the scapulae and will also decrease as the hand is moved distally to the lower posterior chest. Fremitus is increased when there is consolidation of the lung tissue, such as in pneumonia. Decreased fremitus occurs as a result of obstructed transmission of vibrations to the chest wall.[5] Examples of obstructions include pleural effusion, pneumothorax, or emphysema, which are discussed later in this chapter.

Percussion

Percussion is the process of assessing sounds transmitted through body organs and cavities and is generated by tapping. Percussion involves striking one object (e.g., the fingers or hand) against another to produce vibrations and subsequent sound waves. The techniques of percussion are the same regardless of the structure being percussed and include either direct or indirect percussion.

Direct percussion involves lightly striking the chest with the ulnar aspect of the fist. Indirect percussion involves the finger of one hand acting as the hammer, striking the finger of the other hand that is resting on the area of the chest being percussed.

Practice is necessary to become proficient with percussion technique. The downward snap of the striking finger originates from the wrist, not the forearm or shoulder. The tap is sharp and rapid with the tip of the finger, not the pad. The ulnar surface of the fist may also be used for percussion and is generally used to elicit tenderness over solid organs, such as the liver or kidneys. Percussion-generated sounds may be recognized by different characteristics, including intensity, pitch, and location. The general percussion tone is loud over air, is less loud

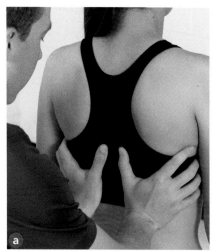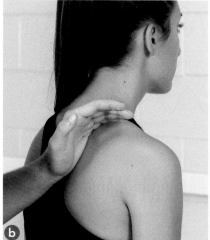

FIGURE 6.4   *(a)* Palpation of the chest for symmetrical expansion. *(b)* Tactile fremitus.

over fluid, and is soft over solid areas. Common sounds produced by percussion are listed in table 6.1. It is often difficult to quantify percussion tones, especially for the novice examiner. The examiner should practice identifying tones from various parts of the body to learn how to quantify them, specifically noting the change from one tone to another when moving from percussing a known air-filled body part (e.g., the lungs) to the abdomen, to muscle, or over bone.

The examiner uses a systematic sequence of percussion, alternating from one side of the chest to the other to compare sounds (figure 6.5) and starting at the apices of the lungs at the top of the shoulders. The predominant sound found at the top of the shoulders will be resonant. Progressing inferiorly, the examiner percusses the chest at approximately 5 cm intervals in the intercostal spaces. In a healthy adult lung, resonance will be the predominant sound. Hyperresonance is found when too much air is present, such as in pneumothorax or emphysema.

A flat note will occur over bone (e.g., over the scapula) or where there is abnormal density in the lungs, which is seen in pneumonia or pleural effusion.[5] Dullness will also be found when percussing the inferior posterior chest wall over the liver and abdominal viscera (figure 6.6).

Auscultation

Auscultation is the skilled listening by a trained ear for sounds produced by the body. Most body sounds, including those of the heart, lung, and bowel, are not typically audible without the use of a stethoscope. Auscultation takes practice so that the sounds can be identified and isolated from each other.

Certain basic principles apply to auscultation regardless of the system being examined:

- Perform auscultation after history, observation, and palpation in order to gather as much information as possible from other sources first.

TABLE 6.1   Sounds Produced by Percussion

Sound	Pitch	Intensity	Quality	Duration	Common location
Tympany	High	Loud	Drumlike	Moderate	Gastric bubble or intestine
Resonance	Low	Moderate to loud	Hollow	Long	Normal lung tissue
Hyperresonance	Very low	Very loud	Booming	Longer than resonance	Emphysematous lung
Dull	High	Soft to moderate	Thudlike	Moderate	Dense organs (liver, spleen)
Flat	High	Soft	Flat	Short	Muscle, bone

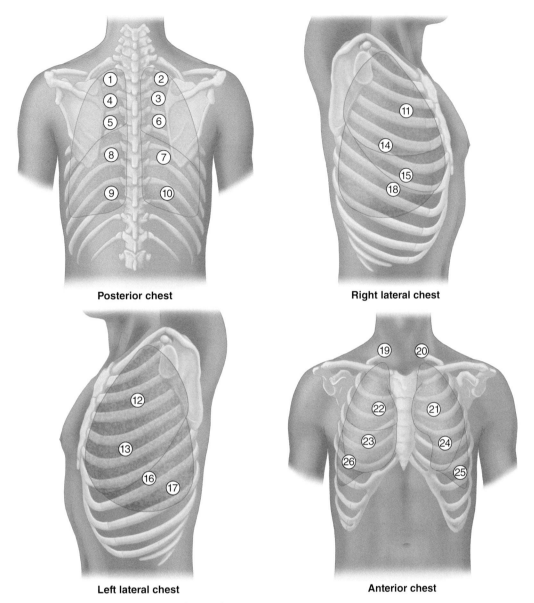

FIGURE 6.5   Suggested percussion and auscultation sequence.

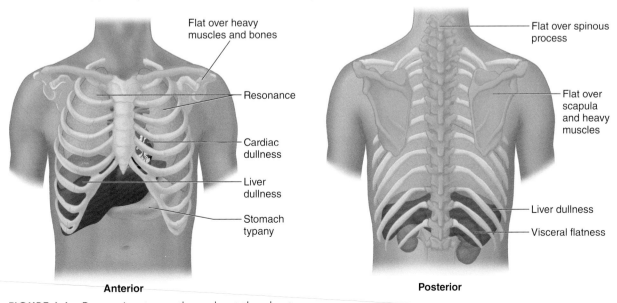

FIGURE 6.6   Percussion tones throughout the chest.

- Perform auscultation in a quiet environment.
- Listen for the presence or absence of sounds as well as their frequency, loudness, quality, and duration.
- Make sure the earpieces of the stethoscope fit comfortably, following the angles of the ear canal.
- Point the earpieces of the stethoscope toward the face.

The examiner uses the part of the stethoscope that best relays the pitch of the sound sought. The diaphragm is used for high-pitched sounds, such as bowel, lung, and normal heart sounds, whereas the bell is used for low-pitched sounds. Abnormal heart and vascular sounds have a lower pitch and may be heard better with the bell.[5] Common characteristics of sounds heard during auscultation are listed here:

- Frequency: Number of sound wave cycles generated per second by a vibrating object. The higher the frequency, the higher the pitch of a sound and vice versa.
- Loudness: Amplitude of a sound wave. Auscultated sounds are described as *loud* or *soft*.
- Quality: Sounds of similar frequency and loudness from different sources. Terms such as *blowing* or *gurgling* describe quality of sound.
- Duration: Length of time sound vibrations last. Duration of sound is *short*, *medium*, or *long*.

Characteristics of Normal and Abnormal Breath Sounds

Characteristic qualities, such as intensity, pitch, quality, and duration in both inspiration and expiration, help the medical professional assess breath sounds.

The diaphragm of the stethoscope is used on bare skin to auscultate the lungs. The examiner must listen systematically at each position throughout inspiration and expiration, should compare the sounds side to side,[1,5] and

Clinical Tips

Listening to Heart and Lung Sounds

Think musically when listening to and describing sounds heard during percussion and auscultation. Just as it took time to train the fingers to feel subtle differences during palpation, it takes time to train the ear to hear subtle differences with percussion and auscultation. Remember, the diaphragm of the stethoscope is best for higher-pitched sounds.

should evaluate the lungs in the anterior, posterior, and lateral aspects to ensure that each lobe is properly examined. Figure 6.7 shows the surface markings of the lobes of the lung. The examiner is always mindful of which lobe is being examined: The front of the chest primarily provides access to the upper lobes, whereas auscultation of the back mainly exposes the lower lobes. To hear the right middle lobe, it may be best for the patient to raise an arm slightly while the examiner places the stethoscope on the midline of the right lateral chest.

One useful technique involves listening in the same sequence used in percussion from left side to right at symmetrical locations to make comparisons as the examiner moves downward from the apex to the base of the lungs. When the athletic trainer listens to the lungs, three different sounds can be appreciated in healthy individuals, depending on the position of the stethoscope (figure 6.8):

- **Bronchial breath sounds** are loud, high pitched, and predominantly expiratory. These sounds represent air moving through large airways and sound more tubular. They are normally heard only over the trachea in the anterior chest midline.
- **Bronchovesicular breath sounds** are heard when air moves through medium-sized airways such as the mainstem bronchi, and they can be heard both anteriorly and posteriorly, toward the center of the thorax. These sounds are of medium pitch and moderate intensity. Inspiratory and expiratory phases are approximately equal.
- **Vesicular breath sounds** predominate in most of the peripheral lung tissue and represent air as it moves into the smaller airways, such as the bronchioles and lung **parenchyma**. These sounds are soft, low-pitched noises that involve mostly inspiration.

When disease affects the lungs, normal breath sounds are altered, depending on the condition (table 6.2). Fluid in the pleural space may make breath sounds distant or even absent; however, fluid within the lung parenchyma, such as in pulmonary edema or pneumonia, may accentuate breath sounds because sound is transmitted more quickly through liquids than through air. Similarly, consolidated masses within the lungs, such as those caused by pneumonia, will transmit louder sounds. Most of the abnormal breath sounds will be superimposed on normal breath sounds and are called **adventitious breath sounds**.

Crackles, or rales, are adventitious sounds that occur because of airflow disruption in the smaller airways, usually by fluid. These brief, discontinuous noises can be either low or high pitched depending on their location within the respiratory tree. Crackles commonly resemble the noise made when several strands of hair are rubbed together between the thumb and index finger held close to the ear.

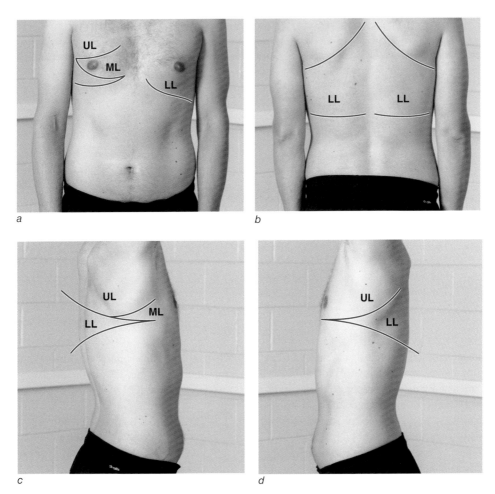

FIGURE 6.7   Surface markings of the lobes of the lung. *(a)* Anterior. *(b)* Posterior. *(c)* Right lateral. *(d)* Left lateral. LL = lower lobe; ML = middle lobe; UL = upper lobe.

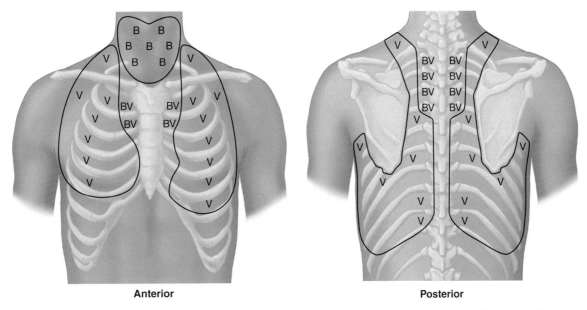

FIGURE 6.8   Normal auscultation sounds. B = bronchial (tracheal); BV = bronchovesicular; V = vesicular.

TABLE 6.2 **Physical Findings Associated With Common Respiratory Conditions**

Condition	Inspection	Palpation	Percussion	Auscultation
Asthma	Tachypnea Dyspnea	Tachycardia	Occasional hyperresonance	Prolonged expiration Wheezes Diminished lung sounds
Bronchitis	Occasional tachypnea Occasional shallow breathing Often no deviation from normal	Tactile fremitus	Resonance	Occasional crackles Occasional expiratory wheezes
Pneumonia	Tachypnea	Increased fremitus in presence of consolidation	Dullness if consolidation is great	Variety of crackles Bronchial breath sounds Egophony, bronchophony
Pneumothorax	Tachycardia Cyanosis Respiratory distress Tracheal deviation	Diminished to absent fremitus Tachycardia	Hyperresonance	Diminished to absent breath sounds Sternal and precordial clicks and crackling Diminished to absent whispered voice sounds

Wheezes are adventitious sounds that indicate airway obstruction from mucus, spasm, or even a foreign body. These sounds are usually more pronounced during expiration and can be either high-pitched, musical noises in the smaller airways (e.g., asthma) or low pitched in the larger airways (e.g., bronchitis). Such low-pitched, sonorous wheezes are also referred to as **rhonchi**. The **stridor** sound is also caused by airway obstruction and can often be confused with wheezes. The obstruction in stridor generally occurs in the central airways, such as the trachea or larynx, and is more pronounced during inspiration as opposed to the expiratory-predominant wheeze.[1,5] **Croup** is a condition that typically produces stridor. **Pleural rubs** are sounds that occur outside the respiratory tree and result from friction between visceral and parietal pleura in conditions that cause pleural inflammation, such as pleurisy or pleuritis. Because these sounds are usually low pitched, they can be heard in both inspiration and expiration and resemble the sound made when two balloons are rubbed together.

Abnormalities can also be detected by listening to the transmission of speech while auscultating the lungs. Transmitted speech is normally muffled and is best heard toward the midline. In pneumonia, changes in vocal resonance occur when consolidation is present. **Bronchophony** occurs when speech becomes clearer and louder. In the extreme, namely, **whispered pectoriloquy**, whispered speech can be heard clearly through the stethoscope. Consolidation of lung tissue also produces **egophony**, in which a spoken "e" is heard as "a." Conversely, any obstruction of the respiratory tree causes diminished vocal resonance.

The athletic trainer must become familiar with normal breath sounds through auscultation, thus better realizing when adventitious sounds are present in the lungs. Here is a summary of the steps in the evaluation of a patient's respiratory system:

History

- Determine onset and duration of symptoms.
- Ask about cough, shortness of breath, and chest pain.
- Obtain history of previous respiratory infections.
- Obtain smoking and environmental exposure history.
- Obtain family history.

Clinical Tips

Loudness of Sounds in the Lungs

The loudness of sounds within the lungs can be confusing for students learning to auscultate. Consider the following:

- Fluid in the pleural space may make breath sounds distant or even absent.
- Fluid within the lung parenchyma, such as in pulmonary edema or pneumonia, may accentuate breath sounds because sound is transmitted more quickly through liquids than through air.
- Consolidated masses within the lungs, such as those caused by pneumonia, will transmit louder sounds.
- Think of air as being an insulator to sounds and fluid as a transmitter of sound.

Inspection

- Check rate, rhythm, and effort of respirations.
- Assess skin color and condition.
- Check posture associated with breathing (note use of accessory muscles).

Palpation

- Palpate any point tenderness or masses.
- Confirm symmetrical expansion.
- Palpate for tactile fremitus.

Percussion

- Percuss over lungs, starting at the apex.

Auscultation

- Assess breath sounds, comparing side to side over all lobes of lung.
- Auscultate both anterior and posterior chest.
- Listen for normal breath sounds and note any abnormal breath sounds.
- Listen for sounds with speaking, such as egophony and bronchophony.

In addition, the athletic trainer must be vigilant in recognizing the signs and symptoms of respiratory disorders.

The following sections discuss the pathological conditions of the respiratory system, beginning with the signs and symptoms of each disorder and including differential diagnosis, referral and diagnostic tests, treatment, implications for return to participation, and prevention.

Asthma and Exercise-Induced Bronchospasm

Airway disease is the most frequently encountered chronic respiratory condition in adolescents, affecting an estimated 8% of children and youths younger than age 18 yr in the United States.[6] Several terms are often used to describe airway disease, especially if a definitive diagnosis has not yet been determined. *Asthma*, *exercise-induced asthma (EIA)*, and *exercise-induced bronchospasm (EIB)* have been used interchangeably for many years; however, *EIA* is no longer a recommended term.[6,7] EIB is defined as a transient narrowing of the lower airways after exercise in the presence or absence of clinically recognized asthma. Exercise triggers bronchoconstriction but does not induce the clinical syndrome of asthma.[8]

Asthma occurs outside of exercise or strenuous activity and generally has two components that lead to obstruction: inflammation and spasm. Inflammation, characterized by mucosal edema and increased secretions, along with bronchospasm of smooth muscle, results in an increase in airway resistance and impeded airflow.

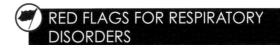

RED FLAGS FOR RESPIRATORY DISORDERS

- Labored breathing with the use of accessory muscles (not associated with exercise)
- Adventitious breath sounds
- Hemoptysis
- Orthopnea
- Dyspnea of rapid onset
- Prolonged cough
- Deviated trachea

Allergens, stress, anxiety, smoke and other environmental pollutants, cold ambient temperatures, and even exercise commonly trigger hyperreactivity of the airways.[6,9] Asthma often begins in childhood and has various degrees of severity and progression. Some people require daily oral or inhaled medications, whereas others need only sporadic or intermittent treatment. Many patients do not have asthmatic symptoms except during strenuous exercise. Despite its various presentations, asthma can be life-threatening if not treated promptly and adequately.

Signs and Symptoms

Patients with airway disease (i.e., asthma and EIB) experience episodic, paroxysmal attacks of shortness of breath and wheezing as well as other symptoms, such as chest tightness and a dry cough. These episodes can be transient, lasting a few minutes to hours, or prolonged over several days. Severe attacks can be associated with substantial respiratory distress and tachypnea. Wheezing may be audible to the unaided ear in some cases. Mild cases may present as only a chronic cough (cough variant asthma). In the general population, particularly among individuals with asthma, cough is a common symptom. In athletes, exercise-induced cough is a particularly frequent symptom that presents after activity and is often termed *locker-room cough*.[10]

In patients suspected of having EIB, another important differential diagnosis is **exercise-induced laryngeal obstruction (EILO)**, in which wheezing and dyspnea are caused by transient obstruction of the upper airways during exercise.[11,12] EIB should be suspected in any patient who complains of shortness of breath, dyspnea, cough, chest congestion, or tightness with exertion. Symptoms of EIB usually occur 10 to 15 min after onset of strenuous exercise and are defined by a decrease of 15% or more in forced expiratory volume within the first second (FEV_1) during exercise spirometry. EIB is more common in winter sport athletes who compete in cold ambient temperatures.[13]

Asthma and EIB should be differentiated from other upper and lower respiratory diseases, such as acute sinusitis, otitis media (middle ear infection), bronchitis, or even pneumonia, particularly in the context of other constitutional symptoms, such as fever, chills, or night sweats. More serious cardiac causes, such as arrhythmia and pericarditis, may also need to be excluded, including EILO, croup, infiltrative lung disease, and even foreign body aspiration. If fatigue is the only presenting symptom, deconditioning may also be a cause. In addition, environmental allergies can account for many of the nonspecific symptoms that mimic EIB.[13,14] The examiner must always consider cardiac failure, chronic obstructive pulmonary disease (COPD), or airway tumors as differential diagnoses in older patients, especially smokers. Determining whether the condition is asthma (occurs at rest) or EIB (only occurs with exercise) is helpful.[3,15] The Global Initiative for Asthma (GINA) guidelines outline several symptoms that increase or decrease the probability of a patient having asthma. For example, symptoms that worsen at night or in the early morning, that vary over time and in intensity, and that are triggered by exercise, irritants, and allergens increase the probability of asthma.[16]

Both respiratory rate and heart rate may be elevated on examination, depending on the severity of the condition. In particular, the use of accessory muscles of respiration may be seen during respiratory distress. The sternocleidomastoid, trapezius, and levator muscles contract during respiratory distress, giving patients the appearance of lifting their shoulders as they breathe. On auscultation, wheezes are usually present, particularly during expiration. The expiratory phase is also prolonged as airway resistance is increased. Breath sounds can be diminished.

Referral and Diagnostic Tests

Resting spirometry measurements are generally poor predictors of variable airflow obstruction in athletes, because their lung function at rest is typically greater than that of the general population. If both the patient history and examination suggest asthma, response to empirical treatment with a β-agonist such as albuterol is often diagnostic. A decrease in predicted FEV_1 measured by spirometry, particularly in response to **cholinergics** such as methacholine (i.e., the methacholine challenge test), is considered the gold standard for diagnosis.[6] The physical examination is usually normal in an athlete with EIB. Some athletes may experience symptoms that develop several hours after exercise. This late-phase response is attributable to the activity of inflammatory mediators. Use of repeated spirometry after exercise can be helpful in the diagnosis of EIB. Most commonly, an exercise challenge or bronchial provocation test is used to determine the diagnosis of EIB.[16] Because of the lack of simple, standardized diagnostic methods, underdiagnosis and misdiagnosis of EIB are common. Symptom-based questionnaires have been used to assist with diagnosis of EIB but have not been validated to date. Figure 6.9 presents a decision tree commonly used for the diagnosis of EIB. Alternatively, many physicians choose to just evaluate the patient's response to an empirical trial of a β-agonist before exercise.

Treatment and Return to Participation

Inhaled β-agonists, both long and short acting, are mainstays in the treatment of asthma. Other medications used to treat asthma include oral and inhaled steroids, mast cell stabilizers such as cromolyn, leukotriene modifiers, and theophylline.[17,18] Treatment recommendations generally follow a stepwise approach in the use of both rescue and maintenance medications as disease severity dictates.[19] A large body of evidence supports use of the long-acting antimuscarinic tiotropium bromide (e.g., Spiriva) for asthma, and this medication is now recommended in current international GINA guidelines for chronic treatment of patients older than age 12 yr with the most severe and frequently exacerbated forms of the disease.[14] Refer to chapter 4 for a complete description of asthma medications and indications. In addition to pharmacotherapy, attention must be given to the avoidance of known triggers and the treatment of concomitant allergies. Although strenuous exercise can provoke airway disease, several studies have shown that regular exercise and improvement

Clinical Tips

Using a Peak Flow Meter

A peak flow meter provides a quick record of pulmonary function and can be used to help assess asthma severity or medication effectiveness. Here is how a patient should use a peak flow meter:

1. Stand or sit up straight.
2. Place the mouthpiece onto the peak flow meter.
3. Slide the indicator to the base of the meter.
4. Exhale completely.
5. Take a deep breath.
6. Place the mouthpiece in the mouth and seal the lips tightly around the mouthpiece.
7. Blow out as hard and fast as possible once.
8. Reset the indicator.
9. Repeat steps 4 through 7.
10. Record the higher of the two numbers.
11. Assess forced expiratory volume.

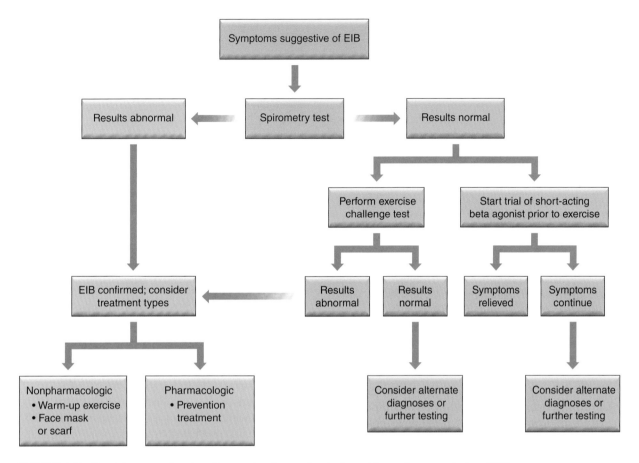

FIGURE 6.9   Decision tree for the diagnosis of exercise-induced bronchoconstriction (EIB).

in physical fitness (specifically pulmonary function) may reduce symptoms and airway irritability.[16,20]

In general, patients and athletes with mild asthma may participate in most sports. However, because cold ambient temperatures exacerbate asthma symptoms, many prefer sports that involve competition in warm, temperate climates, such as track and field. Individuals with moderate to severe asthma are unlikely to be involved in vigorous athletic activities because the disease often limits performance. Patients with acute exacerbations of asthma should refrain from activity until the acute attack resolves and they no longer need rescue medications (e.g., albuterol) regularly.

Treatment for EIB is similar to that for asthma, with the patient using a metered-dose inhaler to administer a β_2-agonist (e.g., albuterol) 15 to 30 min before exercise onset. A patient who has asthma symptoms outside the exercise setting or uses a β_2-agonist more than three times per week should be treated with a regular inhaled corticosteroid. For proper use of a metered-dose inhaler, see chapter 4.

Studies show promise with the use of long-acting β_2-agonists (e.g., salmeterol) and leukotriene inhibitors (e.g., montelukast; Singulair). Other nonpharmacological

strategies include pre–warm-up bursts of physical activity at 80% to 90% of the individual's maximal workload to induce a refractory period that lasts up to 3 h after the initial EIB attack.[16,21] Dietary interventions and strategies to humidify inspired air may also be beneficial.

For a patient experiencing a severe asthma attack or ineffective inhaler treatment, a nebulizer (or *atomizer*) may be used. The nebulizer machine vaporizes liquid medication into a fine mist that is inhaled into the lungs via a mouthpiece or mask. Although studies have shown that both inhalers and nebulizers tend to be equally effective in delivering medication, nebulizers are preferred in more serious rescue situations when the patient is experiencing a severe asthma attack. Nebulizers can administer a higher dose of medication, but inhalers are easier to use, preferred for their portability and low cost, and considered suitable for everyday use. Medications typically administered with a nebulizer include albuterol and ipratropium (Atrovent).

Patients with controlled EIB need not be excluded or discouraged from participating in sports. Effective strategies, both pharmacological and nonpharmacological, exist that can allow an athlete to compete, even at an elite level.

Acute Respiratory Illnesses

Several acute respiratory illnesses are mainly caused by viral infection, and most present with similar symptoms. Common acute respiratory illnesses include influenza (types A and B), severe acute respiratory syndrome coronavirus 2 (SARS-CoV-2) and resultant coronavirus disease 2019 (COVID-19), and respiratory syncytial virus (RSV). In this chapter, these illnesses are grouped together because of their similar signs and symptoms. Often, the specific acute respiratory illness cannot be confirmed via clinical examination and antigen tests are necessary to ascertain its exact nature.

Influenza, generally known as the flu, is a common viral infection. Outbreaks of influenza in the United States usually occur during the fall and winter months. Since 2010, an estimated 12,000 to 61,000 people have died from influenza annually in the United States. Various influenza strains (mainly types A and B) can cause epidemic outbreaks and lead to thousands of hospitalizations each year. In recent years, however, other strains have emerged, including avian and swine influenza (see chapter 14).

SARS-CoV-2, COVID-19, and RSV also have several influenza-like symptoms and usually cannot be differentiated from influenza type A or B without rapid molecular assay testing. There is some evidence that influenza A may lead to increased susceptibility to SARS-CoV-2 and more severe disease.[23] RSV can infect all age groups but is most dangerous in infants and older adults; its symptoms are similar to rhinovirus (the common cold) but can include fever and wheezing. Chapter 14 further describes the spread and effects of SARS-CoV-2 and other types of influenza.

This chapter focuses mainly on signs and symptoms of acute respiratory illnesses and patient referral. People most susceptible to severe complications are considered high risk and include older adults, individuals who live in close quarters (e.g., students), and those with compromised immune systems, diabetes, or chronic heart, lung, or kidney disease. Influenza is transmitted from person to person via contagious droplets that spread when an infected person sneezes or coughs (figure 6.10).

Signs and Symptoms

Milder forms of influenza can be confused with other viral URIs, such as the common cold; however, patients with influenza are generally sicker. Onset of influenza symptoms is rapid and can include high fever, headache, muscle ache, cough, chest pain, shortness of breath, fatigue, loss of appetite, nasal congestion, and sore throat. One clue that aids diagnosis is the reported contact with others diagnosed with influenza. Complications may include secondary bacterial infections, such as sinusitis or pneumonia. Influenza also can cause pneumonia and encephalitis (infection of the brain).

Influenza must be differentiated from SARS-CoV-2, RSV, sinusitis, bronchitis, pneumonia, and other URIs. Compared with influenza type A, symptoms of SARS-CoV-2 infection may take longer to develop. Young adults with RSV may experience mild symptoms similar to the common cold, although the virus is more common in infants and young children and their symptoms are more severe. Fever is a hallmark among patients with influenza, SARS-CoV-2, and RSV, whereas those with sinusitis are typically **afebrile**. COVID-19 spreads more easily than influenza, can cause more severe illness in

---

CONDITION HIGHLIGHT

Exercise-Induced Bronchospasm

A meta-analysis of the literature from 2010 to 2020 reported an EIB prevalence of approximately 23% in athletes; however, this varies depending on the population studied and occurs more often in males than in females.[22] This prevalence is estimated to be 30% to 70% in elite or Olympic-level athletes, but reports vary depending on the environment in which the sport is performed, the type of sport, and the maximum intensity achieved.[16] Exercise-induced cough is particularly prevalent in swimmers and winter sport athletes and occurs more often during winter training.[16] Other risk factors contributing to EIB prevalence include allergic rhinitis, history of allergies or wheeze, or history of asthma in a close relative.[16]

The differential diagnosis is often broad. Patients may not present with any asthma-like symptoms; rather, they may complain of locker-room cough or decreased performance and endurance. Figure 6.9 presents an algorithm that is commonly used to diagnose EIB. Pharmacological and nonpharmacological interventions, including strategies for inspired air humidification, use of intensive warm-up to invoke a refractory period, and treatment with short-acting β_2-agonists prior to exercise, should be considered.

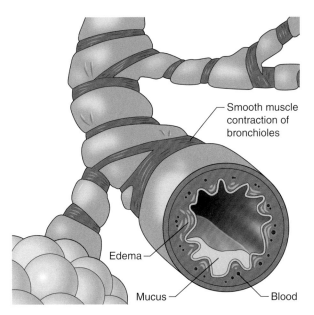

Smooth muscle contraction of bronchioles

Edema

Mucus

Blood

FIGURE 6.10 Influenza causes interstitial inflammation of the bronchiolar and alveolar tissues.

vulnerable populations, and may present with cardiac or other symptoms (see chapter 7). Although COVID-19 has some differences in clinical features compared with influenza and RSV, their presentation and comorbidities overlap significantly (table 6.3).[24]

Referral and Diagnostic Tests

Diagnosis is usually made on clinical grounds, but influenza and COVID-19 cannot be differentiated clinically. Rapid testing for SARS-CoV-2 infection is now common because of the COVID-19 pandemic. To differentiate between SARS-CoV-2, influenza, and RSV infection, the athletic trainer should use a specific rapid test or a combination polymerase chain reaction (PCR) collection kit to immediately test symptomatic patients and individuals in close contact with someone diagnosed with influenza or SARS-CoV-2. Rapid tests provide quick results, whereas combination PCR tests must be sent to a laboratory for analysis. Additional laboratory tests, including a complete blood count (CBC), can be used to delineate viral versus bacterial infection, and blood and sputum cultures obtained in severe illness can isolate pathogens and determine the presence of bacteremia.[25] Chest radiographs should be ordered if pneumonia is suspected on clinical examination.

Treatment and Return to Participation

For generally healthy individuals, treatment for influenza, COVID-19, and RSV is mostly supportive and includes bed rest, analgesics for muscle aches and pains, and increased fluid intake for mild illness. The patient should be sent home to rest and should avoid contact with other individuals to limit disease spread. If influ-

TABLE 6.3   Signs and Symptoms of Influenza, SARS-CoV-2, and RSV

	Influenza	SARS-CoV-2	RSV
Symptom onset	May come on suddenly	Presents 2-14 d after exposure and can be mild to severe	Often occurs in stages and not all at once; mostly in infants and young children
Fever	X	X	X
Cough	X	X	X
Fatigue	X	X	
Sore throat	X	X	
Runny or stuffy nose	X	X	X
Myalgias	X	X	
Headache	X	X	
Sneezing			X
Wheezing			X
Loss of taste or smell		X	
Vomiting	More common in children	X	
Diarrhea	More common in children	X	

Note: RSV = respiratory syncytial virus; SARS-CoV-2 = severe acute respiratory syndrome coronavirus 2.

enza is diagnosed within 48 h of symptom onset, several antiviral medications may shorten the symptom duration by approximately 1 d in high-risk groups. These medications include oseltamivir (Tamiflu), zanamivir (Relenza), peramivir (Rapivab), and baloxavir marboxil (Xofluza).[26] The recommended antivirals change yearly, depending on the most common strain of influenza within the population. In most individuals who are otherwise healthy, influenza fully resolves within 7 to 10 d.

Some antiviral agents, such as nirmatrelvir (Paxlovid), can be administered to patients with SARS-CoV-2 infection. However, health care providers should consult the latest U.S. Centers for Disease Control and Prevention (CDC) treatment recommendations, because they are updated frequently. COVID-19 may take longer to fully resolve; however, the patient may return to low-level activities when they feel able and are no longer contagious. Among individuals in high-risk groups, both influenza and COVID-19 may be severe and can lead to complications, including pneumonia. Patients recovering from influenza are usually fit to return to activity in 1 to 2 wk, but they must be afebrile and have no respiratory compromise at rest, such as shortness of breath or pleuritic chest pain.

Prevention is the best approach in the management of influenza. Depending on the supply of vaccine, the athletic trainer should encourage all patients to be immunized yearly against common strains of influenza. Immunization typically begins in late October and early November. Individuals at high risk are generally immunized first. The influenza vaccine has a variable success rate from season to season, generally ranging from 60% to 70% in people with normal immune systems. See chapter 14 for more information on recommended vaccination schedules. Vaccinations are available for intramuscular or intradermal injection or for intranasal administration, and the nasal spray form can be given to children as young as 6 mo.[26] The main challenge for the athletic trainer is to reduce exposure among patients and athletes, especially during travel. Use of face masks to reduce virus transmission is now common in medical facilities and other close quarters. Other means of prevention, especially for the athletic population, include handwashing and not sharing drinking receptacles or bench towels.

Upper Respiratory Infections

URI is a diagnosis typically given to any number of self-limited viral infections affecting the upper respiratory tract, including the nasopharynx, trachea, and bronchi. Common pathogens include **rhinovirus**, which produces the common cold, as well as adenovirus and parainfluenza. These viruses are highly transmissible through contact with infected respiratory droplets expelled by coughing or sneezing; therefore, entire households are usually affected.

Signs and Symptoms

URI symptoms may include fever, which usually resolves in 24 to 48 h, cough, nasal congestion, sore throat, and runny nose. Symptoms are generally mild and do not limit normal daily activities. Sore throat and fever are usually the first to present, with cough usually the last to resolve. Secondary bacterial infections such as otitis media (i.e., middle ear infection) and sinusitis may result if mucosal inflammation persists. Viral URI symptoms often last 7 to 10 d.

Viral URIs are diagnosed clinically and many times to the exclusion of other, more severe conditions, such as influenza and bacterial infections. Diagnostic testing is usually not indicated or useful.[27]

Referral and Diagnostic Tests

When symptoms include high fever, dark or purulent nasal discharge, or a duration longer than 7 to 10 d, patients should be referred to a physician for evaluation of other potential causes, including a secondary bacterial infection.

Treatment and Return to Participation

The athletic trainer should assure patients that URIs are self-limited. Treatment is mainly supportive. Medications such as over-the-counter cough suppressants, decongestants, antihistamines, and expectorants can alleviate symptoms. Patients should be encouraged to stay hydrated so secretions remain loose, and this is particularly important for athletes because fluid losses associated with exertion may exacerbate symptoms. Handwashing and not sharing drinking containers and towels are particularly important in preventing URI transmission. Athletes may participate in sports if they are afebrile and able to drink plenty of fluids.

Bronchitis

Bronchitis refers to any inflammatory condition of the bronchial passages and generally presents as acute or chronic. The chronic condition, COPD, is discussed

RED FLAGS OF CONSTITUTIONAL SYMPTOMS

- Fever greater than 100 °F
- Chills
- Night sweats

later in this chapter. In acute bronchitis, the inflammation most commonly results from self-limited viral infections. Acute bronchitis is rarely caused by bacterial infections in healthy people. Bacterial infections occur more commonly in smokers and in patients with COPD with underlying impairment of bronchial ciliary motility. Acute bronchitis can also occur as a noninfectious condition in response to environmental allergens.

Signs and Symptoms

A productive cough is the most common sign in a patient with acute bronchitis. The sputum is usually clear but can have a yellowish tinge. Chest congestion or tightness, along with some mild shortness of breath, may be present. If the cause is infectious, constitutional symptoms, such as fever, chills, or night sweats, may be present although transient. Because most cases (90%) are viral in origin, acute bronchitis commonly presents with URI and associated symptoms of runny nose, nasal congestion, and sore throat. The common cold typically lasts 7 to 10 d, whereas symptoms of acute bronchitis typically persist for longer. The causative pathogen for bronchitis is rarely identified. Physical examination of the chest is often normal, but occasionally rhonchi and crackles can be heard.

Bronchitis must be differentiated from underlying pneumonia, which can present similarly. Respiratory symptoms tend to be more severe with pneumonia, whereas constitutional symptoms, such as chills and fever, are less severe and more self-limited in cases of acute infectious bronchitis. Underlying allergic rhinitis as well as sinusitis may also present with a persistent cough secondary to postnasal drainage. In athletes with intermittent bouts of bronchitis, the diagnosis of asthma, either intrinsic or exercise induced, needs to be considered.

Referral and Diagnostic Tests

Although no diagnostic tests other than clinical examination are used to diagnose bronchitis, specific tests may help to exclude other causes. Chest radiographs, as well as a CBC to look for elevations in white blood cells, are useful in diagnosing pneumonia.[28] A computed tomography (CT) scan of the sinuses may reveal underlying sinusitis, and an empirical trial of an antihistamine can help distinguish allergic causes. Testing for influenza may be considered when risk is thought to be intermediate and the patient presents within 36 h of symptom onset. Because most cases of bronchitis are self-limited, referral for medical evaluation is indicated if symptoms do not resolve.

Treatment and Return to Participation

Treatment for bronchitis is supportive in most cases. Mucolytics, cough suppressants, and nonsteroidal anti-inflammatory drugs (NSAIDs) are helpful in reducing symptom severity. Fluids to keep secretions loose are also essential. Because of the risk of antibiotic resistance, antibiotics should not be routinely used in the treatment of acute bronchitis. Clinical data support the view that antibiotics do not significantly change the course of acute bronchitis, and they may provide only minimal benefit compared with the risk of antibiotic use itself. Physician education has led to a significant reduction in antibiotic prescribing for patients with bronchitis.[29]

Acute viral cases of bronchitis may last 7 to 10 d. Athletes with acute bronchitis may be allowed to play as tolerated if their fever has resolved. Because a small increase in expectorated secretions is possible, attention to fluid status and adequate hydration is essential in minimizing the risk of dehydration.

Chronic Obstructive Pulmonary Disease

COPD is characterized by nonreversible airway obstruction and is closely related to asthma, a type of reversible obstructive pulmonary disease. This disease is typically found in long-term smokers, and diagnosis is broadly divided into two main categories: emphysema and chronic bronchitis.

Emphysema is characterized by destruction of the alveoli and pulmonary capillary beds. As a result, there is a decreased ability to oxygenate blood as the lung loses its elastic recoil properties. The body also compensates with lowered cardiac output and hyperventilation. In contrast, chronic bronchitis is defined by excessive mucus production with upper airway obstruction. Damage to the airway lining impairs the mucociliary response that clears bacteria and mucus. Because of the severe respiratory impairment associated with COPD, this disease is rarely seen in the athletic population.

Signs and Symptoms

Patients with COPD tend to be older with a long-standing history of cigarette smoking. Individuals with emphysema have high respiratory rates and a ruddy skin tone attributable to muscle wasting, which makes peripheral capillaries more visible. These patients are thus said to have the "pink puffer" variant of COPD. On examination, the chest is more rounded or barrel shaped because of hyperinflation. Diffuse wheezing and decreased breath sounds can be heard on auscultation. In contrast, patients with chronic bronchitis have the typical productive "smoker's cough." Because these individuals often present with signs of right heart failure, such as edema and cyanosis, they are said to have the "blue bloater" variant of COPD. Coarse rhonchi and wheezing, as well as a markedly prolonged expiratory phase of breathing, are noted on physical examination.

Early in its course, COPD may present similarly to asthma, with wheezing and shortness of breath. Also, acute bronchitis can occur in the setting of COPD—that is, the acute on chronic condition. Patients with COPD, particularly those with emphysema, are at risk of developing pneumothorax. Individuals with chronic bronchitis are more prone to developing pneumonia, which distinguishes itself by persistent constitutional symptoms such as fever. In advanced stages of chronic bronchitis, symptoms are similar to those of congestive heart failure.

Referral and Diagnostic Tests

COPD is generally diagnosed clinically in patients who have long-standing airway obstruction and tobacco abuse. Chest X-rays and CT scans can also be suggestive of the disease. The diagnosis of COPD requires three features:

1. A postbronchodilator FEV_1/forced vital capacity ratio of less than 0.70, confirming irreversibility

2. Appropriate symptoms, including dyspnea, chronic cough, sputum production, or wheezing

3. Significant exposures to noxious stimuli, such as a history of cigarette smoking or other exposure[30]

For patients with clinical findings consistent with COPD absent a history of cigarette smoking, a workup should include investigation for (1) other environmental exposure that may be toxic to the lungs and (2) autoimmune causes and metabolic disorders, such as α_1-antitrypsin deficiency. Patients with COPD who have significant shortness of breath at rest or with minimal activity must be referred to and evaluated by a physician immediately.

Treatment and Return to Participation

Treatment of COPD focuses on addressing the two main processes involved: spasm and inflammation. The identification and reduction of risk factors can be helpful in decreasing exacerbation of symptoms. Agonist medications, either short or long acting, are used to control bronchospasm. Similarly, inhaled anticholinergic medications, such as ipratropium (Atrovent), improve bronchospasm and help control the copious secretion production seen with chronic bronchitis. Glucocorticosteroids, either inhaled or taken orally, are used primarily to treat chronic airway inflammation.[31] Holland and colleagues[32] recommend breathing exercise therapy for the treatment and control of COPD. Oxygen therapy may be needed in more advanced cases, which are typically not seen in the athletic population.[33] Smoking cessation, of course, is paramount to the successful treatment of COPD.

Given that patients with COPD typically do not have the pulmonary reserve to compete in sports, athletic participation is rare. For those with mild disease, participation in sports is permitted as tolerated.[31] Klign and colleagues[34] report that varying exercise modes improves overall endurance in patients with COPD compared with traditional endurance and resistance training. It is recommended that these patients have the disease under control and are compliant with maintenance medications.[31] Precautions must be taken to address any acute COPD flare-up, such as in asthma, by having a short-acting β-agonist (e.g., albuterol) readily available.

Pneumonia

Pneumonia is a diagnosis given to any condition that results in inflammation of the lung parenchyma. Usually, the cause is infectious and can result from a viral, bacterial, or fungal pathogen. Common forms of pneumonia are viral or bacterial and can follow an acute respiratory illness such as influenza or SARS-CoV-2. Fungal infections typically occur in the immunocompromised patient. Patients with pneumonia generally appear ill, although some forms of *walking pneumonia* caused by atypical bacteria, such as *Mycoplasma pneumoniae*, may not be severe. In general, community-acquired pneumonia is easily treatable once properly identified, although hospitalization is sometimes needed in severe cases.

Signs and Symptoms

Patients with pneumonia often have constitutional symptoms that persist if not treated adequately. They may complain of shortness of breath or pleuritic chest pain. A productive cough with dark, discolored sputum is not unusual. If the pneumonia affects the lower lobes of the lungs, diaphragmatic irritation and abdominal pain may be the presenting symptoms.

At physical examination, the respiratory rate may be mildly elevated and breathing may be labored. If there is consolidation, the examiner may detect dullness to percussion over the affected lung field and changes in vocal resonance, such as bronchophony or egophony, on auscultation of the involved areas. Pooling of secretions in the lower lobe can produce adventitious rales at the lung bases along with an occasional wheeze.

Pneumonia can present similarly to other URIs, such as bronchitis and sinusitis. Bronchitis is often confused with pneumonia, particularly when the pneumonia is not severe.[35] Tuberculosis (TB) is also a possibility in a patient who presents with pneumonia of the upper lung lobes. On occasion, pneumonia results from an obstruction by a foreign body or mass in the airway.

Referral and Diagnostic Tests

It is virtually impossible to distinguish viral from bacterial pneumonia on clinical examination alone. Because of the morbidity associated with pneumonia, it is often treated empirically with antibiotics. Any febrile patient who exhibits resting labored breathing with chest pain or cough and presents with signs of consolidation should be referred to a physician. Additional diagnostic tests, such as a chest radiograph, are often ordered by the physician and can aid in confirming the diagnosis. Certain microorganisms, such as viruses and atypical bacteria, may not consolidate, and a normal chest radiograph will result. Sputum cultures taken to isolate specific organisms are usually done when empirical treatment fails. In general, patients should be referred as soon as possible for further evaluation when they are suspected of having pneumonia.

Treatment and Return to Participation

Treatment for pneumonia with first-line antibiotics, such as azithromycin (Zithromax) or clarithromycin (Biaxin), is usually successful. Attention to proper hydration and supportive care with mucolytics and cough suppressants (e.g., guaifenesin and dextromethorphan [Robitussin DM liquid]) are also helpful. Patients who do not improve within 2 to 3 d after initiating treatment should be referred to a physician for reevaluation. Older adults and high-risk patients should be encouraged to ask their physician about the pneumococcal vaccine, which provides protection against the most common strains of pneumonia.

As with any acute infection, participation is restricted until the patient is no longer febrile and their vital signs have returned to normal. In cases of bacterial pneumonia, it is recommended that definitive treatment with antibiotics be initiated before a patient returns to activity. Because of the respiratory compromise that often accompanies acute pneumonia, patients may not feel well enough to return to sports for about 7 to 10 d.

Pleurisy

Pleurisy is a descriptive term for any inflammation of the pleura (i.e., the lining of the lungs) that causes subsequent pain. It is also known as *pleuritis* or *pleuritic chest pain*. Pleurisy may develop in the presence of lung inflammation, such as pneumonia or TB, but it can also develop in association with rheumatic diseases, chest trauma, cancer, and asbestos-related diseases. This condition often results in fluid accumulation at the site of pleural inflammation, known as a *pleural effusion*. The fluid that collects between the lining of the lung and the chest wall may alleviate the chest pain despite worsening of the illness. Large accumulations of fluid can compromise breathing and cause coughing, dyspnea, tachypnea, cyanosis, and intercostal **retractions**.

Signs and Symptoms

The hallmark of pleurisy is chest pain at the site of inflammation; the pain occurs in association with breathing or any movement of the chest wall, such as coughing, sneezing, or laughing. Pain may be referred to the shoulder, and symptoms of coexisting respiratory infection, such as fever, cough, and malaise, may occur.[36] The normally smooth pleural surfaces, now roughened by inflammation, rub together with each breath and can produce a rough, grating sound called a *friction rub*. This sound can be heard easily with a stethoscope or an unassisted ear held to the patient's chest. Other findings on physical examination include rales or rhonchi if there is accompanying pneumonia or bronchitis. If a pleural effusion is present, the examiner also can appreciate decreased breath sounds.

When the diagnosis of pleurisy is possible, the health care professional should always consider primary processes, such as pneumonia, TB, malignancies (e.g., mesothelioma), and autoimmune conditions (e.g., systemic lupus erythematosus, in particular).

Referral and Diagnostic Tests

A diagnosis of pleurisy is based primarily on the clinical examination. Patients with nontraumatic chest pain associated with breathing should be referred to a physician for the evaluation of secondary causes and underlying pathology that is necessary to initiate adequate treatment. Laboratory tests, including a CBC, can help differentiate bacterial from viral infections. A chest radiograph may reveal an underlying pneumonia or mass, which may or may not be malignant. A CT scan of the chest can also be useful to further clarify underlying lung disease, and an ultrasound of the chest can detect fluid associated with pleurisy. If fluid is present, an invasive procedure called a **thoracentesis** may be performed either diagnostically to analyze the fluid or therapeutically to alleviate the symptoms associated with a pleural effusion.

Treatment and Return to Participation

Treatment of pleurisy is directed at the underlying illness. Bacterial infections are treated with appropriate antibiotics. Viral infections normally run their course without medications. NSAIDs are helpful in alleviating pain and inflammation associated with pleurisy. Recovery depends on the nature of the underlying illness but is generally good with treatment. Recuperation from pleurisy caused by malignant disease depends on the type and extent of illness. Early treatment of bacterial respiratory infections can prevent pleurisy. Medications for viral respiratory infections are limited, except for those for influenza type A.

Patients may return to activity once a workup has been completed to rule out a primary condition, such as pneumonia, and once they are afebrile. In addition, patients must refrain from activity if there continues to be any evidence of respiratory compromise at rest or with exertion. When patients resume activity, workloads should be increased gradually over a period of weeks to ensure a safe return.

Spontaneous Pneumothorax and Hemothorax

Pneumothorax results when gas or air is trapped in the chest wall between the parietal and visceral pleura and causes the lung to collapse (figure 6.11). It is deemed spontaneous if the pneumothorax occurs in the absence of a traumatic injury to the chest or lungs.[37] Pneumothorax tends to be more common in tall, thin men in the second and third decades of life and usually results from the rupture of a small **bleb** or an air- or fluid-filled sac called a **bulla**. Other lung diseases commonly associated with spontaneous pneumothorax include TB, pneumonia, asthma, cystic fibrosis, lung cancer, COVID-19, and certain forms of interstitial lung disease.

A more serious condition, known as **hemothorax**, occurs when blood collects in the pleural space. Hemothorax usually results from trauma to the chest wall. Rib fractures that bleed into the plural space are a common cause.[38] Hemothorax may also result from malignancies.

Signs and Symptoms

Spontaneous pneumothorax is characterized by sudden onset of pleuritic chest pain and shortness of breath. Patients are usually tachypneic and have a cough that exacerbates the chest pain.[37] Mild respiratory distress may be apparent, and there may be little chest wall motion on the affected side with breathing. A common sign of pneumothorax is a shift of the trachea away from the affected lung as air pressure pushes the lung toward the midline (figure 6.12). Physical examination of the lungs with a stethoscope reveals decreased or absent breath sounds over the pneumothorax. Hemothorax is also characterized by pleuritic chest pain and dyspnea that worsen rapidly as the chest wall fills with blood. Dullness to percussion in dependent areas can also be appreciated on examination.

A small pneumothorax can easily be missed clinically and sometimes is overlooked as pleurisy, EIB, bronchitis, or a simple URI. Larger pneumothoraces are associated with some degree of respiratory compromise and can present a clinical picture similar to conditions such as pulmonary embolism or foreign body aspiration.

Referral and Diagnostic Tests

Any patient suspected of pneumothorax or hemothorax should be immediately referred to a medical facility. In general, a chest radiograph is conclusive in the diagnosis of pneumothorax, although small pneumothoraces may be overlooked without clinical suspicion. In some cases, air continues to be trapped in the chest cavity through a one-way valve mechanism and can result in a dangerous, life-threatening condition known as **tension pneumothorax**. This condition requires immediate attention

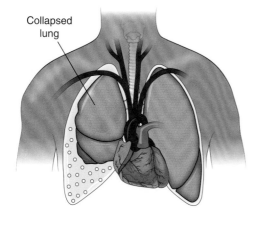

Collapsed lung

Pneumothorax

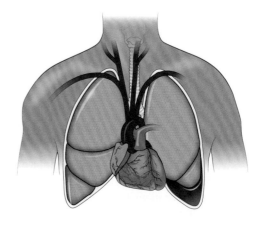

Hemothorax

FIGURE 6.11 Pneumothorax and hemothorax.

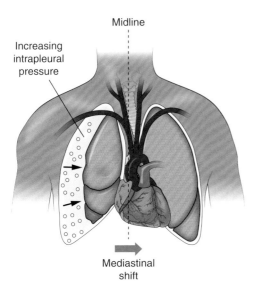

FIGURE 6.12   A common sign of pneumothorax is a shift of the trachea away from the affected lung as air pressure pushes the lung toward the midline.

and needle decompression of the chest. The diagnosis of hemothorax is definitively made when blood is aspirated by thoracentesis.

Treatment and Return to Participation

The physician's treatment objective is to remove the air from the pleural space, allowing the lung to reexpand. Small pneumothoraces may resolve without treatment. Aspiration of air, using a catheter linked to a vacuum bottle, may reexpand the lung. Placement of a chest tube between the ribs into the pleural space allows the evacuation of air from that space when simple aspiration is not successful or the pneumothorax is large.[39] Reexpansion of the lung may take several days with the chest tube left in place. Hospitalization is required for chest tube management. Surgery may be indicated for recurrent episodes.

If hemothorax is suspected, immediate hospitalization for decompression and drainage of blood is required. Exploration for an active bleeding site is mandatory, and other coexisting traumatic injuries to the chest are possible.

Individuals diagnosed with pneumothorax or hemothorax cannot participate in athletics until the condition has resolved radiographically and they are clinically asymptomatic, typically after 8 to 12 wk. Because the recurrence rate of spontaneous pneumothorax can be close to 10%, patients need to be returned conservatively. Approximately 5% of patients are unable to return to their previous level of participation after pneumothorax and thoracotomy.[40] The physician will encourage patients to discontinue smoking and avoid flying in unpressurized aircraft. Moreover, those with increased risks, such as scuba divers and athletes competing at high elevation, need to be counseled carefully and possibly encouraged to discontinue their activities.

Tuberculosis

Pulmonary TB is a highly contagious bacterial infection caused by *Mycobacterium tuberculosis*. The infection involves the lungs primarily but can spread to other organs. TB can develop after an individual inhales droplets sprayed into the air from an infected patient's cough or sneeze. It is characterized by the development of granulomas (granular tumors) in the infected tissues.[41] The primary stage of infection is usually asymptomatic and is otherwise known as latent TB. The CDC reports that in 2022, there were 7,882 reported cases of TB in the United States (a rate of 2.4 cases per 100,000 persons). Those most at risk of developing active TB have a compromised immune system. Among individuals with human immunodeficiency virus (HIV) infection, for example, the rate of progression from latent to active TB may be as high as 162 per 1,000 person-years of observation. Individuals recently infected with *M. tuberculosis* are also at high risk, with a conversion rate of 12.9 cases per 1,000 person-years within the first year.[41] TB may occur within weeks after the primary infection, or it may lie dormant for years before causing active disease. The risk of contracting TB grows with increased contact with infected individuals, in crowded or unsanitary living conditions, and under conditions of poor nutrition.

Signs and Symptoms

Patients are asymptomatic in cases of latent TB. For those with active pulmonary TB, symptoms may be mild and insidious. Fatigue, fever, weight loss, and cough are common symptoms.[42] The cough may produce sputum containing blood (i.e., **hemoptysis**). Other symptoms include chest pain, shortness of breath, and wheezing. Auscultation of the lungs may reveal crackles or wheezing. A pleural effusion may also be found. Enlarged or tender lymph nodes may be present in the neck and other areas. Often, active TB produces some degree of hypoxia and, if present for some time, results in clubbing of the fingers or toes.

Differential diagnoses include community-acquired bacterial pneumonia, fungal pneumonias, primary and metastatic lung malignancies, interstitial lung disease, and HIV-related opportunistic infections. Any patient with a persistent cough and constitutional symptoms should be referred to a physician for follow-up evaluation.

Referral and Diagnostic Tests

Latent TB infection is identified solely with a positive skin test involving a subcuticular injection of a purified protein derivative (PPD), which causes local induration and erythema of the skin when *M. tuberculosis* infection is present.[43] Active TB is diagnosed when the patient with a positive PPD test result has symptoms consistent with pulmonary TB and radiographic evidence of infection. A chest radiograph typically demonstrates granulomatous disease with a predilection for the upper lung fields. Definitive diagnosis of active disease is made with sputum cultures demonstrating acid-fast bacilli.

Treatment and Return to Participation

Despite a low conversion rate to active TB, latent TB is usually treated by **chemoprophylaxis** with medications such as isoniazid and rifampin for several months under physician supervision. Because multidrug-resistant strains of *M. tuberculosis* have emerged, treatment of active TB involves concomitant use of several antibiotics (up to four).[41]

Individuals suspected to have TB must be suspended from activity and referred to a physician immediately. All active TB cases need to be reported to the local health department for tracking and surveillance. Hospitalization may be indicated to prevent disease spread to others until the contagious period has resolved through the patient receiving drug therapy. Normal activity can be continued after the contagious period has passed.

Lung Cancer

Lung cancer is one of the most common cancers in the United States and is the leading cause of death from cancer. Lung cancer primarily affects smokers, although individuals exposed to secondhand smoke have increased risk of the disease. Physical activity has been shown to decrease the risk of certain cancers.[44] Each lung cancer type affects different cells within the lung. Some are more aggressive than others, and some are more responsive to therapy. In general, the prognosis is poor for all types because most lung cancers are not detected until the later stages, usually after involvement of or spread to other organs, including the brain.

Signs and Symptoms

Symptoms of lung cancer develop slowly over time and are often overlooked until the later stages of the disease. Constitutional symptoms predominate and include fever, fatigue, weight loss, and loss of appetite. A cough is usually present with or without bloody sputum. The patient may experience chest pain and shortness of breath. Pneumonia can develop as a secondary consequence. The physical examination is usually nonspecific; however, a pleural effusion can sometimes be detected.

The primary diagnostic dilemma in lung cancer is to determine whether the malignancy is primary or has metastasized from another site. Histological analysis of tissue biopsies can usually reveal the source. Clinical presentation of lung cancer may be like that of many chronic lung diseases, including TB, interstitial lung disease, and COPD. On radiographs, lung cancers may resemble benign granulomas, consolidated pneumonias, or even lung abscesses.

Referral and Diagnostic Tests

Chest radiographs can detect possible malignancies that can be more clearly visualized by CT scans if necessary. A definitive diagnosis is made when cells obtained by bronchoscopy or biopsy are found to be malignant. Other laboratory test abnormalities that may suggest lung cancer include elevated serum (blood) calcium and alkaline phosphatase, decreased serum sodium (i.e., hyponatremia), and abnormal serum levels of carcinoembryonic antigen.[45]

Treatment and Return to Participation

Treatment of lung cancer depends on its type and stage at diagnosis. (For more information on cancer staging, refer to chapter 13.) Options to treat lung cancer may include radiation therapy, chemotherapy, or surgical excision. In the most advanced cases, **palliative therapy** is the only viable option. Overall survival depends on the disease stage. For limited disease, cure rates may be as high as 25%, whereas cure rates for advanced stages are less than 5%.[44]

Summary

Health care providers must remember that chest pain and dyspnea may indicate a respiratory condition but also can point to a cardiovascular problem. Clinicians' ability to perform a thorough examination of the respiratory system will help them distinguish less serious conditions from those that need immediate attention. It takes considerable practice to recognize characteristics of normal and abnormal breath sounds. Many websites and other resources include both audio and animated replication of these breath sounds.

Familiarity with the signs and symptoms, differential diagnoses, and common treatments of respiratory conditions such as asthma, bronchitis, pneumonia, URI, and influenza is also paramount. Understanding of common treatments, implications of illness and treatment on sports participation, and prevention techniques enables athletic trainers to provide the best medical care and follow-up for their patients. Awareness of conditions that less commonly affect athletic patients, such as hemothorax or pneumothorax, emphysema, TB, and lung cancer, is important because the athletic trainer is often the first person the patient seeks help from when experiencing respiratory system problems. Recognizing an abnormal respiratory condition can facilitate quick referral for a patient who otherwise might not seek further medical assistance.

Apply It!

Go to HK*Propel* to complete the case studies for this chapter.

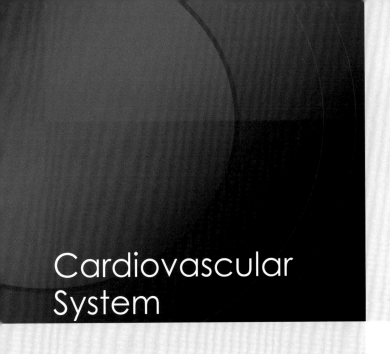

Cardiovascular System

OBJECTIVES

At the completion of this chapter the reader should be able to do the following:

1. Understand the anatomy and physiology of the cardiovascular system.

2. Discuss cardiovascular adaptations to exercise.

3. Identify various cardiac arrhythmias.

4. Identify signs and symptoms of cardiovascular abnormalities.

5. Recognize when to refer an athlete to a physician for further cardiovascular evaluation.

Cardiovascular disorders in physically active individuals have taken on particular importance because of their potential for catastrophic consequences during exercise. Although these tragedies bring notable publicity, many people with cardiac conditions can safely participate in myriad physical activities. The athletic trainer must be knowledgeable about and able to distinguish between the normal physiological changes of the heart seen with exercise training and the pathological cardiac conditions that can result in exercise-related sudden death.

Vascular conditions, such as hypertension and deep vein thrombosis (DVT), result in and can precipitate potentially fatal conditions such as myocardial infarction (heart attack) and pulmonary embolus. Early referral for diagnosis and treatment can limit harmful complications. Hematological conditions ranging from anemia to sickle cell trait are also discussed in this chapter. Promptly referring patients to a physician for these conditions can enhance athletic performance and might even save a life.

Overview of Anatomy and Physiology

The heart is a strong, muscular organ made up of four chambers, two atria and two ventricles, which are responsible for pumping the blood that circulates through the body. Blood from the right side of the heart flows to the lungs, and simultaneously blood from the left side of the heart is pumped into the body. The two sides of this muscular pump are separated by the septum and work in a parallel manner. The right-side atrium and ventricle pump the pulmonary circuit. The left-side atrium and ventricle pump the systemic circuit.

Four valves help to direct the flow. The tricuspid valve separates the right atrium and right ventricle; the mitral valve lies between the left atrium and left ventricle. Another set of valves connects the ventricles to the distal circulation.

On the right side of the heart, the pulmonary valve is connected to the pulmonary artery; on the left side, the aortic valve controls flow to the aorta (figure 7.1). Blood flow returning to the heart from the body enters the right atrium: pulmonic blood into the left atrium via the pulmonary vein and systemic blood into the right atrium via the superior and inferior vena cava.

The heart is positioned in the chest like an acorn, pointing inferiorly and to the left. The anterior surface of the heart consists primarily of the right ventricle. A sliver of the left ventricle makes up the left border and the apex or inferior end of the anterior cardiac surface. Many times, the heartbeat can be palpated at this apical end located on the left side (the fifth rib interspace at the nipple line).

The systemic vasculature is a pipeline that delivers blood to the organs and tissues throughout the body. Arteries carry blood to the tissues via a high-pressure system, and veins return blood to the atria under much lower pressure. With each contraction of the ventricle, a pressure wave (i.e., the pulse) is created, moving through the arteries.

Pulse palpation can provide useful clinical information. The intensity, contour, and regularity of the pulse

---

Clinical Tips

Measuring Heart Rate

Heart rate can be measured by counting the pulse for 15 s and multiplying by 4. A heart rate at rest that is less than 60 beats/min (common in athletes) is termed *bradycardia*.

---

are just as important as the rate. The pulse diminishes with inspiration, but this may not be perceptible. Weak, decreased pulses may indicate shock, heart failure, or a mechanical obstruction such as **aortic stenosis**. Strong, bounding pulses are common after exercise but at rest may be a sign of anemia, **hyperthyroidism**, or anxiety. A double-peak pulse is called a **bisferiens pulse** and can be detected in hypertrophic cardiomyopathy (HCM) or aortic regurgitation.

Understanding how the cardiovascular system responds to exercise requires an understanding of basic cardiovascular physiology at rest. The right and left sides of the heart work together, pumping 5 to 6 L of blood per minute at rest (i.e., cardiac output). The heart pumps

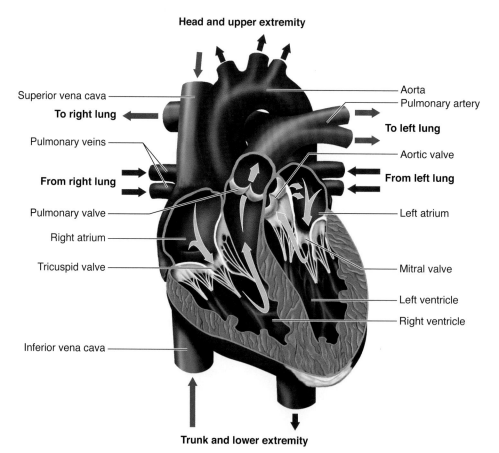

FIGURE 7.1   Anatomy of the cardiac chambers and the course of blood flow through the chambers.

in a rhythmic cycle. Both ventricles contract during sys-tole and relax during diastole. During the relaxed stage, they are passively filled with blood by atrial contraction. Pressures are rising and falling during this cardiac cycle, which permits the heart valves to open and close.

Cardiac muscle is unique because it can contract within itself and operates on a serial electrical system, free from stimuli external to the heart. An electrical impulse begins at the sinoatrial (SA) node within the upper walls of the right atrium. This impulse travels through both atria to the atrioventricular (AV) node in the atrial septum. After a brief delay, the electrical impulse is promulgated to the bundle of His along the ventricular septum to the Purkinje fibers through the inferior and lateral ventricles (figure 7.2). Information on the diagnostic tool, the elec-trocardiogram (ECG), is found in chapter 2.

When the ventricles begin to contract, the pressure increases, closing the mitral and tricuspid valves. A sound is produced, which is called the first heart sound, or S1. As the pressure continues to rise, it forces the aortic and pulmonic valves to open. Once the blood is expelled, the ventricular pressure drops and the aortic and pulmonic valves close. The sound of this closure is the second heart sound, or S2. Because of pressure differences between the right and left sides of the heart, this sound splits into two components during inspiration but is one sound during expiration.

As the ventricles relax, the pressure drops and allows the mitral and tricuspid valves to open. The rush of blood into the ventricles can cause a sound in children and young adults that is called S3. There is a fourth heart sound, or S4, that marks atrial contraction and immediately precedes S1 of the next cardiac cycle. In older adults, S3 and S4 can be pathological heart sounds. *Pathological* is a term used to indicate a condition that involves or is caused by a disease or condition.[1] Other pathological sounds, such as snaps and clicks, may also be heard via auscultation.

Another sound that is often heard is a murmur caused by turbulent blood flow or valvular vibration. Heart murmurs can be benign or pathological. Pathological conditions include leaky (i.e., regurgitation) or stiff (i.e., stenosis) valves, holes between chambers (i.e., septal defects), and metabolic conditions, such as anemia. Mur-murs can occur during or throughout systole, diastole, or both. They can be localized to a particular valvular area, or they may be diffuse. The sound, called a **bruit**, can transmit into the carotid vasculature. Besides location and radiation, murmurs can vary in intensity, pitch, and quality. They can be loud or soft, harsh or blowing, and high or low pitched in character. Respiration or position-ing of the patient can alter the murmur.

Benign murmurs are common in children and young adults. A common cause of a benign murmur is increased

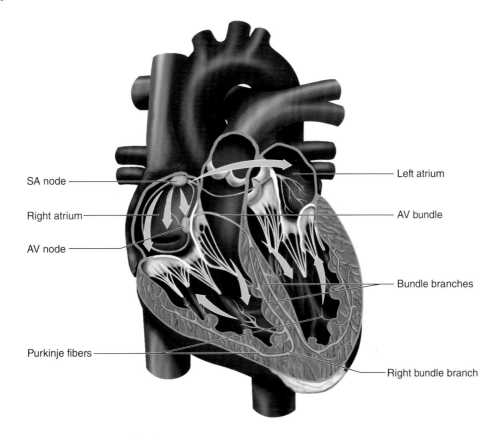

FIGURE 7.2   Electrical activity of the heart.

venous return and subsequent flow through the pulmonic valve. These types of murmurs are most commonly heard at the upper left sternal border or pulmonic area and vary with position (i.e., the loudest when supine, the quietest when standing). Often they are found incidentally on examination. Over time, they may disappear.

When the left ventricle contracts, a volume of blood called the *stroke volume* is ejected into the aorta and through peripheral circulation. *Blood pressure* describes the pressure that the blood is subjected to with each contraction. It has a peak, which is the systolic measurement, and a trough, which is the diastolic measurement. The difference between the systolic and diastolic pressures is known as the *pulse pressure*. The average blood pressure in adults is 120/80 mmHg.

High blood pressure, or *hypertension*, is defined as either systolic or diastolic pressure at or above 130/89 mmHg.[2] Conversely, *hypotension*, or *low blood pressure*, is defined as either systolic or diastolic pressure at or below 90/60 mmHg. Children have lower blood pressure than adults. In fact, a blood pressure of 120/80 mmHg in an 8-year-old suggests hypertension.[3] During dehydration from illness or heat, a drop in blood pressure caused by decreased plasma volume can occur. A fall in systolic blood pressure of 20 mmHg or more when accompanied by symptoms such as lightheadedness or fainting is called *orthostatic hypotension*. When this happens, the patient's blood pressure should be checked in the supine, sitting, and standing positions.

Blood volume is just one factor that influences blood pressure. Cardiac output, peripheral resistance, blood viscosity, and the elasticity of the large arteries can cause variations in systolic pressure, diastolic pressure, or both. Because of the potential variability in blood pressure, proper measurement is important. Making sure the patient is calm and relaxed, using the proper size cuff, supporting the patient's arm, and keeping the blood pressure cuff level with the heart are all important points to remember when measuring blood pressure. Chapter 1 gives instructions on how to take blood pressure.

Cardiovascular Adaptations to Exercise

The heart and cardiovascular system adjust to activity, and well-trained individuals gain tremendous health benefits from the adaptations. Resting heart rate and blood pressure drop with aerobic training and return more quickly to preactivity rates after exercise at a high intensity. The cardiac muscle enlarges with training, but it will return to pretraining size when athletes decondition.

Review of Exercise Physiology

Exercise is usually defined in terms of metabolic characteristics: dynamic or aerobic exercise versus static or anaerobic exercise.[4] Most exercise is a composite of both types. Endurance running and swimming are examples of dynamic exercise, whereas sprint running and power weightlifting are examples of static exercise.

In immediate outcomes, dynamic exercise results in increased cardiac output. Both components of cardiac output, stroke volume and heart rate, are increased. Enhanced cardiac contractility and increased venous return to the heart increase stroke volume. Blood flow is redistributed to the heart and skeletal muscles at the expense of the viscera while remaining constant to the brain. Vascular resistance is decreased because of vasodilation in the skeletal muscle, but blood pressure does not decrease because of the increased cardiac output.[4-6] Pulse pressure is widened during dynamic exercise. Maximal dynamic exercise results in a four- to sixfold increase in cardiac output, a threefold increase in heart rate, and a twofold increase in stroke volume.[5,6]

Heart rate and blood pressure increase in static exercise. The pressure increase can be dramatic, with systolic pressure exceeding 250 mmHg.[5,6] High blood pressure is required to maintain blood flow to exercising muscles whose vessels are being occluded because of the intense muscle contraction. Stroke volume, ejection fraction, and systemic vascular resistance remain unchanged. The higher pressures result in a higher cardiac workload compared with dynamic exercise.

Over the long term, dynamic exercise training results in increased cardiac output. The maximal heart rate cannot change with training, so increased cardiac output is the result of increased stroke volume. The heart adapts to the dynamic work by increasing in size, called *hypertrophy*. With this hypertrophy comes ventricular cavity dilation caused by the chronic volume loading. The increased diastolic volume permits greater stroke volume for less work. These changes can occur in athletes across the life span, including master-level athletes.[4]

Because stroke volume is increased at rest while cardiac output is maintained, a decreased resting heart rate occurs. This decrease in heart rate also occurs at submaximal workloads. Therefore, highly aerobically trained athletes have decreased resting heart rates, or bradycardia, compared with their less trained counterparts.

Blood pressure during ongoing dynamic exercise training in elite athletes has been commonly thought to decrease. This has not been supported in many research studies.[4,6] Scientific evidence, however, supports lowered blood pressure in sedentary adults after they engage in dynamic exercise training.[5]

Long-term, static exercise training also causes cardiovascular adaptations. In untrained individuals, small decreases in heart rate and blood pressure are observed.[4,6] Heavy weight training has been commonly believed to cause hypertension, but this has not been shown in bodybuilders.[4] In individuals with hypertension, however, chronic heavy weight training is not recommended. Pressure overload from chronic resistance training can cause cardiac hypertrophy without the chamber enlargement seen with dynamic exercise. Septal and posterior left ventricular wall thickening may also be seen.

Athlete's Heart

The term **athlete's heart** refers to the physiological and morphological adaptations mentioned previously, which an athlete's cardiovascular system may undergo as a result of ongoing exercise training.[7] Some of these adaptations can be confused with pathological cardiac conditions. It is important to allow healthy individuals the privilege of sport participation; it is even more important to distinguish athlete's heart from pathological disease and to minimize the risk of sudden cardiac death.

Both long-term dynamic and static exercise training can result in cardiac hypertrophy; these changes can occur after just a few weeks of training. Because heart wall thickness can be variable, sometimes as thick as 19 mm,[8] one way to evaluate whether the cardiac changes are pathological is to detrain the athlete. If the wall thickness shrinks, the previous hypertrophy was probably attributable to the benign effects of athlete's heart. A hypertrophic ventricle that does not diminish in size with detraining indicates possible cardiac disease or an idiopathic anomaly.

Preparticipation Examination

As discussed in chapter 1, the preparticipation examination (PPE) sheds light on any medical problems that may affect athletic participation. The American Academy of Family Physicians recommends an initial evaluation for first-time participation in school or college athletics, with annual follow-up questions in certain areas. One area of concern on both the initial and subsequent annual evaluations is cardiac health. The American Heart Association recommends that practitioners use the 14-point standardized screening guidelines, in conjunction with the multisociety-endorsed PPE, as part of the comprehensive physical to detect cardiovascular abnormalities.[9,10] Recommended questions for PPEs, including those related to potential cardiac problems, are listed here:

- Have you ever passed out during or after exercise?
- Have you ever been dizzy during or after exercise?
- Have you ever had chest pain during or after exercise?
- Do you get tired more quickly than your friends do during exercise?
- Have you ever had racing of your heart or skipped heartbeats?
- Have you had high blood pressure or high cholesterol?
- Have you ever been told you have a heart murmur?
- Has any family member or relative died of heart problems or sudden cardiac death before the age of 50 yr?
- Have you had a severe viral infection (e.g., myocarditis or mononucleosis) within the past month?
- Has a physician ever denied or restricted your participation in sports for any heart problems?

These questions are designed to alert the practitioner to potential life-threatening anomalies related to the heart and especially to sudden death events. Any patient who complains of symptoms consistent with these questions should be referred to a physician, preferably a cardiologist, before continuing activity, regardless of whether the patient has already passed a PPE.

General Evaluation of the Cardiovascular System

When the clinician is assessing for cardiac sounds, the patient needs to be in a still and quiet environment. The most important aspect of cardiac auscultation is to develop a routine and listen to five specific areas of the chest (figure 7.3) while the patient is in one position (e.g., sitting), and then to repeat the sequence of auscultation while the patient is supine (figure 7.4) and again with the patient lying in a lateral recumbent position. The five auscultatory areas are as follows:

1. Aortic valve: second right intercostal space at the right sternal border
2. Pulmonic valve: second left intercostal space at the left sternal border
3. Second pulmonic valve: third intercostal space at the left sternal border
4. Tricuspid valve: fourth intercostal space along the lower-left sternal border
5. Mitral valve: fifth intercostal space at the apex of the heart (midclavicular line)

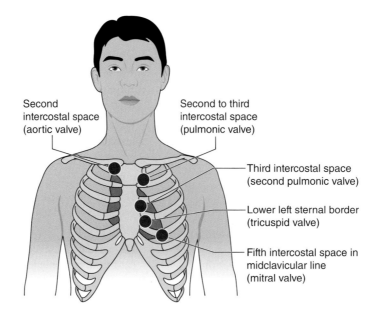

Second intercostal space (aortic valve)

Second to third intercostal space (pulmonic valve)

Third intercostal space (second pulmonic valve)

Lower left sternal border (tricuspid valve)

Fifth intercostal space in midclavicular line (mitral valve)

FIGURE 7.3 Frontal view showing the five traditional designated areas for auscultation of the heart.

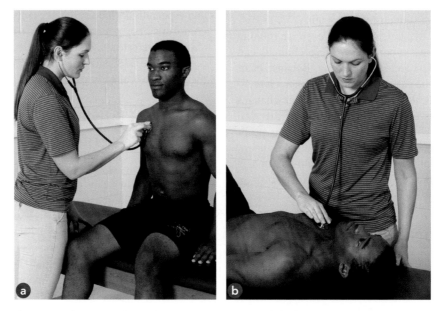

FIGURE 7.4 Cardiac auscultation with (a) the patient sitting and (b) the patient supine.

If the examination is not caused by an emergent situation, the clinician warms the diaphragm of the stethoscope before placing it on the patient's bare chest. When auscultating, the clinician explains what is being done before placing the stethoscope and always follows proper draping protocol when working with female patients. Cardiac sounds can be assessed on female patients wearing a sports bra if the stethoscope is placed on the skin under the clothing.

Accurate cardiac auscultation takes time. The examiner pauses at each auscultatory area to completely hear and isolate the sounds of each valve opening and closing.

This skill requires patience, practice, and a quiet area. The examiner listens for the normal rate and rhythm of the heart in each auscultatory area and then specifically listens for the sounds associated with systole (i.e., contraction of the ventricles) followed by diastole (i.e., relaxation of the ventricles). Diastole is a longer interval than systole.[3] When auscultating in each area, the examiner should also make sure to listen for adventitious or extra sounds or noises. The examiner should be aware that if patients are asked to hold their breath during expiration, S1 may be more predominant; holding the breath on inspiration will cause S2 to be more distinct.

The physical examination of the patient can be variable and nonspecific. In many high-performance athletes, particularly those who practice endurance sports, an increase in parasympathetic tone may cause resting bradycardia. Resting heart rates have been recorded as low as 25 beats/min in elite endurance athletes. Resting blood pressure usually is not changed, but it may be lowered. Third and fourth heart sounds may be present and are of no clinical significance as an isolated finding. Palpation may reveal a left ventricular impulse that is displaced to the left and prolonged. Because of the cardiac hypertrophy, 3% to 50% of high-performance athletes may have a mild midsystolic heart murmur.[10,11] These benign flow murmurs are best heard in the supine position and often disappear on standing.

The ECG in an individual with athlete's heart can mimic many pathological conditions. The increased vagal tone and resultant bradycardia seen in trained athletes are associated with a greater incidence of benign arrhythmias, such as **premature atrial contraction (PAC)** and **premature ventricular contraction (PVC)**, than in the general population.[10] Complete, or third-degree, **atrioventricular (AV) blocks**, however, are rare and need to be investigated for pathology. High voltage on the ECG is common and can skew the determination of hypertrophy. The most common change seen in the athletic heart is early repolarization of the ventricles. On the ECG, this is evidenced by characteristic ST- and T-wave changes.[12]

Pathological Conditions of the Cardiac System

This section reviews various pathological cardiac conditions that may be seen in patients. Rare congenital cardiac conditions are beyond the scope of this chapter. The most recent recommendations for determining eligibility for competition by athletes with cardiovascular abnormalities were published from the 36th Bethesda Conference in April 2015.

Sudden Cardiac Death

Death by sudden cardiac arrest (SCA) is a rare event in the young patient.[13] In the United States, elite athletes are viewed as near invincible because of their incredible physical feats. Nevertheless, it is reported that 45% of all catastrophic deaths in scholastic and collegiate athletes in 2019-2020 were attributable to SCA.[14,15] In 2021, 73% of the sudden deaths in middle school football players were attributed to SCA.[14] Additionally, 88.2% of catastrophic injuries or deaths among high school and collegiate athletes in 2019 to 2020 were attributable to SCA.[15]

Whenever a tragedy of this magnitude occurs, the public reacts with disbelief, and medical knowledge is

Clinical Tips

Potential Causes of Sudden Death

Sudden collapse in athletes could be caused by heatstroke, cardiac events, sickle cell trait collapse, or injury. Understanding the presentation of each will facilitate rapid response and the appropriate disposition.

called into question. Studies tracking these deaths during sports have used data from governing organizations, such as the National Federation of State High School Associations and the National Collegiate Athletics Association (NCAA), and from state and federally funded research groups for data collection, such as the National Center for Catastrophic Sport Injury Research (NCCSIR) based in Chapel Hill, North Carolina. According to the NCCSIR, there were 30 indirect (exertion/medical) catastrophic incidents assigned to a cardiac event in high school through college football athletes in the 2019 to 2020 academic year.[15] Sudden death cases in young women are rare, and the most common cause of sudden cardiac death is congenital cardiac disease.

The prevalence of sudden cardiac death in young athletes (age <35 yr) is estimated to be between 1 in 5,200 for NCAA Division I basketball players versus 1 in 53,703 for athletes in general.[16] This prevalence is much higher than statistics reported in a more general population of active individuals.[17] Male athletes, especially Black athletes, have a higher rate of SCA than do female, Caucasian, or Hispanic athletes. Men's basketball, soccer, and football have more incidences of SCA than other sports.[16,17] These data indicate that active people are not immune to cardiovascular events that may result in death.

Causes

HCM is the most common cause of sudden cardiac death in the young athlete, and it accounts for up to 50% of cases. Other significant causes of sudden cardiac death in the young athlete are coronary artery anomalies, increased cardiac mass, aortic rupture, myocarditis, and aortic stenosis.[17] Rare causes include dilated cardiomyopathy, atherosclerotic coronary artery disease, mitral valve prolapse (MVP), isolated arrhythmias such as long QT syndrome (LQTS) and Wolff-Parkinson-White (WPW) syndrome, and **arrhythmogenic right ventricular dysplasia**.[17]

In the older athlete, coronary artery disease is the most common cause of sudden death, and sudden death owing to coronary artery abnormalities is more common in middle school–aged athletes.[17] Rarely is sudden death in the older athlete caused by HCM, MPV, or acquired valvular conditions.[11,18,19]

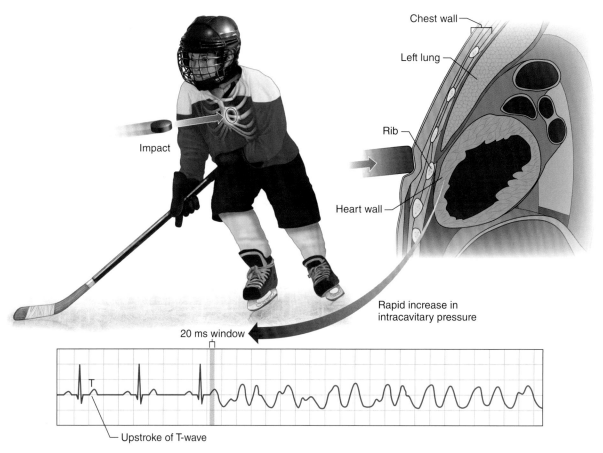

Chest wall

Left lung

Rib

Heart wall

Impact

Rapid increase in
intracavitary pressure

20 ms window

T

Upstroke of T-wave

FIGURE 7.5 The type of injury associated with commotio cordis is a blow to the chest wall that interrupts the usual cardiac rhythm.

Traumatic sudden cardiac death has not captured as much attention because its epidemiology is more difficult to track. However, it is a growing problem that strikes without warning. Between 1996 and 2007, a reported 180 cases of blunt-force death in the United States were attributed to commotio cordis.[20] Most cases involved children with a mean age of 13 yr, with 95% of the deaths occurring in males.[21]

Commotio cordis refers to trauma to the chest wall that interrupts the electrical impulse in the heart. If the cardiac rhythm is not promptly normalized, the individual dies. Typically, the ribs or sternum are not broken, although some contusions may be found. Research has found that a chest blow occurring during the vulnerable phase of repolarization, just prior to the T-wave peak in the cardiac cycle, can induce ventricular fibrillation.[20-23]

Although children and teenagers with thin chest walls are most vulnerable to commotio cordis (figure 7.5), deaths have been reported in adults. Sports such as baseball, ice hockey, lacrosse, and softball, which have hard projectiles that can strike the chest, have been associated with the greatest number of deaths. Commotio cordis also has occurred in sports such as soccer, football, lacrosse, rugby, and karate, in which the blow came from a soft projectile or a collision. It appears that the timing of the incident, rather than the degree of impact of the object, is the causative factor.[21,22] Commotio cordis is the only significant cause of traumatic sudden cardiac death in athletes.

RED FLAGS FOR TRAUMATIC SUDDEN CARDIAC DEATH

Sports with projectiles that can hit the chest at an inopportune time in the cardiac rhythm cycle have been known to cause commotio cordis in young athletes. These sports include baseball, softball, hockey, lacrosse, soccer, football, and karate.

Clinical Tips

Emergency Planning

Every athletic site should have planned access to an AED, to an emergency medical service, and to an established emergency action plan and should have medical personnel trained to respond to sudden collapse.

Prevention

Because death can be the outcome, prevention has become the focus of attention for commotio cordis. Changes in practice have ranged from protective padding to softer balls used in Little League and softball. Because this may not completely resolve the problem, another solution is defibrillation in conjunction with cardiopulmonary resuscitation (CPR). Defibrillation interrupts the heart rhythm so the heart can "reboot" into a normal rhythm.

The American Heart Association states that more than 350,000 cardiac arrests occur annually outside of the hospital, and that communities with comprehensive CPR and automated external defibrillator (AED) training achieve 40% survival rates for cardiac arrest victims. If defibrillation is performed within 3 min, the likelihood of survival is high. For every minute of delay, the chance of survival drops by as much as 10%.[13,106]

The advent of the AED has provided greater public access to lifesaving technology. These devices can be operated by trained laypeople and are increasingly affordable in all sectors. The AED is portable, rechargeable, simple to operate, and easy to maintain. The American Red Cross, the American Heart Association, and the National Safety Council offer AED certification courses in addition to CPR courses for the lay public. The NCAA Sports Medicine Guidelines require providing planned access to an AED and mandating CPR and first-aid certifications for all who work with athlete practices, competition, and skill sessions. In high schools, only 33 of U.S. states are required to have high school coaches certified in CPR.[24] Athletic trainers are required to maintain emergency cardiac certification, including AED use, but this is only helpful if the school hires a board-certified athletic trainer to provide medical care for their athletes. To provide rapid cardiac assessment of and care to those in cardiac fibrillation, AED access must be available near activity areas. Patients who suffer sudden collapse and have agonal or gasping breathing should be treated emergently because they are suffering from a cardiac event.[13,25] An AED should be applied as soon as possible for heart rhythm analysis and possible defibrillation.

Hypertrophic Cardiomyopathy

In the United States, **hypertrophic cardiomyopathy (HCM)** is the leading cause of sudden cardiac death in athletes younger than age 35 yr. This genetic disorder is characterized by an abnormally hypertrophied but nondilated left ventricle in the absence of physiological conditions, such as physical training, or pathological conditions, like aortic stenosis or hypertension resulting in left ventricular hypertrophy (figure 7.6). More than 400 specific gene mutations have been identified to date, and autosomal dominant transmission of this disorder

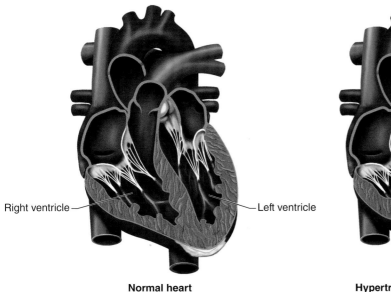
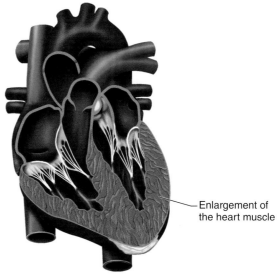

Right ventricle — — Left ventricle

— Enlargement of the heart muscle

Normal heart

Hypertrophic cardiomyopathy

FIGURE 7.6 Hypertrophic cardiomyopathy is characterized by an enlarged left ventricle and ventricular septum walls.

has been described. Therefore, familial history of sudden death at a young age is a critical part of history questioning during the PPE. Over the years, HCM has evolved from an extremely rare untreatable genetic condition to a common genetic disease with management strategies to help achieve quality of life.[18] The prevalence of HCM is estimated at 1 in 500 in the general population and is higher in males of African American descent, at least in collegiate athletes.[17,26]

The walls of the left ventricle thicken in a variable pattern in HCM. As often as 28% of the time, physical obstruction of blood flow occurs during systole. Up to 80% of individuals with HCM have abnormally small coronary arteries that may cause myocardial ischemia.[26,27] Cellular abnormalities include myofibrillar disorganization and death with resultant fibrotic scarring.

Although outflow obstruction can occur, the presence of left ventricular diastolic dysfunction is more common. Either outflow obstruction or diastolic dysfunction can impair exercise performance even in the least symptomatic person.[18,28,29] Both decreased wall distensibility and incomplete myocardial relaxation contribute to altered left ventricular filling, which leads to left atrial dilation and potential development of emboli.[30] Regional myocardial ischemia likely occurs because of the abnormally small coronary arteries and inadequate capillary density.[30] Adding random fibrosis of the cardiac musculature produces a combination of ischemia, fibrosis, and impaired vasodilator reserve that can lead to arrhythmia and sudden death.

Signs and Symptoms

Symptoms of HCM are fatigue, dyspnea, exertional angina, and syncope or near syncope. These symptoms may not correlate with the degree of ventricular hypertrophy or be predictive for sudden death.[9,11,31,32] Physical examination can provide valuable information, but the findings are not consistent. On palpation, an increased left ventricular impulse may be felt. Pulses may be **bifid** in character and exhibit a brisk upstroke. On cardiac auscultation, a classic, harsh precordial ejection murmur may be heard at the left lower sternal border toward the apex. The murmur increases with standing or the Valsalva maneuver and diminishes with squatting; however, a murmur is not always present.

It is important to consider differential diagnoses before determining clinical HCM. The clinical symptoms alone of exertional angina, syncope, and near syncope point to many conditions that could cause sudden death. They also can be related to benign conditions, such as dehydration or vasovagal syncope, or noncardiac conditions, such as asthma or gastroesophageal reflux disease. The potential for a serious, life-threatening condition, however, warrants an immediate referral.

Referral and Diagnostic Tests

Athletes with symptoms of exertional angina, syncope, or near syncope should be referred immediately to a cardiologist for evaluation. Fatigue and dyspnea uncharacteristic for a particular athlete warrant concern and certainly physician referral when accompanied by a heart murmur.

Standard laboratory tests, such as a resting 12-lead ECG or chest radiograph, have limited utility in screening for HCM. The most useful diagnostic test is echocardiography, or magnetic resonance imaging (MRI) with gadolinium contrast.[31,33] Increased left ventricular wall thickness (>15 mm) is the most helpful diagnostic parameter. The majority of male athletes and all female

---

CONDITION HIGHLIGHT

Hypertrophic Cardiomyopathy

Cardiovascular anomaly is the most common cause for sudden death in athletes. Most of these deaths are attributed to HCM.[18] HCM presents with a hypertrophic ventricle wall, typically the left, with the chamber size remaining normal (see figure 7.6). Since it is well documented that athletes, especially endurance athletes, benefit from an enlarged left ventricle as a result of their training, their condition can also be confused with HCM. Signs and symptoms of HCM, such as shortness of breath and fatigue, can be dismissed by the athlete as deconditioning or fatigue. HCM is an inherited disorder, and it is unusual for an electrocardiogram to provide definitive evidence of the structural defect. Family history of death at a young age, symptoms consistent with HCM, and an echocardiogram demonstrating an enlarged ventricle with normal cavity all provide more definitive evidence that should be followed up with a cardiologist before allowing athletic participation. People with HMC are typically limited to low-intensity sports, but there is a suggestion that those with a family history of sudden death at a young age as a result of HCM are strong candidates for an implantable cardioverter defibrillator (ICD) to allow for a more normal life.[18,33] It should be noted that no athlete with HCM should receive an ICD for the sole purpose of athletic competition.

athletes have a ventricular wall thickness of 12 mm or less.[27,34] Therefore, the range from 13 to 15 mm may pose a diagnostic dilemma because it is possible to have physiological hypertrophy in this wall thickness range; however, this hypertrophy has been reported only in male cyclists and rowers.[27,34] Another sign of HCM that can be seen on an echocardiogram is a ventricular septum or free wall thickness ratio greater than 1:3. Asymmetric wall thickening and decreased left ventricular diastolic cavity dimension (<45 mm) may also be present. In addition, the echo may reveal abnormal diastolic filling with decreased early filling and increased late filling and abnormal ultrasonic myocardial reflex activity in the athlete with HCM.[30]

Discontinuing athletic activities for a few weeks to 1 mo for the athlete with these symptoms may help clinicians to determine whether the problem is HCM or simply athlete's heart.[30] Hypertrophy of the ventricular wall will not resolve with detraining in a person with HCM.

As a diagnostic tool for HCM, echocardiography is the gold standard. Its value as a screening tool, however, is limited by its relative expense. If echocardiography were used as a preparticipation screening tool, the cost to prevent one death from HCM would exceed hundreds of millions of dollars. In the future, genetic markers may hold the greatest promise as effective screening tests, with more than 1,500 mutants in 11 major genes and more than 400 specific mutations now implicated in the pathogenesis of clinically diagnosed HCM.[18]

Treatment and Return to Participation

In 2015, medical experts met to determine safe standards for athletic participation for athletes with cardiac conditions. The collection of these papers is referred to as the *36th Bethesda Conference*. One of their many highlights was a classification of sports based on static (burst actions) and dynamic (aerobic) activities and their effect on the heart. In 2015, these papers were updated, and they continue to be specific to the competitive athlete and are the collective scientific statements of both the American Heart Association and the American College of Cardiology. These are summarized in table 7.1 and will be referred to often throughout this chapter. On the basis of the 2015 recommendations, athletes with HCM should be restricted from participation in all competitive sports, with the possible exception of low-intensity (class I [low static]) sports such as bowling, cricket, curling, golf, riflery, and yoga.[35] Furthermore, the placement of an ICD in a patient with HCM does not change the competitive sports recommendations for this disease.

The clinical significance and natural history of individuals who are genotype positive–phenotype negative

remains unresolved. However, no compelling data are available at present with which to preclude these patients from competitive sports, particularly in the absence of cardiac symptoms or a family history of sudden death.

Prevention

Detection of HCM can be difficult, but the patient's medical history, discovered in the PPE, is invaluable. A comprehensive medical history can reveal an autosomal dominant transmission pattern, a family history of cardiac disease, or a record of other premature sudden death in family members. Unfortunately, medical histories have not been as useful as expected because of the variability of expression of the trait. Nonetheless, the athletic trainer and the physician should ask about a family history of cardiovascular disease in every athletic PPE, as discussed previously.

Obstacles in the United States to implementing additional screening tests (i.e., ECGs, echocardiograms, or cardiovascular MRI scans) include the particularly large population of athletes to screen, major cost–benefit considerations, and the recognition that it is impossible to eliminate all risks associated with competitive sports. Although the number of large NCAA Division I programs using noninvasive cardiac testing (e.g., ECG or echocardiograms in the PPE) continues to increase, it is not yet common.[29,31,36]

Coronary Artery Abnormalities

Congenital coronary anomalies are a much less frequent cause of sudden death than HCM in athletes. They are characterized by either an aberrant (i.e., deviating or abnormal) coronary artery takeoff or the complete absence of a coronary artery.[37] Most reports rank coronary anomalies as the second leading cause of sudden death in athletes,[34,38,39] with most events happening during or just after strenuous exercise.[40]

Myocardial bridging refers to when the epicardial coronary artery becomes surrounded by myocardium for a portion of its course. This tunneling is seen in up to 25% of hearts at the time of autopsy after sudden death and usually involves the left anterior descending artery. Rarely does a congenital aberration result in clinical pathology, but the vascular compression from the ventricle during systole has been reported as an exercise-related cause of sudden death.[40] Tunneling of the coronary artery for more than 3 mm underneath the epicardium is the greatest risk factor for cardiac events.[41]

Acquired coronary artery abnormalities that have been associated with exercise-related sudden death are atherosclerotic coronary artery disease, Kawasaki's disease, and coronary artery vasospasm.

TABLE 7.1   **Classification of Sports Based on Peak Static and Dynamic Components During Competition**

Classification	Low dynamic (A) (>50%)	Moderate dynamic (B) (50%-75%)	High dynamic (C) (>75%)
Low static (I) (<10%)	Bowling Cricket Curling Golf Riflery Yoga	Baseball Softball Fencing Table tennis Volleyball	Badminton Cross-country skiing (classic technique) Field hockey* Orienteering Racquetball/squash* Race walking Distance running Soccer*
Moderate static (II) (10%-20%)	Archery Auto racing*† Diving*† Equestrian*† Motorcycling*†	American football*† Field events (jumping) Figure skating Rodeo*† Sprint running Surfing Synchronized swimming "Ultra" racing	Basketball* Ice hockey* Cross-country skiing (skating technique) Lacrosse* Mid-distance running Swimming† Team handball Tennis
High static (III) (>30%)	Bobsledding/luge*† Field events (throw) Gymnastics*† Martial arts Sailing Waterskiing*† Weightlifting*† Windsurfing*†	Bodybuilding*† Downhill skiing*† Snowboarding*† Wrestling*	Boxing* Canoeing/kayaking Cycling*† Decathlon Rowing Speed skating*† Triathlon*†

*Danger of body collision.

†Increased risk if syncope occurs.

Adapted by permission from B.D. Levine, A.L. Baggish, R.K. Kovacs, et al., "Eligibility and Disqualification Recommendations for Competitive Athletes With Cardiovascular Abnormalities: Task Force 1: Classification of Sports: Dynamic, Static, and Impact: A Scientific Statement From the American Heart Association and American College of Cardiology," *Journal of the American College of Cardiology* 66, no. 21 (2015): 2350-2355.

Signs and Symptoms

Symptoms preceding death from coronary artery anomalies are infrequent but include anginal chest pain with exertion, exertional syncope, near syncope with exertion, or exertional dyspnea. If there is any symptom with myocardial bridging, it is usually angina because of myocardial ischemia.[42]

Referral and Diagnostic Tests

Any patient presenting with unexplained exertional chest pain or an exertional syncopal episode must be referred immediately to a physician. An echocardiogram may demonstrate the anomalous takeoff. However, **cardioangiography** is usually required for a conclusive diagnosis (figure 7.7). This procedure is accomplished via a cardiac catheterization, whereby a flexible catheter is introduced via an upper or lower extremity vein. Through the catheter, medication can be administered (e.g., the dye in figure 7.7), tissue can be examined, and some procedures, such as placement of stents and angioplasty, can be performed.

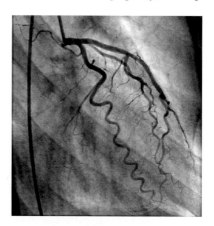

FIGURE 7.7   Cardioangiography showing a coronary stenosis caused by spasm.

© Katie Walsh Flanagan

Treatment and Return to Participation

At present, no medical treatment exists that can permit continued athletic competition for patients with congenital coronary anomalies, although the individual may benefit from β-adrenergic or calcium-blocking agents. In myocardial bridging, surgical resection may resolve the ischemia and allow a safe return to play.

It is recommended that the patient with an anomalous coronary artery retire from competitive sports participation.[43] If possible, surgery to re-create the abnormal artery should be performed; if after 3 to 6 mo the athlete is nonischemic during maximal exercise testing, then sport participation may be permitted.[43]

If there is no evidence of myocardial ischemia after surgery in a patient with myocardial bridging, the patient may also participate in all sports.[41] Any evidence of ischemia, regardless of the cause, will restrict the patient to low-intensity competitive sports (class I [low static]) such as golf or bowling.[41]

Special Concerns in the Mature Athlete

Whereas atherosclerotic coronary disease resulting in myocardial infarction is the overwhelming cause of sudden death in athletes older than age 35 yr, it is much less common in younger populations.[39] The tragic death of Olympic skater Sergei Grinkov at age 28 yr, however, demonstrates that it can occur. Usually, major risk factors for coronary artery disease are present, such as family history, hypercholesterolemia, and hypertension.

Coronary artery vasospasm is a rare cause of exercise-related sudden death. Although most athletes who experience vasospasm have some evidence of atherosclerosis, vasospasm has been reported in individuals with normal coronary arteries.[41] Patients whose vasospasms can be controlled with extended-release nitroglycerin and calcium-channel blockers have no restrictions on participation.[41] However, athletes with silent ischemia as a result of coronary artery vasospasm, who do not present with pain to warn them of ischemia, are limited to low dynamic and low to moderate static competitive sports along with the other cardiac conditions.[41]

Diagnosis of myocardial infarction is beyond the scope of this chapter but is mentioned here because of its relationship with coronary artery disease. When coronary arteries are ineffective in getting blood and oxygen to distal aspects of the myocardium, the tissue dies, resulting in myocardial infarction. Common symptoms of myocardial infarction include crushing substernal chest pain that can radiate into the left arm, neck, and jaw as well as diaphoresis, nausea, vomiting, and dyspnea. Sometimes these symptoms are nonspecific and easily mistaken for indigestion. Often a history of angina can be elicited from the patient.

While waiting for emergency transport, the patient may take an aspirin or prescribed nitroglycerin if available. The patient is given nothing by mouth if unconscious or unable to swallow. Oxygen can also be given if available. The athletic trainer must be prepared to perform CPR and defibrillate.

In older patients with coronary artery disease, several factors are considered when determining the risk of sudden death. These include resting ventricular function, exercise-induced ischemia, exercise-induced ventricular arrhythmia, and a degree of coronary artery stenosis.[41,43] Evidence of abnormalities places the individual at significant risk and requires restriction to low-intensity competitive sports, such as golf or bowling.[41] Reevaluation is recommended every 6 mo. The individual with minimal risk who has evidence of coronary artery disease may be advised to avoid intensely competitive activities, whereas other activity recommendations are evaluated yearly.[41]

Special Concerns in the Adolescent Athlete

Kawasaki's disease is a rare, inflammatory condition of unknown origin that usually occurs in young childhood. This acute, self-limited vasculitis is the most common cause of pediatric acquired heart disease in the United States.[43] If recognized and treated quickly during the acute phase, the cardiac sequelae can be reduced. Cardiac complications include coronary artery **aneurysm** in up to 20% of untreated patients.[107] Coronary artery aneurysms can predispose to myocardial ischemia, myocardial infarction, and SCA.[41]

Patients with a history of Kawasaki's disease who have no evidence of cardiac involvement, or who have transient coronary artery aneurysms and no exercise-induced ischemia or arrythmias, may participate fully in all sports 8 wk after recovery from illness. However, it is recommended that risk assessments are performed in increments of 3 to 5 yr.[41] Minor residual abnormalities after resolution of coronary aneurysms may limit patients to participation in sports such as golf, bowling, baseball, volleyball, and doubles tennis.[35] Unresolved aneurysms or stenoses place patients at significant risk of sudden death, and only sports such as golf and bowling are recommended.[41] Patients with large coronary aneurysms should continue with antiplatelet and perhaps anticoagulant therapies and be reevaluated annually via stress testing. These patients, along with those with myocardial infarction, should follow the guidelines for activity with atherosclerotic coronary artery disease. Patients with no evidence of exercise-induced ischemia or arrhythmias can return to or participate in low- to moderate-intensity static and dynamic competitive sports.[35]

To date, no guidelines for young patients with coronary artery disease are available. Any decision to permit athletic participation must be based on the extent of increased risk that a cardiac event will occur.[41] Athletes with these conditions must be under appropriate medical and surgical care.

Marfan Syndrome

Marfan syndrome is an autosomal dominant, heritable disorder of connective tissue and involves multiple organs and systems, including the cardiovascular, pulmonary, skeletal, ocular, and integumentary systems.[44] Aortic dissection and rupture, along with severe aortic regurgitation, account for the majority of deaths in adolescents and adults with Marfan syndrome.[45] The aorta typically has three flaps (tricuspid), but a bicuspid aortic valve is also common in Marfan syndrome. Maron and other researchers reported that approximately 5% of sudden death events in young athletes are attributable to aortic rupture secondary to Marfan syndrome.[34,38] Increased blood pressure, coupled with aortic stresses of exercise, raises the chances of a catastrophic cardiac event, which is why most people with Marfan syndrome are limited in their athletic participation.

The prevalence of Marfan syndrome ranges from 1 in 5,000 to 1 to 2 in 10,000.[45] There is no racial or ethnic predilection; male and female individuals are equally affected. There is a 50% chance that a person with Marfan syndrome will pass along the trait, but at least 25% to 35% of cases occur sporadically without a family history.[45]

Signs and Symptoms

Typically, people with Marfan syndrome have a tall stature, long and thin limbs, and an arm span-to-height ratio greater than 1.05 (figure 7.8). They have ligamentous laxity and are prone to scoliosis.[47] It is critical to note that multiple variations can be seen in other organ systems affected by Marfan syndrome. It can be very difficult to make a definitive diagnosis, particularly if there is no family history. Table 7.2 contains the requirements for diagnosis. Conclusive diagnosis usually requires confirmation by several specialists under the direction of a primary care physician. Many common clinical manifestations worsen with growth, such as **pectus deformity** and scoliosis; diagnosis is sometimes delayed until adolescence or early adulthood when scoliosis becomes obvious. Rarely, a spontaneous, nontraumatic pneumothorax can be a telltale diagnostic sign. Differential diagnoses for Marfan syndrome include any of the conditions listed in table 7.2 as well as endocrine disorders.

There is no single sign of Marfan syndrome; the diagnosis is based on determination of major signs over

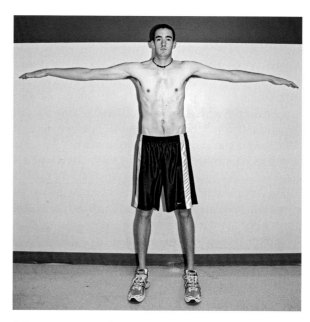

FIGURE 7.8 Marfan syndrome is characterized by an overly tall and thin physical stature with hypermobile joints, sternal deformity, and an arm span that exceeds the person's height.

© Katie Walsh Flanagan

at least two different body systems, with minor involvement in an additional system and attributes in the family history.[45] The five systems that can be affected by Marfan syndrome are the skeletal, ocular, cardiovascular, pulmonary, and skin (integumentary) systems (see table 7.2). A diagnosis for a patient with a negative family history must contain the skeletal system and one other system with at least one major involvement.

The major cardiovascular system criteria are dilation of the ascending aorta and dissection of the ascending aorta; minor criteria include MVP.[45] Any of these can predispose an individual to sudden death. Before the advent of echocardiography, such abnormalities were estimated to occur in 40% to 60% of patients.[46] It is now well established that more than 95% of patients with Marfan syndrome have cardiovascular abnormalities. Because it is impossible to determine whether a person has a potentially lethal cardiac abnormality without special studies, the athletic trainer and team physician need to promptly refer anyone suspected of having Marfan syndrome to appropriate specialists for further evaluation.

In a patient with Marfan syndrome, the mitral valve can have multiple abnormalities that may lead to MVP and to moderate or severe **mitral regurgitation** (figure 7.9). Regurgitation is evidenced on examination by **apical systolic murmurs**.

Aortic root and sinus dilation may be present at birth, whereas dilation of the ascending aorta usually does

TABLE 7.2   **Marfan Syndrome Diagnostic Criteria**

System	Major involvement*	Minor involvement
Skeletal	Pectus excavatum requiring surgery Arm span-to-height ratio >1.05 Positive wrist sign (thumb and index finger overlap when encircling the opposite wrist) Thoracolumbar scoliosis of more than 20° Pectus carinatum Spondylolisthesis Progressive collapse of hindfoot	Moderate pectus excavatum Hypermobile joints Dental crowding owing to high arched palate
Cardiovascular	Dilated ascending aorta, involving sinuses of Valsalva Dissection of ascending aorta	MVP Dilatation of pulmonary artery Dilation or dissection of descending thoracic or abdominal aorta (if age <50 yr) Calcification of mitral valve annulus (if age <40 yr)
Pulmonary	None listed	Spontaneous pneumothorax Apical blebs
Ocular	Lens dislocation (ectopia lentis)	Myopia caused by hypoplastic iris or ciliary muscles Abnormally flat cornea
Skin and integument	Widening of the dura in the spinal cord in the lumbosacral region	Recurrent hernia Skin stretch marks (striae atrophicae) not associated with pregnancy
Family history	Parent, child, or sibling with MFS Presence of mutation of *FBN1* known to cause MFS Presence of haplotype around *FBN1*	None

Note: FBN1 = fibrillin-1; MFS = Marfan syndrome; MVP = mitral valve prolapse.

*This is not a complete list of attributes for diagnosis, but the most common ones are presented.

Based on Asif (2015); Akerman et al. (2015); Braverman et al. (2015); Inna (2022).

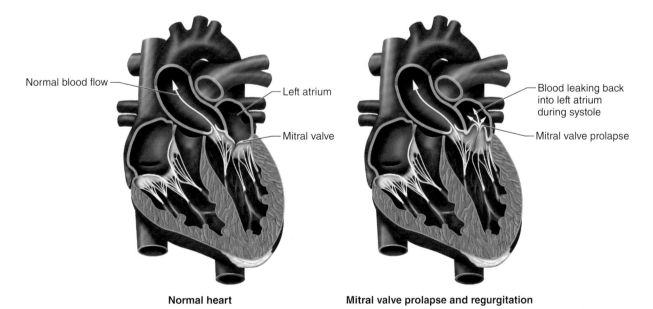

Normal heart   **Mitral valve prolapse and regurgitation**

FIGURE 7.9   Mitral valve prolapse and mitral valve regurgitation.

not begin until the child is older.[47] The rate of dilation is unpredictable, so it is wise to assess any enlargement beyond the time of long bone epiphyseal closure ascribed to pathological dilation.[47] The aortic root must dilate 50 to 55 mm to produce audible aortic regurgitation characterized by a diastolic murmur at the upper right sternal border. In a study of 3,781 athletes age 19 ± 5 yr, those with no inherited thoracic aortic disease had aortic dimensions similar to a control population, and only 11 athletes (5 men and 6 women) had an aortic root diameter over the 99th percentile.[102] Prophylactic surgical repair of the aortic root is usually recommended when the root diameter reaches 55 mm.[48]

The most dramatic cardiovascular manifestation is **aortic dissection**, which occurs in about two-thirds of cases.[49] Gurevitz and colleagues presented a case study of a 54-year-old extreme athlete (marathons, Iron Man races) who had no challenges exercising, yet an aortic dilation was discovered during a preoperative physical for a scheduled hand surgery.[103] During the emergency cardiac surgery, the aortic root and ascending aorta were replaced and the aortic valve was repaired. Following recovery, the patient resumed regular activity.[103] The greater the degree of aortic dilation, the greater the risk of dissection.

With the many potential manifestations seen with Marfan syndrome, a multidisciplinary approach to management is usually optimal. Musculoskeletal manifestations may require surgical intervention if cardiopulmonary compromise or progressive spinal curvature beyond 45° occurs.

Ocular screening is conducted annually. Ectopia lentis was found in 49% of patients with Marfan syndrome; 68% of these patients had bilateral extropia.[50] An athlete should not be barred from participation because of dislocated lenses, but contact sports are restricted because of an increased risk for retinal detachment.[45,50]

Treatment and Return to Participation

From a cardiovascular perspective, individuals with Marfan syndrome are restricted from participation in sports that risk body collision.[44] Athletes without a family history of sudden death and no personal evidence of mitral regurgitation or aortic root dilation may participate in class I (low static) and class II (moderate static) sports such as archery, diving, golf, bowling, cricket, curling, riflery, and yoga (see table 7.1); otherwise, only low-intensity competitive sports (class I [low static]) are permitted.[35,44] Serial 6 mo echocardiographic evaluation is required for continued sport participation.[43] These recommendations apply whether or not a β-blocker is used to help mitigate aortic root enlargement.

Prevention

An annual evaluation is the minimal requirement, and this includes a complete cardiac examination with echocardiography and possibly a cardiovascular MRI or CT scan. MRI or transesophageal echocardiography is used to evaluate or monitor aortic dissection. More frequent examination is required when the aortic diameter increases. Quarterly monitoring of the aorta once the root has reached 50 mm is suggested because the risk of dissection significantly increases at this point.[45,48] Research suggests that prophylactic β-blocker therapy may slow the rate of aortic dilation.[45] Once the aortic root diameter has reached 55 to 60 mm, surgical evaluation for aortoplasty, graft repair, or aortic valve replacement is advised.[48] Anticoagulants may be required, depending on the procedure performed.

Special Concerns in the Preadolescent and Adolescent Athlete

In children, mitral regurgitation may be a more significant problem than aortic root dilation. If mitral regurgitation is severe, mitral valve repair may be necessary, although the long-term results are not known. Mitral valve repair obviates the need for anticoagulation. This can allow the child to engage in mild to moderate physical activity. Some competitive sports and activities with potential for body collision must be avoided.[44,48] Depending on the situation, the child may need to be excused from all physical education activities. However, athletes with Marfan syndrome and bicuspid aortic valve (but no aortic dilation) can participate in all competitive sports, and it is reasonable for many to participate in class I (low static) and class II (moderate static) sports (see table 7.1), depending on the comorbidities of the syndrome.[44]

Myocarditis

Myocarditis is an inflammatory acute or chronic disease process of the cardiac myocytes, often resulting from enteroviral infections, most commonly coxsackievirus B. It can also occur in reaction to toxic agents or drugs such as cocaine.[18,23,51] It traditionally has been regarded as an important cause of unexplained sudden death in young people, and 5% to 22% of sudden cardiac deaths are attributed to it.[51] Cardiac dysfunction arises from inflammation of the myocardium, with necrosis or degeneration of adjacent **myocytes**. Healed or active areas of such inflammation may be a pathological substrate for cardiac arrhythmias, and physical activity may trigger a catastrophic event.[19]

Clinical Tips

Myocarditis and Pericarditis and COVID-19

Data from the COVID-19 pandemic are continuing to emerge. There have been published research correlations linking cardiac inflammatory responses (myocarditis or pericarditis) with messenger RNA vaccination (Pfizer and Moderna) for COVID-19 and, to a lesser degree, with the disease itself.[53-57] This is important information for athletic trainers. These signs and symptoms can begin during return-to-play training after disease resolution or after vaccination. Athletes who present with signs and symptoms of cardiac inflammatory conditions after COVID-19 illness or vaccination must be referred immediately to a physician.

Signs and Symptoms

Early in the course of myocarditis, the patient may experience what is thought to be a generalized viral illness with fever, body aches, nausea, vomiting, and diarrhea. However, the illness may be subclinical, and the patient can be asymptomatic aside from some mild fatigue. In a previously healthy person, symptoms of unexplained **congestive heart failure (CHF)** can herald myocarditis. These symptoms may include increased fatigue, chest pain, dyspnea, pitting edema, syncope, **palpitations**, and exercise intolerance. Sometimes the patient is asymptomatic, and sudden death may be the initial presentation.[52] **Pericarditis** is an inflammation of the pericardium surrounding the heart and may present with similar symptoms to myocarditis. Pericarditis is inflammation in the protective membrane surrounding the heart, not in the heart muscle. It is typically caused by a virus and can be either infectious or noninfectious. Athletes fully recovered from pericarditis can return to full activity after test results, including echocardiography and serum markers for inflammation, have returned to normal.[18]

The patient experiencing CHF gains weight, exhibits tachycardia, and hyperventilates. Auscultation often reveals a prominent S3 heart sound and rales in the lung bases.

Referral and Diagnostic Tests

An athlete who is having difficulty recovering from what appears to be a routine viral illness needs to be referred to a physician. Clinical tests such as a chest radiograph, ECG, and echocardiogram may demonstrate arrhythmias or acute CHF. Nuclear imaging can be used to pinpoint areas of acute inflammation. For cases in which the diagnosis is in question, endomyocardial biopsy is considered.[18]

Treatment and Return to Participation

Treatment of myocarditis involves using diuretics and antiarrhythmic drugs and is usually directed at preventing or treating CHF. Vasodilators and angiotensin-converting enzyme inhibitors are also used.[52] More than 30% of patients with myocarditis recover and return to full activity. One-third will experience residual problems, and the final third will need cardiac transplantation. Athletes suspected of having myocarditis need to refrain from all sports activity for 3 to 6 mo (a convalescent period) and then undergo an evaluation of cardiac status and ventricular function at rest and with exercise.[58] If cardiac function and dimensions have returned to normal, including cardiac serum inflammatory markers, and there are no clinically relevant arrhythmias, the athlete may return to competition.[18] Insufficient data are available to justify performance of an endomyocardial biopsy as a precondition for return to activity after a 6 mo recuperative period.

Prevention

Although the incidence of myocarditis is relatively small, the prognostic outcome for the majority of cases is poor. Health care providers should discourage ill athletes from participating in sport practice and events, particularly athletes with febrile illnesses. Such care not only will reduce the spread of infection but also may decrease the risk of contracting myocarditis.

RED FLAGS FOR MYOCARDITIS

- Body aches
- Chest pain
- Dyspnea
- Fever, night sweats
- Nausea
- Vomiting
- Diarrhea
- Mild fatigue
- Pitting edema
- Syncope
- Palpitations
- Exercise intolerance

Congenital Aortic Stenosis

Congenital aortic valve stenosis (AS) is most commonly related to a bicuspid valve malformation. The pathophysiology arises from impaired left ventricular outflow with compensatory hypertrophy of the interventricular septum and left ventricular free wall (figure 7.10). Of the recorded athletic deaths attributable to AS, the majority were Caucasian males, and death most often occurred during or immediately following exercise.[44,59] Other causes of aortic stenosis are rheumatic heart disease and degenerative calcific changes.[59]

Signs and Symptoms

A history of exercise-induced dyspnea or angina coupled with decreasing exercise tolerance are indicative of AS.[59] Patients may also develop significant myocardial ischemia and left ventricular dysfunction from the increased pressure workload of the heart. This can result in hypotension and exertional syncope, which may be accompanied by lethal arrhythmias. Another cardiac and noncardiac condition to consider that may present in this fashion is HCM. However, the characteristic murmur is definitive.

Referral and Diagnostic Tests

Patients with fatigue, dizziness, chest pain, syncope, or pallor on exertion require medical follow-up.[59] AS can be readily identified on clinical examination by its characteristic loud crescendo–decrescendo systolic murmur heard at the upper right sternal border (i.e., aortic area).

Treatment and Return to Participation

Untreated athletes with mild AS can participate in all sports if they have a normal ECG, exercise tolerance, and no history of exercise-associated chest pain, syncope, or arrhythmia with symptoms.[59] Athletes with moderate AS can participate in low static, low to moderate dynamic exercises and moderate static, low dynamic exercises (classes IA, IB, and A [moderate static]; see table 7.1) if they have mild or no left ventricular hypertrophy by echocardiography, no left ventricular strain on ECG, a normal exercise test, and absence of exercise-associated symptoms. However, athletes with severe AS or symptomatic patients with moderate AS are not candidates for competitive sport.[43,59]

Mitral Valve Prolapse

MVP is one of the most common cardiac abnormalities and is seen in approximately 2% to 3% of individuals, usually women.[60] Although MVP is typically benign, it can lead to serious complications, especially if there is significant mitral regurgitation. Although MVP is mentioned as a cause of exercise-induced sudden death, reports of sudden death are rare.[60] The etiology of MVP is unknown.

Signs and Symptoms

Symptoms include chest pain, heart palpitations, uncharacteristic shortness of breath, exercise intolerance, dyspnea, and fatigue. On occasion, patients complain of syncope or near syncope.

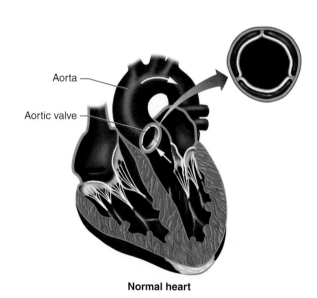

Normal heart

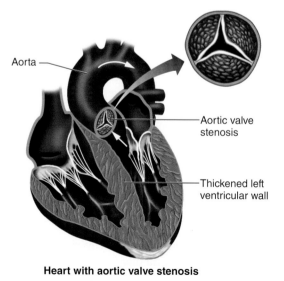

Heart with aortic valve stenosis

FIGURE 7.10 Aortic valve stenosis.

Referral and Diagnostic Tests

Any of the previously mentioned symptoms warrant referral to a physician. Diagnosis can often be made on the auscultative findings of a mid- to late-systolic apical click along with a systolic murmur. Patient positioning is important because both the click and the murmur vary with the patient's position. Squatting accentuates the click, and standing or Valsalva's maneuver increases the murmur (see figure 9.14). Echocardiography can confirm the diagnosis and record the presence of or degree of mitral regurgitation. Patients who complain of palpitations or syncope require cardiac event (Holter) monitoring. A Holter monitor is a portable device that records the ECG over a 24 h or longer period. It has leads with electrodes that are attached to the patient's chest, and it feeds information to a cell phone–sized receiver (figure 7.11).

Treatment and Return to Participation

No treatment is needed in asymptomatic individuals, and athletic participation is unrestricted. Symptomatic individuals may need antiarrhythmic treatment. Arrhythmias

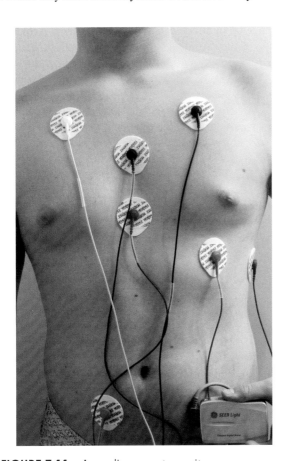

FIGURE 7.11   A cardiac event monitor.

Photo courtesy of Kathleen Knott / Johns Hopkins University.

are closely associated with MVP and are generally the cause of palpitations reported by patients. Although many arrhythmias have been associated with MVP, ventricular arrhythmias cause the most concern because, although rare, they have been assumed to cause sudden death.[18]

Participation in all competitive sports is allowed if the athlete with MVP does not show evidence of family history of sudden death attributable to MVP, moderate to severe mitral regurgitation, prior embolic event, or syncope caused by arrhythmia. If any of these conditions are detected, the athlete may participate only in class I (low static) sports, such as golf and bowling (see table 7.1).[19,61]

Arrhythmias

The electrical pathway that synchronizes and controls the contraction of the atria and the ventricles can malfunction without warning. Most of these malfunctions are innocent, but some are pathological. Arrhythmias can recur frequently or disappear for years, and they vary with activity. Most benign arrhythmias in the athlete are attributable to increased vagal tone and disappear with exercise. Pathological arrhythmias can compromise blood flow and blood pressure. Some can result in sudden death. It is now well understood that a subset of arrhythmias and heart blocks is inherently safe in athletic participation if certain criteria are met.

As discussed earlier, the electrical activity of the heart is generated via the SA node that the ECG depicts as two events, depolarization (contraction) and repolarization (relaxation).

Arrhythmias are divided into two groups depending on the structures they affect: supraventricular and ventricular. WPW syndrome and LQTS are associated with sudden death and are discussed here. Also discussed are supraventricular tachycardia (SVT) and ventricular tachycardia (VT). Other abnormal arrhythmic conditions are beyond the scope of this chapter.

A patient with a suspected rhythm or conduction disturbance needs to undergo a 12-lead ECG (see figure 2.9), echocardiography, stress test, and prolonged ambulatory ECG recordings (using a cardiac event/Holter monitor) as warranted. If this evaluation reveals no evidence of structural heart disease and the patient has no symptoms, the American Heart Association and the American College of Cardiology deem a number of conditions acceptable for full participation in sports.[58]

Wolff-Parkinson-White Syndrome

Wolff-Parkinson-White (WPW) syndrome manifestations include ventricular preexcitation and tachycardia resulting from electrical conduction over accessory pathways. WPW syndrome occurs in 0.1% to 3% of the population and is characterized by a short PR interval

Arrhythmic Conditions

Arrhythmic conditions requiring no limitation of activity in asymptomatic patients without structural heart disease include the following:

- Sinus bradycardia
- Sick sinus syndrome
- Sinus tachycardia
- Premature atrial contractions (PACs)
- Sinus arrhythmia
- First-degree heart block
- Sinus arrest
- Second-degree heart block, type I (Mobitz I)
- Sinus node exit block
- Sinus node reentry
- Wandering pacemaker
- Atrial tachycardia
- Premature ventricular contractions (PVCs)

(<0.12 s) and a prolonged QRS complex (>0.12 s) with a distinctive early depolarization, the delta wave.

It is fortunate that the incidence of WPW in athletes is very low, for it is rarely provoked by exercise testing. Sudden death as the initial manifestation of WPW is rare but well documented, and it appears to be confined to those patients with accessory pathways that have short refractory periods. In some patients, the occurrence of secondary ventricular fibrillation after paroxysmal WPW tachycardia has been occasionally reported.[58]

Referral and Diagnostic Tests

Patients with symptoms of palpitations, near syncope, syncope, or periods of impaired consciousness must have an assessment of functional capabilities and electrophysiological properties of the accessory pathway, in addition to a standard cardiac evaluation.[62]

Treatment and Return to Participation

Surgical treatment for symptomatic WPW is common. If a short refractory period is found, **radiofrequency catheter ablation** is often considered. This technique, carried out via a cardiac catheterization, which is performed via a catheter inserted through the upper or lower extremity veins, simply destroys the accessory pathway of the ventricle, thereby allowing the heart to resume its normal electrophysiological characteristics.[58]

Asymptomatic athletes older than age 20 yr who are without structural disease are unrestricted for athletic participation; younger patients may require more in-depth evaluation before they play in moderate- to high-intensity competitive sports.[58] Athletes with atrial fibrillation or flutter with a resting rate less than 240 beats/min without syncope or near syncope are at low risk of sudden death and can participate fully. Patients with higher rates or symptoms are limited to class I (low static) activities and should consider ablation.[58,61] After ablation, asymptomatic athletes with no inducible arrhythmia, normal AV conduction, and no spontaneous recurrence of tachycardia for several days are cleared for full participation.[58]

Long QT Syndrome

Long QT syndrome (LQTS) is usually a congenital disorder, characterized by a ventricular repolarization abnormality (i.e., QT prolongation) that can be idiopathic or acquired (figure 7.12). It affects 1 in 2,000 to 1 in 5,000 people and has a low rate of death in athletes.[63] Affected individuals may be at high risk of syncope and ventricular arrhythmias. The idiopathic form is inherited (congenital) in both an autosomal dominant manner and an autosomal recessive manner. Five genes are responsible for inherited varieties of LQTS. Seventy-five percent of individuals with LQTS have one of these varieties and, surprisingly, they have different triggers. One gene is triggered by physical exertion, another by rest and inactivity, and still another by auditory or emotional triggers.[63] Acquired forms of the disorder are usually the result of drug or electrolyte abnormalities. Regardless of how one has developed LQTS, all affected patients share similar signs and symptoms.

LQTS is rare in the general population and almost unknown in athletes.[19] Most patients are identified when a family member experiences syncope or sudden death.[64,104]

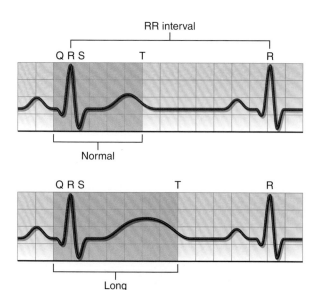

FIGURE 7.12 An ECG of the long QT syndrome (LQTS).

Evaluation for LQTS, particularly in a child, is prompted by unexplained seizures or syncope.[104]

Signs and Symptoms

Patients experience a varied clinical course from no symptoms to syncope with sudden death. Syncope is almost always a result of transient malignant arrhythmia, usually a **torsades de pointes** type of polymorphic VT.

Referral and Diagnostic Tests

Any athlete with exertional syncope or near syncope needs a prompt physical evaluation. The diagnosis of LQTS can be based on an electrocardiogram, but many asymptomatic people have normal ECGs. The corrected QT interval (QTc) must meet specific criteria to be considered prolonged but is affected by sex, age, and heart rate.[58] Borderline prolongation must be interpreted carefully, looking for reproducibility and other evidence of abnormal repolarization, such as prominent U waves and alterations in the T wave.[65] In 10% to 15% of athletes, the QT interval is prolonged, particularly in endurance athletes, but no relationship between QT prolongation and ventricular arrhythmias in athletes has been observed.[104] Tests such as cardiac event monitoring, echocardiography, and exercise stress testing may be useful for confirming the diagnosis in equivocal cases.[105] Genetic testing for the five cardiac ion-channel genes responsible for 75% of LQTS is now available commercially.

Treatment and Return to Participation

β-blockers are the most effective antiarrhythmic agents for LQTS. In acquired LQTS, identifying and correcting the agent or abnormality may be all that is necessary for resolution. Although the risk of sudden cardiac death is not zero in such individuals, there are no compelling data

---

Clinical Tips

LQTS Precautionary Measures

LQTS precautionary measures are outlined by the American Heart Association and the American College of Cardiology:[11,58]

- Avoidance of QT-prolonging drugs
- Hydration replenishment
- Electrolyte replenishment
- Avoiding dehydration
- Avoid febrile-related hyperthermia
- Avoid exertional heat exhaustion/heatstroke
- Access to a personal AED
- EAP specific to venue for patient with LQTS

Clinical Tips

AEDs and Asystole

It is important to note that AEDs are programmed to recognize VT and determine a shock is necessary to reorganize the cardiac pattern into normal sinus rhythm. The AED will not recognize a person in systole (without any heart activity); therefore, it will not instruct to shock the patient. It is critical to continue CPR until unable, or advanced life support takes over.

---

available to justify excluding athletes with LQTS from competitive activities. Because of the strong association between swimming and type 1 LQTS, these athletes should refrain from competitive swimming. Patients with LQTS and an ICD or pacemaker should not engage in sports with a danger of bodily collision because such trauma may damage the pacemaker system. Asymptomatic athletes with no documented arrythmias have no activity restrictions, except swimming and diving, if precautionary measures are in place. Once symptomatic athletes with LQTS-documented arrhythmias become asymptomatic for 3 mo, they are permitted full athletic activity (save for swimming and diving) if they maintain treatment and precautionary measures. There are no athletic restrictions for patients with genotype positive/phenotype negative genes, except for swimming and diving.[65,66]

Syncope

Syncope, or fainting, can be a challenging and frustrating condition for both the practitioner and the patient. The many causes of syncope range from benign conditions, such as vasovagal reaction, to life-threatening conditions, such as HCM or cardiac arrythmia disorders. In many cases, no definitive cause can be established.

Signs and Symptoms

The most frequent cause of syncope in young people is neurocardiogenic (i.e., vasovagal) in response to a trigger. For this chapter, the focus is on underlying cardiac pathology syncope, but there are numerous triggers, such as changing positions (e.g., prolonged sitting to standing), stress during or immediately following office medical procedures (e.g., biopsy, sutures), pain, severe emotions, extreme temperatures, use of certain drugs, or lack of sleep, hydration, or food. Symptoms are a prodrome of nausea, dizziness, blurred vision, and diaphoresis. The mechanism of neurocardiogenic syncope is believed to be the result of activated cardiac mechanoreceptors set off by forceful systolic contraction, causing increased vagal stimulation with resultant bradycardia and hypotension. Decreased venous return from abrupt postural changes in susceptible individuals as well as intense catecholamine release, as seen in anxious, fearful, or panic situations, can result in neurocardiogenic syncope. Athletic trainers may see a vasovagal response in the athlete who reacts to pain, observes an injection, or receives minor surgery. These are all anxiety-producing situations, and the athlete (or coach) can be apparently healthy one minute and suddenly collapsed on the floor the next. These causes are different from syncope caused by an organic or physiological abnormality. Nevertheless, the immediate treatment is similar.

Referral and Diagnostic Tests

Any case of exertional syncope or near syncope, including postexercise events, requires evaluation by a physician. A thorough history and physical examination are essential in assessment of the patient with syncope. The history of the syncopal event may dictate what laboratory tests are indicated to confirm the diagnosis. Standard laboratory tests include orthostatic vital signs, hemoglobin and hematocrit, blood glucose, electrolytes, and a resting ECG. Situations that call for a more extensive cardiac assessment are exercise-induced syncope without definitive etiology, a family history of premature sudden cardiac death, or physical examination findings of a significant heart murmur or Marfan syndrome. An athlete with a history suggestive of neurological syncope or an abnormal neurological examination receives an extensive neurological assessment as well.

Most cases of neurocardiogenic syncope do not require an extensive workup if the patient is young and the history is consistent with vasovagal reaction. However, Vettor and Zipes state that those who experience exercise-induced syncope must be evaluated for underlying cardiac pathology prior to return to exercise.[67]

Treatment and Return to Participation

Immediate treatment for a patient who has sustained syncope is to evaluate the airway, breathing, and circulation

---

Clinical Tips

Syncope and Sudden Collapse

Syncope is defined as a brief lapse in consciousness, whereas *sudden collapse* may occur during activity and has life-threatening sequelae. Any athlete who slumps over or falls to the ground must be evaluated for airway, breathing, circulation, and consciousness.

(i.e., ABC) status. If the patient is pale, sweating, and has good airway, breathing, and circulation, the immediate treatment is to raise the feet, thereby assisting the venous return to the vital organs, particularly the heart and brain. Further assessment continues as the patient regains consciousness and can assist with the medical history, including drug or supplement ingestion. In addition to the aforementioned cardiac anomalies, the individual may simply have skipped a meal, been dehydrated, or been exhausted.

Secondary treatment for syncope depends on its etiology. If the syncope is cardiac in origin (e.g., LQTS), β-blocker medication and disqualification from sport are in order. In other cardiac conditions, such as WPW syndrome, ablation of the accessory pathway cures the problem, and the patient can return to full athletic participation. If the syncope is neurological in origin (e.g., epilepsy), medical treatment may permit full to modified athletic participation. If the cause of the syncope is asthma related, medical treatment may permit full to modified athletic participation. If the syncope is vasovagal, correcting the problem can be as simple as improving nutrition or hydration or adding salt to the diet to regain electrolytes lost through perspiration and to maintain electrolyte balance.

In the athlete, syncope is a serious condition that requires a thorough evaluation. Straightforward episodes of vasovagal or **orthostatic syncope** dictate a cost-effective assessment. Questionable cases and those with syncope predicated by exercise must be examined for cardiac or neurological etiologies. Return to participation is dictated by the etiology of the syncope and how well the underlying problem can be controlled or eliminated. Vasovagal syncope is not cause for any athletic restriction, nor is syncope controlled by medication. Athletes with underlying structural cardiac conditions that led to syncope should be limited to the classification of participation outlined in the 2015 Task Force 1 of the "Eligibility and Disqualify Recommendations for Competitive Athletes with Cardiovascular Abnormalities" series.[58,61] Athletes with idiopathic syncope may not participate in sports in which transient loss of consciousness is detrimental.

Prevention

Prevention depends on what is causing the syncope. Maintaining proper nutrition, sleeping habits, and hydration can usually prevent vasovagal syncope. When exercising in the heat, the athlete who does not usually salt their food might benefit from some additional salt in the diet, because electrolytes lost through sweat could be the culprit causing the syncope.

Hypertension

Systemic hypertension is the most common cardiovascular disorder among athletes. Most of the time there is no identifiable cause. The elevated blood pressure (>129/80 mmHg in adults) results from increases in total peripheral resistance mediated by changes in plasma epinephrine and norepinephrine along with the **renin–angiotensin system**.[2] It is estimated that 25% of the global population has hypertension, with estimates of rising to 29% by 2025.[68] Systolic blood pressure tends to rise with age, with men sustaining higher blood pressure readings until age 45 yr, where women tend to have higher percentages of hypertension than do men. Whereas Black individuals have higher percentages of hypertension (50%) than non-Hispanic White individuals (23%), Mexican American individuals have lower percentages than both (20%).[68]

Untreated hypertension can lead to serious consequences, such as heart disease, atherosclerosis, renal disease, visual changes, and neurological impairment. It is also a major independent factor for coronary artery disease for all people regardless of sex, race, ethnicity, or age.[69] Therefore, hypertension should be identified as soon as possible and treated appropriately.

Signs and Symptoms

Although most cases are asymptomatic, hypertension is more likely to occur in people with a family history of the disease. It is also more common in those who are obese and in African American individuals. Symptoms on presentation can include headaches, malaise, visual problems, and exercise intolerance.

Referral and Diagnostic Tests

Annual blood pressure screening is an essential part of early diagnosis. Usually, three separate measurements that demonstrate elevated blood pressure—seated, standing, and supine—are needed to confirm the diagnosis (see chapter 1). Updated and more stringent diagnostic guidelines were issued by the American College of Cardiology and the American Heart Association in 2022 (see table 1.2). Proper conditions, positioning, and equipment minimize false-positive measurements. Clinical findings that may be detected in those with hypertension include cardiac hypertrophy, tachycardia, decreased pulses, bruits, retinal changes, thyroid abnormalities, and tremors.

When evaluating a patient with suspected hypertension, the examiner obtains a thorough history of diet, exercise, weight, and supplements and medication use.[2] High sodium intake can contribute to hypertension. It is important to consider exercise history as well because even an athlete can overtrain, resulting in blood pressure changes or deconditioning between seasons. Both situations cause susceptibility if there is a familial tendency toward hypertension. Body weight is often elevated, which is commonly seen in specific sports (linemen in football, throwers in track and field, wrestlers, and judo athletes) and can contribute to the problem. Many drugs can contribute to or exacerbate hypertension. Common offenders include caffeine, nasal decongestants, nicotine, appetite suppressants, and nonsteroidal anti-inflammatory drugs (NSAIDs). In addition, many drugs banned for those participating in athletic competition, such as ephedrine, cocaine, steroids, erythropoietin, and amphetamines, elevate blood pressure.[70]

Assessment includes taking serial blood pressure readings out of the office over a period to confirm that the heightened reading is not an artifact of being in a physician's office. The physician orders an ECG to evaluate for cardiac hypertrophy, urine tests for blood and protein, and blood work that specifically checks lipid levels, electrolytes, liver and kidney function, and markers of glucose intolerance and diabetes mellitus. Thyroid function is assessed as needed. If there are cardiac concerns, an exercise stress test may be indicated in addition to the ECG. Underlying organ damage must be evaluated.[70]

Treatment and Return to Participation

Treatment can be nonpharmacological or pharmacological and generally is based on a step approach. Strategies such as smoking cessation, diet and weight control, alcohol moderation, and exercise all have a role in the management of hypertension.[69] For most people, medications are needed to effectively lower and maintain blood pressure. This may be especially true in athletes, as they are already exercising, rarely smoke, and typically have their weight under control. With this in mind, lifestyle changes are encouraged and may limit the number of medications required for blood pressure control.

The several classes of hypertension drugs act in different ways. For the active patient, **angiotensin-converting enzyme (ACE) inhibitors** are the drugs of choice because they have fewer side effects with exercise. Commonly prescribed diuretics increase the chance for dehydration and heat illness. β-blockers restrict exercise capacity, exacerbate asthma, and are banned in certain competitive sports.

Patients with stage 1 hypertension (see table 1.2) can participate in all sports if there is no evidence of end-organ damage or heart disease; however, they should have a blood pressure assessment every 2 to 4 mo. Activities are focused on dynamic exercise, but static activities are not prohibited. Blood pressure needs to be under control or in the mild range (<140/90 to 159/99 mmHg) before an athlete engages in highly competitive sports or highly strenuous physical training. Blood pressure for a hypertensive athlete should be checked every 2 to 4 mo.[71]

Patients within stage 2 hypertension (>160/100 mmHg) are restricted from strenuous exercise, especially high static sports such as weightlifting, boxing, and wrestling, until their blood pressure can be controlled. Dynamic physical activities, however, are encouraged because few data suggest that strenuous dynamic exercise in persons with severe hypertension will lead to progression of the hypertension or exercise-induced sudden death.[70]

Prevention

Prevention of hypertension includes careful monitoring to make sure it remains consistently within safe participation guidelines. The NCAA mandates annual blood pressure assessment as a critical aspect of the PPE,[72] as does the American Heart Association and American College of Cardiology.[9,11,32] Early recognition of consistently elevated blood pressure can be addressed with nutrition, exercise, and, if need be, pharmacological interventions discussed earlier. The Dietary Approaches to Stop Hypertension (DASH) diet has been called the "greatest impact on young and middle-aged adults with stage 1 hypertension."[73] Further, it is estimated that the 8.8 million U.S. adults with untreated hypertension could benefit from the DASH diet, physical activity, and weight loss.[73]

Deep Vein Thrombosis

Deep vein thrombosis (DVT) is a condition in which a blood clot becomes lodged in a large vein. This results in venous blockage with stasis distal to the clot. Most of these clots occur in the lower legs (figure 7.13). However, DVT can occur in any limb. For instance, subclavian vein thrombosis, although rare, has been reported in baseball pitchers.[74]

Many factors contribute to the formation of DVT. In an active population, DVT is usually caused by trauma to the extremity from injury or surgery. Other less common causes include prolonged sitting (e.g., plane, bus, or car), hypercoagulability disorders such as **factor V Leiden anticoagulant gene mutation**, pregnancy, and **polycythemia**. Women who use oral contraceptives, particularly women who smoke, also have an increased risk of blood clots.[75] When DVT migrates to the lungs and becomes a **pulmonary embolism (PE)**, it is often fatal and attributes to as many as 300,000 fatalities a year.[76]

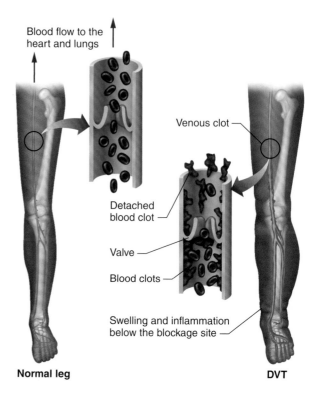

FIGURE 7.13 Although a deep vein thrombosis (DVT) commonly occurs in the lower leg, a swollen foot can be a sign of a DVT anywhere in the leg.

It is possible to confuse DVT with a more superficial **thrombophlebitis**, **postphlebitic syndrome**, ruptured Baker's cyst, or even cellulitis, as they all have similar presentations with a swollen extremity. Even the common problem of calf muscle strain may be confused with DVT. Usually the mechanism of injury can help differentiate a strain from DVT. If the patient has had recent surgery, traveled long distances while sitting down, or been subject to a known trauma, DVT is highly possible.

Signs and Symptoms

The symptoms of DVT are often nonspecific; some DVTs are actually asymptomatic. The key symptoms are limb pain, tenderness, and swelling. In the leg, these symptoms are worsened by standing and walking. On examination, there is usually distal edema of the affected extremity. This can be confirmed by comparison with the contralateral extremity. In the lower leg, the examiner squeezes a passively dorsiflexed calf, as a test for Homans' sign, realizing the test is not specific for DVT nor is it commonly present with DVT.[77] Measuring the patient's temperature can be important because fever may be the clue to DVT proximal to the knee, which is closely associated with the often-fatal pulmonary embolus. The Wells' Clinical Prediction Rule for DVTs,[78,79] which provides a score for predisposing factors, signs, and symptoms of DVT, has been validated as being useful for patients at low risk of a blood clot.[79] Pitting edema, calf swelling greater than 3 cm, and tenderness along distribution of the affected veins and collateral superficial veins are all score-worthy signs of DVT.[78] The thrombus is generally confirmed through Doppler ultrasound testing but may require invasive **contrast venography**.

Treatment and Return to Participation

Treatment requires anticoagulation, which can be started on an outpatient basis but may require hospitalization. After adequate anticoagulation is reached with heparin, the patient usually must keep taking other anticoagulants, such as warfarin (Coumadin), for 3 mo or more.[80] Anticoagulants must be monitored and adjusted following blood tests every week or so until the medication level is stabilized. Another, more expensive, injectable drug, enoxaparin (Lovenox), is also available and requires less monitoring than other anticoagulants. Note that mixing alcoholic beverages with anticoagulant medications is dangerous; alcohol can increase the blood-thinning properties of these drugs. Serious, if not deadly, ramifications can be caused by such combinations, and they need to be fully explained to the patient. Patients also need to be aware that NSAIDs (aspirin, naproxen, ibuprofen, etc.) alter the blood-clotting process and may exacerbate bleeding time. While patients are taking anticoagulants, collision or contact sports are not advised. In addition to medications, the patient's diet needs to include adequate but not excessive vitamin K.

Athletes undergoing continued anticoagulation therapy should not participate in collision or contact sports. Once anticoagulation is completed and if hypercoagulable evaluation is negative, a gradual return to play may be granted with careful monitoring for recurrence.

Prevention

Simple prevention is difficult, with the exception that all individuals should avoid prolonged sitting, such as when traveling by plane, train, bus, or automobile. As women age, they may need to consider an alternative form of contraception to birth control pills. Postsurgical and hypercoagulability situations require subspecialty care. Prompt recognition of symptoms by the athletic trainer is essential to initiate proper care of DVTs and to prevent catastrophic results.

Pulmonary Embolus

A PE can be a catastrophic complication of DVT. PE occurs when a blood clot becomes lodged in one of the pulmonary blood vessels. If the vessel is large enough, gas exchange can be interrupted long enough for death to occur before the clot can be dissolved (figure 7.14). Injury and trauma can also elicit a hypercoagulability response in otherwise healthy patients.[81]

Signs and Symptoms

Symptoms are not specific and can lead to a delay in diagnosis. Common symptoms include acute dyspnea and chest pain. Coughing, or coughing up blood (hemoptysis), are also signs of a PE.[75] If the embolism is large, the patient may experience a sense of impending doom. Fatigue and exercise intolerance may occur. Common clinical findings include tachycardia and tachypnea. Low-grade fever may develop, and hemoptysis may ensue.

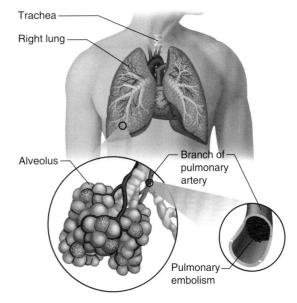

FIGURE 7.14 Pulmonary embolisms cause life-threatening emergencies when they occlude pulmonary vessels.

There may be signs of DVT, although many instances of PE occur without warning. There have been published findings of athletes suffering from PEs. One study followed five seasons of basketball players in the literature and found 15 suspected PEs, mainly male individuals;[82] two articles presented baseball players with PEs;[83,34] and one study each affecting a female gymnast athlete[85] and softball player.[86] These findings illustrate that although they are rare, PEs do occur in the athletic realm.

Because the symptoms of a PE are nonspecific, many serious differential diagnoses must be considered. Cardiovascular conditions range from angina and pericarditis to aortic aneurysm and myocardial infarction. Pulmonary illnesses include pneumonia, pneumothorax, and pleuritis. Gastrointestinal pathologies, such as ulcers, gastritis, and esophageal rupture, can produce atypical chest pain and warrant consideration.

Referral and Diagnostic Tests

When a PE is suspected because of acute dyspnea or chest pain, the patient needs emergent medical attention. A high index of suspicion is often needed to diagnose a PE because standard tests are of limited value. Special hospital studies, such as ultrasound, computed tomography scan, **ventilation–perfusion scan**, or pulmonary arteriography, are performed to confirm the diagnosis.

Treatment and Return to Participation

As for DVT, anticoagulation treatment is the mainstay of medical therapy, and hospitalization may be required in the early stages of treatment. Ninety percent of those treated with anticoagulants recover with no ascertainable sequelae of DVT.[80] At least 3 mo of anticoagulation therapy is needed. Continuation of therapy depends on the risk factors for recurrence. Athletic participation is limited in the same manner as for DVT.

Prevention

In most cases, the cause of the PE is not determined. For those with a defined cause such as hypercoagulability, long-term anticoagulation may be necessary.[80] An individual at risk of PE but unable to use anticoagulants may require a filtering device inserted into the vena cava; the device catches clots to keep a life-threatening clot from reaching the lungs. In both instances, athletic participation is significantly restricted depending on the activity and the level of participation. A study providing early prophylactic anticoagulation medication to those hospitalized following trauma, including those with long bone fractures of the lower extremity and severe head or chest trauma, did not demonstrate that the early intervention prevented early PE.[81]

Peripheral Arterial Disease

Peripheral arterial disease (PAD), also called *peripheral arterial occlusive disease*, is typically caused by atherosclerosis, usually presents after age 50 yr, and is more common in older adults. Risk factors include smoking, hypertension, diabetes, and **hyperlipidemia**.[87] In the heart, coronary artery disease is a subclassification of PAD.

Signs and Symptoms

The hallmark of PAD is intermittent **claudication**, which is a reproducible ischemic muscle, leading to cramping, weakness, pain, or numbness in the affected muscles. Most commonly, this is in the lower leg and is provoked by exercise of a given intensity and duration. In the beginning, the symptoms are relieved by rest. However, as PAD progresses, pain can also occur at rest. The key signs are diminished or absent pulses, arterial bruits, dry skin, and ulcerations on the heels and toes that are slow to heal.

PAD could be mistaken for many common problems, such as shin splints, muscle cramps, or arthritis. Lumbar spinal stenosis causes pseudoclaudication, symptoms of which occur with walking or prolonged standing and are relieved by sitting and flexing the spine. Individuals with these conditions do not have any pulse abnormalities or skin changes from arterial insufficiency. Claudication can also occur as the result of vein damage; this causes venous stasis, edema, and pain while resting. Other arterial diseases, such as arteritis and **Raynaud's disease** (see chapter 13), can mimic PAD. Neurological causes of peripheral pain, such as lumbar disc disease or diabetic peripheral neuropathy, may be confused with PAD. Another condition to rule out is compartment syndrome of the lower leg, which has both acute and exertional onset.

Referral and Diagnostic Tests

Clinical suspicion of PAD warrants referral to a physician for assessment. The athletic trainer becomes suspicious when an athlete complains of cramping or weakness in the lower extremities that worsens with exercise. One way to test for PAD is to measure the ankle–brachial index.[88,89] This test determines the ratio of ankle to brachial systolic blood pressures. The gold standard test is invasive angiography.

Treatment and Return to Participation

Treatment focuses on correcting the contributing factors, such as smoking, hypertension, and hyperlipidemia. To decrease the risk of stroke or heart attack, a daily aspirin is recommended.[87] Regular exercise with breaks when symptoms occur may be more beneficial than any medication. Initiating a walking program and gradually adding other physical activities, such as biking or swimming, are excellent for the patient with PAD. Surgical referral for arterial bypass is an important consideration for these patients, as PAD can digress to necessary limb amputation. Treating or resolving the risk factors can decrease the potential for deterioration. Return to participation depends on the type and level of activity. Risk factor modification is the best preventive strategy for patients with a propensity for PAD.

Anemia

Anemia refers to a decreased number of red blood cells or a decreased hemoglobin concentration in the blood. It is a common medical condition, and it can be a sign of a chronic disease such as cancer. The size of the red blood cell differentiates anemias into three general categories: microcytic, normocytic, and macrocytic.

Microcytic anemias include iron deficiency, **thalassemia**, lead poisoning, **sideroblastic anemia**, and anemias of chronic disease. Normocytic anemias include blood loss, hemolysis, chronic disease, dilutional pseudoanemia, and sickle cell disease. Macrocytic anemias include nutritional anemias related to deficiency of vitamins B_{12} and folate, drug-induced aplastic and **hemolytic anemias**, malignancy, and other hemolytic anemias such as enzyme deficiencies or red blood cell membrane defects.

In the athlete, decreased hemoglobin is usually the result of iron deficiency, exertional hemolysis, or dilutional pseudoanemia. These disorders are more common in endurance athletes, particularly females.[90] In a study of nearly 300 athletes (age 10-17 yr), 16% had anemia, with the sports of judo (37%) and basketball (34%) having the highest prevalence. The investigators found a significant correlation between anemia and short stature, suggesting that anemia may affect growth via poor oxygen distribution to growing tissues.[91] Because many other conditions can result in anemia and treatments can vary, it is important to be certain of the diagnosis.

Iron deficiency anemia is the most common true anemia seen in athletes. It is rare in male athletes unless they experience a gastrointestinal bleed, whereas as many as 5% of female athletes have iron deficiency anemia and up to 16% of female athletes are iron deficient.[90] This is attributable to menstrual blood loss combined with inadequate dietary iron intake.

Dilutional pseudoanemia has been labeled *sports anemia*. It is not a true anemia. The volume of red blood cells is normal, but the increased plasma that comes about from endurance training appears to dilute the hemoglobin levels.[90]

Signs and Symptoms

Anemia can produce symptoms of weakness, fatigue, dizziness, and headache. Patients are often asymptomatic if the anemia developed slowly. Decreased performance typically brings the anemia to the athlete's attention. Clinical findings include tachycardia, **orthostatic hypotension**, dyspnea, tachypnea, and pallor. Vertigo, tinnitus, syncope, thirst, difficulty sleeping, and chest pain have also been reported.[92] Mouth and tongue abnormalities suggest nutritional deficiencies. Less common clinical findings, such as jaundice and **hepatosplenomegaly**, indicate serious pathology and require urgent medical referral.[92]

Craving ice or constantly eating crunchy, raw vegetables may suggest iron deficiency anemia.[90] NSAIDs can cause gastrointestinal irritation with resultant blood loss, and continual alcohol use can cause similar findings.

Antibiotic use (e.g., penicillin, sulfa, cephalosporin) can trigger hemolytic anemia and acute illnesses such as infectious mononucleosis or mycoplasma pneumonia. In very rare instances, antibiotic use may trigger hemolytic anemia as a result of the immune system creating antibodies against red blood cell antigens. For more information on antibiotic adverse effects, see chapter 4.

Dilutional pseudoanemia can be indistinguishable from very mild iron deficiency anemia.[90] Because lead poisoning and sideroblastic anemia are extremely rare in the athlete, a microcytic anemia is usually a choice between iron deficiency and thalassemia. Other conditions to consider are exertional hemolysis and systemic illnesses such as infectious mononucleosis. The symptoms of hypothyroidism or depression also can mimic those of anemia.

Referral and Diagnostic Tests

A patient who presents with symptoms of fatigue and loss of energy and who bruises easily should be referred to a physician for a complete blood count (CBC) as well as other tests. Initial tests also include a peripheral blood smear. The CBC measures hemoglobin concentration. The typical cutoff criterion for anemia is below 14 g/dL for men and below 12 g/dL for women (see table 2.4).[90]

As previously mentioned, the size of the red blood cell classifies the anemia into one of three general categories: microcytic, normocytic, and macrocytic. The mean corpuscular volume (MCV), which is one of the tests contained in the CBC, allows for this classification. Microcytic anemia is defined by an MCV of less than 75 fL. An MCV of 75 to 95 fL defines normocytic anemia; and an MCV of greater than 98 fL defines macrocytic anemia. The degree of abnormality in the MCV can provide a clue to the diagnosis. Although both iron deficiency and thalassemia conditions have a low MCV, an MCV of less than 60 fL is more suggestive of thalassemia than iron deficiency anemia. Table 2.4 lists normal values for the CBC.

Looking at the size, shape, and color of the red blood cells provides valuable information to determine the type of anemia. Using the previous example of iron deficiency and thalassemia, the peripheral blood smear for both conditions will show microcytic cells. The cells in iron deficiency are hypochromic compared with the normochromic cells seen in thalassemia.

Many tests can be ordered to determine the presence of anemia:

- *Stool blood:* Can be done in the physician's office, or the patient can collect stool on special cards at home; can determine microscopic blood in the stool, which indicates a gastrointestinal source
- *Serum ferritin:* A measure of tissue iron stores, which are low (<12 ng/dL) in iron deficiency anemia and normal to elevated in other microcytic anemias; serum ferritin can be low and the individual not be anemic; although some authorities think that decreased ferritin is associated with decreased exercise performance, scientific evidence does not support this claim
- *Serum iron:* Decreased in iron deficiency anemia and in anemia of chronic disease; elevated in thalassemia and sideroblastic anemia
- *Total iron-binding capacity (TIBC):* Increased in iron deficiency anemia and may be normal or increased in thalassemia; decreased in anemia of chronic disease and can be decreased in sideroblastic anemia
- *Reticulocyte count:* A marker of red blood cell production; should be elevated in anemia, but it is inappropriately low in iron deficiency anemia
- *Hemoglobin electrophoresis:* Can be ordered to identify genetic hemoglobinopathies, such as thalassemia or sickle cell disease
- *Vitamin B$_{12}$ or folate:* May be decreased in the malnourished athlete (e.g., with an eating disorder) with macrocytic anemia
- *Bone marrow biopsy:* Invasive test reserved to determine very serious anemias, such as **aplastic anemia** that can be caused by drugs such as NSAIDs or antibiotics

Treatment and Return to Participation

Iron deficiency anemia is not difficult to treat. However, before treatment, one must identify and correct any source of abnormal blood loss. Historically, the way to rectify anemia was to supplement orally via iron pills. It has been reported that taking ferrous sulfate of up to 65 mg/d (iron pill) can impair iron absorption for at least the next 24 h. A response is expected within 2 wk, showing a weekly increase in hemoglobin. When the hemoglobin is back to normal (typically in 3-6 wk), daily iron therapy is continued for another 3 to 6 mo to reestablish iron stores.[90,93]

When it is difficult to decide between dilutional pseudoanemia and iron deficiency anemia, an empirical trial of iron therapy is tried. If the hemoglobin has increased after 1 to 2 mo of therapy, then the patient has iron deficiency anemia. In thalassemia minor, no treatment is required. In fact, iron therapy can be harmful.

Dilutional pseudoanemia does no harm, and competition is not restricted. Because iron-deficiency anemia can impair athletic performance, training and competition are limited to what the athlete can tolerate. Full training and competition are dictated by the athlete's degree of anemia and the demands of the sport.

Prevention

Prevention of iron deficiency anemia focuses on consuming adequate amounts of iron in the diet. Here are foods that are rich in iron:

- Organ meat (e.g., liver, heart, kidney)
- Lean red meat
- Dark poultry
- Shellfish (e.g., oysters, clams, shrimp)
- Eggs
- Legumes (e.g., beans, dried peas, lentils)
- Leafy green vegetables
- Iron-fortified cereals

The best source of iron is lean red meat. Although some vegetables, such as spinach and beans, contain iron, these sources are not as bioavailable. Also, some foods, such as breads, pastas, and cereals, are iron fortified. To enhance absorption, advise the patient to avoid coffee or tea and to drink orange juice or other drinks with vitamin C. In addition, cooking in cast iron cookware can provide some iron leaching into the food.

Hemolysis

Exertional hemolysis is defined as the intravascular breakdown of red blood cells as a result of the rigors of physical activity—in other words, premature destruction of red blood cells. Initially reported in runners, it was called *foot strike hemolysis* because it was believed to occur from the physical pounding of the soles of the feet. However, the process has been seen in a variety of sports from weightlifting to swimming.

Hemolysis may result in anemia and decreased iron stores. Hemoglobin released in the plasma binds to haptoglobin, which carries it to the liver for salvage. When hemoglobin stores are saturated, it may be secreted into the urine with iron. It would be rare for hemolysis to present with signs and symptoms because it typically displays as asymptomatic microscopic hematuria.

Signs and Symptoms

In a patient with substantial hemolysis, symptoms of mild anemia, such as fatigue and weakness, may be present. It is more likely that the patient will be asymptomatic. In anemia, dark-colored urine suggests **hemoglobinuria**. In **hemolysis**, it is more likely that the urine will have a combination of myoglobin from muscle breakdown and some hemoglobin, particularly if the inciting activity is intense or prolonged.[90,94] Because clinically significant exertional hemolysis is extremely rare, its diagnosis is one of exclusion. Pathological causes of hemolytic anemia, including red cell trauma from other sources such as cardiac valvular disease, enzyme defects, toxin and metabolic disorders, and paroxysmal nocturnal hemoglobinuria, are differential diagnoses and need to be excluded.

Referral and Diagnostic Tests

A physician orders the following diagnostic tests to confirm hemolysis: A CBC usually shows normal to mildly decreased hemoglobin and red cell concentrations, MCV is elevated but rarely exceeds 108 fL, blood smear is normal, reticulocyte count is elevated, and the serum haptoglobin concentration is low.[90,94] Examination of the urine may detect the presence of hemoglobin.

Treatment and Return to Participation

In most cases of exertional hemolysis, there is no anemia. Therefore, no treatment is needed if the person has adequate iron stores. Excellent prognosis and full return to participation are the norm for athletes who have exertional hemolysis. Prevention is important in the rare case of a problem.

Prevention

Prevention of hemolysis depends on the mechanism of injury. If excessive impact is to blame, then steps need to be taken to reduce it. Examples include better-cushioned shoes, softer running surfaces, and varying the activity with cross-training.

Sickle Cell Trait and Sickle Cell Anemia

Sickle cell trait (SCT) is caused by a genetic defect in the hemoglobin of the affected person. The altered hemoglobin, called hemoglobin S, causes a chronic hemolytic anemia because the abnormally sickle-shaped defective red blood cells (figure 7.15) logjam, producing ischemia in distal areas. This is characterized by decreased red blood cell survival, microvascular occlusions from sickling in which the cells stick together, and increased susceptibility to certain infections. These complications result in significant morbidity and a decreased life expectancy.[95,96] It is estimated that 8% of the U.S. population has SCT, and the largest percentage of this group are people of African ancestry.[97]

People with SCT have the abnormal gene from one parent, whereas those with **sickle cell anemia**, also termed *sickle cell disease*, have abnormal genes from both parents. In the athlete with sickle cell anemia, the average hemoglobin concentration is 50% to 66% of normal counts, which is prohibitive for binding oxygen to the red blood cells. Until recently, only in very rare instances would a person with sickle cell anemia be able to participate in sports and that would be restricted to the least physically demanding. The challenge with allowing athletes with sickle cell anemia to participate is that there were no evidence-based data to deem it safe with confidence.[96-99] In controlled studies, it was demonstrated that

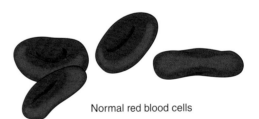

Normal red blood cells

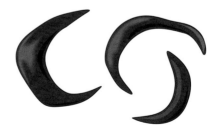

Sickle cells

FIGURE 7.15 Comparison of normal red blood cells and sickle cells.

both children and adults with sickle cell anemia had substantially lower cardiovascular fitness than people without sickle cell anemia; however, Liem stated that "safety data from several studies in both adults and children with SCA [sickle cell anemia] that use maximal cardiopulmonary exercise testing to measure fitness suggest that exercising with increasing intensity until exhaustion appears to be safe and does not result in adverse events."[99] Newer data show a distinct benefit with regular exercise in the athlete with sickle cell anemia, but it is a careful balance that requires individual planning and careful monitoring.[99]

People with SCT are not prohibited from athletic participation. Those with the trait are not anemic, and they have a normal life expectancy. Approximately 1 in 12 African American individuals has SCT. In contrast, only 1 in 10,000 Caucasians carries the trait.

Unfortunately, there have been some rare deaths in athletes with SCT associated with extreme environmental conditions, such as altitude or hot, humid conditions, in combination with high-intensity workouts. In a 38 yr period, there were 25,664 sickle cell anemia-related deaths in Black Americans.[98] The study found that acute causes of death were more common in younger age groups. In 2021, there were two exertion-related deaths in scholastic and collegiate football athletes as a result of complications from SCT.[14] Ischemia resulting from sickling may cause **rhabdomyolysis**, **lactic acidosis**, and shock.[72] To differentiate exercise-induced rhabdomyolysis (caused by repeated high-intensity physical exertion) and rhabdomyolysis, a new acronym was formed: ECAST, which is exercise collapse associated with SCT.[99] People with SCT are prone to heat illness because they have an inability to concentrate their urine, which makes them prone to dehydration. It is not known if this has been a factor in these rare deaths. All 50 states test for SCT at birth, and confirmation of this status is mandated by the NCAA prior to participation in athletics.[72,95] The presence of SCT is not prohibitive in athletics, but knowledge of it can preemptively allow education and awareness that could prevent a sickling collapse. Athletic trainers should be aware of the sickle cell status of their athletes and be proactive in preventing a sickling crisis.

Signs and Symptoms

The signs and symptoms of sickle cell anemia or trait often present in specific environments. Early, preseason practice in a hot, humid environment or events at high altitude tend to lead to attacks in a previously undiagnosed athlete. In addition, intensive exercise such as sprinting and intervals can be the trigger, and sickling can begin as soon as 2 to 3 min into intense, all-out exertion.[72,96,100] Often the athlete develops an ischemic-like pain from working muscles robbed of blood supply, similar to the pain of intermittent claudication when leg arteries are

narrowed by atherosclerosis. With sickling, the athlete's legs become weak and wobbly (without a prodrome of muscle twinges) and can no longer hold up the patient. On examination, the muscles look and feel normal as opposed to heat cramping, which presents with more excruciating pain and large, rock-hard muscles in full contraction.[101] This is an emergency situation. The collapse of an athlete from sickle cell anemia or trait, if not witnessed, can be confused with heat cramps, heatstroke, malignant hyperthermia, syncope, or cardiac arrest.

Referral and Diagnostic Tests

Athletes suffering from heatstroke usually do not collapse within the first 30 min of practice, and those suffering from cardiac collapse are typically unable to communicate. Collapse as a result of sickling is sudden; it occurs early in an intense activity, and the victim can verbally articulate. SCT collapse requires oxygen and emergency transport to a hospital equipped to handle such an emergency. If prompt diagnosis and management are not undertaken, the athlete may go into shock, experience multisystem organ failure, and die. Diagnosis of SCT can be made with a Sickledex test, with confirmation by **hemoglobin electrophoresis**.

Treatment and Return to Participation

The athletic trainer should confirm athletes' sickle cell status in the PPE via documentation of the test. Recognition, emergent first aid (ABCs, oxygen), administration of high-flow oxygen (15 lpm) with a nonrebreather mask, and transport to the hospital emergency department for

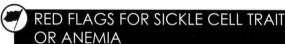

RED FLAGS FOR SICKLE CELL TRAIT OR ANEMIA

- Heat intolerance
- Severe muscular cramping
- Affected muscles feel normal, not hard or contracted
- Hyperventilation
- Tachycardia
- Hypotension
- Symptomatic indicators in high-altitude environments
- Symptomatic indicators after intense exercise
- Sudden onset, early in the practice or training session

appropriate care are necessary and may decrease the likelihood of the patient going into acute renal failure or multisystem organ failure.

If the athlete survives an episode of complete sickle cell anemia or trait collapse, restriction from similar exercise settings or environmental conditions is warranted. This is an individual case-by-case situation and may mean that the athlete is disqualified from that competitive sport.

Prevention

The following are some guidelines for working with athletes with SCT:

- Athletes should build up slowly in training with paced progressions, allowing longer periods of rest and recovery between repetitions.

- Encourage participation in preseason strength and conditioning programs to enhance the preparedness of athletes for performance testing, which should be sport specific. Exclude participation in performance tests such as timed/repeat sprints.

- Athletes should cease activity with the onset of symptoms.

- Allow athletes with SCT to set their own pace.

- Encourage the athlete to participate in a year-round strength and conditioning program that is consistent with the individual's needs, goals, abilities, and sport-specific demands. Extended recovery between repetitions of sprints and/or interval training should be allowed.

- Carefully monitor athletes with SCT who are new to altitude.

- Ambient heat stress, dehydration, asthma, illness, and altitude predispose the athlete with sickle cell anemia to the onset of crisis with physical exertion.

The medical staff must adjust work/rest cycles for environmental heat stress, emphasize hydration, control asthma, withhold participation when the athlete is ill, and watch closely at high altitudes.[34,100,101] Since 2009, the NCAA has mandated that all athletes be confirmed for status of SCT.[72] Those involved with the athlete, including peers, parents, and coaches, need to understand the warning signs of collapse and the consequences of inaction. Health care professionals need to consider screening other physically active patients for SCT, which is relatively inexpensive.

Summary

Conditions that affect the cardiovascular system can have catastrophic sequelae in athletes and physically active individuals. Appreciating the anatomy and physiology of the cardiovascular system is one way to understand the demands placed on this system. Another is to understand the various cardiac arrhythmias and abnormalities, their effect on the human body, and the implications of both on strenuous activity. This chapter highlights some cardiovascular abnormalities that can create problems for athletic participation, how to recognize them, and when to refer a patient who exhibits them to a physician.

The preparticipation history and examination are critical to the identification of cardiovascular problems. The initial examination offers the best opportunity to seek additional medical evaluation. Having access to AEDs and trained personnel is crucial, as is knowledge of the venue-specific emergency plan. Many athletes with cardiovascular conditions have long and productive careers within safe parameters because of early discovery and proper treatment of their conditions.

Apply It!

Go to HK*Propel* to complete the case studies for this chapter.

Gastrointestinal System

At the completion of this chapter the reader should be able to do the following:

1. Describe the basic anatomy of the abdomen and the gastrointestinal system.

2. Perform a basic examination of the gastrointestinal system, including history, inspection, auscultation, percussion, and palpation.

3. Recognize conditions of the gastrointestinal system that require referral.

4. Describe appropriate initial management of common disorders of the gastrointestinal tract.

5. Recognize conditions of the gastrointestinal system that may preclude the patient from participation, and recognize which symptoms are self-limiting.

Health care providers often hear complaints about abdominal pain or discomfort. Nausea, diarrhea, and constipation account for some of these complaints, whereas heartburn and gastroesophageal reflux account for others. For the physically active, common causes of gastrointestinal complaints include the stress of hectic schedules and travel for competition and the consumption of greasy or spicy foods. Gastrointestinal disorders are often transient; although they may affect performance or the ability to compete, they usually are not serious. Fortunately, because they work closely with athletes and patients, athletic trainers can identify more serious gastrointestinal conditions that require further medical evaluation and treatment.

This chapter reviews the anatomy and physiology of the gastrointestinal system and procedures for evaluating the abdominal area, including auscultation, palpation, and percussion. This chapter also presents common disorders of the gastrointestinal system, including signs and symptoms, diagnostic tests, and differential diagnoses. Treatment of selected conditions and implications for athletic participation are also discussed.

Overview of Anatomy and Physiology

The gastrointestinal system is composed primarily of a long tube between the mouth and the anus that serves to process food and fluids (figure 8.1). The alimentary tract performs several vital functions, from the ingestion of solids and liquids, to the absorption and balancing of electrolytes, and, finally, to waste production and excretion. For athletes, it is unlikely that sport will cause significant gastrointestinal problems; yet gastrointestinal problems are common, and they can affect athletic performance.

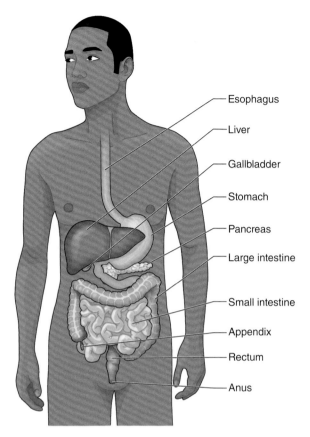

FIGURE 8.1 The gastrointestinal system is composed of a long tube between the mouth and the anus that serves to process food and fluids.

The major organs of the gastrointestinal tract start with the esophagus, which connects the mouth to the stomach via a muscular band called the *gastroesophageal junction* or lower esophageal sphincter. The mouth and teeth, although part of the gastrointestinal tract, are discussed in chapter 12. Within the pouch of the stomach, hydrochloric acid and enzymes, such as pepsin and gastric lipase, serve to break down food for later absorption in the intestines. The stomach empties through another muscular ring, the pyloric sphincter, into the duodenum, the first portion of the small intestine.

The small intestine is about 21 ft long, and it comprises the duodenum, jejunum, and ileum. The small intestine completes the digestive breakdown of food with enzymes produced by the pancreas and liver. Nutrients are absorbed throughout the length of the small intestine as it coils back and forth and joins the large intestine in the lower right portion of the abdomen. This connection also has the ileocecal valve, which is designed to prevent fecal material in the large intestine from backing up into the small intestine. There is a small blind pouch called the *cecum* at this end of the large intestine, and the small wormlike (vermiform) appendix originates from the base of the pouch. The large intestine or colon serves to absorb

water and produce neutralizing mucus as it ascends up the right side of the abdomen (the ascending colon), traverses across the upper abdomen (the transverse colon), and then descends down the left side (the descending colon). The colon also hosts numerous bacteria that further decompose food residue. As the descending colon comes to an end at the lower right side of the abdomen, it produces an S-shaped curve called the *sigmoid colon*. This in turn empties into the rectum, and together they serve as the primary storage location for solid or semisolid waste. Finally, the rectum ends with the sophisticated musculature of the anal canal and then the anus.

Among the many important organs in the abdomen, the gastrointestinal tract includes the liver, gallbladder, pancreas, and spleen as well as the kidneys and related structures (figure 8.2). Each of these essential organs helps digestive and absorptive functions of the gastrointestinal system.

The liver is a large organ located under the right diaphragm that has the following crucial functions in metabolism: storing vitamins and iron, filtering toxins from the blood, and producing critical blood proteins. Bile is produced in the liver and stored in the saclike gallbladder, where it is periodically released into the duodenum to help in the absorption of fats. The pancreas sits below the stomach and assists digestion by producing several enzymes that are also released into the duodenum. In addition, the pancreas produces the essential hormones insulin and glucagon that are released into the bloodstream to maintain blood sugar (i.e., glucose) levels.

Most abdominal organs and the inner lining of the abdominal cavity are covered with a protective membrane called the *peritoneum*. When the peritoneum becomes inflamed or irritated by blood or infection, the entire abdomen can become very tender, and the muscles of the abdominal wall may become rigid. Individual sensory nerves do not innervate each organ within the peritoneum, which is why abdominal pain is not necessarily specific to the origin (location) of pathology.

The rectus abdominis muscle and the internal and external oblique muscles serve to protect the organs of the abdominal cavity (figure 8.3). Just like muscles elsewhere in the body, they can be injured by overuse, acute strain, or contusions. For the patient with abdominal pain, distinguishing whether the pain is from the internal organs or the overlying muscles is important. Sometimes this distinction can be difficult, or there may be problems with both.

When referring to the abdomen, clinicians will typically divide it into quadrants. The midline extends from the center of the sternum through the pubic bone, and the horizontal line extends through the umbilicus. This creates right and left upper and lower quadrants, commonly referred to as the RUQ, LUQ, RLQ, and LLQ, respectively. Here are structures that are within these quadrants:

The image labels (top to bottom): Esophagus, Liver, Gallbladder, Stomach, Pancreas, Large intestine, Small intestine, Appendix, Rectum, Anus

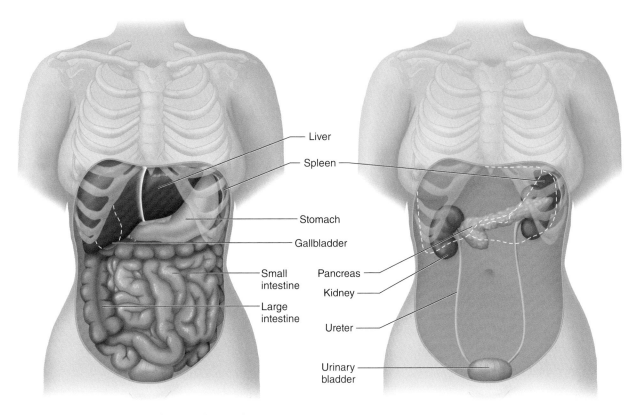

FIGURE 8.2   Structures of the abdominal cavity.

Right upper quadrant

Liver

Gallbladder

Duodenum

Head of pancreas

Right adrenal gland

Portion of right kidney

Portions of ascending and transverse colon

Left upper quadrant

Left lobe of liver

Spleen

Stomach

Body of pancreas

Left adrenal gland

Portion of left kidney

Portions of ascending and transverse colon

Right lower quadrant

Lower pole of right kidney

Cecum and appendix

Portion of ascending colon

Bladder

Ovary

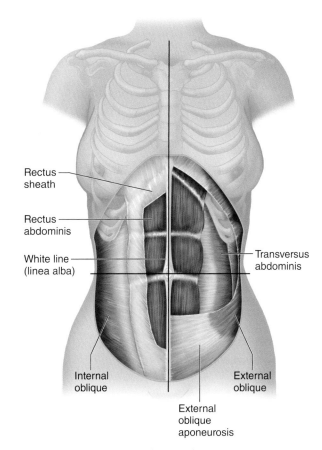

FIGURE 8.3   Abdominal musculature.

Uterus (if enlarged)

Right spermatic cord

Right ureter

Left lower quadrant

Lower pole of left kidney

Sigmoid colon

Portion of descending colon

Bladder

Ovary

Uterus (if enlarged)

Left spermatic cord

Left ureter

This distinction becomes important and helpful in diagnosing many conditions.[1] Appendicitis, for example, will typically cause RLQ pain, whereas constipation can cause LLQ pain. Here are common causes of abdominal pain in different anatomical locations:

Right upper quadrant

Cholecystitis

Duodenal ulcer

Hepatitis

Pneumonia

Left upper quadrant

Abdominal aortic aneurysm

Gastric ulcer

Pneumonia

Splenic laceration or rupture

Periumbilical

Abdominal aortic aneurysm

Diverticulitis

Early appendicitis

Intestinal obstruction

Right lower quadrant

Appendicitis

Ectopic pregnancy

Hernia

Ovarian cysts

Pelvic infection

Renal stone

Left lower quadrant

Constipation

Diverticulitis

Ectopic pregnancy

Hernia

Ovarian cysts

Pelvic infection

Other clinicians may use the nine-region classification, which uses two imaginary horizontal lines and vertical lines to divide the abdomen into regions (figure 8.4). Anatomical correlates of the nine regions of the abdomen are listed here:

Epigastric region

Pyloric end of stomach

Duodenum

Pancreas

Portion of liver

Umbilical region

Omentum

Mesentery

Lower part of duodenum

Jejunum and ileum

Hypogastric region

Ileum

Bladder

Uterus (in pregnancy)

Right hypochondriac region

Right lobe of liver

Gallbladder

Portion of duodenum

Hepatic flexure of colon

Portion of right kidney

Suprarenal gland

Left hypochondriac region

Stomach

Spleen

Tail of pancreas

Splenic flexure of colon

Upper pole of left kidney

Suprarenal gland

Right lumbar region

Ascending colon

Lower half of right kidney

Portion of duodenum and jejunum

Left lumbar region

Descending colon

Lower half of left kidney

Portion of jejunum and ileum

Right iliac region

Cecum

Appendix

Lower end of ileum

Right ureter

Right spermatic cord

Right ovary

Left iliac region

Sigmoid colon

Left ureter

Left spermatic cord

Left ovary

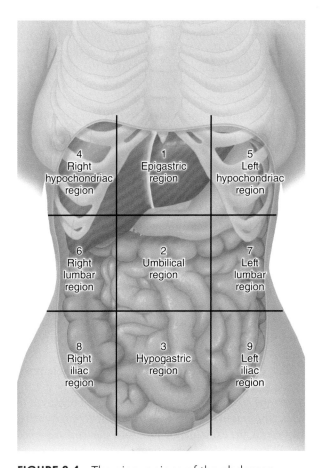

FIGURE 8.4   The nine regions of the abdomen.

Evaluation of Abdominal Pain

The patient with abdominal pain may not have a problem with their gastrointestinal tract. Many possible conditions, including diseases of the heart, lungs, kidneys, and musculoskeletal system, can present as abdominal pain. Some differential diagnoses for abdominal pain include the following:

- Muscle contusions
- Gastroenteritis
- Appendicitis
- Peptic ulcer disease
- Cholecystitis
- Splenic rupture
- Diverticulitis
- Pelvic inflammatory disease
- Pancreatitis
- Other conditions: myocardial infarction, pneumonia, pericarditis, pneumothorax, kidney disease, reproductive system problems

Key questions to ask the patient to evaluate abdominal pain are as follows:

- Onset of pain: Sudden or gradual?
- Duration of pain: Present for hours? Days? Weeks?
- Temporal factors: Constant pain or intermittent?
- Relationship to meals: Better with food or worse?
- Quality of pain: Burning, cramping, stabbing?
- Radiation of pain: Does it seem to spread up or down?
- Severity of pain: Determine by use of pain scale
- Aggravating or alleviating factors: Better lying down or sitting up? Have over-the-counter medicines, such as antacids or others, been tried?
- Associated symptoms: Nausea, vomiting, diarrhea, constipation, fever?
- Last bowel movement?
- Medications or supplements that may cause symptoms?

For female patients, it is important to obtain an appropriate menstrual cycle history. Pain that is perceived as being abdominal may be from the reproductive system, such as ovarian cysts, menstrual cramps, pelvic infection, or complications of pregnancy.

CONDITION HIGHLIGHT

Stitch in the Side

A condition that has frustrated athletes and health care providers is exercise-related transient abdominal pain (ETAP), commonly called a *side stitch*. It is characterized as a sharp, acute, cramping sensation in the abdomen that occurs during exercise. Complaints of ETAP are more common in 10K runners compared with longer-distance runners. In a 2000 study of people across six sports, athletes participating in swimming (75%), running (69%), and horseback riding (62%) were most likely to report having experienced a side stitch in the past year.[2] Theories for the cause of the pain include ischemia of the diaphragm, stress on subdiaphragmatic ligaments, and irritation of the parietal peritoneum.[3]

All proposed treatments to date are anecdotal, and prevention tips are inconsistent. Better-conditioned athletes report fewer instances of ETAP, so one can rationalize that if individuals can continue to increase their fitness, the incidence of ETAP should decrease. Age also seems to be protective in ETAP, with older athletes reporting fewer incidences of ETAP than younger athletes.[2]

As with other conditions, the examiner must determine whether any trauma is involved and obtain the details of that injury. A past medical history or family history of gastrointestinal problems can also help in the diagnosis, as can social history factors such as alcohol intake.[4] Taking a thorough history, including training regimen or use of training logs, may be helpful in diagnosing the endurance athlete with gastrointestinal complaints.[5,6] Signs or symptoms that may indicate a severe or life-threatening condition constitute red flags with abdominal pain (see the Red Flags for Abdominal Pain sidebar). Beyond the obvious issues that are always red flags, such as unstable vital signs or altered mental status, these findings are serious enough that either a physician should be contacted immediately or the patient should be taken to an emergency department.

Physical examination of the abdomen involves the skills of inspection, auscultation, palpation, and percussion. Inspection consists of carefully examining the abdomen when the patient is lying comfortably supine. Initially, the examiner notes the presence of scars that may indicate prior surgery, thus reducing concern about acute appendicitis or gallstones, and looks for obvious bruising or contusions as well as swelling or distention. A yellowish tint can indicate jaundice from liver disease,

or a faint bluish discoloration around the umbilicus may indicate intraabdominal bleeding. The examiner watches the movement of the abdomen as the patient breathes in and out for asymmetry that can indicate intraabdominal masses or hernia.

In distinguishing abdominal muscle pain from problems of the abdominal organs, it is helpful to have the patient tense the muscles by doing a partial sit-up. As the patient's head is raised from the table, the muscles are held taut and muscle pain is aggravated, so this can help pinpoint a problem that is muscular.

Auscultation is always performed before palpation in the examination of the abdomen. In the examination of the heart and lungs, palpation is done before auscultation; however, palpation of the abdomen may create abdominal sounds that were not there before palpation. Auscultation should reveal the normal clicks and gurgling of bowel sounds that may be heard anywhere from a few times to dozens of times every minute. Chapter 1 covers use of the stethoscope and basic auscultation techniques. The examiner needs to be alert to abnormal sounds, such as high-pitched tinkling sounds or rushing water sounds, as well as the potentially absent sounds that can indicate intraabdominal pathology. Some patients may have quieter abdomens; bowel sounds are not considered absent until the examiner has listened continuously for 5 min with no sound heard.

Percussion is a skill that requires considerable practice; it is not covered in detail in this text. It may be used to assess the size and density of the abdominal organs or to detect the presence of air or fluid in the abdominal cavity. In general, the examination follows a standard sequence for abdominal percussion (figure 8.5) or percussion to determine the size of the liver (figure 8.6). As indicated in chapter 1, percussion may be direct or indirect.

The examiner should practice percussing normal tympanic and dull sounds of the four quadrants exhibited by various positions of percussion. Tympany is the

---

RED FLAGS FOR ABDOMINAL PAIN

- Vomiting bright-red blood or black material that looks like coffee grounds
- Fever of 38.3 °C (101 °F) or greater, accompanied by severe abdominal pain
- Persistent vomiting, such that the person cannot keep any fluids down for more than 24 to 36 h (in younger patients, the time window is shorter)

predominant sound throughout the abdomen and hollow organs because of the air contained in the stomach and intestines (table 8.1). A dull sound is present over solid masses adjacent to hollow organs.

Examiners use indirect percussion to tell when they are directly over solid organs or hollow organs of the abdomen. A change in sound from tympanic to dull is easier to detect, so examiners usually start over an area known to be normally tympanic. Percussion is most commonly performed to determine the size of the liver and spleen. Examiners must understand the surface anatomy of the liver (figure 8.7) in order to assess the liver through indirect percussion.

The patient lies supine during palpation. If the patient has difficulty relaxing the abdominal muscles to allow the examiner to adequately palpate deeply, the knees may be bent slightly to encourage relaxation of the abdominal muscles. Palpation is used to assess masses or areas of tenderness at both the superficial and deep levels.[1]

At first, the abdomen is palpated lightly (pressing only about 1 cm deep) in all quadrants to assess for muscular tenderness or rigidity as well as any superficial masses. The palmar aspect of the fingers is used in a steady, even fashion, avoiding any sharp or sudden jabbing motions. Pain or resistance to even this light palpation generally indicates either injury or inflammation of the abdominal musculature or peritoneal lining.

If significant tenderness is not present with light palpation, the examiner presses more firmly and deeply and continues to press as deeply as the patient will comfortably allow, generally to a depth of at least 3 or 4 cm (figure 8.8). In this manner, the examiner may be able to feel the edges of the liver in the RUQ (figure 8.9) or an enlarged spleen in the LUQ. Tenderness in the RLQ

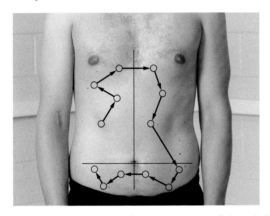

FIGURE 8.5   Sequence for percussion of the abdomen.

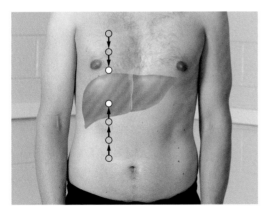

FIGURE 8.6   Percussion sequence to determine liver size.

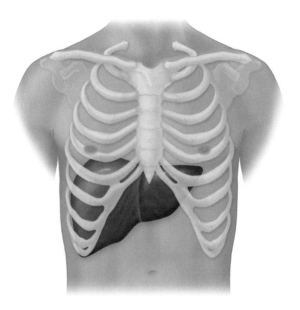

FIGURE 8.7   Surface anatomy of the liver.

TABLE 8.1   **Percussion Notes of the Abdomen**

Sound	Description	Location
Tympanic	Drumlike high-pitched, hollow sound	Over air-filled structures
Hyperresonant	Low-pitched, hollow quality between that of tympany and resonance	Distended bowel, hyperinflated lung, emphysema, or pneumothorax
Resonance	Sustained note of moderate pitch	Over normal lung tissue
Dullness	Short, soft, high-pitched sound with little resonance	Over solid organs such as the liver

with deep palpation may indicate appendicitis, pelvic problems, or ovarian problems in a female patient.

To palpate the liver more adequately, the athletic trainer stands on the right side of the patient with the left hand placed under the patient. The left hand presses up at the 11th or 12th rib, causing the liver to be lifted toward the anterior abdominal wall. The right hand simultaneously palpates the liver. The clinician asks the patient to breathe regularly and then tries to feel the edge of the liver with the right hand as the patient breathes (figure 8.10). The edge of the liver should be smooth and firm. Palpation of the liver does not normally cause pain, so the clinician should be suspicious if direct palpation of the liver is painful for the patient. Often the liver is not palpable except in a very thin person or if it is enlarged.

The examiner pays special attention to the spleen while palpating the LUQ. The same basic technique may be used as when palpating the liver: namely, to reach across the patient with the right hand, placing it beneath the costovertebral angle (figure 8.11). The fingers of one hand are placed just below the patient's left costal margin to lift the spleen anteriorly. The patient takes a deep breath while the examiner moves the fingers of the other hand up and under the ribs toward the spleen. The inspiring breath will push an enlarged spleen down to meet the fingers of the other hand; the examiner may be able to feel the spleen just below the left costal margin. A normal-sized spleen is typically not palpable. Pain with palpation of the spleen indicates that the patient should be referred to a physician.

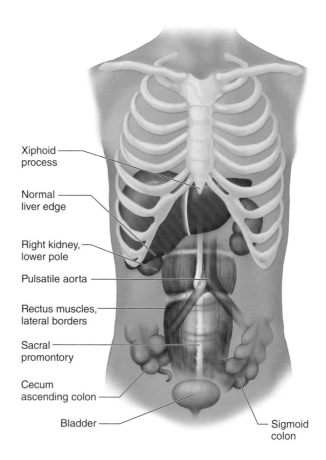

Xiphoid process
Normal liver edge
Right kidney, lower pole
Pulsatile aorta
Rectus muscles, lateral borders
Sacral promontory
Cecum ascending colon
Bladder
Sigmoid colon

FIGURE 8.9 Structures felt by deep palpation of the abdomen.

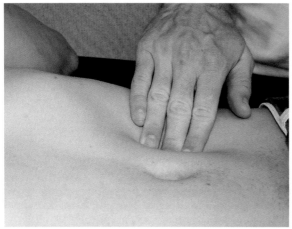

FIGURE 8.8 Deep palpation of the abdomen. If the patient tolerates light palpation of the abdomen, the examiner can press firmly and deeply to the patient's tolerance (3-4 cm) and try to feel the edges of the abdominal organs.

© Micki Cuppett

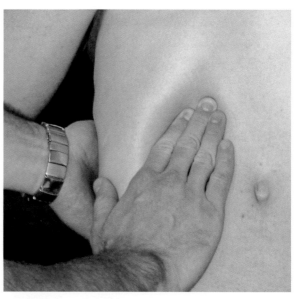

FIGURE 8.10 Palpation of the liver.

© Micki Cuppett

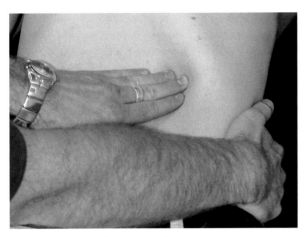

FIGURE 8.11   Palpation of the spleen.

© Micki Cuppett

Evaluation of the Athlete With Acute, Traumatic Abdominal Pain

As with any traumatic injury, an assessment of the mechanism of injury is important. A sharp blow with the end of a hockey stick is obviously more likely to cause damage than a blow with an elbow. Fortunately, the abdominal organs are generally well protected, and most trauma results only in contusions to the muscles. After the clinician has confirmed that there is no damage to the underlying organs, these injuries can be treated just like any other muscle contusion.

The spleen is the most commonly injured solid abdominal organ.[7] The spleen that is not enlarged is generally well protected by the lower ribs on the left. When trauma results in rib fracture, however, the ribs can lacerate the spleen. The spleen can become enlarged (i.e., splenomegaly) from various causes; most commonly, the enlargement resulting from **infectious mononucleosis** is temporary and lasts a few weeks. This enlargement will cause the spleen to extend downward beyond the protection of the ribs and make it vulnerable to direct trauma that can cause splenic contusion or laceration. (See chapter 14 for more information about mononucleosis.)

Less commonly, the liver can also be lacerated or contused by direct trauma. The pancreas is deep enough in the abdomen that contusion is rare, but it should be suspected if there is persistent abdominal pain with radiation through to the back. Injury to the hollow organs (i.e., stomach, intestines) is rare and generally occurs only when there is enough force to cause crushing damage against the spine.

When a patient sustains an injury to the abdomen, the health care provider initially assesses the overall status and vital signs. Unfortunately, sideline evaluations can be normal or reveal only vague, nonspecific findings even in patients with significant injuries. If there is diffuse abdominal tenderness or rigidity, pain in the back without trauma to the back, low blood pressure, or rapid heart rate or if the mechanism of injury suggests injury to the liver or spleen, then the patient must be seen by a physician before resuming play.

Clinical Tips

Abdominal Examination

History
- Pain: onset, duration, quality, severity, radiation
- Associated symptoms: nausea, vomiting, diarrhea, constipation, fever, fatigue, painful urination
- Aggravating or alleviating factors
- Medications
- Appetite and food intolerance
- Bowel habits

Observation
- Shape and symmetry
- Assessment of skin and scars

Auscultation
Note: Perform before percussion and palpation of the abdomen!
- Bowel sounds
- Vascular sounds

Percussion
- The four quadrants
- Liver span and spleen

Palpation
- Light palpation to assess tenderness in all four quadrants
- Deeper palpation for masses in all four quadrants
- Palpation of spleen, liver, kidneys, and McBurney's point

Nausea, Vomiting, and Diarrhea

Nausea, vomiting, and diarrhea can result from several conditions, including self-limited viral illness, food poisoning, side effects of medications, dietary indiscretions, or stress. They may also be signs of more serious conditions, such as appendicitis, pancreatitis, or pelvic inflammatory disease. In most cases, however, nausea, vomiting, and diarrhea are self-limiting conditions that can be managed with over-the-counter medicines and common-sense precautions.

An important consideration is the severity and duration of symptoms of nausea, vomiting, or diarrhea in terms of the patient's hydration status. With mild or intermittent symptoms, most people will still take in enough oral fluids that they can go for several days without significant concerns about dehydration. However, when symptoms are more severe, then intravenous fluids may be needed to treat dehydration that could develop over 24 to 36 h. When these symptoms have been present for more than 24 to 36 h or are accompanied by significant pain or fever, the patient is referred to a physician.

The characteristics of the vomited material must be determined. Undigested food or minimal amounts of yellow to green stomach acid or bile are common and not worrisome. If the patient has been persistently vomiting bilious material or has noted any blood, dark coffee ground–like material, or foul-smelling stool-like material, then urgent referral is needed.

Similarly, for the patient with diarrhea, it is important to obtain a description of the stool characteristics. Loose or watery brown stools are most common and reflect a more benign process. If the diarrhea is bloody or maroon in color or seems to be more like mucus than water, then referral is needed.

Treatment

The patient who feels nauseated or queasy but has not been vomiting and has little or no pain or fever can safely and effectively take over-the-counter **antiemetic agents** containing a high-concentration carbohydrate and phosphoric acid solution, such as Nausetrol or Emetrol. When used as directed on the label, these agents can safely treat the symptoms and will not mask a more serious condition. If they fail, numerous prescription medicines can be used, including promethazine (Phenergan) and prochlorperazine (Compazine).

Once the patient has started vomiting, the stomach must be given enough time to settle down between vomiting spells. A common scenario is the person who vomits, then feels better, and decides to drink some water or other fluids in order to both quench thirst and avoid dehydration. If this happens too soon after the last vomiting spell, the hypersensitive stomach will start the vomiting again. This behavior of drinking too quickly is very common in the person who "just can't stop vomiting." After any spell of vomiting, the person should not drink anything at all, not even a sip of water, for about 1 h (sometimes 2 h). Once the stomach has remained quiet for that time, then one of the over-the-counter or prescription antinausea (or antiemetic) medicines listed previously can be used. The patient who can tolerate these medicines can slowly advance to sips of water or electrolyte solutions (e.g., Gatorade, Powerade, or Pedialyte). Finally, the patient can add more carbohydrates to the diet in the form of grains and fruits as tolerated. The BRAT (bananas, rice, applesauce, toast) diet has long been used in children with nausea, vomiting, and diarrhea. These foods are tolerated well by both children and adults and may be helpful in quieting the gastrointestinal tract while recovering from nausea, vomiting, and diarrhea. Acidic, spicy, or greasy foods should be avoided for 1 or 2 d to be certain the patient can tolerate them and to prevent a recurrence of vomiting.

The mainstay for the treatment of diarrhea is hydration, but loperamide (Imodium) obtained over the counter can be very effective in the control of diarrheic episodes. Loperamide can decrease stool frequency and volume to allow the patient to continue a somewhat normal routine. It may, however, have side effects of drowsiness and dizziness that may impair performance. Use of antidiarrheals when invasive pathogens are suspected is controversial because they can delay the clearance of pathogens from the bowel, thereby prolonging the disease. However, in the afebrile patient with a nonbloody stool, antidiarrheals can be a very effective and safe method of treatment.[8,9] The patient must hydrate with electrolyte solution and water as discussed previously and adhere to a bland diet until symptoms subside.

Return to Participation

The decision on when to return a patient to participation depends on the sport in question and the severity and duration of symptoms. It is unlikely that mild illnesses that cause nausea, vomiting, or diarrhea in the absence of fever will be significantly aggravated by athletic activity;

Clinical Tips

Vomiting

The patient who is vomiting should not drink anything at all for about 1 h to allow the stomach time to quiet down. If the stomach remains quiet for 1 h or so, only then should the patient progress to sips of liquid.

rather, athletic performance may be significantly impaired by the illness. A mild case of nausea, vomiting, or diarrhea may have little effect on most sports participants. For sports in which stamina plays a greater role, such as cross country running, the athlete may see a significant impairment of performance with mild to moderate symptoms; the same symptoms may have little to no effect on the athlete for whom performance time is relatively short, such as in weightlifting or gymnastics.[8] A good rule of thumb for most patients with afebrile illnesses is to avoid activities when there are symptoms below the neck (e.g., chest congestion, vomiting, diarrhea) and play as tolerated when symptoms remain above the neck (e.g., headache, sore throat, earache). In cases where antibiotics are used, the patient should wait a minimum of 24 h prior to gradual return to play.[8]

Viral Gastroenteritis

Viral **gastroenteritis**, or acute gastroenteritis, is a very common condition caused by any one of several viruses, including adenovirus, astrovirus, echovirus, and Norwalk agent.[9] These viruses cause a self-limited inflammation of the stomach and intestines that is usually completely resolved within 2 to 3 d. These infections are contagious and can spread through a family or college dormitory or by the actions of food handlers.

Signs and Symptoms

Signs and symptoms of viral gastroenteritis include watery diarrhea, nausea with or without vomiting, and fever. The affected patient may also have diffuse aches, pains, and chills. Management includes general supportive measures and attention to hydration as noted previously.

Treatment and Return to Participation

Over-the-counter loperamide is very effective for diarrhea but may have side effects of drowsiness and dizziness that can significantly affect performance. Referral is considered if there is no response to over-the-counter medicines, if symptoms persist for more than 48 h, or if the patient has an accompanying high fever. The patient can return to normal activity whenever symptoms are resolved and hydration is adequate. With usual good hygiene, the risk of spread to fellow athletes or coworkers is extremely low.

Food Poisoning or Bacterial Diarrhea

The term *food poisoning* is often overused. People who experience sudden onset of gastrointestinal symptoms often attribute them to something they ate or drank. Food poisoning generally should be suspected when multiple people who ate the same food become ill at about the same time. Sampling and culturing the person's stool can confirm the diagnosis. Food poisoning typically occurs when food is improperly handled, cooked, stored, or refrigerated. In some cases, the problem is the bacterium itself; in other cases, it may be from the toxin or toxins produced by the bacterium. The most common causes are *Campylobacter*, *Salmonella*, and *Staphylococcus* species, but several other bacteria can also cause problems, including *Shigella* species, *Bacillus cereus*, *Yersinia* species, and *Escherichia coli*.[10]

Signs and Symptoms

Bacterial diarrhea is typically more severe and lasts longer than viral gastroenteritis. It may cause higher fevers or severe abdominal cramps and is more likely to result in weight loss and dehydration. Depending on the bacterium, onset may occur 4 to 6 h after eating the contaminated food (e.g., *Staphylococcus*) or 3 to 10 d later (e.g., *Salmonella*). This variable duration obviously makes it difficult to pinpoint a specific food.

Treatment and Return to Participation

Initial management of diarrhea can include over-the-counter medicines as for viral gastroenteritis. If the patient is significantly ill or there is blood in the stool, then referral is needed for thorough evaluation and treatment. This may include stool specimens and antibiotics. If several patients become ill at the same time, then it may be important to trace back to a shared meal as the source. If the culprit was simply poor refrigeration of a single food, then the problem may resolve on its own. However, the source may be a food worker with a contagious infection that may spread until treated. The patient may return to normal activity, including athletic participation, when symptoms resolve completely and strength and hydration return to normal.

Parasitic Infection

Parasitic infections of the gastrointestinal tract are less common than bacterial or viral infections but may still cause significant problems. The most common parasites are single-celled organisms called protozoa. *Giardia* is a common waterborne protozoan that is found worldwide, especially in people who drink from more remote streams when hiking or camping. *Entamoeba* species are parasitic protozoa that are also found worldwide but are much more common in tropical regions.[11] In addition, tapeworms, roundworms, and flukes can be parasitic in humans. These infestations are uncommon, and discussion is beyond the scope of this text.

Signs and Symptoms

Giardia-induced diarrhea is characterized by the significant gas that typically results. The diarrhea may be acute or chronic and intermittent. The diarrhea is often explosive in nature, with patients complaining of dull abdominal cramping and bloating with gas and flatulence. *Entamoeba* may cause a variety of symptoms from chronic intermittent diarrhea, abdominal pain, and weight loss to profound bloody diarrhea and fever.[10]

Treatment and Return to Participation

The athletic trainer must recognize that parasitic infections are different from self-limited viral and bacterial diarrhea, and patients must be promptly referred for the appropriate antibiotic treatments. The treating physician makes decisions about return to participation.

Stress-Induced Gastrointestinal Symptoms

It is well known that stress can cause a wide variety of gastrointestinal symptoms from diffuse abdominal pain and cramps to heartburn, nausea, vomiting, diarrhea, constipation, and anorexia.[5,12,13] The diagnosis of stress-induced or functional gastrointestinal problems is one of exclusion. The patient is thoroughly evaluated for other causes of symptoms, and only when these have been excluded can the problem be considered stress induced. Even highly stressed people can develop other, easily treatable conditions; therefore, the health care provider must not be too quick to attribute symptoms to stress.

Treatment and Return to Participation

If the patient has been thoroughly evaluated and other causes have been ruled out, the athletic trainer can play an important role in the management of stress-induced gastrointestinal symptoms. It is very important to under-

stand and to remind the patient that the symptoms are not imaginary. Medical research has increasingly helped in understanding the vital connection between the mind and the body: Biochemicals of the brain can become imbalanced, causing major depression or symptoms of anxiety. These conditions can affect the rest of the body and impair healing or worsen other chronic illnesses. Stress causes very real symptoms of stomach pain, nausea, or even vomiting or diarrhea. The athletic trainer can assist in management by maintaining close communication with the physician, allowing the patient to have time off as needed, or playing or working through the symptoms as needed in each case.

Constipation

Constipation is commonly misunderstood as a simple decrease in the frequency of bowel movements, with many people feeling that they must have a bowel movement every day or something is wrong. A better definition for constipation is a subjective discomfort from difficulty in passing stool or a change in consistency such that stools are excessively hard or small.

Signs and Symptoms

People have a wide range of tolerance, but constipation can cause significant abdominal pain, cramps, and general discomfort.

An initial evaluation to determine the cause of the constipation is helpful. Hundreds of medications, such as narcotic pain relievers, nonsteroidal anti-inflammatory drugs, and antidepressants, and many nutritional supplements can cause temporary or persistent constipation.[14]

Referral and Diagnostic Tests

Referral to a physician is indicated if (1) the patient's symptoms fail to respond to over-the-counter agents or (2) if the problem persists over a period of weeks and the patient cannot participate in normal activities without restriction.

Treatment and Return to Participation

Treatment is best directed at increasing fluid and fiber intake. Fiber intake may be dietary, by means of whole grains and vegetables, or from over-the-counter fiber supplements, such as Metamucil or Citrucel. These fiber supplements can be taken indefinitely as needed. Stronger over-the-counter agents, such as milk of magnesia (magnesium hydroxide) or magnesium citrate, are effective but may be too strong for some people and lead to temporary diarrhea.[10] These medications are for short-term use because long-term use can lead to a form of dependence.

Heartburn and Gastroesophageal Reflux Disease

The terms *heartburn* and *esophageal reflux*, or **gastroesophageal reflux disease (GERD)**, are generally interchangeable and refer to a very common condition in which stomach acid travels up through a dysfunctional lower esophageal sphincter (LES) into the esophagus or even into the back of the throat. Although GERD is more common after age 60 yr, it can affect patients of any age and is estimated to cause frequent symptoms in 14% of adults. More than 60 million people in the United States report having symptoms of GERD at least weekly.[15] LES relaxation results in incomplete closure of the sphincter and can be exacerbated by numerous causes, including foods (e.g., chocolate and high-fat meals) and common medications (e.g., calcium-channel blockers used for hypertension and nitrates used for heart disease). Other causes include family history, obesity, and tight-fitting clothing. Behavioral factors include overeating in general and especially exercising or lying down with a full stomach. Certain foods are also well-known triggers for some people, including mints, alcohol, carbonated beverages, and foods that contain caffeine or are tomato or citric acid based.

Signs and Symptoms

In addition to the heartburn sensation, signs and symptoms of GERD include chest pain (potentially severe), belching, regurgitation of food and acid, chronic cough, and laryngitis. It is essential to remember that not all people with GERD feel a heartburn sensation. Some people experience only a chronic cough or frequent asthmatic attacks from acid that goes up the esophagus and then into the airways. GERD should be considered in any patient with a chronic cough, chronic laryngitis, or atypical asthma. Exercise-induced laryngeal obstruction has been identified in patients with GERD symptoms and

laryngitis.[16] GERD is not simply a nuisance condition. In some cases, after persisting for years, heartburn and GERD can cause significant damage to the esophageal lining (esophagitis), which can increase the risk of esophageal cancer. These complications are rare in people younger than age 40 yr but are more common in those who also smoke cigarettes and drink alcohol.[11]

Referral and Diagnostic Tests

Any patient whose symptoms do not respond to over-the-counter medications or who needs them daily for weeks should be referred for further evaluation. Various diagnostic tests can be performed, including a barium esophagogram or *upper GI series* that involves swallowing barium and having a series of X-rays taken. More commonly, this includes the use of an endoscope to directly visualize the esophageal lining. This is called *esophagogastroduodenoscopy* and is performed as a simple outpatient procedure.

Treatment and Return to Participation

Treatment of GERD is initially directed toward appropriate lifestyle management. Some self-assessment may be needed, so the patient can determine which foods, food quantities, and behaviors cause symptoms and then adjust accordingly. Although over-the-counter medicines can be very effective, avoidance of triggers generally yields similar or better results. Over-the-counter medications work by decreasing stomach acidity and thus diminishing symptoms, not by stopping the reflux. Several effective agents include antacids (e.g., Maalox, Mylanta, Rolaids, Tums) and histamine sH_2 blockers (e.g., cimetidine [Tagamet HB], famotidine [Pepcid AC], ranitidine [Zantac]).[11] The most effective, yet also the most expensive, over-the-counter agents are the proton pump inhibitors (PPIs) omeprazole (Prilosec), lansoprazole (Prevacid), and esomeprazole (Nexium). These agents can prevent symptoms if taken before known triggering behaviors or foods, or they can be taken as needed after symptoms start. PPIs are commonly used; however, some studies have reported that patients taking PPIs for a prolonged period displayed increased risk of cardiovascular disease, gastrointestinal malignancies, and chronic kidney disease.[17] Some patients require stronger prescription medications and higher doses. Symptom failure to respond to over-the-counter medications does not mean the patient does not have GERD.

Heartburn and GERD are rarely severe enough to interfere with athletic activity. Individuals should be reminded not to eat for 2 to 3 h before activity to avoid triggering symptoms.[3,18]

Gastritis and Peptic Ulcer Disease

Gastritis is a diffuse or patchy inflammation of the stomach lining. **Peptic ulcer disease (PUD)** is a more serious condition, in which there is a deeper ulcer in the stomach (i.e., gastric ulcer) or, more commonly, in the duodenum (i.e., duodenal ulcer). Gastritis can have several causes; in otherwise healthy and younger patients, it usually results from (1) processes of erosion and then an ulcer caused by nonsteroidal anti-inflammatory drugs or alcohol or (2) infectious processes caused by the bacterium *Helicobacter pylori*. PUD may also be caused by *H. pylori*.[11] These conditions are more common in people older than age 40 yr but may be seen in children as well. Other factors can contribute to the development of gastritis, including smoking, severe stress, and steroids.

Signs and Symptoms

Symptoms of gastritis include generally mild to moderate persistent mid-abdominal pain, loss of appetite, and nausea. Eating often aggravates the pain. Patients with PUD have similar symptoms but often have more severe pain that worsens a couple of hours after eating but improves with food. Pain can wake the patient from sleep. Both conditions can lead to gastrointestinal bleeding. Gastritis is less likely to cause bleeding, but PUD can sometimes cause severe and dangerous bleeding. If blood passes through the digestive tract, it may present as very dark or black stools with a very sticky, tarlike consistency. Blood in the stomach is also an irritant and may cause vomiting, in which case the condition may present as red blood or coffee ground–like material in the vomitus (i.e., partially digested blood takes on the appearance of dark coffee grounds). On occasion, a patient may have bleeding gastritis or PUD with no apparent gastrointestinal distress; thus, any black, tarry stools or blood or coffee ground–like material in vomit are causes for concern and prompt referral.

Referral and Diagnostic Tests

See the Diagnostic Tests for Gastrointestinal Disorders sidebar.

Treatment and Return to Participation

The over-the-counter antacids, H_2 blockers, and PPIs discussed previously can all provide substantial relief from symptoms of gastritis or PUD. Nonetheless, any patient with gastritis or PUD should see a physician regularly because of the potential for severe complications. Testing

Diagnostic Tests for Gastrointestinal Disorders

- Radiological studies
- Radiograph of abdomen
- Upper gastrointestinal (GI) series (barium swallow)
- Ultrasound
- Computed tomography (CT) scan
- Endoscopy
- Upper endoscopy (esophagogastroduodenoscopy [EGD])
- Lower endoscopy (colonoscopy or flexible sigmoidoscopy)
- Laboratory testing
- Complete blood count (CBC)
- Chemistry panel (sodium, potassium, blood urea nitrogen [BUN], creatinine)
- Serology for *Helicobacter pylori*
- Liver enzymes (alanine transaminase [ALT], aspartate transaminase [AST], γ-glutamyltransferase [GGT], bilirubin)
- Pancreatic enzymes (amylase, lipase)
- Stool studies
- Evaluation for red or white blood cells
- Stool cultures
- Microscopic evaluation for parasites

for and treating potential *H. pylori* infection can bring about a cure and thus avoid the long-term need for acid suppression.

Symptoms can be variable. In most cases, they will not interfere with athletic activity, and the individual can fully participate in sports. However, the individual should not participate if there is unexplained blood or coffee ground–like material in the vomit or black and tarry stools.

Irritable Bowel Syndrome

Irritable bowel syndrome (IBS) is defined as abdominal discomfort or pain associated with altered bowel habits for at least 3 d/mo in the previous 3 mo, with the absence of organic disease. These consensus-based criteria (called the ROME criteria) have been used since 1989.[19] The peak prevalence of IBS is from ages 20 to 39 yr, and it is estimated to affect 5% to 10% of the population. It is 1.5 times more common in women than in men, tends to be familial, and is often triggered by stress.[20] There are various theories as to its underlying cause, with some experts believing that IBS is attributable to an overly sensitive gastrointestinal tract, others reporting an overgrowth of intestinal bacteria, and others believing it to be an underlying neurological disorder that disrupts normal gastrointestinal motility. Although there are no definitive diagnostic tests for this syndrome, the ROME criteria continue to be refined and the identification of potential biomarkers related to the symptoms is encouraging.

Signs and Symptoms

IBS has several different symptoms. Some people have just one or two, whereas others have several symptoms together or different symptoms at various times. Some individuals have diarrhea predominantly, some have the constipation-predominant type, and some have diarrhea alternating with constipation. Others have neither significant constipation nor diarrhea but instead have persistent upper abdominal bloating and generalized discomfort. Some patients have diffuse abdominal pain, with or without fecal urgency (i.e., a sudden sensation of an urgent need for a bowel movement). Some types of abnormalities associated with bowel movements are most common with IBS, and abdominal pain is often relieved by a bowel movement, although some patients have a feeling of incomplete bowel evacuation. Patients may also complain of occasional mucus mixed with stool or abdominal distention and nausea. IBS is also associated with many other chronic pain and mental health disorders, ranging from migraine to fibromyalgia and from depression to anxiety. Differential diagnoses of IBS include celiac disease, colorectal cancer, diverticular disease, gastrointestinal infection, lactose intolerance, or ischemic colitis.

Referral and Diagnostic Tests

No specific test exists for IBS. Thus, any patient with these symptoms is referred for evaluation for other causes, including inflammatory bowel diseases (IBDs; see subsequent sections), celiac disease, tumors, or infections. After a thorough history and physical, testing is then designed to assess for other causes of chronic abdominal distress. Numerous questionnaires have been developed with varying success in determining IBS. The Endurance Athlete Questionnaire has been determined to be a valid and reliable measure of IBS.[20] Routine testing for celiac disease in patients with diarrhea-predominant or mixed-presentation IBS should be considered.[21] Laboratory testing such as complete blood count (CBC), thyroid function studies, and stool studies for parasites are low yield and not recommended in routine diagnostic evaluation of IBS.[19] Red flag features such as anemia, rectal bleeding, nocturnal symptoms, or weight loss may suggest the use of colonoscopy to assess for colon cancer, IBD, celiac disease, or other abdominal diseases.[22]

Treatment and Return to Participation

Management of IBS consists of providing the patient ongoing reassurance and supportive encouragement, as there are no agents shown to control all symptoms. The best responses seem to come from constant vigilance toward a high-fiber diet and stress management. The most distressing symptom is then treated as needed. Diarrhea and constipation can each be managed with over-the-counter medicine, but patients must avoid inadvertently cycling back and forth between the two. Prescription antispasmodic medicines (e.g., dicyclomine) can sometimes be used to control cramping and pain. Behavioral modification can be very helpful as an adjunct to medical treatment.[21]

Clinical Tips

IBD Versus IBS

Many people confuse the terms *inflammatory bowel disease* (IBD) with *irritable bowel syndrome* (IBS), but they are very different and should be easily differentiated through the patient history. People with IBS complain of abdominal cramps with diarrhea or constipation that is relieved with a bowel movement. Those with IBD often report diarrhea, blood in the stool, and weight loss.

Athletes and physically active patients with IBS can fully participate in sports depending on symptom severity. Although some athletes may cope with symptoms during critical games or performances, others may become incapacitated at these times. Professional assessment and management of stress, including techniques such as biofeedback, can be very helpful for these athletes.

Celiac Disease

Celiac disease is an autoimmune disorder that affects the gastrointestinal tract and is thought to be triggered by dietary gluten in affected individuals. The disease is characterized by chronic inflammation of the small intestinal mucosa, which leads to atrophy of the small intestinal villi and subsequent malabsorption.[23] The incidence of celiac disease is increasing partly because of improved detection and recognition; independent of improved diagnosis, this increased incidence could be related to environmental factors that may promote loss of tolerance to dietary gluten. Celiac disease affects approximately 1% of the U.S. population and was originally thought to occur in people of European ancestry. However, the incidence of this disease is now worldwide. It is two to three times more common in women.[24] Celiac disease is *not* a food allergy.

Signs and Symptoms

Typical presentation of celiac disease includes chronic diarrhea with cramping and gas pain. Patients often have weight loss, and adolescents may experience delayed onset of growth or puberty. A history of nervousness and/or depression is often present, as is a family history of autoimmune disease. Other complaints may include bone or joint pain, migraine, weakness, fatigue, and anemia.[25-27] The physical examination is often normal, but the patient may present with abdominal distension or dermatitis herpetiformis.

Referral and Diagnostic Tests

Laboratory tests are performed to differentiate celiac disease and to rule out more common diseases. These tests include a basic metabolic panel, CBC (iron deficiency), thyroid-stimulating hormone (thyroid disease), vitamin D level, and allergy testing. If celiac disease is suspected from history and physical examination, the initial serologic test assesses the tissue transglutaminase (tTG) antibody level. This antibody is found in every tissue in the body and acts to join proteins together. In people with celiac disease, tTG activates specific immune cells and triggers the inflammatory response that leads to atrophy of the villi in the small intestine.[28] The diagnosis is often confirmed with repeat blood tests after the patient has adhered to a gluten-free diet for 4 wk. The TTG–immunoglobulin A test has 95% sensitivity and specificity, provided the patient is consuming a gluten-containing diet at the time of testing, and is therefore the first-line diagnostic test for celiac disease.[23] Endoscopy with biopsies of the duodenal mucosa may be necessary to confirm the diagnosis. Celiac disease should be differentiated from GERD, pancreatic insufficiency, Crohn's disease (CD), or other IBDs.

Treatment and Return to Participation

The general treatment for celiac disease is to remove gluten from the diet. The patient can substitute rice, corn, and soybean flour for products that contain gluten. Periodic blood tests are performed to measure antibody

---

CONDITION HIGHLIGHT

Gluten Sensitivity and Intolerance

Since the early 2000s, the number of people choosing a gluten-free diet (GFD) is much higher than the projected number of patients with celiac disease.[24] This has fueled a global market of gluten-free products and highlights several conditions related to the ingestion of gluten. There are three main forms of gluten reactions: allergic, autoimmune (celiac disease), and immune-mediated conditions (gluten sensitivity).[29] Wheat allergy is an adverse reaction to wheat proteins, with onset in minutes to hours after gluten ingestion. This reaction may affect the skin, gastrointestinal tract, or respiratory tract. Celiac disease or other autoimmune gluten disorders generally present months to years after gluten exposure. There is a third condition in which some people experience distress from eating gluten-containing products and show improvement with a GFD. This condition is distinct from celiac disease and wheat allergies.[26] Gluten sensitivity cannot be distinguished clinically; *serology* tests need to be conducted. Patients with gastrointestinal discomfort or distress after gluten ingestion should be referred for a follow-up blood test and immune-allergy tests.

levels, which normalize with gluten abstinence. Gluten abstinence is required for life, because the immune response to gluten recurs if gluten is consumed again. Usually, no medications are prescribed for celiac disease, but patients may benefit from iron, vitamin, and calcium supplements. The most difficult aspect for the athlete with celiac disease is the dietary restrictions while traveling with the team or with set team meals. The athletic trainer may need to check the gluten-free status of many standard gluten-containing products provided by the athletic department, such as energy drinks or meal replacement bars.[24]

Inflammatory Bowel Diseases

Crohn's disease (CD) and ulcerative colitis (UC) are severe inflammatory diseases of the small intestine and colon; together, they are referred to as **inflammatory bowel diseases (IBDs)**. Although these conditions can occur in families, the underlying cause is unknown. Each condition has certain specific characteristics; for example, CD more commonly affects the small intestine, and UC is more likely to have symptoms beyond the gastrointestinal tract.[30] This text discusses both conditions together.

Signs and Symptoms

CD and UC typically present with chronic diarrhea, abdominal pain, urgency, cramping, and weight loss. The diarrhea is often bloody and can lead to anemia. Some patients also develop other symptoms beyond the gastrointestinal tract, including arthritis and eye and skin conditions.

Referral and Diagnostic Tests

Any patient with bloody diarrhea or persistent gastrointestinal symptoms needs to be referred to a physician. Evaluation will routinely include direct visualization of the colon by means of colonoscopy, and often a biopsy of a small piece of the bowel wall is used to make the diagnosis. Laboratory testing can also reveal anemia and other evidence of inflammation that accompanies these conditions.[31]

Treatment and Return to Participation

UC and CD require regular and close management by a physician. These diseases are commonly treated with methotrexate and thiopurines to help control symptoms. These medications have considerable negative side effects, including headache, anorexia, weight loss, alopecia, and muscle weakness, none of which are conducive to athletic participation. Newer biologic medications

have improved the outlook for patients with CD and UC. These medications are immunosuppressive, so patients must be closely monitored for additional health problems. In addition, even when symptoms seem controlled, the patient needs to be monitored for potential complications, including an increased risk of colon cancer.[10]

Athletic performance will vary depending on the disease severity and the degree of control with medications. The disease state may or may not interfere with participation, depending on whether it is currently flaring or well controlled. Physical activity is a lifestyle modification often used with patients with CD, but the amount of physical activity is much less than the exercise intensity of a competitive athlete.[32] In addition, medications used to treat these diseases can cause problems and side effects, such as severe headaches, depression, or fatigue. Because approximately 25% of patients with CD are diagnosed before age 20 yr, their nutritional status must be closely monitored and supplemented as necessary to prevent malnutrition and delayed growth. As a result of poor nutrient absorption, the patient's diet must be supplemented with iron, vitamin D, calcium, and other essential nutrients for growth.[33]

Appendicitis

Acute abdominal pain accounts for 7% to 10% of all emergency department visits, and acute **appendicitis** is the most common reason for urgent abdominal surgery in the United States, with about 9% of the population requiring an appendectomy at some point in their life.[34] Appendicitis is caused by an acute obstruction and inflammation of the appendix, but the diagnosis remains challenging.[35]

Signs and Symptoms

Many signs and symptoms point toward appendicitis, and the diagnosis is usually suspected based on several symptoms and then confirmed at surgery. Pain from appendicitis generally starts as a nonspecific discomfort

RED FLAGS FOR APPENDICITIS

- Diffuse epigastric or periumbilical pain early
- Pain localization to right lower quadrant (RLQ) within 12 to 18 h
- Point of maximal tenderness at McBurney's point
- Low-grade fever
- Nausea or vomiting

located around the umbilicus or in the midline epigastric region. A patient typically progresses from anorexia, with the complete loss of appetite, to abdominal pain to nausea and mild vomiting. Patients may have a slight fever and either constipation or diarrhea. As the pain progresses, it usually begins to localize to the RLQ.[36] As it progresses, the patient often lies motionless with the right thigh drawn up, and attempts to straighten the thigh increase the pain. The patient's abdomen may be very tender to even light touch around McBurney's point in the RLQ, halfway between the right anterior superior iliac spine and the umbilicus, and it may be very rigid (figure 8.12). The diagnosis of acute appendicitis is made in approximately 90% of the patients presenting with these symptoms.

Other conditions can mimic appendicitis. Some are benign, but others, such as acute pelvic inflammatory disease, can be serious.

Referral and Diagnostic Tests

Appendicitis is a surgical emergency because of the risk for appendix rupture and severe intraabdominal infection that can result. Any patient with sudden and severe RLQ pain and tenderness associated with anorexia, nausea, or vomiting should be sent to the emergency department of the closest hospital. Although some cases may progress over a few days, it is more typical to see progression over several hours.[35] Athletes at away games who are more than a couple hours from home may need to be seen in the emergency department at an away hospital and should not wait until they get home.

Treatment and Return to Participation

Even with advanced diagnostics, such as computed tomography (CT) scans, it is not always possible to

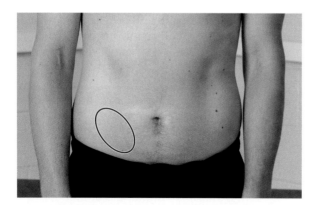

FIGURE 8.12 McBurney's point: Tenderness at this point, halfway between the umbilicus and the right anterior superior iliac spine (ASIS), generally indicates appendicitis when accompanied by fever and nausea.

diagnose appendicitis until surgery, and it is expected and understood that some cases of suspected appendicitis will have a normal appendix surgically removed. **Laparoscopic** appendectomy remains the most common treatment; however, increasing evidence suggests that broad-spectrum antibiotics can be used for the treatment of uncomplicated acute appendicitis in approximately 70% of patients.[36] Timing of the return to participation is best deferred to the surgeon. It depends on the sport in question, the type of surgical procedure performed (open versus laparoscopic versus nonsurgical treatment), and the extent of potential surgical complications.

Cholecystitis and Cholelithiasis

Inflammation of the gallbladder is called **cholecystitis** and is mostly caused by gallstones, or **cholelithiasis**. Gallstones are common, occurring in about 8% to 10% of the U.S. population. They are more common in individuals older than age 30 yr, in women, and in American Indian and Hispanic individuals.[11] Rising trends in obesity and metabolic syndrome have contributed to an increase in diagnosis. Several risk factors are associated with cholelithiasis, including obesity, pregnancy, and obesity during pregnancy.[37]

Signs and Symptoms

Gallstones often cause no symptoms at all, but they are the underlying cause of more than 90% of cholecystitis cases. Symptoms are generally caused by a stone blocking the bile duct that drains the gallbladder. The patient may have intermittent RUQ pain, nausea, vomiting, or simply indigestion. Symptoms are often worse after consuming a high-fat meal; they may be mild and minimally distressful or sudden and very severe. If the duct is blocked for a prolonged time, the patient may develop jaundice or severe pain and fever. On examination of the abdomen, the patient typically has tenderness in the RUQ and may exhibit a sudden stopping or arrest of inspiration when the examiner deeply palpates the liver while the patient takes a deep breath.[37] This is called **Murphy's sign**.

Referral and Diagnostic Tests

Any patient with significant RUQ pain and tenderness needs to be seen by a physician. Laboratory tests, including white blood cell count and liver enzymes, may help with the diagnosis, but the gold standard for diagnosis of cholelithiasis is diagnostic ultrasound. The ultrasound can also indicate thickening of the gallbladder wall with cholecystitis.[37]

Treatment and Return to Participation

Gallstones and cholecystitis are treated surgically by removing the gallbladder (i.e., cholecystectomy). This procedure can usually be done with laparoscopic surgery, with a short overnight hospital stay and a return to most activities within a few days. Sometimes open surgery is needed, and then the patient may be hospitalized for several days and may recover slowly over weeks.

Overall, prognosis is excellent for cholecystitis and cholelithiasis. Return to play after surgery depends on the type of surgery, and the decision is best left to the surgeon. For many patients, however, symptoms of gallstones may be mild and intermittent, and the patient can simply remain on a very low-fat diet to get through the season and then have elective surgery after the season ends.

Colorectal Cancer

Colon cancer is a common neoplasm arising from the lining of the large intestine. In the United States, colon cancer is currently the second leading type of cancer (behind skin cancer). According to the American Cancer Society, 106,180 new cases of colon cancer were predicted in 2022, with 44,850 new cases of rectal cancer diagnosed.[38] Colon cancer incidence increases with age, with a peak incidence in the seventh decade of life.[39]

Many risk factors are known to increase the incidence of colorectal cancer. The lifetime risk of colorectal cancer is about 1 in 50 in the general population, but the risk increases two to three times for those with a first-degree relative with colon cancer.[40] Younger patients with colorectal cancer tend to have a more aggressive form of the disease compared with older adult patients. Several other risk factors increase the likelihood of developing colon cancer, including hereditary polyposis syndromes, obesity, IBD or other intestinal diseases, type 2 diabetes, dietary factors such as heavy consumption of processed and red meat, and lack of physical activity.[38] The incidence of colorectal cancer has decreased since 2000, owing to a concerted effort to screen using a colonoscopy or stool-based test.

Signs and Symptoms

The signs and symptoms of colon cancer vary widely. Patients may present with vague abdominal pain, weight loss, red blood or maroon-colored stool, anemia, or a change in bowel habits from diarrhea to constipation or to changes in stool caliber.

Referral and Diagnostic Tests

If colon cancer is suspected or abnormal bowel movements are ongoing, referral should be made to a physician capable of performing a colonoscopy. After the diagnosis of colon cancer is made, referral should be made to a colorectal surgeon if colon resection needs to be performed. Referral may also be made to an oncologist, depending on the disease stage.

Treatment and Return to Participation

Treatment for colorectal cancer depends entirely on the stage at diagnosis. Early cancers that have not spread can be treated by surgical removal of the cancerous growth or of that portion of the colon. More advanced cancers that have spread to local lymph nodes or distant organs involve surgical resection as well as adjunctive radiation, chemotherapy, or both.

The importance of early diagnosis in colon cancer cannot be overemphasized. When diagnosed early, more than 90% of patients with colon cancer can be "cured" (or have a five-year survival rate of >90%).[39] Unfortunately, many cases are not found until they are advanced and spreading through the body. The decision of return to participation depends on the type of treatment. For simple removal of a cancerous polyp, the patient may return to full activity right away. If part of the colon is removed, the surgeon needs to make the decision based on the extent of the patient's cancer, the surgery involved, and the patient's recovery rate.

Summary

Athletic trainers must remember that not all abdominal distress is caused by gastrointestinal disease; they must be alert to possible cardiac, pulmonary, and reproductive system causes of symptoms in the abdomen. Other than appendicitis, most gastrointestinal problems in physically active individuals are not true emergencies. The athletic trainer can initially manage symptoms safely with over-the-counter medications, and eventually with referral to the physician only if the over-the-counter medications do not elicit an adequate response. Severe gastrointestinal symptoms with accompanying high fever, however, need to be assessed by a physician.

Gastrointestinal problems may or may not interfere with performance, and return to participation is generally based on symptom severity. In addition, many gastrointestinal disorders are chronic and intermittent in nature. The athletic trainer can help the patient in managing these symptoms as needed.

Apply It!

Go to HK*Propel* to complete the case studies for this chapter.

Genitourinary and Gynecological Systems

Although injury to the genitourinary and gynecological systems is rare in athletics, disorders of these systems are common in the athletic population. This chapter focuses on these systems and discusses how an athletic trainer might recognize and refer patients with these conditions to a physician. Although athletic trainers do not perform most of the evaluations mentioned in this chapter, they have a relationship with their patients whereby they may be able to gather enough symptomatic data to warrant referral to a physician. In addition, knowledge of the types of diagnostic tests performed will better enable the athletic trainer to explain them to patients.

Overview of Anatomy and Physiology

The genitourinary system is common to both males and females, with few exceptions. Here we discuss the basic anatomy and physiology of the genitourinary system before diverging into the anatomical differences between males and females. Following the anatomy discussion is an overview of the physiology of ovulation, menstruation, and pregnancy.

Anatomy of the Kidneys, Ureters, and Urinary Bladder

The kidneys act to remove excess water, salts, and products of metabolism from the blood in order to maintain proper acid–base status. The body's waste products are then conveyed in the urine to the urinary bladder by the ureters. Normally, a person has two kidneys, two ureters, and a single urinary bladder (see figure 8.2). The kidneys lie posterior to the peritoneum in the retroperitoneal space on the posterior abdominal wall, alongside the spine and against the psoas major muscles. The kidneys are bean-shaped organs whose upper poles are protected by the

At the completion of this chapter the reader should be able to do the following:

1. Explain the anatomy of the genitourinary and gynecological systems.

2. Explain the physiology of ovulation and menstruation.

3. Describe common genitourinary and gynecological disorders that athletic trainers encounter in the care of physically active individuals.

4. Differentiate conditions of the genitourinary and gynecological systems that warrant referral.

5. Summarize preventive strategies for genitourinary and gynecological disorders and for sexually transmitted infections (STIs).

6. Refer patients with signs or symptoms of an STI to a physician.

7. Describe the physiological changes that occur in pregnancy.

8. Recommend limitations for pregnant patients.

lower bony thorax, and each has an associated adrenal gland superior to it. Because of the large size of the right lobe of the liver, the right kidney lies at a slightly lower level than the left. In muscular individuals and those with well-developed abdominal musculature, the kidneys are generally not palpable on examination.

The anatomy surrounding the two kidneys differs from an anterior perspective. The right kidney is associated with the liver and is separated from it by the hepatorenal recess. The left kidney is associated with the left adrenal gland, stomach, spleen, pancreas, a portion of the small bowel, and the descending colon. In the posterior, both kidneys lie well protected by the costovertebral angle between the 12th rib and the vertebral spine (figure 9.1). They are also attached superiorly to the diaphragm and move slightly on respiration.

The kidneys are enclosed in a strong fibrous capsule that is surrounded by a layer of fat called **perirenal fat**. The unique characteristics of the density of the kidney itself and the perirenal fat allow for the kidneys to be visualized on abdominal radiographs. The kidney is a solid organ with a thick cortex under the fibrous capsule (figure 9.2). Filtration begins at the medulla, continues on the interior in the calix structures, and ends in the collection area before the ureter.

The ureters are muscular ducts, or tubes, that carry urine from the kidneys to the urinary bladder. Urine passes from the kidneys through the ureters by peristaltic waves of muscular contraction. The ureters are approximately 25 cm long and are retroperitoneal. Each descends almost vertically along the psoas major muscle just anterior to the tips of the transverse processes of the lumbar vertebrae (L2-L5). In the female, the ureters and uterine arteries are closely associated. The uterine artery crosses the ureter at the side of the cervix; therefore, during a surgical procedure to remove the uterus and cervix, the ureter may be inadvertently damaged.

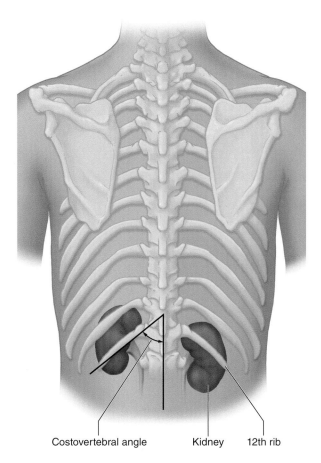

FIGURE 9.1 Posterior view of the kidneys protected within the costovertebral angle between the 12th rib and the spine.

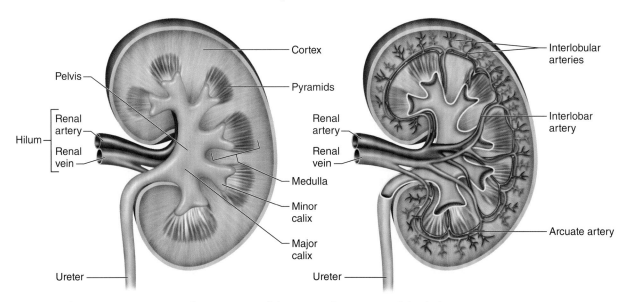

FIGURE 9.2 Cross section reveals two views of the internal structure of the kidney.

The urinary bladder is a muscular sac or vesicle that functions to store urine (figure 9.3). Its shape, size, position, and relation to other structures vary with the amount of urine it contains. The urinary bladder is composed chiefly of smooth muscle. In the adult, the empty urinary bladder lies posterior to the symphysis pubis within the pelvis. As it fills, it ascends into the lower abdomen. A full bladder may reach as high as the level of the umbilicus. The ureters enter at the superolateral aspect of each side of the bladder. The bladder is then drained by a single urethra that empties from the central inferior aspect.

The blood supply to the kidneys is provided by the right and left renal arteries, respectively. These branch off from the descending aorta at nearly right angles. Venous drainage is provided by the right and left renal veins that empty into the inferior vena cava. Blood supply to the ureters is more complex, but it is principally supplied by arterial branches from the renal, aortic, common iliac, vesicular, or uterine arteries. The main arteries supplying the urinary bladder are branches of the internal iliac arteries. In the female, however, branches of the uterine and vaginal arteries also provide a portion of the blood supply to the bladder. Venous drainage occurs via the vesicular venous plexus that drains to the internal iliac vein.

The urinary bladder is supplied by parasympathetic motor fibers to the detrusor muscle of the bladder and sensory fibers. The sensory fibers are stimulated by stretching of the bladder, causing a sensation of fullness and activating the micturition, or urination, reflex. Micturition is preceded by contraction of the diaphragm and abdominal wall. The neck of the bladder descends, the detrusor muscle contracts by reflex, and urine is voluntarily expelled from the bladder.

Anatomy of the Urethra

The urethra is a fibromuscular tube that conducts urine from the bladder (and semen from the ductus deferens in the male) to the exterior. The urethra originates at the central lower portion of the urinary bladder, traverses the pelvis, and terminates at the external urethral orifice.

The female urethra is approximately 4 cm long. It is closely associated, often fused, with the anterior vaginal wall. The urethral orifice is located between the clitoris (anteriorly) and the vagina (posteriorly).

The male urethra is considerably longer, averaging 20 cm in length. The male urethra consists of three parts: prostatic, membranous, and spongy. The proximal prostatic portion descends through the prostate gland. The membranous portion of the urethra descends from the lower portion of the prostate to the bulb of the penis. This portion of the urethra is surrounded by a sphincter (i.e., muscle). The lowermost portion of the membranous urethra is most susceptible to rupture or penetration by a catheter. The spongy portion of the urethra lies in the corpus spongiosum and traverses the bulb, shaft, and glans of the penis, terminating at the external urethral orifice or meatus.

Male Genital Anatomy

The male genital organs comprise the penis, ejaculatory duct, prostate gland, bulbourethral gland (Cowper's gland), and paired testes, each with an epididymis, ductus or vas deferens, and seminal vesicle (figure 9.4). Spermatozoa, formed in the testes and stored in the epididymides, are contained in the semen, which is secreted by the testes and epididymides, seminal vesicles,

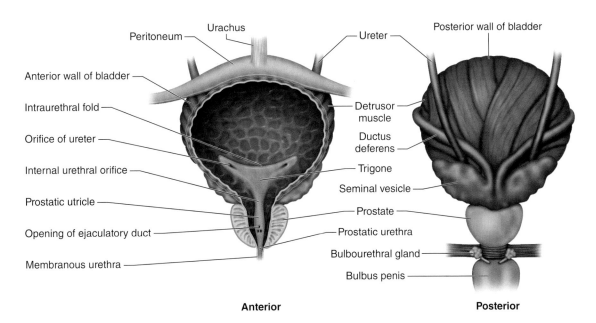

FIGURE 9.3   Anatomy of the urinary bladder in a male.

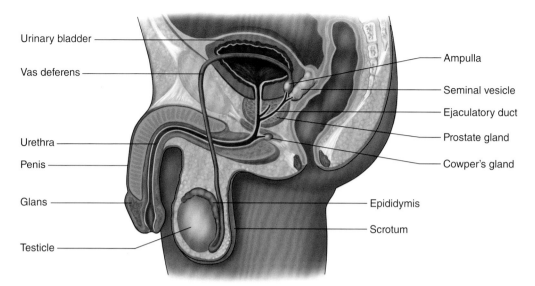

FIGURE 9.4   Anatomy of the male genitourinary system.

prostate, and bulbourethral glands. The sperm, on leaving the epididymides, pass through the ductus deferens and ejaculatory ducts to reach the urethra and pass through the external urethral orifice.

The testes are paired ovoid glands located in the scrotum and are responsible for producing spermatozoa and steroid hormones. They reside away from the core of the body to maintain a slightly lower temperature of approximately –17.2 to –16.7 °C (1-2 °F) below that of the body proper. The left testicle often lies slightly lower than the right testicle in the scrotum. The epididymis is associated with the posterior portion of each testicle. The testes and epididymides are covered by a dual-layered tunica vaginalis testis, which is derived prenatally from the processus vaginalis of the peritoneum (figure 9.5). The potential cavity between these two layers or some part of the processus vaginalis may become distended with fluid, forming a hydrocele.

The testes and epididymides receive their blood supply from the testicular artery, and venous drainage occurs via the pampiniform plexus, which forms the bulk of the spermatic cord. The veins of the pampiniform plexus can become varicose, leading to the formation of a varicocele. Lymphatic drainage from the testes empties into the lower aortic lymph nodes.

The scrotum is a cutaneous pouch that houses the testicles and epididymides. A median raphe indicates the subdivision of the scrotum by a septum into right and left compartments. Smooth muscle, known as the dartos muscle, is firmly attached to the overlying skin. The dartos muscle contracts in response to cold, exercise, and sexual stimulation. Loose connective tissue underlying the dartos allows free movement and is the site for the accumulation of edema.

The prostate gland is a fibromuscular pelvic organ surrounding the male urethra and containing glands that contribute to the semen. It is located behind the symphysis pubis and directly in front of the rectum, which is where it can be palpated by a digital rectal examination (DRE). Venous drainage and lymphatic drainage of the prostate are important because these contribute to the distinct areas for the spread of prostate cancer. Venous drainage occurs via the prostatic venous plexus that drains into the internal iliac vein and communicates with the vertebral plexus, thereby allowing **metastatic** spread of prostate cancer to the vertebrae. Lymphatic drainage terminates in the internal and external iliac lymph nodes.

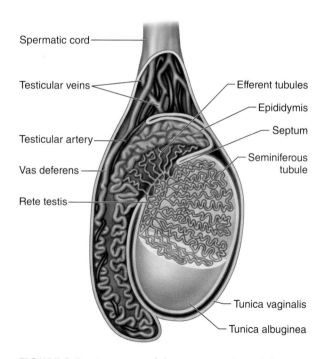

FIGURE 9.5   Anatomy of the testis and epididymis.

Female Genital Anatomy

The female genital organs comprise the ovaries, fallopian tubes, uterus, vagina, and external genitalia, specifically the mons pubis, labia majora and minora, vestibule of the vagina, bulb of the vestibule, vestibular glands, and clitoris (figure 9.6).

The ovaries are paired organs that produce oocytes (eggs) and secrete steroid hormones. The ovaries are situated on the lateral wall of the pelvis, where they can be palpated bimanually. The paired fallopian tubes allow the passage of oocytes from the ovaries as well as spermatozoa from male ejaculation, and a fallopian tube is the usual site of fertilization. From there, it conveys the early embryo to the uterus. Fallopian tubes are also where tubal pregnancies occur, and they are susceptible to scarring associated with ascending infections (e.g., pelvic inflammatory disease [PID]), which can ultimately render the tube unable to transmit either oocytes or spermatozoa, resulting in infertility.

The uterus is a muscular organ that lies within the pelvis (figure 9.7). The uterus accepts the fertilized egg and is the site for implantation and development of the fetus. The upper uterine segment receives the fallopian tubes. The lower uterine segment terminates in the cervix, which opens to the vagina. The uterus has three distinct layers: a mucosa or endometrium, a muscular coat or myometrium, and a serosa or perimetrium.

The vagina lies posterior to the urinary bladder and anterior to the rectum. It serves as a receptacle for the penis, as the lower end of the birth canal, and as the excretory duct for the products of menstruation. The anterior and posterior walls of the vagina are approximately 7.5 and 9 cm long, respectively. The opening of the vagina into the vestibule may be partially closed by a membrane

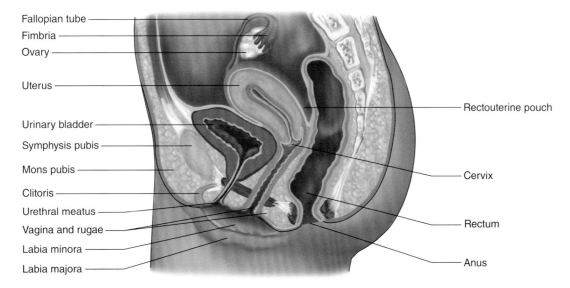

FIGURE 9.6   Anatomy of the female genitourinary system, lateral view.

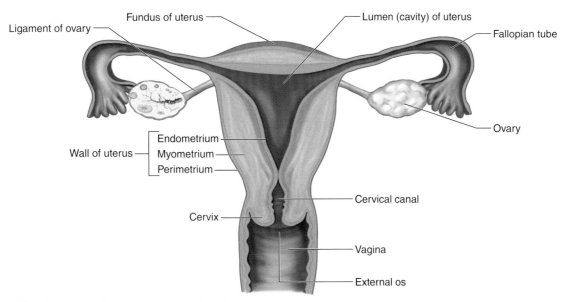

FIGURE 9.7   Anatomy of the uterus, anterior view.

called the hymen. The opening is located posterior to the urethral orifice and anterior to the anus. The vagina and cervix can be inspected through a speculum placed in the vagina. A Papanicolaou (Pap) smear is taken from the cervix to aid in the detection of cervical cancer.

Blood supply to the ovaries (i.e., to the ovarian arteries arising from the lower abdominal aorta), fallopian tubes (via the ovarian and uterine arteries), and uterus (via the uterine artery) forms a complex **anastomosis**. The vagina and cervix are supplied by branches from the internal iliac arteries. Venous drainage for the ovaries is distinct for each side. The right ovarian vein drains to the inferior vena cava, whereas the left ovarian vein empties into the left renal vein. The veins of the fallopian tubes drain into the ovarian and uterine veins. The uterine veins form a uterine venous plexus on each side of the cervix and drain to the internal iliac veins. The uterine venous plexus connects with the superior rectal vein, forming a portal–systemic anastomosis. The vaginal veins form the vaginal venous plexuses and lie along the sides of the vagina, draining into the internal iliac veins. Lymphatic drainage, again, is related to the metastatic spread of cancer. The ovaries drain to the lumbar lymph nodes. The fallopian tubes have their lymphatic drainage directed to the lower lumbar lymph nodes with the ovaries and uterus. The uterus drains to the lower aortic and external iliac lymph nodes. The superior and middle portions of the vagina drain into the external and iliac lymph nodes, and the lower portion of the vagina drains into the superficial inguinal lymph nodes. The cervix drains to the external and internal iliac nodes and sacral lymph nodes.

Physiology of Ovulation and Menstruation

Normal menstrual cycles depend on an intact hypothalamic–pituitary axis, functioning ovaries, and a normal outflow tract. The menstrual cycle, which averages 28 d, requires a well-coordinated series of events (figure 9.8).

Clinical Tips

Evaluation of the Genitourinary System

When evaluating the genitourinary system, a person of the patient's gender should also be in the room. Ask only questions pertinent to the suspected condition. For example, if a possible pregnancy or anorexia is a concern, it is appropriate to ask the patient for the date of the latest menstrual period but inappropriate to ask for date of last sexual relations.

The normal menstrual cycle is divided into two parts: a proliferative, or follicular, phase and a secretory, or luteal, phase. During the follicular phase, estrogen and luteinizing hormone (LH) levels increase as follicle-stimulating hormone (FSH) levels decrease. The endometrium thickens during this phase. Before ovulation, estrogen sharply declines, followed by a surge in LH and a steady rise in progesterone. It is shortly after this that ovulation occurs, followed by a slight increase in core body temperature. The remnant of the follicle (i.e., corpus luteum) supplies the progesterone for the second half of the cycle. During this time, the endometrium prepares itself for implantation. If fertilization and implantation do not occur, the corpus luteum involutes and progesterone levels decline, prompting menses, which is the discharge of the endometrium from the uterus through the vagina.

Physiological Changes of Pregnancy

Noteworthy physiological changes occur in pregnancy. Cardiac output, defined as stroke volume (SV) × heart rate (HR), increases during pregnancy as a result of increases in both SV and HR. Plasma volume also increases with pregnancy.[1,92,100,101] The high flow of blood exiting the heart can often create a benign heart murmur. Blood pressure, defined as cardiac output × systemic vascular resistance (SVR), decreases because of a decrease in SVR. In a previous study, healthy women who exercised during pregnancy experienced reduced resting HR and increased endothelial cells in umbilical cord blood.[1]

Respiratory changes also occur in pregnancy and result in increased tidal volume, which translates into increased minute ventilation at rest despite a normal respiratory rate. Of note, the forced expiratory volume in 1 s (FEV_1) does not change, which is important for patients with asthma because peak flow meter values would not need to be altered. Overall airway resistance is also decreased in pregnancy.

Physiological responses to exercise are somewhat different in pregnancy than in nonpregnancy. For example, respiratory rates increase with mild exercise in pregnant females, whereas their maximal oxygen consumption ($\dot{V}O_2max$) is lower. The respiratory quotient ($\dot{V}CO_2/\dot{V}O_2$) is also increased in pregnant females who exercise, suggesting a possible greater dependence on carbohydrates as the preferred fuel source. This may also explain why hypoglycemia can develop more rapidly during prolonged strenuous exercise in pregnant females. In addition, the core temperature is higher in pregnancy, which requires caution in the expectant mother who exercises, especially in hotter climates.

Anatomical considerations because of the enlarging uterus result in common changes in pregnancy. Urinary

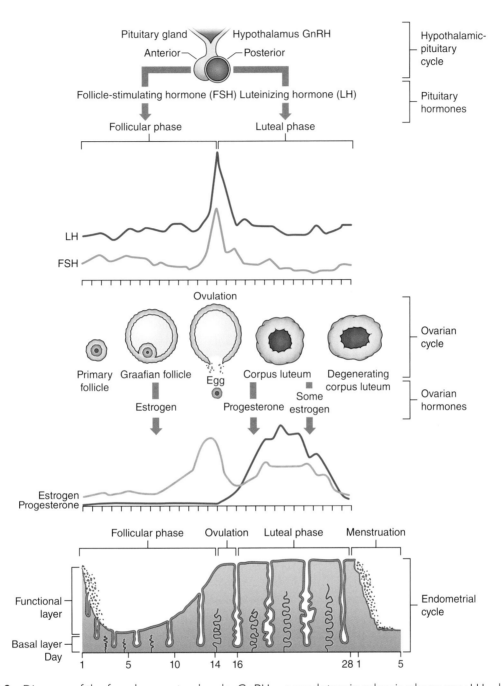

FIGURE 9.8   Diagram of the female menstrual cycle. GnRH = gonadotropin-releasing hormone; LH = luteinizing hormone; FSH = follicle-stimulating hormone.

frequency increases during pregnancy as a result of pressure from the uterus on the urinary bladder. Low back pain is another common complaint and again results from the growing uterus. In this scenario, however, changes in biomechanics lead to increased lumbar lordosis that is more commonly the cause of low back discomfort. Lower extremity edema may also develop and is more common later in pregnancy.

Evaluation of the Genitourinary and Gynecological Systems

Evaluation of the genitourinary and gynecological systems by the athletic trainer begins with a thorough and complete history. Maintaining a clear and professional demeanor with the patient is key, as is using correct medical terminology and anatomical terms. It is strongly advisable and a good professional practice to have a person of the patient's gender present when taking the history to increase the patient's comfort. Ask pertinent history questions, and ask about signs, symptoms, onset, and other details that can assist in a diagnosis. The goal is to collect enough information to refer the patient to the correct provider. Visual inspection and palpation of the genitourinary and gynecological systems is best left to the medical professionals who have expertise and specialize in these areas. These providers may order distinctive tests based on their findings, and they only need the history, not other evaluative information, to assist them.

Pathological Conditions of the Genitourinary System

Kidney Stones

The incidence of kidney stones has risen 40% since the 1990s.[5] Kidney stones, also known as renal or urinary calculi or *nephrolithiasis*, arise in the kidney when urine becomes supersaturated with a salt capable of forming solid crystals. Although they are commonly referred to as *kidney stones*, these calculi may be found in the ureters, urinary bladder, or urethra as well. Renal calculi are commonly composed of calcium oxalate (50%), calcium phosphate (10%-20%), struvite (7%), and cystine (3%).[2] In the United States, the lifetime prevalence for kidney stones is 13% in males and 7% in females. There is a reported five-year recurrence rate of 35% to 50% following an initial kidney stone.[3] Caucasian males are affected more commonly than African American males, although African American males have a higher incidence of associated infection with renal calculi. Females of all races have been noted to have a higher incidence of infected **hydronephrosis**. The age of onset of symptomatic renal calculi is generally in the third or fourth decade.

Most stones pass spontaneously, but some patients require hospitalization for unremitting pain, dehydration, associated urinary tract infection (UTI), or inability to pass the stone.

Signs and Symptoms

Most kidney stones originate within the kidney and proceed distally, creating various degrees of urinary obstruction as they become lodged in the narrow canal areas. Acute passage of a kidney stone from the kidney through the ureter gives rise to pain so excruciating that it has been likened to that of childbirth. The location and the quality of pain are related to the position of the stone within the urinary tract. The severity of pain is related to the degree of obstruction, the presence of ureteral spasm, and the presence of any associated infection. The pain typically begins suddenly at night or in the early morning, but it can follow heavy exercise and may present with a more gradual onset.[4] The pain is typically described as unilateral flank pain that radiates to the groin.[2] The patient with a kidney stone is often writhing in pain, moving about and unable to lie still. Nausea and vomiting are common. Examination demonstrates flank tenderness, costovertebral angle tenderness, and, occasionally, testicular pain, notably in the absence of any testicular tenderness. The abdominal examination is often normal, although bowel sounds may be hypoactive because of a mild ileus. The presence of fever raises the possibility of an infectious complication and warrants immediate referral.[5,6]

Types of Kidney Stones

Each of the following five commonly identified types of kidney stones has its own causes:

1. *Calcium stones* are composed of calcium oxide, calcium phosphate, calcium oxalate, and uric acid. Common causes of calcium stones include hyperparathyroidism, increased gut absorption of calcium, a renal phosphate leak, hyperuricosuria, hyperoxaluria, hypocitraturia, and hypomagnesemia.

2. *Struvite stones* are composed of magnesium ammonium phosphate. These stones are associated with chronic urinary tract infections secondary to gram-negative rods.

3. *Uric acid stones* are associated with high purine intake (a diet rich in organ meats, legumes, fish, meat extracts, or gravies), gout, and malignancy.

4. *Cystine stones* are caused by an intrinsic metabolic defect resulting in failure of renal tubular reabsorption of cystine, ornithine, lysine, and arginine.

5. *Indinavir stones* typically appear in patients with human immunodeficiency virus (HIV) who are treated with the protease inhibitor indinavir (Crixivan). These stones are composed entirely of the protease inhibitor.

Once a kidney stone passes to the urinary bladder, it may be asymptomatic and passed during urination. During passage of the stone through the urethra, the patient usually notes burning and some blood-tinged urine depending on the stone size.

The list of differential diagnoses for kidney stones is long, and this diagnosis often depends on the side of the body involved and on the patient's sex and age. Differential diagnoses include UTI, **pyelonephritis**, urinary obstruction, renal vein thrombosis, testicular torsion, PID, ectopic pregnancy, bowel obstruction, appendicitis, cholecystitis, **biliary colic**, and constipation.[4,5] Among those older than age 60 yr, an **abdominal aortic aneurysm (AAA)** may also be included as a differential diagnosis.[5,7] In a series of 134 patients with symptomatic AAA presenting to the emergency department, 18% had an initial misdiagnosis of a kidney stone.[8]

Referral and Diagnostic Tests

Patients with symptoms suggestive of a kidney stone should be referred immediately to a physician if this is the first episode. Any patient with new or recurrent presentation and an associated fever needs to be referred immediately for physician evaluation and a urology consultation. Also, a patient with recurrent symptoms who cannot tolerate oral fluids and has unrelenting pain with a history of renal failure or a single kidney should be referred for immediate physician evaluation and possible observation or hospitalization.

The mainstay of diagnostic testing for kidney stones is a urinalysis. Blood is often visible in the urine and may be detectable in more than 90% of symptomatic individuals using both a urine dipstick test and microscopy. Urine pH can also be helpful, because a urine pH greater than 7 suggests the presence of urea-splitting organisms and struvite stones. Alternatively, a urine pH less than 5 suggests the presence of uric acid stones. The presence of pyuria (>5 white blood cells [WBCs] per high-power field) in a centrifuged urine specimen should prompt a careful search for an associated infection.[2] (Normal urine values are listed in table 2.3.) In these cases, a complete blood count (CBC) and differential, serum creatinine, and urine culture are in order.

Imaging studies may also be performed and are often done to confirm the initial diagnosis. The imaging study most often used is the renal colic computed tomography (CT) scan.[4,6] This is a rapid test with sensitivity in the range of 95% to 100%. The kidney-ureter-bladder radiograph is often used in conjunction with the CT scan.[5] Radiographs may demonstrate a radiopaque stone. Radiographs are occasionally used to monitor the passage of a stone under certain circumstances. Ultrasonography is also widely used and has similar sensitivity to a CT scan, although the CT scan is less operator dependent. It should be noted that there is no exposure to radiation in ultrasonography; therefore, this is an ideal imaging tool for pregnant females. An **intravenous pyelogram (IVP)** may be used in the diagnosis of kidney stones but has essentially been replaced by CT.

Treatment and Return to Participation

The crux of treatment for the uncomplicated passage of a kidney stone is pain management and maintenance of adequate hydration. Pain management is often obtained with nonsteroidal anti-inflammatory drugs (NSAIDs) or narcotic analgesics, such as morphine sulfate or meperidine (Demerol);[4] however, newer recommendations prefer NSAIDs over opiates.[5] An antiemetic medication also may be added when nausea is present and deters the use of oral analgesics or hydration. Use of forced oral or intravenous fluids has not been shown to alter outcomes or to improve stone passage; therefore, the focus should remain on hydration maintenance. A strainer is useful for filtering the urine during passage to collect the stone for analysis. Antibiotics are necessary in the presence of an associated infection.

The overall prognosis for kidney stones is very good. Fifty percent of stones pass uneventfully within 48 h.[2] Recurrence rates increase with time, but treatment options to reduce the risk of recurrence are available based on the type of stone present. Return to participation can follow kidney stone passage and adequate rehydration. However, even after diagnosis of a kidney stone, any patient who develops fever, increasing pain, or emesis should be referred for immediate physician evaluation.

Prevention

Individuals who have had a kidney stone may benefit from maintaining adequate hydration and avoiding dehydration,[3,9] which may decrease the chance of urinary saturation with stone-forming salts. Obesity, diabetes, hyperparathyroidism, intestinal malabsorption, and anatomical abnormalities have been reported to contribute to kidney stone recurrence.[5] Daily consumption of coffee, tea, beer, or wine may decrease the risk of stone formation, whereas daily apple or grapefruit juice consumption may increase this risk. Sodium intake should be restricted to help prevent recurrence. Increasing the amount of dietary bran may decrease bowel transit time and limit the formation of urinary calculi.[2] It should be noted that although nearly 60% of kidney stones are calcium derivatives, dietary intake of calcium should not be eliminated or reduced below a reasonable level.[3]

Sports Hematuria

Sports hematuria is the benign, self-limiting presence of three or more red blood cells per high-power field in a centrifuged urine specimen and is directly associated with exercise or activity. Sports hematuria is asymptomatic and has been documented to occur in both contact and noncontact sports. The degree of hematuria is believed to be related to exercise intensity and duration. In most circumstances, hematuria will resolve within 72 h of onset in individuals without any coexisting urinary tract pathology.[10,11] Previous studies reported that active people younger than age 30 yr had higher incidences of postexertional hematuria than did older participants.[10-13]

The incidence of sports hematuria is estimated to be as high as 80% in swimming, lacrosse, and track and field, 55% in football and rowing, and 20% in marathon runners. Researchers have identified several possible causes of sports hematuria, such as increased glomerular permeability, direct or indirect trauma to the kidneys, renal ischemia, dehydration, and hemolyzing factor release, all of which seem to be related to both exercise duration and intensity.[10,11,14]

Signs and Symptoms

By definition, sports hematuria is asymptomatic. Hematuria may be discovered during a routine urinalysis, such as that performed during a physical or preparticipation examination. On occasion, athletes present with gross hematuria (i.e., visible presence of blood in the urine) after a prolonged and strenuous workout. However, microscopic hematuria is not visibly apparent but is noted during a dipstick or urine analysis. Regardless of how hematuria is determined, sports hematuria generally resolves within 72 h without any further intervention than rest. One study with 500 runners noted that postexertional hematuria continued to 7 d in some (12%) and beyond 7 d in 7% of participants.[14] Three patients with persistent hematuria (>14 d) had other kidney pathologies.[14]

The differential diagnosis includes distinguishing true hematuria from false-positive urine blood dipstick results. True hematuria may result from a UTI, urethritis, interstitial nephritis, renal papillary necrosis, nephrolithiasis (kidney stone), polycystic kidney disease, kidney laceration, neoplasm (arising from any structure in the urinary tract), urinary bladder cancer, and prostatitis in males.[2] A false-positive urine dipstick result for blood may be attributable to medication intake (e.g., phenazopyridine, rifampin, nitrofurantoin, phenytoin), food dyes, menses, and myoglobin in the urine. Also, menstruating females may present with hematuria that is menstrual blood. It is appropriate to ask female patients presenting with hematuria whether they are currently menstruating. However, the health care provider should not dismiss signs or symptoms that could indicate a concurrent condition.

Referral and Diagnostic Tests

Asymptomatic hematuria observed in a patient during routine testing should be reviewed by a physician. These individuals are generally retested at 24 to 72 h to document resolution. Any patient with symptomatic hematuria or systemic symptoms is referred to a physician for immediate evaluation.[14]

Although sports hematuria is a benign condition, not all hematuria is benign; therefore, the evaluation must include some basic tests. A urinalysis or dipstick test demonstrates the presence of blood in the urine. Because drugs, dyes, and myoglobin can mimic hematuria by causing a false-positive result on the urine dipstick, microscopic examination of a spun urine specimen will confirm the presence of red blood cells. If symptoms of dysuria (i.e., painful urination) are present, a urine culture may be performed. If the patient has a history of hypertension, renal disease, repeated UTI, or pyelonephritis, an initial serum creatinine test may be performed. If hematuria persists beyond 72 h, further evaluation is generally warranted. Additional tests include a renal ultrasound, CT scan, and possible **cystoscopy**.

Treatment and Return to Participation

Treatment of sports hematuria is simply rest for 24 to 72 h. Resolution is the rule, and it should be documented with a repeat urinalysis after rest. Prognosis is excellent because sports hematuria is benign and self-limiting.[11]

Urinary Tract Infection

UTI is the most common bacterial infection seen in U.S. ambulatory care settings, and it occurs in either the upper or lower urinary tract.[2] These infections most commonly involve the urinary bladder (cystitis), but they can also involve the urethra, ureters, and kidneys (i.e., pyelonephritis). UTIs are a leading cause of morbidity and health care expenditures in persons of all ages.

Anyone can develop a UTI; however, sexually active young women are at highest risk. Several factors have been attributed to this increased risk, such as a short urethra, sexual activity, delays in micturition (particularly after intercourse), and use of diaphragms and spermicides.[18] Approximately 25% to 49% of U.S. women age 20 to 40 yr have had at least one UTI.[15] Fortunately, the risk of complicated UTI in this population is very low, although up to 20% of young women with a UTI will develop recurrent UTIs.[16]

UTIs are less common in men than in women but can occur. Catheter-associated UTIs are also known to occur.[17]

Signs and Symptoms

In most people, a UTI is signaled by a constellation of symptoms, including dysuria, increased urination frequency, and voiding small amounts of urine relative to the patient's normal pattern. On occasion, lower pelvic discomfort or cramping may also be present. The presence of gross hematuria, abnormal vaginal bleeding, or fever warrants prompt physician attention.

Differential diagnoses for UTI include urethritis, noninfectious cystitis, pyelonephritis, vulvovaginitis, sexually transmitted infections (STIs), dehydration, mittelschmerz, endometriosis, and **balanitis**.

Referral and Diagnostic Tests

Because of the relative discomfort associated with a UTI and the possibility of developing an ascending infection, symptomatic patients need to be referred to a physician for evaluation and treatment.

The diagnosis of an uncomplicated UTI is often made based on the history, physical examination, and urine specimen examination. A urine dipstick test is the most reliable tool for determining a UTI. The presence of nitrates or leukocytes confirms the diagnosis. A urine specimen can also be examined specifically for the presence of leukocyte esterase, nitrite (a surrogate marker for bacteria), and leukocytes on microscopic examination. A urine Gram stain can also aid in the identification of bacteria. The finding of a single bacterial organism, under high-power oil immersion, on an unspun urine specimen correlates with a count of more than 100,000 colony-forming units (CFU)/mL on urine culture.[15,17] Because of its limited added value in determining treatment for most uncomplicated UTIs, a urine culture may not be performed in the initial evaluation. Evaluation of a recurrent, complicated, or catheter-associated UTI often necessitates obtaining a urine culture.[2,18]

Urine culture results must be viewed considering certain threshold values shown to correlate with significant **bacteriuria**. In young women, a urine culture producing more than 100,000 CFU/mL is considered positive because of its high specificity for diagnosis of a true infection. In men, a urine culture yielding more than 1,000 CFU/mL is considered positive; in catheterized patients, this value falls to more than 100 CFU/mL.

The use of additional urological testing for anatomical abnormalities is generally unrewarding. However, a urological evaluation should still be performed in prepubescent children, in male adolescents with a first UTI, and in men with pyelonephritis or recurrent UTI.[17]

Clinical Tips

Significance of Dipsticks

Ready access to and knowledge of how to correctly use urinary dipsticks is critical in the early diagnosis of a urinary system condition. When properly used, the dipstick can quickly determine the presence of hematuria, infection, or dehydration, among other maladies.

Treatment and Return to Participation

UTIs are treated with antibiotics. An uncomplicated infection can be treated with trimethoprim-sulfamethoxazole (Bactrim), ciprofloxacin (Cipro), or cephalexin (Keflex) for a short (3 d) course. Recurrent UTIs should be treated with a longer course (7-10 d) of antibiotics, with antibiotic choice based on the urine culture results. (For more on antibiotics, see chapter 4.) If a female patient experiences more than three UTIs in a year, prophylactic antibiotics may be used to prevent recurrence. Studies have demonstrated the effectiveness of prophylactic antibiotic use after coitus, when given continually at a lower dose than treatment dose, for recurrent UTIs.[15] Complicated UTIs require a longer course of treatment and should be treated for 10 to 14 d.

The prognosis for an uncomplicated UTI is excellent and generally does not preclude participation. For the few patients who develop a complicated UTI, return-to-play decisions need to be based on their unique complication. Individuals with fever or poor fluid intake as a result of nausea or vomiting should be observed and should return to play only after symptoms resolve with treatment.

Prevention

A few simple actions may help prevent recurrent UTIs. Patients should avoid delays in urination and limit the use of either diaphragms or spermicides. Wearing breathable (cotton) underwear also reduces the chances of UTI. Some data support the effectiveness of cranberry (*Vaccinium macrocarpon*) supplements in preventing and treating UTIs.[19,20] Other urban myths, such as postcoital voiding, increasing fluid consumption, and avoiding bubble baths, have shown no reproducible evidence in preventing UTIs.[18]

Urethritis and Cystitis

Urethritis is an inflammation of the urethra, whereas cystitis is an inflammation of the urinary bladder and ureters. Both conditions are subcategories of UTIs. Both present with similar signs and symptoms and are caused by irritation of the urinary system (bladder, ureters, and/or urethra). The term *urethritis* is sometimes used to describe a syndrome of STIs, but it can have both infectious and noninfectious causes. (STIs are discussed later in this chapter.) Infectious causes of urethritis are typically sexually transmitted. The two most common categories of infection linked to urethritis are (1) gonococcal urethritis (GU), caused by *Neisseria gonorrhoeae*, and (2) nongonococcal urethritis (NGU), caused by *Chlamydia trachomatis, Ureaplasma urealyticum, Mycoplasma hominis,* and *Trichomonas vaginalis*.[21] Less common infectious causes of urethritis include herpes genitalis and syphilis, which may also be associated with communicable conditions such as epididymitis, **orchitis**, prostatitis, or UTIs. The incidence of GU is in decline. Conversely, the incidence of NGU is rising and is notably higher during the summer months. Urethritis affects males and females equally, although up to 50% of females may be asymptomatic; the infection is more common in homosexual males than heterosexuals or homosexual females. Infectious urethritis may occur in any sexually active person, but the incidence is highest among people age 20 to 24 yr.[2,21]

Signs and Symptoms

Signs and symptoms of urethritis are similar to those of a UTI. Symptom onset typically occurs between 4 and 14 d after contact with a partner with the infection. Urethral discharge may be present and may be yellow, green, brown, or blood tinged. Dysuria is usually localized to the urethral orifice and is worst with a first-morning void. Urethral itching or hematuria may be present, but up to 25% of individuals with urethritis have no signs or symptoms.[22] Males may report heaviness or aching in the testicles, although associated tenderness should suggest orchitis or epididymitis. Females may report worsening of symptoms with menses. The presence of fever, chills, sweats, or nausea suggests a more systemic infection and warrants immediate referral to a physician.[23]

Differential diagnoses for urethritis are best considered by sex. In both males and females, these diagnoses include recent kidney stone passage and STIs such as chlamydia, gonorrhea, herpes, mycoplasma, syphilis, and trichomoniasis. Other etiology without sex considerations that need to be ruled out include dermatological diseases involving the urethral orifice (e.g., contact dermatitis secondary to spermicides), molluscum contagiosum, urethral stricture, urethral trauma, urethral warts, urethral diverticulum, and urethral cancer. Differential diagnoses affecting females include rigorous sexual intercourse (*honeymoon cystitis*), **oophoritis**, PID, salpingitis, vaginitis, and vulvovaginitis. Differential diagnoses exclusive to males are epididymitis and chronic bacterial prostatitis.[23]

Referral and Diagnostic Tests

Patients suspected of having urethritis or cystitis are referred to a physician for diagnosis and treatment. To avoid further irritation or possible infection of others, the patient should be counseled to refrain from sexual intercourse until they have consulted a physician.

The diagnosis of urethritis is most often based on history and examination. A urinalysis is not particularly helpful in establishing the diagnosis but may be helpful in excluding cystitis or pyelonephritis. Microscopic examination of the specimen will reveal pyuria (>8 WBCs/μL) and possible microscopic hematuria. A dipstick test is specific for WBCs (>10 WBCs/μL).[22,23] Further testing should be done if STI is suspected.

More than 30% of individuals with NGU do not have leukocytes in their urine. A urethral culture may be performed to determine the presence of gonococcus or chlamydia. In cases of confirmed GU or NGU, testing for syphilis, hepatitis B virus (HBV), and human immunodeficiency virus (HIV) is encouraged.[2] Females of childbearing age who have experienced unprotected intercourse must undergo a pregnancy test before treatment.

Treatment and Return to Participation

Antibiotics are the mainstay of treatment for urethritis to prevent morbidity and to reduce transmission to others. Symptoms will resolve in all patients with urethritis over time regardless of treatment. The choice of antibiotic is based on the likelihood of whether the infection is GU or NGU. Current recommendations are to treat for both GU and NGU. Azithromycin in a single 2 g dose treats both GU and NGU, is the treatment of choice for urethritis, and is well tolerated. Intramuscular ceftriaxone or oral cefixime, ciprofloxacin, or ofloxacin can be used in single doses to treat GU only. Doxycycline can be taken for 7 d to treat NGU only. In the case of recurrent NGU, a prolonged course of erythromycin for 14 to 28 d is recommended.[2] Antibiotic treatment is recommended for sexual partners of patients with culture-positive urethritis, including for *Trichomonas* infection. For males with NGU, all sex partners within the 60 d preceding diagnosis should be referred for evaluation and treatment. Prevention of reinfection includes abstinence from sexual activity until the patient and partners have been effectively treated.[23,24]

The overall prognosis for urethritis is excellent. Antibiotics help to decrease any associated morbidity and prevent further transmission. Patients with urethritis are counseled to abstain from sexual intercourse until all partners have been treated, and they are further encouraged to use barrier devices (e.g., condoms) when engaging in sexual intercourse with multiple partners. Uncomplicated urethritis should not interfere with an individual's ability to train or compete.

Prevention

Prevention of urethritis equates to education. Sexually active patients are encouraged to use barrier methods during intercourse. Education about STI risk factors can be beneficial. Risk factors include intercourse at a young age, unprotected intercourse, multiple sexual partners, intercourse with partners known to have infections, and drug abuse. Early diagnosis and early treatment of patients with urethritis, along with identification and treatment of all partners, helps to limit transmission.

Sexually Transmitted Infections

Sexually transmitted diseases (STDs) and STIs are sexually transmittable infections as they pass via sexual contact, but some may occur in the absence of sexual activity. The term *STI* is typically preferred to *STD*, as it covers a broader range and includes people who have an STI and may infect others but may not have signs of a disease (table 9.1). STIs are unique in that they tend to affect males and females differently, and their presentations differ depending on sex. Males tend to present more regularly with signs and symptoms of an STI, whereas females do not, chiefly because their anatomy may preclude obvious symptoms. Many females may forgo medical evaluation and self-treat if they suspect

a UTI. General signs and symptoms of STIs are similar in both sexes, including dysuria (i.e., painful urination), urge to void but production of small volume, and urethral discharge, itching, and burning.

Catch-all terms associated with STIs are **nongonococcal** or **nonspecific urethritis** (**NGU** or **NSU**). Both occur in males and females and are caused by organisms that are not necessarily sexually transmitted. The signs and symptoms of both are similar to other STIs, in that patients present with dysuria, a frequent need to void, and discharge. These symptoms can be less intense than those of other STIs and can occur up to 6 wk after exposure, unlike the 2 to 8 d incubation period for gonorrhea. A number of causative agents include *Escherichia coli*, herpes simplex, trauma, chemical contact, or chlamydia. NGU is not a true STI. Undetected, this infection can spread to the testes, epididymis, prostate, and seminal vesicles in males. In females, the inflammation can spread to the labia, ovaries, uterus, and fallopian tubes, producing PID.[25]

Prevention

Most STIs can be prevented by using barrier protection (e.g., a condom) during sexual intercourse, knowing the medical history of the sex partner, and avoiding risky behaviors that include multiple sex partners, unsafe sexual practices, and excessive alcohol consumption, which may lead to risky behaviors. Some STIs, such as herpes, can be contagious even with barrier use, because the barrier must completely cover the lesion to deter the infection.

TABLE 9.1   **Sexually Transmitted Diseases and Infections**

Disease	Incubation	Transmission	Signs and symptoms	Treatment	Long term
HIV	1-6 mo	Sexually transmitted	Malaise, fever	Zidovudine for maintenance	AIDS
HPV	1-6 mo	Sexually transmitted	Genital warts	Symptomatic	Chronic carrier
Syphilis	1-13 wk	Sexual contact	Chancre, dermatological signs, constitutional symptoms	Penicillin	Incapacitating cardiovascular disease, often with neurological signs
Gonorrhea	Males: 2-14 d Females: 7-21 d	Sexually transmitted	Dysuria, discharge, frequency of voiding	Ceftriaxone, doxycycline	Hydrocele and abscesses in males; salpingitis in females
Chlamydia	7-28 d	Sexually transmitted	Dysuria, meatal itching, asymptomatic	Tetracycline or doxycycline	Pelvic inflammatory disease if left untreated
Herpes simplex virus 2	4-7 d	Sexual contact	Lesions	Acyclovir	Chronic carrier

Note: AIDS = acquired immunodeficiency syndrome; HIV = human immunodeficiency virus; HPV = human papillomavirus.

Patients must understand that having a STI does not provide immunity from another infection in the manner seen with childhood diseases discussed in chapter 14. The surest way to avoid STIs is to abstain from sexual relations or to maintain mutually monogamous sexual intimacy with an STI-free partner. An individual with a STI should abstain from sexual contact until the treatment course has been completed and all lesions have healed completely.[22]

Concerns With Adolescents and Public Health Implications

Patients younger than age 18 yr who are sexually active and report their anxiety about a possible STI to the athletic trainer are of special concern. In addition to state statutory rape laws, each state has specific laws regarding the reporting of this type of medical information to another person, parent, or guardian. The athletic trainer should consult the school counselor or nurse about applicable laws. The health of the athlete is of utmost importance. The treating physician has the obligation to report infectious diseases to the appropriate agency, but athletic trainers must be aware of the ramifications for youths with STIs.

Human Immunodeficiency Virus and Acquired Immunodeficiency Syndrome

HIV is bloodborne and is usually transmitted through sexual intercourse, shared intravenous materials, transplantation of infected organs, or from mother to child during birth or breastfeeding.[27] HIV is the precursor to acquired immunodeficiency syndrome (AIDS), the late-stage result of HIV infection. HIV may remain dormant for years after infection; however, it is estimated that 90% of patients with HIV eventually develop AIDS if left untreated.[2]

HIV transmission via saliva, urine, tears, insect bites (including mosquitoes), or bronchial secretions has not been recorded, but the virus has been found in these fluids.[2] HIV transmission through sexual contact is rarer compared with HBV transmission because HIV is not as hardy, but this should not preclude caution. The presence of a concurrent STI increases the likelihood of acquiring HIV.[27]

The incubation period for HIV can last several months or years before symptom onset, but most individuals with HIV will obtain a positive test result within 6 mo. Some patients develop a self-limiting mononucleosis-like illness weeks to months after HIV exposure, but the acute illness lasts only a few weeks and is often dismissed. Antiretroviral therapy (ART) is highly recommended for patients with HIV infection to reduce their likelihood of acquiring AIDS and to prevent HIV transmission to others. Patients with HIV must be educated that plasma HIV RNA (viral load) of less than 200 copies/mL with ART can prevent sexual transmission of the virus.[97]

In 2022, the CDC reported a peak in HIV infection rates in the United States for people ages 25 to 29 yr. Infection rates for American Indian, Alaska Native, and Asian individuals also increased, whereas those for Hispanic and Latino and White individuals remained stable. African American individuals had the highest number of new cases in 2020 compared with all other ethnicities. In 2020, males accounted for 81% of all HIV diagnoses among adults and adolescents.[28]

CONDITION HIGHLIGHT

Herpes Simplex Virus

Herpes simplex virus (HSV) has two forms: HSV-1 (oral herpes, often called *fever blisters* or *cold sores*) and HSV-2 (genital herpes). According to the Centers for Disease Control and Prevention (CDC), HSV is among the most prevalent STIs. In the United States, by age 30 yr, 50% of people from higher socioeconomic backgrounds and 80% of those from lower socioeconomic backgrounds are seropositive, but seropositivity does not indicate that these people are symptomatic.[26] HSV-1 transmission usually occurs through oral secretions or sores, and the virus is spread via kissing or sharing cups or utensils, toothbrushes, and so on. HSV-1 can cause genital herpes, but most cases of HSV-2 are caused by infection from HSV-1. Both types can be transmitted even if sores are not present. HSV-2 can be passed to infants via childbirth. Although many patients have no overt signs of HSV, the typical presentation is lesions with vesicles (blisters). Other signs and symptoms include fever (102-104 °F), lymphadenopathy, and listlessness. Illness, stress, fatigue, sunlight, menstruation, and physical trauma to the affected area can trigger a herpes outbreak in individuals with the virus. There is no cure for herpes, but drugs such as famciclovir (Famvir), acyclovir (Zovirax), and valaciclovir (Valtrex) are used to treat herpes symptoms.

Generally, individuals are not in danger of contracting HIV unless they engage in risky activities (e.g., sexual behaviors, needle sharing). The U.S. Preventive Services Task Force strongly recommends HIV testing for all adolescents and adults at increased risk of HIV infection, including pregnant females. Health care workers with HIV may be required to notify their employers of their status and may be restricted in the types of procedures they can perform.[27] Of particular concern are pregnant females with HIV. In a joint statement, the American College of Obstetricians and Gynecologists and the American Academy of Pediatrics put forth a policy in 2011 that strongly supports universal HIV testing as a component of prenatal care, and it has been jointly reaffirmed annually since then.[29] Extensive studies have been performed and great strides have been made in improving prevention of mother-to-child perinatal HIV transmission.[30]

Signs and Symptoms

After infection, a broad variety of clinical issues may occur. *AIDS-related complex* (ARC) is the term used for patients with HIV who have not yet developed opportunistic infections associated with AIDS. General signs and symptoms of ARC include malaise, intermittent fever, diarrhea, anemia, weight loss, lymphadenopathy, **hairy leukoplakia**, and **thrush**. Some life-threatening cancers, including Kaposi's sarcoma, non-Hodgkin's lymphoma, and lymphoma of the brain, may be acquired through AIDS-related infection in patients who never manifested ARC symptoms.[2,22]

AIDS itself is considered an opportunistic infection, settling on whole-body systems or organs. Signs and symptoms are presented chiefly via other known pathologies but are in fact caused by AIDS. Associated illnesses include encephalitis, meningitis, tuberculosis, central nervous system (CNS) infections, vascular and digestive complications, peripheral neuropathies, and renal pathologies.[27]

Because HIV and AIDS can manifest as a multiorgan system problem, the list of differential diagnoses is lengthy. These diagnoses range from malaise and simple gastrointestinal disturbances to pneumonia, cancer, or complex regional pain syndrome.

Referral and Diagnostic Tests

Individuals who present with unexplainable fatigue or slow-healing wounds are referred to a physician for further evaluation. If a patient has reason to warrant HIV testing, a blood test is necessary to confirm the virus. A high-sensitivity enzyme-linked immunoabsorbent assay is used for screening.[27] False-positive results are known to occur, so reactive tests are supplemented by additional studies, such as the **Western blot** or the indirect fluorescent antibody test. At-home or so-called rapid tests for HIV are commercially available but not all are approved by the Food and Drug Administration (FDA). Consumers must understand that both false-positive and false-negative results are possible.

Treatment and Return to Participation

Clinical trials have begun for an experimental HIV vaccine that uses messenger RNA technology similar to that used to create COVID-19 vaccines.[98] However, more research is warranted, because the initial clinical trial results reported that the vaccine was ineffective.[99] Both HIV and AIDS weaken the immune system, so treatment comprises symptom management to maintain overall health and avoid invasion by opportunistic infections. Highly active antiretroviral therapy (HAART) is the principal method of preventing immune deterioration.[27] Long-term HAART yields gradual improvement in immune response and, coupled with other prophylactic medications, can retard or stabilize HIV infection.[31]

An athlete with HIV is not banned from participation, and the chance of transmission via sports is negligible if health care providers practice approved bloodborne pathogen policies. The illnesses associated with AIDS may preclude athletic endeavors, but the decision is up to the individual athlete and the physician. Because HIV attacks the immune system, athletes with the virus should keep their distance from sick teammates.

The National Collegiate Athletics Association (NCAA) does not require college athletes with HIV to report or acknowledge infection to the organization or on health screenings. However, HIV is reportable to the local health authority, and the United States and most countries require mandatory reporting of AIDS.[32]

Genital Warts

Genital warts are caused by human papillomavirus (HPV) and are typically acquired via sexual contact. They are also called *venereal warts* or *condylomata acuminata* and result in a fibrous overgrowth of the dermis. There are more than 100 identified strains of HPV, any of which can cause genital warts. These warts tend to grow rapidly in areas of the skin and mucous membranes that experience heavy perspiration or poor hygiene, and they often accompany other STIs.[33] Since the early 2000s, the prevalence of HPV has increased to twice the rate of genital herpes in the United States, and young adults (ages 15-25 yr) account for nearly one-half of all infections each year. The association between HPV and genital herpes is disconcerting because HPV has an association with cancer that herpes does not share. Several types of

HPV cause cervical cancer (as discussed in the Ovarian and Cervical Cancer section). The incubation period for HPV is 1 to 6 mo.

Women with a history of specific types of genital warts need to be monitored over time because these warts can develop into an invasive cervical carcinoma. In addition, some types of genital warts have developed into bladder cancer. Genital warts are not common before puberty or after menopause.[33] HPV also causes nongenital warts, such as the common and plantar warts (see chapter 16).

Signs and Symptoms

Genital warts look like common warts: that is, they are typically painless, minute, pink or red, soft, moist outgrowths that can appear in clusters. They can resemble cauliflower and are found in warm, moist areas of the body. In women, they are found on the vulva, vaginal walls, cervix, and perineum. Males with HPV may present with warts in the urethra or penile shaft, and homosexual men may present with warts in the perianal area or rectum. Genital warts do not resemble acne or express any discharge.

Differential diagnoses for genital warts include secondary syphilis, cervical cancer, and skin tags.

Referral and Diagnostic Tests

Patients with wart-like genital growths are referred to a physician for assessment. Genital warts are diagnosed based on their appearance; however, lingering or unusual warts must be differentiated from secondary syphilis by biopsy. Women with cervical warts must obtain a clear Pap smear before undergoing any further diagnostic tests on warts.

Treatment and Return to Participation

Although genital warts are typically removed by electrocauterization, cryotherapy, laser, or, if necessary, surgical excision, these remedies are not infallible. There is no single curative treatment, and only visible warts are usually treated. Urethral warts are removed via resectoscope with the patient under general anesthesia and via circumcision of males to prevent recurrence.[33] Urethral lesions also need to be monitored for the rare occasion of urethral obstruction. Direct injection of interferon-α may remove genital warts that have returned after previous removal but will not reduce the rate of return. HPV and genital warts do not prohibit sport participation.

In 2006, the FDA approved a vaccine for four HPV types that cause cervical cancer. The vaccine is approved for both male and female youths and young adults (as discussed in the Ovarian and Cervical Cancer section).

Syphilis

Syphilis, a sexually acquired disease caused by the organism *Treponema pallidum*, has systemic ramifications. The disease has been called the "great imitator" because so many of its symptoms reflect other diseases.[2] Although syphilis is preventable and curable, new cases are seen in the United States each year. A 2022 CDC report shows an upward trend, with 133,945 total cases in 2020 compared with 36,000 reported cases in 2010, including nearly 41,655 primary and secondary cases in 2020 compared with 10,000 in 2006.[34] Although no particular group is without representation, homosexual men are the fastest growing population, with 53% of the new diagnoses.

Syphilis presents with a series of clinical manifestations interrupted by years of latency. No body system is protected from the disease, and a mother with syphilis can transmit it to the fetus. Acquired, not congenital, syphilis is discussed here. Unlike HBV, *T. pallidum* is an unstable organism that cannot live long outside its human host. Transmission occurs from person to person via direct contact with a syphilis sore.[35] Syphilis has an incubation period of 1 to 13 wk, but it is more typical to develop signs and symptoms between weeks 3 and 4 postinfection. Within hours of exposure, *T. pallidum* infiltrates the lymphatic system and subsequently moves throughout the entire body. The CNS is affected during the secondary stage of the disease.

Signs and Symptoms

There are four distinct stages of syphilis (see the Stages of Acquired Syphilis sidebar); signs and symptoms depend on the disease stage. Primary syphilis begins with a chancre or sore at the point of contact with a person with the disease. This occurs most often on the external genitalia and mouth.[35] The chancre may be a single firm, round, painless sore or multiple sores. These sores form a painless ulcer and exude a clear serum. More often, a person with syphilis is unaware because the sores heal on their own untreated, and many patients are asymptomatic for years. Untreated, however, the syphilis infection progresses to the secondary stage.

Signs of secondary syphilis include skin rash and mucous membrane lesions that can appear 4 to 12 wk after infection. Although most rashes are antipyretic, they are rough and red with reddish brown spots. Sixty to eighty percent of people with syphilis present with secondary rashes on the palms or soles (figure 9.9), but rashes can develop anywhere on the body and may be so subtle that they are overlooked.[2,36] These rashes often heal spontaneously, only to reappear. Other signs and symptoms associated with the secondary stage include fever, lymphomegaly, pharyngitis, myalgia, malaise, headache, weight loss, and patchy hair loss.[22] Again, if left untreated, secondary syphilis progresses to latent-stage syphilis.

The early latent period of the disease is usually a time without symptoms; it may last the remainder of the patient's life or may spontaneously relapse. This period begins approximately 1 yr after infection and may be treated by penicillin given for a reason other than syphilis.

Late latent (or tertiary) syphilis is the final stage of this devastating disease. When other body systems are affected by syphilis infection, profound sequelae, including cardiovascular, neurological, musculoskeletal, and visual system deterioration, occur. Untreated syphilis can cause death.[35] In addition, patients with syphilis have a fivefold increased risk of HIV infection.[2]

The differential diagnoses for primary syphilis include genital herpes, scabies, ulceration, and trauma. Alternative diagnoses for secondary syphilis, which presents primarily as a dermatological reaction, include dermatitis, drug reaction rash, rubella, mononucleosis, ringworm, warts, and fungal infection. Latent stages of syphilis are more troublesome because they can manifest in any body organ or system and go undetected until serological tests for *T. pallidum* have been performed.[35]

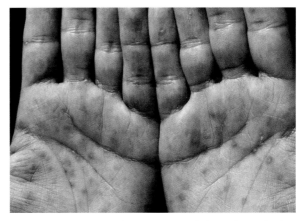

FIGURE 9.9   Secondary-stage syphilis rash on the hands.
Martin M. Rotker / Science Source

Referral and Diagnostic Tests

Primary syphilis is diagnosed from exudates removed from the chancre, followed by serological workup if the results are unremarkable.

The serological test for syphilis (STS) is the most common screening tool used for diagnosis. The STS is

Stages of Acquired Syphilis

Primary Stage

Usually within 3 wk of exposure

- Chancre
- Contagious

Secondary Stage

Usually 4 to 12 wk after exposure

- Dermatological presentations, including rash and mucous membrane erosion
- Cerebrospinal fluid (CSF) abnormalities
- Lymphadenopathy
- Contagious

Early Latent Stage

- Up to 1 yr after exposure
- Usually asymptomatic
- May never progress to later stage

Late Latent Stage (or Tertiary)

- More than 1 yr after exposure
- Symptomatic but not contagious
- Cardiovascular syphilis marked by aortic insufficiency, coronary stenosis, or aortic aneurysm
- Neurosyphilis marked by personality changes, hyperactive reflexes, decreased memory, slurred speech, optic atrophy, seizures, or hemiparesis

often used by allied health workers to determine whether subsequent evaluation is warranted.

Treatment and Return to Participation

Treatment for primary and secondary syphilis includes the physician taking a full sexual history from the patient, including all sexual partners during the past 3 mo in the case of primary syphilis and during the past 12 mo for secondary infections.

Penicillin is the appropriate medication for all forms of syphilis, and a single intramuscular injection of penicillin will cure a patient who has had syphilis less than 1 yr.[35] If the patient is allergic to penicillin, erythromycin or tetracycline can be administered at a dosage of 500 mg every 6 h for 15 d (see chapter 4).

Syphilis is a reportable disease, and the patient's sexual partners must be notified by the reporting agency, tested, and given treatment.

Gonorrhea

Gonorrhea is sexually transmitted, is caused by a gram-negative organism, *N. gonorrhoeae*, and is a major cause of PID in women. The disease can affect the epithelium of the urethra, cervix, rectum, pharynx, and conjunctiva. Incidence rates have been increasing since 2009, with the CDC reporting nearly 678,000 cases in 2020 compared with more than 350,000 new cases 6 yr prior in 2014.[37] Adults age 20 yr or older, primarily men, have the highest incidence of gonorrhea. Reported rates of infection increased in most racial and Hispanic ethnic groups, with the greatest observed increase in non-Hispanic African American individuals and non-Hispanic people of multiple races.[37] The infection has a relatively short incubation period of 2 to 21 d. Transmission almost always is via direct sexual contact, with rare exceptions of transmission from mothers to infants during vaginal birth and from health care personnel to patients through broken skin.

If gonorrhea is left untreated, serious, sex-related complications may include male postgonococcal urethritis, epididymitis, and prostatitis. Women can develop PID or **salpingitis**, an inflammation of the fallopian tube, and both can lead to acute pain, infection, possible tubal scarring and adhesions, and resultant infertility (figure 9.10).

Both men and women may develop systemic or disseminated gonococcal infection, which presents with malaise, mild febrile illness, pustular lesions, and arthritis. Systemic disease is associated with bacteremia that may manifest as ocular infections, septic arthritis, skin lesions, and tenosynovitis.

Signs and Symptoms

Men and women with gonorrhea have differing presentations and complications. Women may not seek treatment as quickly as men because their symptoms are mild and may be more easily dismissed. In men, symptoms begin as discomfort in the urethra, moving quickly to dysuria and a purulent, yellow-green urethral discharge. Women's symptoms include dysuria, frequency of voiding, painful intercourse, mid- and lower abdominal pain, and vaginal discharge.[2,38]

Differential diagnoses for gonorrhea include syphilis, chlamydia, UTI, or injury. For women, infection resulting from a lost or forgotten tampon is another differential diagnosis.

Referral and Diagnostic Tests

Individuals manifesting symptoms consistent with gonorrhea are immediately referred to a physician. A patient suspected of having gonorrhea is also tested for syphilis (STS) before initiating treatment. Gonorrhea may occur concurrently with other STIs, so it is important to treat

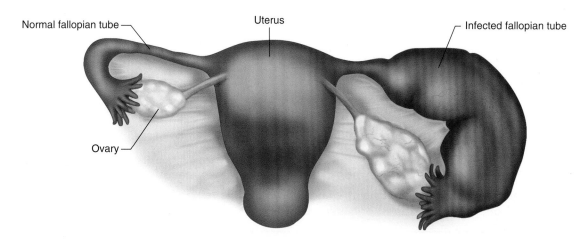

FIGURE 9.10 Salpingitis is an inflamed or infected fallopian tube that can result from unresolved gonorrhea.

them all. Specific tests for gonorrhea include a urethral swab of the discharge, which confirms the disease in 90% of men with the infection but only in 60% of women.[22,36] Culture with exudates from the urethra, cervix, rectum, and pharynx can confirm diagnosis.

Treatment and Return to Participation

Because strains of drug-resistant gonorrhea have emerged, the use of penicillin has been challenged. The current drug of choice is ceftriaxone (125 mg intramuscularly), but because this STI often occurs in conjunction with chlamydia, the latter also must be treated.[24,38] The referring physician will typically use a combination of medications, keeping in mind the complexity of treating two STIs and the challenge of drug resistance.

As with syphilis, all of the patient's sexual contacts must be located, cultured, and treated.

Chlamydia

Chlamydia includes all members of the genus *Chlamydia*, gram-negative bacteria with a unique developmental cycle within host cells. Almost every species of bird and mammal is infected with chlamydia and it can produce a broad spectrum of diseases because of its parasitic reproductive process. Chlamydia causes many different diseases in humans, largely in the eye, respiratory system, and genital tract. The strain of chlamydia most commonly associated with an STI is *C. trachomatis*, and it is the most frequently reported STI in the United States.[21] Chlamydial infection is the most common reportable disease in the United States, with 4 million new infections in 2018, and it tends to be linked with other STIs such as gonorrhea, NGU, and syphilis.[21,39] Approximately one-half of NGU cases are caused by *C. trachomatis*, which has an incubation period of 2 to 3 wk. The infection is on the rise, and its prevalence in the United States is highest among people age 15 to 24 yr.[21]

The primary danger from chlamydia is the possible repercussion from untreated disease. Females are more likely to be asymptomatic; sequelae include risk of infertility, ectopic pregnancy, PID, and chronic pelvic pain.[39] Males risk urethral infection, epididymitis, infertility, and reactive arthritis (formerly Reiter's syndrome).[2]

Signs and Symptoms

The signs and symptoms of chlamydia are consistent with those of other STIs, but patients with the disease may remain asymptomatic. Chlamydia presents with urethral discharge, dysuria, fever, and meatal itching.

Other STIs, such as gonorrhea and NGU, need to be ruled out when chlamydia is suspected. In addition, differential diagnoses include UTI, yeast infection, and dermatitis.

Referral and Diagnostic Tests

Diagnosis of chlamydia is based on cultured secretions obtained by swabbing the infected area. Physicians have found little benefit from serology for this diagnosis.[39]

Treatment and Return to Participation

Because chlamydia is often concurrent with gonorrhea and tends to persist after gonorrhea is successfully treated, physicians should evaluate and provide remedies for both diseases. Untreated, chlamydia can lead to infertility, PID, ectopic pregnancy, and chronic pelvic pain.[39] Chlamydia is resistant to penicillin and cephalosporins and must be treated with azithromycin, tetracycline, erythromycin, or doxycycline to be eradicated. The U.S. Preventive Services Task Force recommends routine screening of young women for chlamydia to prevent the sequelae that can follow the disease. Chlamydia must be reported to the local health authority in most states.[36] The U.S. Preventive Services Task Force recommends routine screening for chlamydial infections in sexually active females age 24 yr or younger and in older women at increased risk of infection.[39]

Pathological Conditions Related to the Male Genitourinary System

Testicular Torsion

The testicle is covered by the tunica vaginalis, which attaches to the posterolateral surface of the testicle and allows for limited mobility. If the testicle can twist or freely rotate (i.e., torsion; see figure 9.11), venous occlusion can occur, which subsequently leads to arterial ischemia, causing infarction of the testicle.

The incidence of testicular torsion in males younger than 25 yr is approximately 1 per 4,000. The highest incidence is among males age 12 to 16 yr, but it can occur at any age.[40] Torsion predominantly affects the left testicle. Recall that typically, the left testicle lies slightly lower than the right. A subgroup of individuals has a higher frequency of testicular torsion because of a congenital extremely narrow attachment of the epididymis to the tunica vaginalis (**bell clapper deformity**). This attachment allows the testicle to rotate freely on the spermatic cord within the scrotal sac.[41] This congenital abnormality is found in as many as 12% of males.[42] Testicular torsion can also occur after exercise, sexual activity, or trauma,

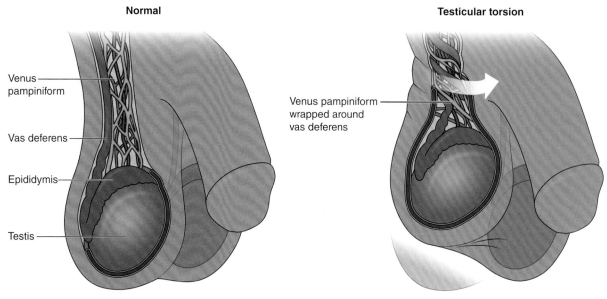

FIGURE 9.11   Testicular torsion.

or it may develop at rest. Previous studies (56 and 64 patients, respectively) demonstrated that incidences of testicular torsion are higher in warmer temperatures, which suggests that colder weather contributes to a reduced frequency of these types of injuries.[43,44] Other than early identification of the bell clapper deformity, no preventive measures can prevent a testicular torsion. Wearing an athletic supporter or tighter-fitting undergarments may lower the risk of torsion.

Signs and Symptoms

The history of testicular torsion includes the sudden onset of severe unilateral scrotal pain. The most common symptoms include scrotal swelling, abdominal pain, nausea, and vomiting. Younger patients may be reluctant to disclose scrotal pain, and they may present with lower abdominal pain.[45] Less frequently a fever or urinary frequency may be documented. Examination of the scrotum reveals a tender and painful testicle that is often elevated in relationship to the contralateral testicle. The involved testicle often is in a horizontal position rather than its usual vertical orientation. The testicle may be enlarged with scrotal swelling and erythema. In general, elevation of the involved testicle provides no relief of pain as compared with epididymitis, in which pain relief is notable with elevation of the involved testicle.

Referral and Diagnostic Tests

Testicular torsion is a urological emergency. Patient history and physical examination may not confirm testicular torsion, and imaging studies (including ultrasonography and nuclear scans) may be helpful in confirming the diagnosis.[40,46]

The possibility of testicular torsion requires immediate and emergent evaluation by the physician or immediate referral to an emergency department. Diagnosis and treatment within 6 h of pain onset results in an 80% to 100% salvage rate for the affected testicle.[40] Beyond this time frame, the salvage rate steadily decreases and approaches 0% at 12 h.[45]

Imaging studies can provide useful information but because testicular torsion is a clinical diagnosis, treatment should not be delayed for imaging if the diagnosis is clear. For cases in which the diagnosis is less clear, color Doppler ultrasonography can be performed.[47,48] A color Doppler is used to assess arterial blood flow to the testicle. A radionuclide scan can also be performed to assess arterial blood flow, with decreased uptake indicating a lack of blood flow to the testicle.

Because testicular torsion is a urological emergency, there is little room for error in diagnosis. The differential diagnoses, however, should include epididymitis, orchitis,

Clinical Tips

Testicular Torsion in Youth

Adolescent and younger patients often report vague thigh or knee pain when referring to testicular pain. Whether this is attributable to an inability or unwillingness to focus on their testicular issue, athletic trainers should maintain an index of suspicion for testicular torsion if patients have a mechanism consistent with this trauma. This is especially true in the absence of clinical findings of thigh or knee pathology.

RED FLAGS FOR TESTICULAR TORSION

Testicular torsion is a urological emergency requiring immediate medical attention. It presents as follows:

- Scrotal swelling
- Abdominal pain
- Nausea and vomiting
- Tender testicle
- Elevated testicle compared with uninvolved testicle
- Possible horizontal rather than vertical orientation

hydrocele, varicocele, hernia, and acute appendicitis. Traumatic hematoma and testicular carcinoma should also be considered differential diagnoses for testicular torsion.[45,46]

Treatment and Return to Participation

Early diagnosis and referral are key to successful treatment. Once testicular torsion is diagnosed, the physician can attempt a manual reduction. Because most testicular torsion involves a "turning in" toward the midline, the process of detorsion involves rotating the affected testicle 180° from medial to lateral. The physician may need to repeat the rotation two or three times for a complete detorsion. Success is determined by a marked decrease in pain. Detorsion can be accomplished manually in 25% to 80% of affected individuals.[45,46] If manual detorsion is not successful, surgery is indicated for definitive treatment and involves detorsion and orchiopexy, which is surgical fixation of the testicle.

The prognosis for testicular torsion depends on rapid referral and diagnosis. If detorsion is obtained within 6 h of symptom onset, nearly 100% of torsive testicles can be salvaged. A delay in treatment up to 12 h results in decreasing rates of salvage. Return to participation is based on the result of the torsion and physician clearance.

Hydrocele

Hydroceles are fluid collections within the tunica vaginalis of the scrotum or along the spermatic cord (figure 9.12). Most hydroceles are developmental in origin because of persistence of a patent processus vaginalis. However, for unknown reasons, hydroceles can also develop as a result of an imbalance between scrotal fluid production and absorption. It is estimated that approximately 6% of men have a clinically apparent hydrocele.[2]

Signs and Symptoms

Hydroceles are usually asymptomatic. Increased fluid collections, however, can cause scrotal aching. A hydrocele typically manifests as a nontender fullness in the hemiscrotum and is palpable just anterior to the testicle. They can be congenital, and they may also resolve spontaneously.[22] Inability to clearly delineate or palpate the testicular structures or the presence of tenderness raises the possibility of an alternative diagnosis.

Both hydroceles and varicoceles are differential diagnoses for each other. In addition, differential diagnoses include the following:

- Epididymitis
- Orchitis
- Testicular tumor
- Testicular torsion

For hydrocele, another differential diagnosis is an inguinal hernia. For varicocele, another differential diagnosis is spermatic vein compression.

Referral and Diagnostic Tests

Athletic trainers should immediately refer any male with painful scrotal swelling to a physician. Although a hydrocele is not an emergency, nontender scrotal swelling that is consistent with a hydrocele needs to be examined by a physician to document its presence. An experienced physician can confirm the diagnosis of a hydrocele. In some cases, an ultrasound may be performed to confirm the diagnosis.[49,50]

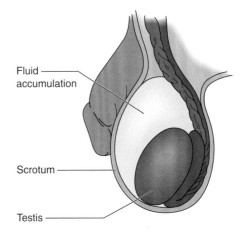

Fluid accumulation

Scrotum

Testis

FIGURE 9.12   Hydrocele is a painless swelling in the scrotum.

Treatment and Return to Participation

Asymptomatic adults with an isolated hydrocele can be observed indefinitely or until they become symptomatic. Surgical intervention is warranted for the following indications:[49,50]

- Inability to distinguish a hydrocele from an inguinal hernia
- Failure to resolve spontaneously after an appropriate interval of observation
- Inability to clearly examine the testes
- Association of hydroceles with suggestive pathology, such as testicular torsion or tumor

Return to participation may take 2 to 6 wk after a simple hydrocele repair. The presence of a hydrocele does not preclude participation in athletics. If the hydrocele is symptomatic or has been surgically repaired, the treating physician will decide on return to play.

Varicocele

A varicocele is a dilation of the pampiniform venous plexus and the internal spermatic vein within the scrotum (figure 9.13). The etiology of a varicocele is unclear. Varicoceles occur in approximately 20% of men; however, about 40% of infertile men may have a varicocele.[51] Varicoceles are the most common correctable cause of male infertility.[52]

Signs and Symptoms

Approximately 80% to 90% of varicoceles occur on the left side of the scrotum because of anatomical vascular differences.[51] Men are generally asymptomatic but occasionally report an aching pain or heaviness in the scrotum. Physical examination demonstrates a soft thickening just above the testicle and has been described as feeling like a "bag of worms." In a previous study, radiological testing discovered bilateral varicoceles in 35% to 40% of men with a unilateral palpable varicocele.[51] Varicoceles are staged according to size:

- *Large:* Those easily identified by inspection alone
- *Moderate:* Those identified by palpation without the Valsalva maneuver
- *Small:* Those identified by palpation, using the Valsalva maneuver to increase intraabdominal pressure, which will impede venous drainage and increase varicocele size

Referral and Diagnostic Tests

Development of a new varicocele or sudden onset of testicular swelling or pain requires immediate physician evaluation. Any male with a known varicocele who develops increasing testicular pain also warrants physician evaluation. Referral to a urologist for a surgical opinion is indicated when there is significant testicular pain, impairment of testicular function as evidenced by decreased semen quality, or testicular atrophy (volume <20 mL or length <4 cm).[53]

Diagnosis of a varicocele is typically clear by physical examination. The Valsalva maneuver may aid diagnosis (figure 9.14). If the physical examination is equivocal, a Doppler ultrasonogram may be performed to demonstrate the varicocele. Individuals who have a new or sudden-onset varicocele or a nonreducible varicocele in the recumbent position may warrant abdominal CT to evaluate for renal or vascular pathology as a cause of spermatic vein compression.[52,53]

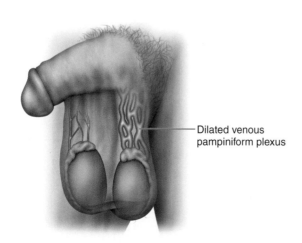

FIGURE 9.13 Varicocele in the spermatic cord.

Dilated venous pampiniform plexus

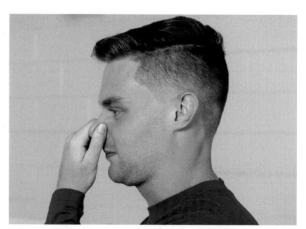

FIGURE 9.14 In the Valsalva maneuver, the patient is asked to exhale against a closed epiglottis (bearing down).

Treatment and Return to Participation

There is no medical treatment per se for an asymptomatic varicocele. Surgical treatment via laparoscopy, if warranted, involves microscopic ligation of the involved veins to prevent continued abnormal blood flow.[52]

The presence of a varicocele poses no known risks to the athlete involved in individual or team sports. After surgical correction of a varicocele, return to play is generally within 2 to 6 wk but depends on the athlete's circumstances and the surgeon's recommendations. Use of a protective cup is recommended for involvement in contact or collision sports if early return is allowed.[51]

Testicular Cancer

Testicular cancer is an abnormal growth of cells in the testicles. It is most common in men ages 20 to 34 yr and typically affects a single testicle. Because of its high cure rate if diagnosed early, most men with testicular cancer are cured. Although the number of new cases of testicular cancer has risen steadily since 1975, so too has the survival rate, which is now 95%.[54]

In 2022, nearly 9,000 men were diagnosed with testicular cancer, and 460 men died of the disease that year, according to the National Cancer Institute.[54] The diagnosis of testicular cancer is rising in all ethnic groups, but the greatest increase is in non-Hispanic American Indian or Alaskan Native men.[54] Testicular germ cell tumors account for 90% of the cancers,[55] are highly inheritable, and are one reason this cancer is increasing.[56] Conditions associated with an increased risk of testicular cancer include cryptorchidism (i.e., failure of one or both testicles to descend into the scrotum during development), family history of testicular cancer, maternal exposure to diethylstilbestrol while pregnant, testicular atrophy, and some possible environmental and drug exposures.[54]

Signs and Symptoms

Any new or unexpected change in the testicles should prompt an evaluation by a physician. The most common findings noted by the individual or during the testicular self-examination (TSE) include a solid, firm mass, painless swelling, a growth, or pain in the testicle.[55] Less commonly, a sense of heaviness or prolonged aching in the testicles may be noted.

Referral and Diagnostic Tests

Any male with an abnormal testicular examination, a new painless testicular growth, swelling, or testicular pain should be referred to a physician for further evaluation. Physical examination of the testicles by the athlete or a physician can determine whether a palpable mass or swelling is present. An ultrasound of the scrotum and testicles is then performed to document the presence or absence of an abnormality. Patients of reproductive age who are suspected of having testicular cancer should be counseled on their choice to bank their sperm before surgery, as long-term consequences of radiotherapy or chemotherapy on testicular function are not well understood.[57] Confirmatory testing is by tissue diagnosis most commonly obtained by radical orchiectomy (i.e., surgical removal of the testicle and spermatic cord). In the presence of testicular cancer, a chest radiograph and CT scan of the abdomen and pelvis are performed to evaluate for metastatic spread of the disease.[57]

The differential diagnoses for testicular cancer include orchitis, epididymitis, hydrocele, and varicocele.

Treatment and Return to Participation

The initial treatment for testicular cancer is a radical orchiectomy involving the testicle and spermatic cord. Therapy is then based on tumor type (i.e., **seminoma**, nonseminoma, or other), cancer stage, microscopic appearance, tumor location and extension, and both physician and patient preference. Treatment options include chemotherapy, radiation therapy, and surgical resection of the lymph node or nodes.[55] Overall treatment success is high for testicular cancer. Follow-up care is essential, is based on tumor type, and involves periodic chest radiographs, CT scans, and blood tests for tumor markers.

Cure rates for testicular cancer are high, ranging from greater than 80% for more disseminated cancers to nearly 100% for cancers localized to the testicle. During treatment, individual participation in athletics may be limited because of pain or discomfort. Specific decisions about the degree of involvement in athletics will be made by the treating physician in conjunction with the athlete. After complete recovery, patients can obtain a testicular prosthesis via surgical implantation. After successful treatment of testicular cancer, there are no contraindications to participation in athletics, although the use of a support cup is recommended in contact or collision sports to protect the remaining testicle.[55,57]

RED FLAGS FOR TESTICULAR CANCER

- Painless testicular swelling
- Testicular growth
- Painful testicle
- Palpable firm, solid mass within the testicle

Prevention

There is no known way to prevent testicular cancer. Recommendations are for men (particularly those ages 16-45 yr) to perform monthly TSEs. These consist of examining and palpating the scrotum for lumps or swelling and bringing any abnormality to a physician's attention. Here is how to complete a TSE:

- Stand in front of a mirror and look for scrotal swelling.
- Examine each testicle individually with both hands, fingers under the testicle, while rolling the testicle gently with the thumbs, palpating for lumps or swelling (figure 9.15).
- Palpate the epididymis superior and posterior to each testicle.
- Perform once each month, preferably after a shower; the heat of the shower will enable the scrotal skin to relax and be more pliable.

A monthly TSE can help in the early recognition and diagnosis of testicular cancer, thereby improving overall survival. In a large international systematic review, researchers discovered that few men were informed about the danger of testicular cancer and fewer performed regular TSEs.[58] Specifically, they reported that the African Americans in their study were the least informed about testicular cancer and TSEs. The researchers cited education as paramount to prevention, and they noted that organizations can assist with education. For example, the Testicular Cancer Awareness Foundation used 89% of its funding to educate young men to perform routine self-examinations.[58] A study has tasked the U.S. Preventive Services Task Force with increasing awareness for men to do TSE in hopes of more men detecting any testicular abnormalities sooner.[59]

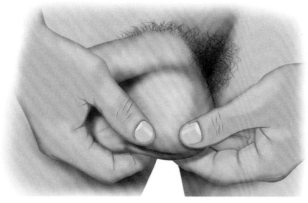

FIGURE 9.15 Testicular self-examination.

Prostate Cancer

As discussed at the beginning of this chapter, the prostate gland is responsible for contributing to the seminal fluid and is located directly anterior to the rectum (see figure 9.4). Prostate cancer is an abnormal growth of cells within the prostate gland. It is the second leading cause of cancer deaths among men in the United States, and African American men have a higher rate of death from prostate cancer compared with all other racial and ethnic groups.[60] The incidence of prostate cancer increases with age, and an estimated 1 in 10 men will develop prostate cancer in their lifetime. Risk factors for the development of prostate cancer include advancing age, family history of prostate or breast cancer, and race.[60] Since 2002, the incidence of prostate cancer and its death rate have steadily and significantly decreased.[60]

Prostate cancer prevention involves risk factor modification and regular prostate screening. Recent advances in genetic testing show promise in identifying prostate cancer risk. Research on polygenic risk scores states that they should be used in conjunction with other assessments to determine risk.[61] Men at risk of developing prostate cancer should consider consuming a diet low in animal fats and chromium and engaging in regular exercise. As with testicular cancer, the U.S. Preventive Services Task Force has issued recommendations for screening for prostate cancer. Their recommendations include using individual-based **prostate-specific antigen (PSA)** testing in men ages 55 to 69 yr.[62] One rationale for individual-based testing (and not mandated routine testing) is the harm resulting from false-positive results in men whose prostate cancer would never have been symptomatic in their lifetime, and the potential lifelong complications of treatment that may not have been necessary.[62] The once-popular DRE (used to palpate the prostate) is no longer as effective as the PSA test, but it is sometimes utilized with PSA testing for symptomatic or susceptible patients.

Signs and Symptoms

No reliable signs or symptoms suggest the early presence of prostate cancer. Advanced or metastatic prostate cancer may result in fatigue associated with anemia, weight loss, hematuria, urinary retention (caused by obstruction), urinary incontinence, back pain, pathological fractures, or spinal cord compression.

Conditions that involve the prostate gland and should be excluded when determining whether the patient has prostate cancer include benign prostatic hypertrophy, both acute and chronic prostatitis, **prostatic calculi**, prostate cysts, and **prostatic tuberculosis**. Other cancers that can mimic prostate cancer include lymphomas.

Referral and Diagnostic Tests

Any male suspected of having prostate cancer should be referred to a physician for evaluation and possible testing.

The early diagnosis of prostate cancer is based on a medical history and a physical examination that includes a PSA blood test and possible DRE to palpate the prostate. As PSA levels rise, so does the risk of prostate cancer. It should be noted that prostate cancer can be detected in about 8% of men when the PSA is 1 ng/mL; with a level of 4 to 10 ng/mL, the chance of prostate cancer is about 25%. In general, biopsies are not recommended unless the PSA is 2.5 to 3 ng/mL.[63] Both malignant and benign cells are produced by PSA, and there is growing evidence that PSA alone is not a strong indicator of prostate cancer; if PSA is used, it must be confirmed by other diagnostic tests specific for prostate cancer. Elevated PSA could indicate prostatitis, UTI, recent sexual activity, or a recent, vigorous DRE.[63]

When cancer is suspected, an ultrasound examination with a transrectal needle biopsy can often provide a definitive tissue diagnosis. However, ultrasound-guided prostate biopsies have been shown to miss 20% to 30% of the cancers and undergrade others.[63] Once prostate cancer is diagnosed, further testing and imaging for cancer staging are performed. These tests generally include a CBC, serum chemistries, liver function tests, PSA, ratio of free PSA to total PSA, alkaline phosphatase, and urinalysis. Imaging studies can include chest radiographs, a CT or magnetic resonance imaging (MRI) scan of the abdomen and pelvis, a ProstaScint scan (i.e., immunoscintigraphy used to detect extraprostatic spread), and a bone scan.

Treatment and Return to Participation

Treatment strategies for prostate cancer are changing with new advances. Treatment options include surgical removal (prostatectomy), radiation (including via external or internal radioactive seeds implanted into the prostate gland), and hormone therapy. Standard treatment for localized prostate cancer ranges from watchful waiting, to active surveillance, to radical prostatectomy, and to radiation therapy. Metastatic cancer is rarely curable.[63] Management of metastatic prostate cancer involves the addition of palliative radiation therapy to sites of painful metastases. The physician outlines specific treatment regimens for the patient.

Mortality rates from prostate cancer are declining in the United States. Early diagnosis can lead to the detec-tion of prostate cancer confined to the prostate gland and subsequently improve survival.[60] The overall prognosis in terms of survival is related to tumor size, lymph node involvement, and the presence or absence of metastases. For small cancers, localized within the prostate gland itself, overall survival is excellent, and a cure may be expected. In contrast, the 10-year survival rate for men with aggressive cancers that have metastasized is 25%.[60]

Patients may return to play during treatment for prostate cancer if they feel well and experience no significant side effects from their treatment regimen.

Pathological Conditions of the Gynecological System

Vaginitis

Vaginitis is an inflammation of the vagina, usually derived from infection. Vaginitis can also be attributable to a fungal condition or caused by an estrogen deficiency.[2] In the sexually active patient, bacterial vaginosis (BV), trichomoniasis, and candidiasis are three common conditions that may account for 90% of all cases of vaginitis.[22]

The normal vaginal environment is relatively stable. High estrogen levels in women of childbearing age help protect the vagina by increasing vaginal thickness. Bacteria are an important component of this environment and help maintain an acidic pH.[22] An abnormality or disruption in this system can create an environment that allows for pathogen growth and subsequent infection. Examples may include frequent douching, use of antibiotics or certain other medications, intercourse, foreign objects in the vagina, STIs, and pregnancy. Chemicals or foreign objects can also cause inflammation of the vagina. In addition, wearing certain undergarments (e.g., thongs) can transport bacteria from the anus, thereby introducing foreign bacteria to the vagina.

Bacterial vaginosis occurs when the normal balance of bacteria in the vagina is disrupted. A shift in the dominance or overgrowth of certain bacteria causes symptoms. BV is not an STI, but it may be more common in sexually experienced persons, and it may occur secondary to sexual intercourse, which can change the vaginal environment.

Candidiasis also is not an STI, but it is more common than BV in the sexually naive person. Candidiasis is often called a *yeast infection*. Women with diabetes or who are immunocompromised are at greater risk of candidiasis. Other risk factors may include pregnancy, obesity, and wearing nonbreathable or close-fitting underwear.

Trichomoniasis is an STI, and prevention consists of abstinence from sexual intercourse or protection with a condom. Prevention of vaginitis caused by BV or *Candida* infection is aided by promotion of a normal vaginal environment, which is facilitated by avoiding douching, wearing breathable cotton underwear, and using condoms during intercourse.

Signs and Symptoms

Vaginal discharge is a common symptom in vaginitis. However, the description of the discharge differs depending on the cause. BV discharge is typically thin, white, or gray in color and malodorous. The patient may also experience vaginal itching.

An individual with *Trichomonas* infection may not have any symptoms, but discharge described as thick, frothy, and green or yellow is not uncommon. The patient may experience discomfort with voiding, although this does not occur in most cases.

Last, individuals with candidiasis or fungal vaginitis may experience a thick white discharge resembling cottage cheese that is associated with itching or burning. This may also involve the vulva and surrounding skin and is thus termed *vulvovaginitis*.[2]

The differential diagnosis for a patient with vaginal discharge includes STIs. Other causes of vaginal inflammation include contact dermatitis, in which the skin reacts to some chemical or object; a retained foreign object, such as toilet tissue, a tampon, or a condom; chemical irritants; and, much less commonly, a neoplasm, such as cervical or vaginal cancer.

Referral and Diagnostic Tests

Any individual with vaginitis benefits from referral to a physician because diagnosis requires a pelvic examination, and treatment typically involves prescription medication.

Initially, a sexually active patient with vaginal discharge is evaluated for STIs in general. Diagnosis of the common causes for vaginitis involves sampling the discharge or vaginal fluid, measuring the pH of the secretions, and performing microscopic examination of the vaginal fluid. Trichomonads can be seen microscopically and are described as "swimming" on the slide. Microscopic findings for BV include "clue cells," which are vacuolated epithelial cells. Demonstration of pseudohyphae and budding yeast on a **potassium hydroxide (KOH) preparation** suggests candidiasis.

Another diagnostic tool, in which KOH is added to the sample, is called the *whiff test*. If the discharge is attributable to BV, a particular fishy odor may be noted. Measurement of the vaginal pH is also helpful with diagnosis. BV and trichomoniasis tend to occur when the pH is less acidic (>4.5). Other, more sophisticated tests are available but not necessarily needed for diagnosis.

Treatment and Return to Participation

Metronidazole is used to treat both BV and trichomoniasis. The patient must abstain from drinking alcohol while taking metronidazole because the combination can cause nausea and vomiting. Treatment for vulvovaginal candidiasis includes the use of antifungal agents, either oral or topical, many of which are available over the counter (see chapter 4).[2] On occasion, vaginitis of fungal origin is resistant to initial therapy, and further evaluation and treatment are required. Including yogurt with active cultures in the diet can help with certain cases of vaginitis, such as those related to a patient taking antibiotics, because yogurt helps promote stabilization of the normal bacterial flora. Partners of individuals with *Trichomonas* infection also need to receive treatment to prevent further spread.

The prognosis is good for common causes of vaginitis, and interference with athletic activity is not typical; therefore, return to play is not usually delayed. Problems related to BV and trichomoniasis, however, can occur during pregnancy and may include the risk of premature labor and premature rupture of membranes. In addition, patients with frequently recurring vulvovaginitis may have an underlying disorder, such as diabetes or a compromised immune system, although other systemic symptoms or complaints would likely be present in these cases.

Special Concerns

None of these causes of vaginitis are reportable to a public agency. However, a partner of a patient with trichomoniasis must be treated to prevent its spread or recurrence.

It is especially important to treat vaginitis caused by BV or trichomoniasis in the pregnant female because it may place her at risk of complications such as premature labor. Complications can be prevented by prompt diagnosis and treatment. The health care provider must encourage any patient with recurrent or chronic vaginitis that resists treatment to be carefully evaluated for underlying causes to ensure that she is receiving the proper treatment.

Pelvic Inflammatory Disease

In generally accepted terms, primary PID is defined as a bacterial infection of the upper genital tract that originates in and ascends from the lower genital tract (figure 9.16). It includes a host of inflammatory disorders such as endometritis, salpingitis, and many STIs. Sites of inflammation or infection include the endometrium,

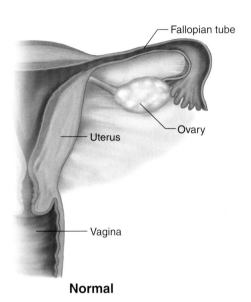

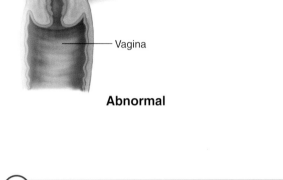

FIGURE 9.16 Pelvic inflammatory disease.

perimetrium, fallopian tubes, ovaries, and pelvic peritoneum. These infections usually are a result of sexually transmitted organisms, such as *C. trachomatis* and *N. gonorrhoeae.* At highest risk are sexually active women younger than age 25 yr, individuals with multiple sex partners, and those with a history of past PID or STI.[64,65]

Signs and Symptoms

Signs and symptoms of PID vary over a large spectrum, from mild or relatively few to severe. Diagnosing even the mildest cases is important, however, because sequelae from the disease can be problematic. Typically, symptoms begin within the first couple of weeks after menses, and subtle findings can include abnormal vaginal bleeding or **dyspareunia** (i.e., painful intercourse). Because no examination finding or laboratory test is optimal in diagnosing PID, the CDC lists the following minimal criteria: lower abdominal tenderness, **adnexal** tenderness, and cervix motion tenderness without evidence of a different, obvious source.[64,65]

To further clarify diagnosis, the CDC also includes the following: fever greater than 38.3 °C (101 °F); elevated erythrocyte sedimentation rate (ESR); elevated C-reactive protein (CRP); presence of leukocytes on a saline preparation of vaginal secretions; abnormal cervical or vaginal discharge, particularly mucopurulent discharge; and documented cervical infection with *N. gonorrhoeae* or *C. trachomatis.* More definitive answers may require surgical sampling of tissue, which is not without its own risks and can lead to false-negative results.

RED FLAGS FOR PELVIC INFLAMMATORY DISEASE

Females with any of the following signs or symptoms should be referred to a physician:

- Abnormal vaginal bleeding
- Lower abdominal tenderness
- Fever
- Abnormal vaginal discharge
- Amenorrhea (≥3 mo)

The differential diagnosis of a female thought to have PID may include inflammation or infection that has occurred near the upper genital tract. Appendicitis, classically described as periumbilical pain that radiates to the right lower quadrant, is another process that is typically diagnosed clinically and may be entertained as a possible cause of symptoms. This, however, would have no particular relationship to menses, and such a diagnosis would be more likely for someone with anorexia, nausea, and vomiting without symptoms of PID. Other possibilities include, but are not limited to, tubal pregnancy, corpus luteal cyst, endometriosis, mittelschmerz (typically described as a dull pain of short duration at mid-cycle), gastroenteritis, and lymphadenitis of the intestinal lymph nodes. A careful history of symptoms, including fever, genitourinary complaints, and onset of pain, especially in relation to the menstrual cycle, and an evaluation for risk factors can provide useful information in the diagnosis of PID.[25,65]

Referral and Diagnostic Tests

Symptoms or health history findings that raise suspicion for PID warrant urgent referral to a physician. If appendicitis or other emergent surgical problems are suspected, immediate referral to a physician or emergency department is necessary.

Every female of reproductive age presenting with pelvic complaints or symptoms requires a pregnancy test to evaluate the possibility of pregnancy. Because of the varying presence of signs and symptoms, it is prudent to obtain a urinalysis to evaluate for urinary tract problems. Other specific tests include a cervical or vaginal smear to be evaluated for the presence of leukocytes, overwhelming bacterial load, or trichomonads and possibly a Gram stain to identify specific organisms. A cervical culture for gonorrhea and chlamydia is performed. Blood tests with a CBC and differential, ESR, and CRP also are performed. If the diagnosis is unclear, a pelvic ultrasound may be performed to evaluate for other abnormalities.[25,64,65]

Treatment and Return to Participation

Treatment of PID must be initiated as soon as the diagnosis is made to prevent long-term sequelae. Assigning the most appropriate antibiotics for the specific condition is critical, but health care providers must also consider patient compliance and accessibility and affordability of the chosen medication.[65] The inpatient versus outpatient setting is controversial; however, it is generally accepted that certain patients need to be treated in a hospital setting:

- Patients who require surgical intervention for an ectopic pregnancy or abscess that requires drainage
- Pregnant patients
- Patients not responding to outpatient therapy
- Patients noncompliant with therapy or follow-up within 48 to 72 h
- Patients who are immunocompromised

Medical treatment for PID includes antibacterials.[64,65] Chapter 4 lists outpatient and inpatient medications geared toward treating the most common bacterial organisms.

Prompt diagnosis and prompt treatment of PID are crucial because of the sequelae, which include infertility, increased risk of ectopic pregnancy, recurrent infections, and chronic pelvic pain. The risk of infertility is relatively high, increases with subsequent infections, and depends on infection severity and therefore the time between infection and treatment initiation.

Before return to participation, adequate antibiotic therapy is instituted, fever is resolved, nausea and vomiting are rectified to ensure adequate hydration status, and pelvic or abdominal pain is minimized. If a surgical procedure was performed, the surgeon determines when return to activity will be allowed.

Prevention

Early diagnosis is important but is not nearly as crucial as prevention. Individuals, both male and female, should understand the problems associated with PID and the importance of preventing transmission of STIs, especially because many who have *N. gonorrhoeae* or *C. trachomatis* may be asymptomatic. The only proven method to prevent the transmission of many STIs, besides abstinence, is correct condom use. It should also be noted that intrauterine device (IUD) use and douching may increase PID risk among females.

Special Concerns

Patients diagnosed with PID should be tested for other STIs, notably HIV and syphilis, and advised to receive HBV vaccinations if they have not been immunized previously. A Pap smear also is performed to look for pathological changes caused by HPV. In addition, the patient's sexual partners need to be evaluated for gonorrhea and chlamydia infection and treated if there was sexual contact within 60 d of the patient's symptoms. The patient should abstain from sexual activity until fully treated. Follow-up testing in 4 to 6 wk for gonorrhea and chlamydia may be warranted and recommended by the physician.[2,65] Last, information about STIs and their prevention needs to be made available to all individuals, and adherence to safe-sex practices is encouraged.

Dysmenorrhea

Dysmenorrhea is described as severe cramps and pain associated with menstruation or painful menstruation and is categorized as either primary or secondary. Primary dysmenorrhea is not associated with gross pathology; rather, it involves a type of prostaglandin that acts to constrict blood vessels in the uterus, causing ischemia and subsequently painful uterine contractions during menstruation. Primary dysmenorrhea is a common gynecological condition, found in 45% to 95% of menstruating women.[66]

Secondary dysmenorrhea, by contrast, is caused by a gross pathological process involving the uterus. This can include endometriosis—in which endometrial tissue is found outside the uterus—PID, uterine fibroids or polyps, pelvic tumors, ectopic pregnancy, and miscarriage. In these cases, the painful uterine contractions are a result of the associated condition.[67]

Signs and Symptoms

Primary dysmenorrhea may be more common in the first few years after menarche and in those whose gravidity and parity status is low. The patient may also have a significant family history for this condition. In addition, smoking, early menarche, and a history of heavy flow and long menstrual periods may be risk factors associated with more severe dysmenorrhea. Symptoms may include not only cramping of the lower abdomen or back, with occasional radiating pain to the thighs, but also nausea, vomiting, diarrhea, headache, and other systemic problems. The pain and associated symptoms typically begin just before or at menses onset and last through the first day or two of menstruation. Physical examination yields no obvious pathology. Dysmenorrhea is highly correlated with absenteeism in school for adolescent girls, and missing class or practice on a reasonably monthly schedule could indicate a suspicion for this condition.[67,68] In a critical review of the literature, authors found that compared with women without dysmenorrhea, women with primary dysmenorrhea had a diminished capacity for pain and were at risk of other chronic pain conditions later in life.[69,70]

Secondary dysmenorrhea may not be as closely tied to menses onset, and symptoms last longer but may still have some relation to the menstrual cycle. Physical examination may or may not provide an etiology, and symptoms may vary depending on the underlying pathology. If a female has been diagnosed with primary dysmenorrhea and treatment, such as NSAIDs or oral contraceptives, has failed, then a pathological cause must be considered, and the patient should be reevaluated. It is important to listen to the patient and get a good history of the frequency and quality of pain. In a study of 144 women with chronic pelvic pain who reported severe dysmenorrhea, 96 (66.7%) had endometriosis.[71]

Differential diagnoses for dysmenorrhea include endometriosis, PID, uterine fibroids or polyps, pelvic tumors, ectopic pregnancy, or miscarriage.

Referral and Diagnostic Tests

Females who experience severe menstrual pain, who have pertinent systemic complaints as mentioned previously, or who have abnormal menstruation routinely need to be referred to a physician for evaluation.

As always, a thorough history and physical examination are warranted with a presentation of dysmenorrhea. A careful health history of the patient's menstrual cycle includes age of onset, length, frequency, flow, and regularity of cycling as well as sexual activity history, family history, and type and severity of associated symptoms. Any female being evaluated for dysmenorrhea warrants a pregnancy test, regardless of sexual history. Depending on the history and physical examination, other diagnostic tests may be necessary. Options include pelvic ultrasound, laparoscopy (direct visualization of the pelvic organs via a surgical procedure), hysteroscopy (view of the inside of the cervix and uterus with an endoscope), and radiological procedures. In some cases, tissue sampling or endometrial biopsy may be required for review by a pathologist.

Treatment and Return to Participation

The management of dysmenorrhea varies according to its etiology. For primary dysmenorrhea, NSAIDs and oral contraceptives have been the mainstays of treatment.[72] NSAIDs should be taken just before menses onset and continued through the first few days of menses. They function to decrease levels of the inciting prostaglandins. Oral contraceptives alone or in combination with NSAIDs can be beneficial. Patients should be cautioned about the long-term adverse effects of NSAIDs, as many athletes and physically active individuals take them often for myriad ailments, not just during menses. Adverse effects of oral contraceptives can include anorexia, thrombosis, nausea, depression, dizziness, weight change, nervousness, varicose veins, breakthrough bleeding, gallbladder disease, and cerebral hemorrhage, among other serious conditions. Risks of oral contraception increase with smoking, and oral contraceptives are contraindicated for patients with a history or family history of breast cancer, vascular diseases, or jaundice; these women should use alternative methods of birth control. A review of 10 studies (686,305 participants) showed a significant relationship linking oral contraceptive use and breast cancer risk.[73]

Treatment for secondary dysmenorrhea depends on the pathological etiology as previously discussed. Secondary dysmenorrhea should be considered in a patient whose primary dysmenorrhea does not respond well to treatment. Older females with dysmenorrhea are more likely to have a secondary or pathological cause for their discomfort and warrant close evaluation.

Dysmenorrhea can certainly be disabling to those affected; however, several treatment options exist for the varying etiologies, and prognosis generally is good. Participation may be limited only by the patient's symptoms, unless the individual is being treated for a certain pathological condition that may, as directed by the physician, exclude her from strenuous physical activity.

Prevention

There is no primary prevention for primary dysmenorrhea. Secondary prevention for primary dysmenorrhea stems from its treatment. Starting NSAIDs before menses, when pain would typically develop, or taking oral contraceptives lends itself to this secondary prevention. For secondary dysmenorrhea, only certain causes, such as PID and STIs, are preventable by employing safe-sex practices.

Amenorrhea

Amenorrhea is typically categorized as primary or secondary. Primary amenorrhea is classically defined as the absence of menarche (i.e., onset of menses) by age 16 yr. If there are no signs of puberty onset (menses, breast development) by age 13 yr, the patient should be referred for a workup for primary amenorrhea.[74] Secondary amenorrhea is less well defined but alludes to the fact that a female's menstruation has stopped after having previously been normal. Depending on the source, secondary amenorrhea may be defined as either (1) the absence of menses for 3, 4, 6, or 12 mo in a previously menstruating female or (2) fewer than three menstrual cycles per year.[2] To add further confusion, **oligomenorrhea** is used to describe menstrual cycles with intervals greater than 36 d but less than 90 d. Because the cause of oligomenorrhea is often the same as for amenorrhea, this section focuses mainly on amenorrhea, with the knowledge that the discussion may apply to many cases of missed menstrual periods in general.

The cause of amenorrhea, both primary and secondary, is highly variable. To understand the various etiologies, a basic review of ovulation is necessary. The ovulatory pathway consists of the hypothalamic–pituitary axis, the ovaries, a feedback loop, the uterus, and a subsequent outflow tract. The hypothalamus secretes gonadotropin-releasing hormone (GnRH), which stimulates the pituitary gland to secrete FSH and LH. These hormones then stimulate the ovaries to produce estrogen and progesterone, which each directly affect the menstrual process (see figure 9.8). Low circulating levels of these hormones, in turn, directly feed back to the hypothalamus, causing it to produce more GnRH. One can therefore imagine both hormonal and anatomical problems that can interfere with normal ovulation.

The source of amenorrhea depends on the cause. In general terms, anatomical defects can occur that are congenital, genetic, or acquired. Ovarian failure can occur prematurely. Chronic anovulation or the absence of ovulation in the presence of estrogen, such as in **polycystic ovarian disease** or certain tumors, can occur. Chronic anovulation also can occur in the absence of estrogen or

in **hypogonadism**, such as occurs with **athletic amenorrhea**, stress, anorexia nervosa, and pituitary tumors. Research has demonstrated that high-intensity training may delay menses onset and contribute to menarche cessation if the athlete has already begun menstruation.[75,76] Female athletes who display the combination of amenorrhea, disordered eating, and low bone density have a condition that used to be termed the *female triad*. The International Olympic Committee recently renamed this condition *relative energy deficiency in sport* or *REDs* because, except for amenorrhea, males suffer from the same energy-deficient condition that creates many medical issues for the athlete.[76] Because bone health is related to estrogen, amenorrhea can affect bone health and contribute to stress fractures.[75,77]

Signs and Symptoms

Signs and symptoms of amenorrhea vary greatly and depend on its etiology. For primary amenorrhea, genetic disorders and anatomical abnormalities of the reproductive system must be considered. A classic example is a genetic defect called **Turner's syndrome**. Patients with Turner's syndrome may present with physical features such as short stature, webbed neck, shield chest, increased carrying angle of the elbows, and other possible findings, in addition to primary amenorrhea.

Problems with the outflow tract can also cause amenorrhea. If there is no exit path for the sloughed endometrial lining, then the patient perceives there is no menses, but she may have severe cramping and pain from retained tissue and blood with each menstrual period. Obstruction can be congenital, such as an imperforate hymen or **labial agglutination**, or it can occur secondarily, such as with **uterine synechiae** or, as seen in **Asherman's syndrome**, scarring after a surgical procedure.

Proceeding further up the ovulatory chain, ovarian failure from various causes can lead to amenorrhea. It can be related to genetic defects, autoimmune disorders, or prior chemotherapy and can be associated with various symptoms. Not uncommonly, a woman may have symptoms similar to those of menopausal women, such as hot flashes, vaginal dryness, and mood changes. The patient may also have systemic symptoms common to particular autoimmune or endocrine disorders. For example, those with hypothyroidism may exhibit fatigue, weight gain, constipation, or cold intolerance.[74]

Problems with the hypothalamic–pituitary axis are varied as well. Deficient, absent, or inappropriate secretion of GnRH from the hypothalamus is common in females, which in turn results in amenorrhea. Not all females are affected, and some have greater risk than others. For the athlete, diet, sport and activity level, and genetic composition may all contribute to athletic amenorrhea.[76,78,79] Diagnosis of athletic amenorrhea is important because a hypoestrogenemic state, such as with athletic amenorrhea and ovarian failure, can adversely affect bone mineral density, leading to fracture. The athletic trainer needs to look for signs or symptoms of disordered eating in the evaluation of the athlete, because this remains a common and well-described entity (see chapter 17).[76,78,79]

Another potential cause for amenorrhea that involves the hypothalamic–pituitary axis is inhibition of GnRH by increased prolactin levels, which can occur as a result of a pituitary tumor that could have neurological manifestations, such as headaches and visual disturbances, as well as a complaint of galactorrhea. Polycystic ovary syndrome is a common condition that is manifested by **hyperandrogenism** (with associated acne and **hirsutism**), obesity, and hyperinsulinemia.[2]

Referral and Diagnostic Tests

Females with primary amenorrhea are referred to a physician for a complete evaluation. A female who has had normal menstrual cycles but who misses three consecutive periods or who is oligomenorrheic needs to be evaluated by a physician. However, missing just one or two menses is not always benign, and one must not allow the number of missed menses to define the line between passiveness and concern.

The workup for amenorrhea involves assessment of the neuroendocrine system, genetics, anatomy of the patient, and a pregnancy test. A complete medical history, including exercise, nutrition, and menstrual history, and a physical examination should be performed. Laboratory evaluation may include a urine pregnancy test and blood tests for thyroid-stimulating hormone, FSH, estradiol, and prolactin. Testing for levels of LH, dehydroepiandrosterone, and testosterone may be indicated depending on the history and physical examination. In addition, the physician may elect to perform a progestin challenge to determine whether the endometrium has been primed by estrogen and if there is a patent outflow tract. With proper estrogen priming of the endometrium, its lining should slough after withdrawal of progesterone, as it would with normal menstruation.[74]

Other laboratory evaluations may include karyotyping to check for any chromosomal abnormalities. This will also provide evidence of the presence or absence of a Y chromosome. Depending on the history, laboratory, and examination findings, neuroimaging may be helpful to look for an intracranial mass, specifically involving the pituitary. Other imaging may include evaluation of the reproductive tract and the gonads.

A bone density assessment should be considered in all females with a prolonged history of oligomenorrhea or more than 6 mo of amenorrhea, particularly in those with a history of disordered eating.[76,78,79]

Treatment and Return to Participation

Treatment of amenorrhea depends on its etiology and the sequelae one is trying to eliminate or prevent. One such problem is low bone mineral density or other effects of a hypoestrogenemic state. Treatment may consist of dietary changes to improve overall energy balance, hormone replacement therapy, and decreased activity.[78] In some cases of amenorrhea, surgery could be required, such as for a patient with a pituitary tumor or an outflow tract abnormality. Treatment for polycystic ovarian disease may include oral contraceptives and medications to control the **hyperinsulinemia**. Knowing the underlying cause of the amenorrhea is key in determining treatment.[78,80]

In the case of athletic amenorrhea, treatment involves both pharmacological and nonpharmacological measures. Oral contraceptives are the mainstay of pharmacological treatment for athletic amenorrhea and should be strongly considered if nonpharmacological measures fail. In the presence of either osteopenia or osteoporosis, nasal calcitonin should be considered. Neither bisphosphonates nor selective estrogen receptor modulators have been well studied in young premenopausal women. Nonpharmacological measures include dietary changes and adjustments in physical activity in order to promote an overall positive energy balance, daily calcium and vitamin D supplementation, nutrition counseling, and screening or treatment for disordered eating.[74,76,80]

As with treatment, prognosis relies on the etiology of amenorrhea. The concern for females with amenorrhea caused by low gonadotropin stimulation is the increased risk of low bone mineral density and its sequelae, such as stress fractures. Correcting the underlying conditions or providing hormone replacement when the cause of the hypoestrogenemia cannot be corrected is important in trying to prevent adverse outcomes for patients.

Because the etiology of amenorrhea is broad, return-to-play recommendations for each type are not presented here. For female athletes with athletic amenorrhea, an intense exercise routine can play a major role, although there may be multiple contributing factors. Simply reducing the athlete's level of activity and ensuring an adequate and well-balanced diet may help her return to a regular menstrual pattern. Therefore, return to play is not prohibited, but it may be limited, at least initially. Such decisions and treatment plans require the involvement and communication of the athlete, athletic trainer, physician, registered dietitian, coach, and perhaps a mental health provider.[76,78]

Special Considerations

As discussed previously, special care must be taken when evaluating an athlete for amenorrhea because of its possible complications. In addition to medical intervention, changes in exercise routine may be required. Nutritional evaluation is also important, especially with athletic amenorrhea or in the presence of an eating disorder. The relevance of age in the return-to-play decision depends on the cause of the amenorrhea and required treatment.

Mittelschmerz

Mittelschmerz is pain secondary to ovulation; hence, it tends to occur at mid-cycle and is also referred to as *intermenstrual pain*.[81] The pain associated with ovulation is thought to be attributable to fluid that is released from the ovary, along with the ovum, during ovulation. This fluid can be irritating to intraabdominal tissue and can cause pain for females.

Signs and Symptoms

Pain can vary in severity and can be sudden, severe, and sharp. The pain tends to be in the lower abdomen, usually occurs on one side, and can be accompanied by light vaginal spotting.[22] This is probably secondary to the unilateral release of the ovum. The affected side may change from one month to the next. Typically, the pain will last minutes to hours and, occasionally, a day or two. Because mittelschmerz is related to ovulation, there will be a history of pain that occurs between menstrual periods.[82]

Lower abdominal pain in a female can pose a diagnostic dilemma because the differential diagnoses can be varied. However, as previously mentioned, a good history can be extremely useful. Certain signs or symptoms are considered serious; periumbilical or right lower quadrant pain associated with nausea, vomiting, or fever should always raise concern for appendicitis. Taking a patient history, including obtaining sexual and menstrual data, and performing a physical examination and possibly imaging and laboratory studies can help in diagnosing PID (see the Pelvic Inflammatory Disease section). Ectopic pregnancy may also be associated with lower abdominal pain and needs to be included in the differential diagnosis, especially if there is a history of PID or prior ectopic pregnancies. Endometriosis, UTI, kidney stones, constipation, and gastroenteritis should also be considered depending on history, onset, and symptoms.

Ovulation must be occurring for a diagnosis of mittelschmerz; therefore, it is not a diagnosis in a woman who is no longer menstruating.

Referral and Diagnostic Tests

A female who presents with new-onset lower abdominal pain or pelvic pain needs to be referred to a physician for evaluation. If the individual's pain is associated with nausea, vomiting, or fever, she should be immediately referred to a physician. She should also be referred if the pain is prolonged (lasts >2 d), if the pain is severe or unrelieved by over-the-counter medications, or if there is a suspicion of pregnancy or STI.

There is no diagnostic test for mittelschmerz; rather, it is a diagnosis of exclusion. A good health history, including menstrual history, is very helpful. Depending on the history and type of pain, a pelvic examination may be warranted to exclude other etiologies. Occasionally, imaging, such as ultrasound, can be helpful in looking at anatomy and ruling out certain structural causes. In addition, one should always have a low threshold for ordering a urine pregnancy test.[82]

Treatment and Return to Participation

The standard treatment for mittelschmerz includes over-the-counter pain medications, such as NSAIDs and acetaminophen (Tylenol). Heating packs can alleviate some of the discomfort. Oral contraceptives prevent pain by preventing ovulation.

The prognosis for mittelschmerz is generally good, and athletic activity is not contraindicated. Although the pain is generally tolerable, it can be significant for some. The use of oral contraceptives has proven useful in relieving the pain of mittelschmerz.[82] Again, pain unrelieved by standard medications may warrant referral to a physician.

Ovarian and Cervical Cancer

Ovarian cancer is a malignant cell growth originating from an ovary; it is the leading cause of death from a gynecological malignancy. Cervical cancer is a malignancy originating from the cervix and has significant morbidity and mortality as well. Cervical cancer is one of the most common cancer types in females, and it has a high cure rate if detected early.[83]

Ovarian cancer is typically seen in older women, with symptoms usually presenting late in its course. Risk appears to be proportional to the number of times a woman ovulates. For example, women who have never had children are at increased risk. Oral contraceptives that prevent ovulation may decrease a woman's risk. Age is another factor and is related to the greater number of ovulatory cycles experienced. Other risks include family history, personal history of breast or colon cancer, and history of prolonged hormone replacement therapy. Multiple sex partners, early sexual activity, STIs, cigarette smoking, and a weak immune system are possible risk factors for cervical cancer.[83,84] Genetic predisposition is an important risk factor, especially with the *BRCA1* or *BRCA2* gene mutation.

HPV plays a significant role in the development of cervical cancer.[85] Several HPV genotypes exist, but only a few are associated with cervical cancer. This may be why sexual activity plays an important role in the development of this malignancy. Risk factors include sexual activity beginning at a young age, a higher number of sexual partners, a history of other STIs, and smoking.

Signs and Symptoms

Signs and symptoms are not usually present with either ovarian or cervical cancer in the early stages, because symptoms may occur only after the tumor has grown large enough to have some mass effect. Unfortunately, by this time, the tumor has likely metastasized to other sites. Symptoms may vary, depending on the tumor size and location and the sites of metastasis. Gastrointestinal disturbances, such as constipation or diarrhea, may occur with either malignancy.[84] Patients may also experience early satiety or unexplained weight changes. Vaginal bleeding and discomfort may occur with cervical cancer, as may urinary complaints. Extension of cervical cancer may obstruct lymphatic and venous drainage, causing lower extremity edema, perhaps unilaterally.[86] Symptoms involving other organs depend on metastatic spread. Symptoms for either cancer can be nonspecific and of little diagnostic value.[86]

Because the symptoms of ovarian or cervical cancer can be vague or nonspecific, the differential diagnoses can be broad. For both ovarian and cervical cancer, a definitive diagnosis is based on tissue biopsy. For ovarian cancer, a benign ovarian mass or complex cystic ovarian disease is considered in the differential diagnosis, as is localized spread of cancer from surrounding tissues. The differential diagnoses for cervical cancer include severe cervical dysplasia, vaginal dysplasia or cancer, and uterine cancer with localized spread to the cervix.[84,86]

Referral and Diagnostic Tests

Any suspicion of malignancy requires referral to a physician for evaluation. A female with a personal or family history of malignancy and with unexplained symptoms as previously described needs to be referred. In addition, females should be encouraged to have routine pelvic examinations and Pap smears as outlined by their physician.

Diagnosing ovarian cancer may prove somewhat difficult. Finding an adnexal or pelvic mass on examination is of concern, especially in an older woman or one with other risk factors for ovarian cancer. Unfortunately, no good screening test is available. Serum tumor markers are used in the initial evaluation of ovarian cancer, but currently they are not appropriate for use as screening tests. Pelvic ultrasound may demonstrate an ovarian mass if suspected or symptoms warrant this examination. Laparoscopy plays an important role in the diagnosis and staging of ovarian cancer because no one laboratory test or imaging technique is sufficient.

The incidence of cervical cancer has decreased, largely because of screening examinations with Pap smear testing in which cervical cells are collected and evaluated for atypical or abnormal appearance. Further evaluation and treatment depends on the results. The U.S. Preventive Services Task Force currently recommends that females be screened with a Pap smear at least every 3 yr (barring any previous abnormal results) beginning no longer than 3 yr after first sexual activity or by age 21 yr, whichever comes first. Some people may not need routine screening, such as women older than age 65 yr who have had normal screenings in the past, or women who have had total hysterectomies but without a history of malignancy or a questionable malignancy. These cases, however, must be individualized and the decision made by the patient in consultation with a physician.[86]

Treatment and Return to Participation

Treatment of ovarian cancer largely depends on the disease stage, which is determined by surgical exploration. There are four stages (I-IV), with stage IV being the least favorable. The degree of tumor extension plays a large role in staging. Therapies include surgical removal of involved tissue and chemotherapy. Invasive cervical cancer therapies include surgery, radiation therapy, and chemotherapy. Here again, the choice depends on the stage of malignancy.[84,86]

Several treatments are available for cervical dysplasia (i.e., precancerous lesions) discovered by Pap smear. Treatment may be as simple as frequent follow-up and repeat Pap smears, or it may include colposcopy with biopsy or removal of the abnormal tissue.

Morbidity and mortality resulting from ovarian and cervical cancers are high because of the nature of the disease process and the lack of symptoms early in the disease course. Screening for cervical cancer by Pap smear has allowed for great progress in preventing invasive disease. Much progress has also been made in the fight to prevent cervical cancer with the advent of Gardasil and Cervarix, which are three-series vaccines designed to help prevent HPV infection.

Athletic participation for women undergoing treatment for ovarian or cervical cancer is limited by the toll of treatment, which can include nausea, vomiting, fatigue, and diarrhea. Treatment requires a multidisciplinary approach, and good communication among all involved is important for the patient's well-being.

Prevention

Many risk factors for ovarian cancer are difficult to avoid. Probably the best forms of prevention are vaccination against HPV and routine medical examinations, with special attention given to patients with risk factors such as a family history and prior medical history of gynecological malignancy.

Cervical cancer has risk factors associated with sexual activity. Therefore, changes in sexual behavior or practices as described previously may decrease risk. Routine examinations, including screening for cervical lesions, cannot be overemphasized. HPV vaccination (e.g., with Gardasil) has added much in the way of cervical cancer prevention. Current CDC age recommendations for administration of HPV vaccine to females are 11 to 12 yr, although it can be given as early as age 9 yr. The vaccine is also recommended for girls and women aged between 13 and 26 yr who have not received the series and have no contraindications.[87,88] The Gardasil vaccine is also approved for males to prevent HPV, and it is recommended that they begin vaccination between ages 9 and 15 yr. Greater effort is needed to educate all patients on the importance of HPV vaccination in the prevention of cervical cancer.

Breast Cancer

The breast consists of glands, blood, lymph tissue, fat, and fibrous or connective tissue (figure 9.17). Underlying the breast is muscle. The lymph tissue drains to nodes in the axillae. To facilitate milk delivery, the breast has numerous milk glands, which open to lobules. Several lobules make up a lobe, and these lobes empty into ducts that deliver the milk to the nipple. The lymphatic system is also an important aspect of the breast (figure 9.18), and it can act as a conduit for cancer to metastasize to other areas.

A neoplasm arising from the breast tissue is a breast cancer in both males and females. Approximately 10% to 15% originate in the ducts of the breast, with another significant portion originating within the lobules. These cells can escape the breast or metastasize and affect other areas of the body. Except for skin cancer, breast cancer is the most diagnosed cancer among U.S. women. In 2019, an estimated 42,280 women died from breast cancer, with 264,121 newly diagnosed cases in women, according to the CDC.[89] The American Cancer Society noted that 2,710 men were diagnosed with breast cancer in 2022, and 530 of them succumbed to the disease.[90]

Risk factors associated with breast cancer include sex, age, prior or family history of breast cancer, and genetics. One's overall exposure to estrogen, either physiological or by replacement, may increase the risk of breast cancer. Therefore, women who have taken hormone replacement

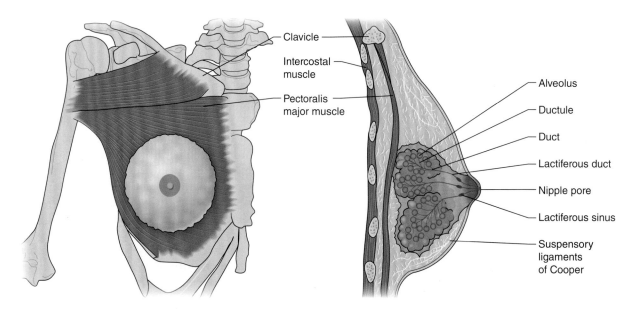

FIGURE 9.17 Anatomy of the female breast.

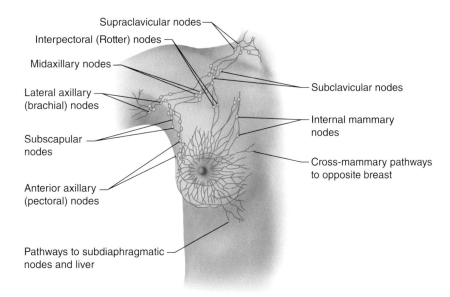

Supraclavicular nodes

Interpectoral (Rotter) nodes

Midaxillary nodes

Lateral axillary (brachial) nodes

Subscapular nodes

Anterior axillary (pectoral) nodes

Pathways to subdiaphragmatic nodes and liver

Subclavicular nodes

Internal mammary nodes

Cross-mammary pathways to opposite breast

FIGURE 9.18   Lymphatic system surrounding the breast.

therapy for several years, women who began menstruation at an early age, women who experienced menopause at a late age, and women who never had children or began childbearing at a later age may all be at increased risk.[91]

The three major types of breast cancer are described based on their location of origin and histology: infiltrating ductal carcinoma or ductal carcinoma **in situ** if localized, infiltrating lobular carcinoma or lobular carcinoma in situ if localized, and inflammatory breast carcinoma.

Signs and Symptoms

Early stages of breast cancer usually are silent. The initial tumor is typically painless, and the first sign may be a breast or axillary lump or mass not previously evaluated, skin puckering, or abnormality noted on a mammogram. Many of these lumps are benign and associated with fibrocystic change, which may be manifested by breast tenderness just before menstruation. In that case, the lump is a fluid-filled cyst, rather than a solid, fixed nodule. Other warning signs include nipple discharge, change in breast size or shape, change in appearance of the skin overlying the breast, and recent inversion of the nipple.[89-91]

Although breast cancer in men is rare, it does occur. Concerns about breast cancer expressed by a male should not be taken lightly.

The finding of a breast mass can be frightening. Not all masses are cancerous, and, in fact, most are probably benign. In the very young person (i.e., before puberty), a lump may appear around the nipple, followed by a similar occurrence on the other side, with both remaining unchanged until sometime during puberty. A fibroadenoma, which is a firm but painless mass, is typically a benign lesion that tends to occur in the young person during the late teens to early 30s. It is typically well circumscribed and mobile on examination. These lumps tend to persist and sometimes calcify. Fibrocystic change is a common benign breast lesion that consists of fluid-filled cysts within the breast tissue. These cysts or lumps are typically tender, especially just before menses, and may be fluctuant on examination.[22]

Referral and Diagnostic Tests

Although many breast lumps are benign and can have characteristic findings, the importance of a medical evaluation of a lump cannot be underestimated. Any individual with any signs or symptoms of a breast or axilla mass or breast changes needs to be referred to a physician.

The diagnosis of breast cancer starts with a thorough medical history and physical examination, including breast palpation by a trained medical provider. In the

RED FLAGS FOR BREAST CANCER

- Nipple discharge, especially when unilateral
- Change in breast size or shape
- Change in appearance of the skin overlying the breast, especially pitting, in which the skin begins to resemble an orange peel
- Inversion of the nipple, especially when recent in onset and unilateral

presence of a suspicious palpable breast mass, imaging of the breasts by mammography, MRI, or ultrasound may help further clarify the malignant potential of the mass. A potential difficulty in younger female athletes involves their relatively dense breast tissue, which may make clear imaging of a mass more difficult.[91]

Other diagnostic tools are more invasive and involve sampling or removing tissue for pathological examination. These tools include fine-needle aspiration, in which a needle is introduced into the lump and cells are aspirated for cytological examination; core needle biopsy, which introduces a large needle to obtain tissue for pathological review; and surgical biopsy, which involves surgical removal of a portion of the mass or the entire lump and surrounding tissue. These tissue samples are used to make a definitive diagnosis.

Treatment and Return to Participation

Treatment for breast cancer largely depends on its progression, which is measured with a staging system. This system assigns stages based on the tumor's size, lymph node involvement, and location of any metastatic spread. For instance, stage 0 is noninvasive cancer, such as ductal carcinoma in situ or lobular carcinoma in situ. This type of cancer is localized but has the potential to spread. Stage IV represents the other end of the spectrum: The cancer has metastasized beyond the breast and its lymph nodes. In addition to staging, other factors are extremely important when treating breast cancer. These include the patient's age; the general state of health, previous medical history, sex, pregnancy status, and menopausal status; and the specifics of the tumor itself, such as the presence of certain receptors on the tumor cells.

Multiple treatments exist, including surgery, chemotherapy, radiation therapy, hormone therapy, and biological therapy. Surgery ranges from the common removal of the mass and surrounding tissue, including a sampling of the axillary lymph nodes, to the uncommon removal of the entire breast and its lymph nodes. Often some other form of therapy is used in addition to surgery, especially if only a portion of the breast is removed. This may include radiation, chemotherapy, or hormone therapy, which are also used before surgery for certain larger cancers that may require shrinkage preoperatively.[89,90]

Prognosis varies from person to person but overall is related to cancer stage. Stage IV obviously offers the worst prognosis for five-year survival. Other factors include those used to determine the treatment, such as the patient's overall health, age, and tumor receptor status. The time to return to participation can range from days to weeks or months and is determined by the overall tumor burden, including metastases, treatment side effects, and the patient's overall condition.[91]

Prevention

Because many risk factors associated with breast cancer are not controllable, screening is very important. Screening includes monthly breast examinations performed by the patient and examinations performed by a medical professional every 2 to 3 yr between the ages of 20 and 40 yr and yearly thereafter. Women should become familiar with the usual appearance of their breasts so they can detect any changes that might be warning signs for breast cancer. A monthly breast self-examination is performed by first palpating for lumps or abnormalities.

Mammography is another screening tool, and the American Cancer Society recommends that it be done yearly after age 40 yr. Recommendations for breast examinations and mammography may need to be altered if the patient has a past medical history or family history of breast cancer. For patients without breast symptoms, mammograms can be offered annually between ages 40 and 54 yr. At age 55 yr, women without breast symptoms can choose to have mammograms every 2 yr, or they can decide to continue with annual evaluations. Screening should continue if the patient is in good health and expected to live another 10 yr or longer.[90] It is important for older patients to seek the advice of their physician regarding screening.

Preemptive breast removal—that is, breast removal for someone without cancer or a lump—may seem extreme but is not uncommon. For example, a person with a strong family history of breast cancer or who is known to carry a gene associated with breast cancer (*BRCA1* or *BRCA2*) may elect to have breast removal to preempt the cancer.

Pregnancy

Normal pregnancy consists of a series of remarkable changes that occur within the female body. Multiple organ systems are affected to support a growing fetus while maintaining the health of the mother. A few of these important normal changes are highlighted here and a single pathological condition, ectopic pregnancy, is discussed.

Before becoming pregnant, a woman should maintain proper nutrition, start the use of prenatal vitamins, and discontinue using or avoid potentially harmful substances such as tobacco, alcohol, and illicit drugs. Folic acid is present in most prenatal vitamins and is important in helping to prevent neural tube defects in the fetus. All pregnant women should take folic acid.

The initial signs and symptoms of pregnancy include a missed menstrual period and breast swelling or tenderness. Nausea and vomiting, known as *morning sickness*, may also be present early in pregnancy and, if severe, may compromise hydration, nutrition, and weight gain. Severe cases of nausea and vomiting, termed *hyperemesis*

Breast Self-Examination

Perform a breast self-examination 7 to 10 d after the first day of the menstrual cycle. Here is how to perform a breast self-examination:

- Stand before a mirror and visually inspect the breast in three positions:
    1. Stand with arms at one's side.
    2. Hold the arms behind the head and press forward.
    3. Place the hands on the hips, rolling the shoulders and elbows forward.
- Raise one arm, and use at least three or four fingers to palpate the other breast using these motions (figure 9.19):
    4. Palpate the breast in a circular motion, covering the whole breast, moving in toward the nipple.
    5. Palpate the breast in toward the nipple.
    6. Palpate the breast in an up-and-down motion.
- Palpate the axillary area because it is rich with lymph nodes and should not contain unusual lumps or masses.
- Squeeze the nipple and look for any discharge.
- Repeat the preceding steps for the other breast.
- Complete this examination both in the shower and while lying supine.

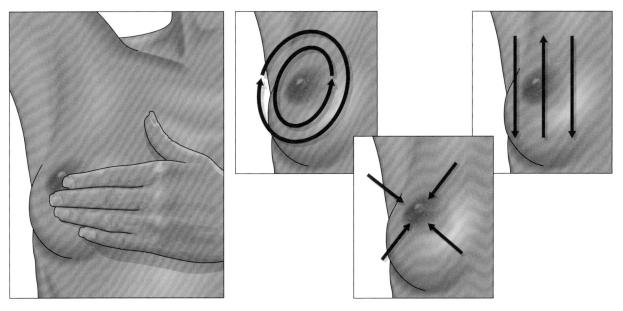

FIGURE 9.19   Breast self-examination.

gravidarum, can lead to hospitalization for fluid replacement, electrolyte correction, and control of emesis. In general, however, symptoms are not this severe and typically subside. In fact, the pregnant woman's fluid status increases during pregnancy. Blood volume increases, as does intracellular and extracellular fluid. Fluid tends to accumulate more during the day, and swelling of the distal extremities is very common.[1]

As described earlier, physiological changes also occur in pregnancy. Plasma volume and cardiac output increase as a result of increased SV and HR. In addition, blood pressure decreases in normal pregnancy because of an overall decrease in SVR. Respiratory changes include an increased tidal volume, increased minute ventilation, and decreased overall airway resistance. Despite these changes, the woman's FEV_1 and respiratory rate usually remain unchanged at rest.[1,92]

Gastroesophageal reflux is another common symptom occurring among pregnant women and is attributable to both anatomical and physiological changes. A patient may note that certain foods aggravate reflux, and avoidance of these foods is prudent. If avoidance of the offending foods does not help, pharmacological therapy may be necessary. This therapy can consist of calcium-containing antacids, histamine (H_2) antagonists, or proton pump inhibitors as prescribed.

Low back pain is a common complaint as well and is largely a result of the woman's altered center of gravity secondary to the enlarging fetus, uterus, and breast tissue. Low back pain is generally more of a problem during the latter stages of pregnancy. Interestingly, although the woman's bones may adjust to the various stresses placed on them, they appear to suffer no ill effects from the high calcium demands of the fetus.

Throughout the course of pregnancy, a woman's breasts enlarge and may become tender. It is also possible for a pregnant woman to notice that she is expressing fluid from her breasts before the birth of her child. The fluid expressed is known as *colostrum* and is a normal change associated with pregnancy.

Exercise and physical activity for healthy women should be encouraged in pregnancy. Women who exercise regularly in pregnancy have the benefits of improved cardiac function, limited weight gain, improved mental health, and decreased time in labor.[1,92,93] Few scientific data address participation in vigorous and competitive sports by the pregnant athlete, but some recommendations are noteworthy. Pregnant athletes should avoid exercise in the supine position as much as possible, particularly after the first trimester. Scuba diving, downhill skiing, contact sports, and the use of hot tubs, steam baths, and saunas place the fetus at potential risk and are discouraged during pregnancy.[94] In addition, pregnant athletes are generally discouraged from participation in contact or collision sports after the 14th week of pregnancy, although this is based on indirect evidence. Furthermore, a pregnant athlete who participates in competitive endurance sports should consider participation at the noncompetitive level for the duration of the pregnancy.

Although exercise during pregnancy is safe in most cases, exercise needs to be discontinued in some situations pending a complete evaluation by a physician.[32,94] The American College of Obstetricians and Gynecologists lists the following contraindications to exercise in pregnancy: vaginal bleeding, pregnancy-induced hypertension, incompetent cervix, preterm labor, premature rupture of membranes, and intrauterine growth restriction. Warning signs that suggest the immediate cessation of exercise include back, pubic, or abdominal pain or dizziness, nausea, uterine contractions, excessive fatigue, and decreased fetal movements.[93,94] When in doubt, the athlete

should discuss these issues with a physician. According to NCAA recommendations,[32] the pregnant athlete should do the following:

- Avoid supine exercise after the first trimester.
- Be discouraged from heavy weightlifting.
- Be discouraged from activities that require the Valsalva maneuver.
- Avoid activities associated with a high risk of falling (gymnastics, horseback riding, or downhill skiing).
- Consider noncompetitive activity if involved in endurance sports.
- Avoid contact sports after the 14th week of pregnancy, even though there are no data regarding contact sports and pregnancy.
- Avoid any physical activity pending evaluation by an obstetrician when the mother has a previously diagnosed medical condition that may affect normal pregnancy, such as uncontrolled diabetes, hypertension, or cervical defects.
- Remain well hydrated.
- Avoid overheating.

Several factors come into play for individuals returning to activity postpartum (after delivery). Pelvic floor injury has occurred in up to 80% of first-time pregnant women, and recovery of specifically the levator ani (the largest muscle in the pelvic floor) can take 6 to 12 mo.[93] Heavy and strenuous physical activity, including sustained Valsalva maneuvers, can adversely affect full recovery. Cardiovascular recovery to prelabor levels can take 12 wk, and nutrition demands must be evaluated,

RED FLAGS FOR TERMINATING EXERCISE WHILE PREGNANT

Signs to terminate exercise while pregnant and follow-up with an obstetrician are as follows:

- Vaginal bleeding
- Shortness of breath before exercise
- Dizziness
- Headache
- Chest pain
- Calf pain or swelling
- Preterm labor
- Decreased fetal movement
- Amniotic fluid leakage
- Muscle weakness

especially if the individual is breastfeeding. Patients who undergo surgical procedures (including caesarean section) have longer recovery times. It is paramount that the patient follow the physician's recommendations for successful full return to participation or competition. Health care providers working with the athlete should know and be mindful of any indicators of postpartum depression and refer the athlete to a physician.[93]

Ectopic Pregnancy

Ectopic pregnancy is an infrequent yet important complication of pregnancy. Ectopic pregnancy occurs when the fertilized egg implants outside the normal endometrial lining of the uterus (figure 9.20). This is lethal for the fetus and can be for the mother as well. Appropriate diagnosis is therefore extremely important. The implantation can occur in many places, but most occur in the ampulla of the fallopian tube, which is the long length of the tube leading to the uterus.

Common causes of ectopic pregnancy include anatomical abnormalities, such as scarring or obstruction of a portion of the egg's path that hinders the normal migration of the fertilized egg to its proper implantation site in the uterus. Some risk factors include a prior ectopic pregnancy, a history of PID, IUD use, a history of tubal ligation, an abnormally formed uterus, and cigarette smoking. Diagnosis of an ectopic pregnancy involves serial measurement of serum β-human chorionic gonadotropin (HCG) levels and pelvic or abdominal imaging with ultrasound.[95]

Signs and Symptoms

Signs and symptoms of ectopic pregnancy include abnormal vaginal bleeding, bleeding outside of the usual menstrual cycle, sudden or sharp abdominal or pelvic pain, dizziness, and possible referred pain to the shoulder.[95,96] Other symptoms may include amenorrhea, vaginal bleeding, and pain. An athlete may have hemodynamic compromise in severe cases when rupture of the fallopian tube and hemorrhage have occurred.

Referral and Diagnostic Tests

Some women may be unaware that they are pregnant, and any signs or symptoms associated with ectopic pregnancy should be followed up with a history of the last menstrual period. The placenta produces a hormone, HCG, which can be detected in the blood or urine of pregnant women. The presence of HCG confirms pregnancy. A pelvic examination and ultrasonography are performed to further confirm the pregnancy and assess the fetal tissue.

Treatment and Return to Participation

Treatment most commonly involves aborting the fetus through administration of methotrexate or surgical intervention. Under favorable circumstances, methotrexate can be considered to avoid the risks and trauma of surgery. This agent stops fetal growth and allows the body to absorb it over time. It is not, however, recommended if the growth of pregnancy is large or the fallopian tube is ruptured.[96] Each method of treatment carries its own risks, however, and is generally prescribed by the obstetrician in conjunction with the woman's personal wishes.

The prognosis for recovery from an ectopic pregnancy is generally very good if the pregnancy is identified early in its course. In the event of either a delayed diagnosis or fallopian tube rupture, the prognosis is considered guarded. Ectopic pregnancy can easily become fatal for the mother. If diagnosis is delayed and rupture occurs, it can result in hemorrhage and hemodynamic collapse.

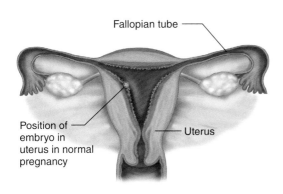

Normal pregnancy

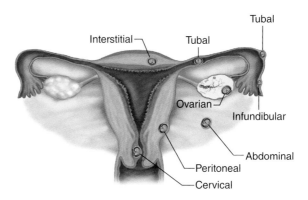

Possible sites of embryo in ectopic pregnancy

FIGURE 9.20   Ectopic pregnancy.

Successful treatment of an ectopic pregnancy may be followed by infertility. Several weeks of follow-up with a physician are required for both medication and surgical interventions, and the patient must be fully recovered before beginning to return to full activity.

Summary

Active patients are unique individuals by nature of their high-intensity exercise and the physical demands placed on their bodies. Yet like everyone else, they can develop any number of genitourinary or gynecological problems. Some of these conditions are unique to athletes, such as sports hematuria and amenorrhea in the athlete, and others are common to athletes and nonathletes alike.

The team of professionals caring for the active population must all be aware of the common medical problems that can occur in this group so they can receive prompt attention and diagnosis. Because of the sensitive nature of these systems and the unique relationship of the athletic trainer to the athlete, familiarity with the signs and symptoms is especially critical to proper assessment and the subsequent early return of the individual to activity or sports.

 Apply It!

Go to HK*Propel* to complete the case studies for this chapter.

Neurological System

At the completion of this chapter the reader should be able to do the following:

1. Describe the anatomy and function of the nervous system.

2. Recognize and assess an athlete with a suspected sport-related concussion.

3. Describe a return-to-play progression for an athlete after sport-related concussion.

4. Recognize and refer a patient with signs or symptoms of a life-threatening neurological condition.

5. Identify conditions that make a person susceptible to migraine and stroke.

6. Recognize the symptoms of complex regional pain syndrome.

7. Describe chronic neurological conditions and their effect on athletic participation.

8. Differentiate when to refer a patient to a physician for further neurological evaluation.

Neurological disorders in the active population are generally divided into two categories: immediately life-threatening conditions, such as encephalitis, meningitis, or stroke, and those with chronic implications, which may include migraine, amyotrophic lateral sclerosis (ALS), complex regional pain syndrome (CRPS), or epilepsy. In addition, there has been increased emphasis on sport-related concussion (SRC) because of the incidence of and possible short- and long-term consequences of concussive injuries. All conditions discussed in this chapter have one basic tenet: Early recognition of symptoms and rapid referral can lead to better outcomes. Infectious neurological conditions, such as encephalitis and meningitis, are discussed in chapter 14; autoimmune neurological conditions, such as multiple sclerosis and Guillain-Barré syndrome, are presented in chapter 13.

Although chronic neurological conditions are less common, they produce symptoms that can interfere with normal daily function and prevent vigorous activity for periods of time. Most have no clear or distinguishable signs, and only the patient's symptoms can guide the clinician to a correct diagnosis. These conditions can also cause emergent situations that require immediate medical referral.

Many symptoms associated with neurological conditions are vague and fleeting and are sometimes passed off as a result of overtraining or fatigue, both of which are common to the athlete. This chapter reviews the pertinent neurological anatomy and highlights signs and symptoms associated with specific neurological conditions. A strong knowledge base, coupled with an inclusive medical history, will enable the athletic trainer to recognize important symptoms and properly refer the patient to a physician.

Overview of Anatomy and Physiology

The neurological system consists of the brain, spinal cord, and nerves that arise from it. Understanding the anatomy and physiology of this system is critical to evaluating conditions specific to it. Depending on the location of the neurological tissue, it may or may not regenerate if damaged. Signs and symptoms of injury or insult to this system typically present some distance from the actual damage and increase the challenge in determining the cause of an injury. Appreciating the anatomy and physiology will enable the practitioner to make a better decision about the cause of the condition and therefore assist with diagnosis and treatment.

Skull

The human skull is made up of two main components: the cerebral cranium, which protects the brain and brainstem, and the anterior facial bony structure. The cerebral cranium consists of these bones: frontal, temporal, parietal, occipital, sphenoid, and ethmoid. The facial skeleton is made up of the mandible, zygomatic, maxillary, and nasal bones (figure 10.1).

Meninges

The meninges lie just under the skull and provide three protective layers: the outermost dura mater, the arachnoid mater, and the pia mater (figure 10.2). The dura mater is a thick, tough, fibrous membrane functionally composed of two layers, with the periosteum against the skull and the inner dura supporting structures of the brain. The real and potential spaces formed between these membranes allow for arteriovenous connections that can be disrupted by hematoma (i.e., accumulation of blood between the spaces) caused by trauma.

Blood supply to the meninges comes from vessels that follow grooves in the skull. Although the periosteum adheres directly to the skull bones, a potential epidural space exists, and ruptured vessels or infection can cause an actual space to form, as seen when a hemorrhage causes an epidural hematoma. In the spine, a true epidural space, separating the dura from the periosteum of the vertebral bones, contains fat and epidural veins.

The inner lining of the dura mater forms folds in the cerebral hemispheres. The membranous plate known as the falx cerebri divides the hemispheres into right and left halves. Another plate formed by the dura, the tentorium cerebelli, separates the cerebral hemispheres from the cerebellum and brainstem.

Large sinuses or cavities that lie within the dura mater allow for the venous return from cerebral veins located between the two layers. The walls of these sinuses are made up primarily of dura. The function of the superior sagittal sinus is to collect venous blood, as well as excess cerebrospinal fluid (CSF), which drains through its arachnoid villi. The blood flows into the transverse sinuses, which also receive blood from other veins of the brain. Together with the sigmoid sinuses, these major venous pathways leaving the brain become the internal jugular vein.

The cavernous sinuses are smaller and receive venous blood from the hypothalamus. They are of clinical importance because the internal carotid artery and several nerves pass through them after entering the cranium at the base of the skull.

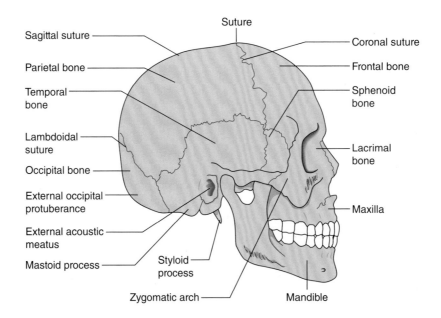

FIGURE 10.1 Bony structures of the head and face.

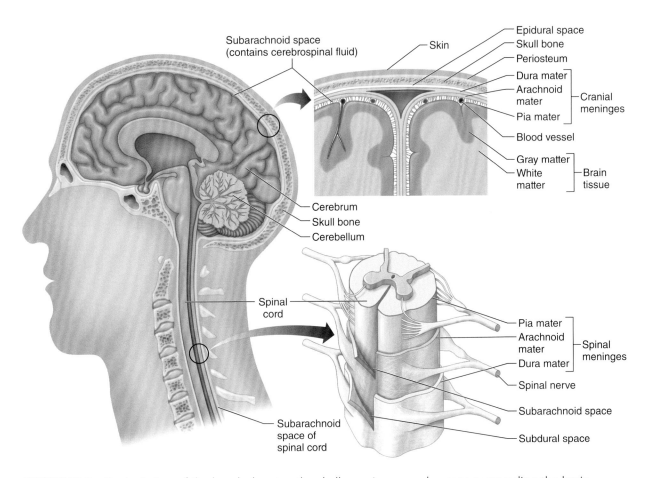

FIGURE 10.2   Sagittal view of the head, showing the skull, meninges, and spaces surrounding the brain.

The arachnoid mater is named for its delicate, spiderweb-like consistency. The arachnoid mater and dura mater are separated by the subdural space, which is a potential space that contains only a small amount of CSF and numerous small veins. If the membrane is disrupted, it can become distended with blood, pus, or other fluids under pathological conditions. The subarachnoid space separates the arachnoid from the pia mater and is filled with fibrous connecting trabeculae, the major arteries, and CSF.

The pia mater is the innermost layer of the meninges and is very thin, adhering directly to the surface of the brain and spinal cord. It follows every fold and enters every crevice, making it difficult to distinguish this membrane from the surface to which it adheres. No potential or actual spaces exist between the pia mater and neural tissue.

Meninges also provide a protective covering to the brainstem and spinal cord, which is why infections affecting the meninges can be detected via a lumbar tap that draws CSF from the membranes covering the spinal cord.

Cerebrum

The two cerebral hemispheres are composed of neural tissue. These hemispheres are divided into four principal lobes: frontal, temporal, parietal, and occipital (figure 10.3). The lobes have been extensively researched in attempts to isolate the locations of specific physiological functions and pathological processes. The most commonly used is Brodmann's classification system, which identifies functional cortices of each lobe by numbers (see figure 10.4).

Frontal Lobe

The frontal lobe contains the primary motor area (area 4), the premotor area (area 6), the frontal eye field (area 8), Broca's speech area (areas 44 and 45), and the frontal association area (areas 9, 10, and 11). The primary motor cortex is highly organized in a somatotopic fashion, with the lips, tongue, face, and hands on the lowest part; moving upward to the trunk, arms, and hips; and ultimately to the feet, lower legs, and genitalia that hang

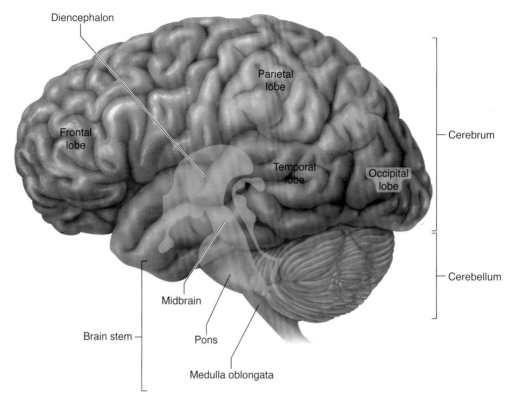

FIGURE 10.3 The four principal lobes of the cerebral cortex.

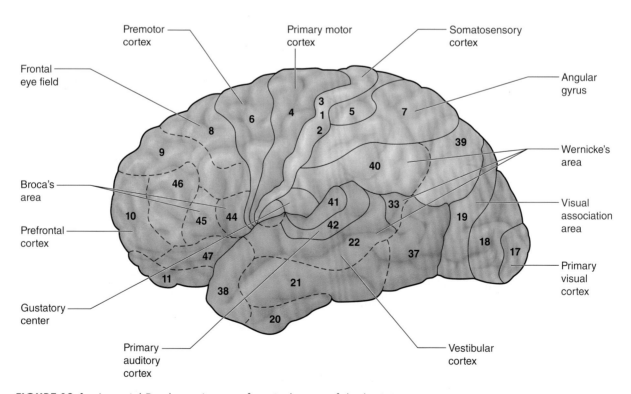

FIGURE 10.4 A partial Brodmann's map of cortical areas of the brain.

over the edge into the interhemispheric fissure. This cortical area is responsible for voluntary movement of the skeletal muscle of the contralateral side of the body. The frontal eye fields coordinate contralateral deviation of the head and eyes.

Clinically, seizure activity within this cortex results in convulsions of the parts of the body represented in the area of electrical disruption. Damage to this cortex can lead to contralateral flaccid paresis or paralysis, and spasticity is usually present if there is concomitant injury to the premotor area. The left hemisphere usually influences and correlates with right hand dominance. Broca's area is located in the dominant hemisphere only. Damage to this area results in Broca's aphasia, also known as *expressive aphasia*, which presents with intact comprehension and impaired expression of speech.

Parietal Lobe

The parietal lobe contains the primary sensory cortex (areas 1, 2, and 3), the sensory association areas (areas 5 and 7), and the cortical taste area embedded in the facial sensory area (areas 1, 2, and 3). The primary sensory cortex, like the motor cortex, is also organized somatotopically. This cortex receives sensory information from the skin and mucosa of the body and face. The types of sensory information processed here include pain, temperature, touch, and proprioception. Pathological injuries to the primary sensory cortex, such as those that occur with a cerebrovascular accident (CVA), also known as stroke, lead to paresthesias, impaired sensation, and, rarely, complete anesthesia of the representative body areas on the contralateral side.

Occipital Lobe

The occipital lobe contains the primary visual cortex (area 17) and the visual association areas (areas 18 and 19). The visual cortex receives information from the ipsilateral half of each retina. Therefore, the right visual cortex receives information from the right half of each retina, which correlates clinically with the left visual field. Irritative lesions to this area, such as seizure or migraine, can lead to visual hallucinations; cortical damage, such as that caused by CVAs, results in contralateral homonymous visual field defects. Pathology of the visual association areas can lead to impairments of spatial orientation and visual disorganization in the same visual field.

Temporal Lobe

The temporal lobe contains the primary auditory cortex (area 41), auditory association area (area 42), temporal association area (represented here by anterior area 22), and Wernicke's speech comprehension area (posterior area 22). The primary auditory cortex receives auditory input from the cochlea of both ears. Irritation of this area can cause buzzing or roaring sounds, and damage can cause hearing deficits ranging from mild, caused by a unilateral lesion, to severe loss or deafness, caused by bilateral lesions. Wernicke's area, like Broca's area, is located in the dominant hemisphere only and is involved in higher auditory processing and in speech comprehension. Injury to this area can lead to word deafness, or **Wernicke's aphasia**.

Although specific areas of the brain may be critical to certain functions, other brain areas can also be involved. These other areas can play a more dominant role when the brain must adapt to neural loss resulting from trauma or disease.

Brainstem

The brainstem acts as the main conduit for information between the brain and the spinal cord by way of three large bundles of fibers called the *cerebellar peduncles*. These bundles contain the ascending and descending tracts carrying motor and sensory information, descending tracts of the autonomic nervous system, and pathways of the monoaminergic system. In addition, the brainstem contains almost all of the cranial nerve nuclei and houses the center that controls respiration, cardiovascular system functions, level of consciousness, sleep, and alertness.

The brainstem comprises the medulla oblongata, the pons, and the midbrain. Each of these areas is associated with neural fibers related to specific body functions. Here is what each of these areas contain:

Medulla Oblongata

- Ascending and descending tracts
- Nuclei of cranial nerves (CN) IX, X, and XII
- Inferior cerebellar peduncles

Pons

- Longitudinal neural tracts
- Raphe nucleus, which is important in pain modulation and in controlling the level of arousal during the sleep–wake cycle
- Nuclei of CN V, VI, and VII
- Auditory pathways
- Middle cerebellar peduncles

Midbrain

- Ascending and descending longitudinal neural tracts
- Nuclei of CN III and IV
- Substantia nigra, which connects with the basal nuclei

- Superior and inferior colliculi, which are involved in the visual and auditory pathways
- Pathways of the monoaminergic system, which interact with the raphe nucleus and its functions
- Periaqueductal gray matter, which contains autonomic pathways and endorphin-producing cells that modulate pain
- Superior cerebellar peduncles

Autonomic Nervous System

The autonomic nervous system innervates glands, smooth muscle, and cardiac muscle. It is divided into the parasympathetic and sympathetic nervous systems. The parasympathetic nervous system is also referred to as *craniosacral* because of its origins in the brainstem and the sacral levels of the spinal cord. The cranial division consists of parasympathetic fibers in four of the cranial nerves (CN III, VII, IX, and X) that innervate the head and the thoracic and abdominal viscera. The sacral division comprises parasympathetic fibers from segments S2 to S4 and innervates the bladder, genitalia, descending colon, and rectum. The sympathetic nervous system is also referred to as *thoracolumbar* because it arises from the thoracic and lumbar areas of the spinal cord. These sympathetic fibers usually travel with the peripheral nerves or along the wall of a blood vessel to their target vessels in skeletal muscle.

The major functions of the parasympathetic and sympathetic nervous systems, which are generally antagonistic, are as follows:

Parasympathetic Nervous System

- Constricts the pupils
- Decreases heart rate
- Increases gastrointestinal peristalsis and secretion
- Expels wastes

Sympathetic Nervous System

- Increases heart rate and breathing
- Dilates blood vessels in skeletal and cardiac muscles and constricts them in the gastrointestinal tract
- Dilates the bronchial passages
- Dilates the pupils
- Erects the hairs for protection and display
- Increases sweat secretion
- Mobilizes glucose

The sympathetic nervous system is responsible for the fight-or-flight response and is catabolic, expending energy as it prepares the body for danger. The parasympathetic nervous system dominates during times of rest.

Disruption of the sympathetic system can lead to several clinical conditions. **Horner's syndrome** is a neurological condition manifested by facial flushing of the affected side, **ipsilateral miosis**, and moderate **ptosis** of an eye. This syndrome is caused by a lesion or tumor at the level of the carotid plexus, cervical sympathetic chain, upper thoracic cord, or brainstem. Sympathetic pathway disruption at the level of the peripheral vascular system can lead to the severe vasoconstrictive episodes characteristic of Raynaud's disease (see chapter 13). Reflex sympathetic dystrophy and causalgia also involve abnormalities at the level of the peripheral blood vessels leading to sympathetic overactivity.

Cerebellum

The cerebellum is located dorsal to the pons and medulla oblongata and consists of two hemispheres connected by the vermis. The cerebellar peduncles connect the cerebellum to the brainstem and contain communicating neural pathways. The cerebellum controls function in the higher-level coordination of voluntary movements and in the maintenance of balance, equilibrium, and muscle tone. Injuries to this structure generally result in the loss of muscle tone (hypotonia) and the loss of muscle coordination (**ataxia**). Other clinical signs of cerebellar disease include nystagmus, **dysmetria**, intention tremor, and **dysdiadochokinesia**.[1]

Spinal Cord

The spinal cord is the body's communication system, transmitting nerve impulses to the brain from the spinal nerves that innervate sensory organs and muscles. The cord is divided into gray and white matter.

Gray Matter

- The gray matter consists of neurons or nerve cells.
- The anterior, or ventral, gray matter contains nerve cells for axons in the ventral roots that carry motor output.
- The intermediolateral gray matter contains nerve cells that carry autonomic nerve fibers.
- The posterior, or dorsal, gray matter contains sensory fibers that convey pain, temperature, proprioception, and touch input.
- These nerve cells are further mapped out into laminae based on the types of information being carried.

White Matter

- The white matter surrounds the gray matter.
- It consists of the ventral, lateral, and dorsal columns, which contain myelinated and unmyelinated nerve fibers.

The dorsal columns comprise the ascending sensory tracts called the *fasciculus gracilis* and the *fasciculus cuneatus*. Together they relay information about touch, proprioception, and two-point discrimination. The lateral columns contain the spinothalamic tracts, dorsal and ventral spinocerebellar tracts, and the spinoreticular pathway. The crossing over, or decussation, that occurs between the axons of the dorsal columns and the spinothalamic tracts in the spinal cord is clinically important. Brain injuries involving these areas lead to contralateral deficits, whereas injuries within the spinal cord result in deficits in ipsilateral touch, proprioception, and contralateral pain perception.

Injuries to the motor tracts result in two different clinical conditions based on the level of injury. Injuries at or peripheral to the anterior horn cells in the spinal cord gray matter present as lower motor neuron syndromes; injuries in the lateral white column or above are associated with upper motor neuron syndromes.

Spinal Nerves

The 31 pairs of spinal nerves in the body arise from the spinal cord as ventral or dorsal roots. The dorsal roots contain sensory fibers carrying pain and temperature information from the muscles; they also contain axons from muscle spindles and skin and joint mechanoreceptors. The ventral roots are composed primarily of motor neuron fibers from skeletal muscle, as well as muscle spindle fibers, autonomic axons, and axons carrying thoracic and abdominal visceral sensory information.

The spinal nerves combine to form the cervical, brachial, lumbar, and sacral plexuses and then innervate the limbs via peripheral nerves (figure 10.5a). Therefore, peripheral nerves generally contain fibers from several different spinal nerves. Dermatomes represent areas of skin supplied by specific spinal nerves. They are clinically significant in diagnosing the sensory area of nerve injury (see the Dermatomes sidebar). Nerve injury must be distinguished from the cutaneous innervation of the periph-

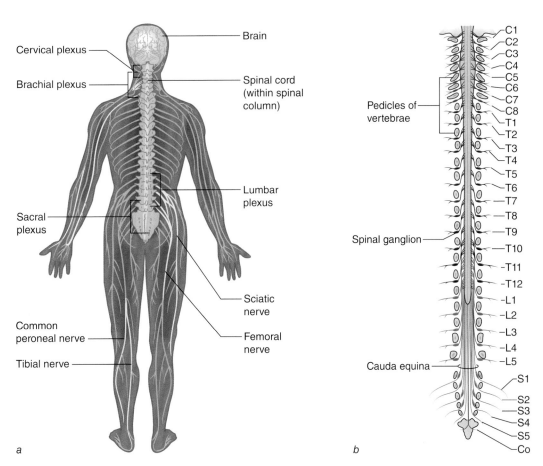

FIGURE 10.5   *(a)* Posterior view of the location of spinal nerves exiting the vertebrae. *(b)* Posterior view of the spine and spinal cord.

Dermatomes

Nerves exit the spinal cord in an orderly manner similar to a ladder. A dermatome is an area of skin supplied mainly by one spinal cord segment through a particular spinal nerve (figure 10.6). Fortunately, dermatomes overlap, so if one nerve is severed, sensations can be transmitted by the nerve above or below it. By following this generalized map of the spinal cord and spinal nerves and their related dermatomes, the clinician can find useful landmarks that aid in assessment.

- The thumb, middle finger, and fifth finger are each in the dermatomes of C6, C7, and C8.
- The head and neck are at the level of C2 and C3.
- The chest is at the levels of C5 through T7.
- The groin is in the region of L1.

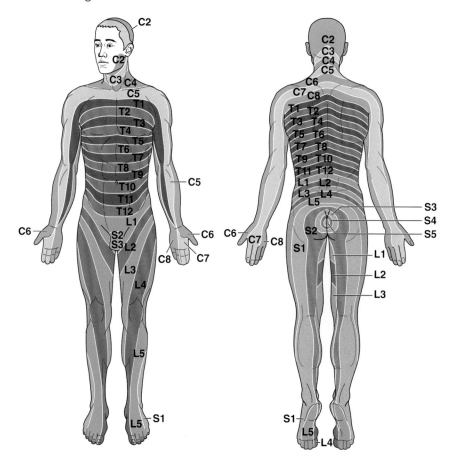

FIGURE 10.6   Anterior and posterior view of dermatomes.

eral nerves. A myotome is a muscle or group of muscles supplied by one ventral (motor) nerve. Motor deficits may be attributed to damage in specific myotomes.

Myelination is a process in which a nerve is enveloped in a myelin sheath. In the peripheral nervous system (PNS), this is accomplished by the encircling of a nerve axon by Schwann cells. Gaps between the Schwann cells are called the *nodes of Ranvier* (figure 10.7), and they expose unmyelinated axons. This is significant because nerve conduction in these myelinated nerves is saltatory,

jumping from node to node, which increases the conduction velocity. This type of myelination ceases just before the interface of the dorsal or ventral nerve root with the spinal cord. At this juncture, between the PNS and the central nervous system (CNS), known as the Oberstein-er-Redlich zone, astrocytes and oligodendrocytes form the myelin covering.

Demyelinating conditions such as multiple sclerosis, which affects the CNS, and Guillain-Barré syndrome, which affects both the PNS and CNS, can lead to varying

Clinical Tips

Upper and Lower Motor Neurons

- *Upper motor neurons* pertain to the brain or spinal cord. Damage to these structures presents as weakness, paralysis, increased muscle tone, spasticity, hyperactive deep tendon reflexes, and the presence of Babinski's reflex. Typically, damaged or destroyed upper motor neurons do not regenerate.

- *Lower motor neurons* pertain to nerve cell bodies, axons, or both. They are located in the anterior horn of the spinal cord and peripheral nerves. Damage to these nerves causes decreased muscle tone, flaccidity, diminished or absent deep tendon reflexes, muscular twitching, and progressive atrophy of the affected muscles. Most lower motor neurons can regenerate if they are located outside of the spinal cord.

degrees of sensory and motor loss. Remyelination often takes place in the PNS; however, it occurs sluggishly, if at all, in the CNS.

Evaluation of the Neurological System

Unlike most other body systems, evaluation of the neurological system depends largely on symptoms, and practitioners should be attuned to patient complaints and comments. Although there can be signs (physical evidence) of a neurological deficit, they are not as common as symptoms. In a thorough evaluation of neurological conditions, clinicians should know the warning signs and listen to the patient's descriptions of symptoms.

Warning Signs of Neurological Diseases

Assessment of the neurological system begins with obtaining the patient's clinical history, coupled with listening carefully to the complaints and terms the patient uses to describe symptoms. In general, neurological diseases can present with either positive or negative manifestations.

- Positive manifestations represent inappropriate excitation of the nervous system. These include hypersensitivity; seizures; movement disorders that include tremors, spasms, and tics; and upper motor neuron signs, such

as spasticity, hypertonicity, and hyperreflexia. Patient descriptions of such positive symptoms may include the following: heaviness, weakness, cramps, slow reaction, tiredness, tremors, visual disturbances, incoordination, a deadened feeling, numbness, tingling, or a pins-and-needles sensation.

- Negative manifestations represent a loss of function. These include paresis, paralysis, hyposensitivity, dementia, aphasia (whether receptive-sensory, expressive-motor, or anomic), syncope, neck stiffness, gait dysfunction, movement disorders, incoordination, sensory ataxia or proprioception loss, and lower motor neuron signs such as hypotonicity–flaccidity, hyporeflexia, and atrophy.

In the case of SRC, the history component of the evaluation is crucial in identifying signs and symptoms, determining the presence or absence of amnesia and loss of consciousness, and evaluating the athlete's mental status.

The physical examination begins with a visual inspection of the spinal column, assessing for deviations, muscular imbalance, or surgical scars. The athlete's musculature, although typically stronger on the dominant side, should not be unilaterally hypertrophic. The health care provider assesses bilaterally for tremors, atrophy, and muscular tone. The dermatomes are bilaterally assessed for sensation as described in chapter 1, followed by bilateral comparison of the reflexes. Evaluation of the cranial nerves (described in the next section) and muscular strength tests follow. Muscular strength tests include both range-of-motion and break tests for the brachial plexus and heel and toe walking for the lower extremities. The practitioner notes any weakness or differences and refers the athlete to a physician when a discrepancy occurs in either. Functional knowledge of the myotomes and dermatomes is instrumental in assessing any neurological issue. The physical examination for SRC should include assessment of cognition and coordination (balance), along with the aforementioned evaluation of strength, myotomes, and dermatomes.

Clinical neurological signs can help in differentiating muscle weakness. The pattern of muscle weakness varies depending on the area of injury within the motor unit: upper motor neuron, lower motor neuron, neuromuscular junction, muscle itself, or manifestation as functional weakness. Upper and lower motor neurons have already been discussed. Neuromuscular junction disorders are characterized by signs of injury that include fatigable weakness, normal or decreased muscle tone, and normal deep tendon reflexes. Decreased or absent reflexes present with injury at the muscle level (myopathy). Functional weakness, in contrast to actual weakness, is associated

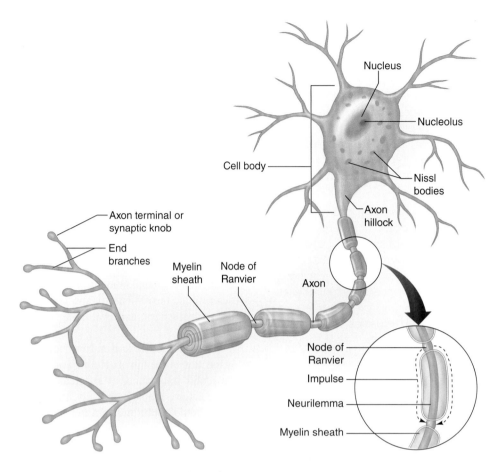

FIGURE 10.7 A neuron. Note the unmyelinated areas in the nodes of Ranvier.

with decreased power in the presence of normal tone, reflexes, and muscle girth.

Understanding the basic anatomy and physiology of the neurological system also helps in identifying injuries to higher neurological systems. Cerebral injuries may present with aphasia, apraxia, paresis, paralysis, sensory deficits, and visual and auditory dysfunction. Cerebellar damage leads to varying degrees of ataxia and incoordination as well as to dysmetria and tremor. Neurological injury to the brainstem may manifest with cranial nerve palsies (CN III-XII). In addition to these symptoms, many other common signs associated with neurological disease have special terminology.

Neurological presentations can range from emergent to urgent to routine in severity and in their need for medical evaluation and management. The Red Flags for Urgent Intervention sidebar provides a framework of warning signs and symptoms that warrant immediate referral to a physician or an emergency department. Indications for referral of specific disorders are addressed in the Pathological Conditions section.

RED FLAGS FOR URGENT INTERVENTION

- Any alteration in the level of consciousness
- Fixed or abnormal pupil reactions, abnormal eye movements, or acute visual impairments
- Any focal neurological symptoms occurring after head trauma
- Paralysis or progressive (either unilateral or bilateral) muscle weakness
- Bowel or bladder incontinence
- Acute severe headache, especially associated with nausea and vomiting or focal neurological deficits
- Prolonged or recurrent generalized seizure

Cranial Nerves and Cranial Nerve Testing

The cranial nerves emerge from the cranium, as opposed to spinal nerves, which emerge from the spinal cord (figure 10.8). The cranial nerves provide sensory and motor innervation to the head and neck, including sensation, voluntary muscle function, and involuntary muscle function. Testing these nerves is essential to ascertaining their integrity and to noting discrepancies that may indicate a medical condition.

Olfactory Nerve (CN I)

The olfactory nerve (CN I) can be tested by placing different-smelling substances underneath a single nostril with the other nostril occluded. Both nares are tested because injuries to this nerve are usually unilateral. The clinical spectrum of pathology can range from normal function to anosmia, in which the patient can discern only ammonia, to organic dysfunction, in which the patient cannot recognize any smells. Use caution when evaluating an athlete who appears to be disoriented. Do not use a noxious odor to provoke a response to CN I in athletes suspected of having a concussion or cervical spine injury.

Optic Nerve (CN II)

The optic nerve (CN II) carries visual information within the complex visual system. The fibers of the optic nerve carrying information from the right half of the retina cross over and join with those same fibers of the contralateral optic nerve. Together, these fibers form the optic tract. The optic tract then forms optic radiations that eventually synapse on the primary visual cortex. Different clinical visual defects occur depending on the area of lesion within the optic pathway. Complete assessment of the optic nerve requires testing the visual fields, acuity, and pupillary light reflex.

To test the visual fields, the health care provider faces the athlete, who is looking straight ahead. The athletic trainer moves the fingers of one hand within the athlete's peripheral vision and monitors the athlete's response regarding which finger is moving. Next, the practitioner focuses on individual eye deficits by repeating this test while the athlete closes one eye. The Snellen eye chart, described in chapter 11, is used to test visual acuity. Alternatively, the athlete may be asked to read something.

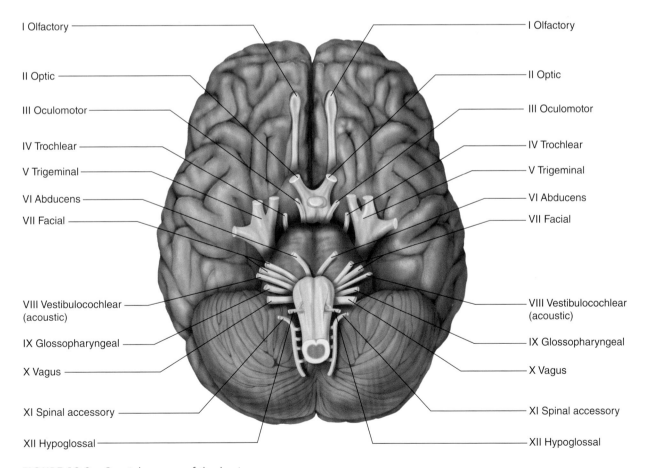

I Olfactory
II Optic
III Oculomotor
IV Trochlear
V Trigeminal
VI Abducens
VII Facial
VIII Vestibulocochlear (acoustic)
IX Glossopharyngeal
X Vagus
XI Spinal accessory
XII Hypoglossal

I Olfactory
II Optic
III Oculomotor
IV Trochlear
V Trigeminal
VI Abducens
VII Facial
VIII Vestibulocochlear (acoustic)
IX Glossopharyngeal
X Vagus
XI Spinal accessory
XII Hypoglossal

FIGURE 10.8   Cranial nerves of the brain.

Oculomotor Nerve (CN III)

The oculomotor nerve (CN III) controls the pupillary light reflex. When light is shone in an athlete's eye, the pupil normally constricts (direct response); the pupil of the other, unstimulated eye should constrict as well (consensual response). Any deviation from this is abnormal. This nerve is also responsible for eye adduction (toward the midline) and downward movement.

Trochlear Nerve (CN IV) and Abducens Nerve (CN VI)

The trochlear (CN IV) and abducens (CN VI) nerves can also be tested by monitoring the movements of the extraocular muscles. The athlete is asked to visually follow a finger, while maintaining a static neck position, as it is slowly moved within the visual field. Then the athletic trainer passes the finger across the midline space toward the athlete's nose, watching for movement of both eyes in toward the midline and testing for convergence. Saccadic eye movements are tested by having the athlete look in each direction and watching the coordination and quality of movement. The trochlear nerve (CN IV) is responsible for upward eye movement, and the abducens nerve (CN VI) coordinates eye movement laterally away from the nose (figure 10.9).

Trigeminal Nerve (CN V) and Facial Nerve (CN VII)

The health care provider tests the response of the trigeminal nerve (CN V) and the facial nerve (CN VII) by observing for symmetry when the athlete bares their teeth and clenches their eyes closed (figure 10.10). Sensory testing of the trigeminal nerve is performed with a light touch and pinprick in the divisions of the trigeminal nerve on both sides. If any abnormalities are found, further tests are warranted. When testing the motor function of the trigeminal nerve, the athletic trainer has the athlete

clench the teeth and then place a hand under the athlete's chin to resist jaw opening. Any noticeable muscle atrophy or elicited muscle weakness indicates an abnormal test. Sensory testing of CN VII and CN IX (glossopharyngeal) appraises the athlete's ability to distinguish taste. For example, the athlete might be asked to tell the difference between sweet and sour.

Vestibulocochlear Nerve (CN VIII)

Testing of the vestibulocochlear nerve (CN VIII) involves auditory testing of hearing and equilibrium. Auditory testing is performed using the Rinne test and the Weber test (see chapter 12). In both tests, a vibrating tuning fork is placed at various points on the patient's head, and the patient is asked to identify which placement is louder. Conductive deafness occurs when conduction of sound is impaired, as opposed to sensorineural deafness, in which there is neurological disruption. Auditory testing may also be conducted by creating a sound, such as snapping the fingers, behind each ear of the patient and looking for a response.

Glossopharyngeal Nerve (CN IX), Vagus Nerve (CN X), and Hypoglossal Nerve (CN XII)

Tests of the glossopharyngeal (CN IX), vagus (CN X), and hypoglossal (CN XII) nerves involve observing the athlete's tongue and mouth anatomy and watching for deviations in tongue movement when the mouth is opened and the tongue stuck out. The athlete is asked to push their tongue against their cheek or a depressor to demonstrate strength. The athletic trainer watches

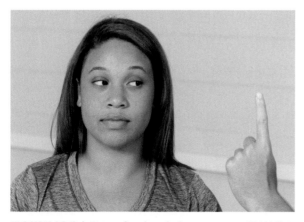

FIGURE 10.9 A test for the abducens nerve (CN VI) is to have the athlete move the eyes laterally, following the finger of the examiner.

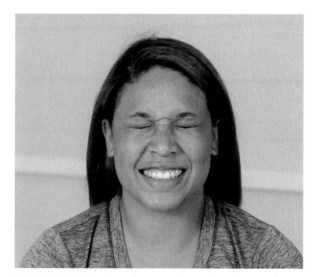

FIGURE 10.10 The trigeminal (CN V) and facial (CN VII) nerves are tested by clenching the teeth and making facial expressions, respectively.

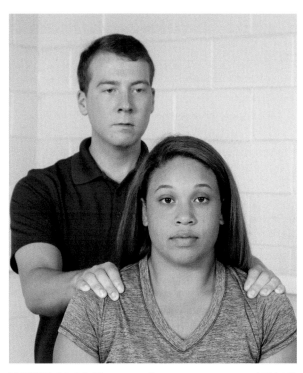

FIGURE 10.11 The spinal accessory nerve (CN XI) is tested by a resisted shrug, which determines the bilateral integrity of the trapezius muscle.

the uvula for deviation from midline as the patient says "aah." The vagus nerve (CN X) controls the gag reflex, which is assessed by touching each side of the pharyngeal wall behind the tonsils and observing movement of the uvula. The vagus nerve is also responsible for movement of the larynx and pharynx, which can be tested together by observing the quality and coordination of movement while the athlete swallows water.

Spinal Accessory Nerve (CN XI)

The athletic trainer tests the spinal accessory nerve (CN XI) by focused examination of the sternocleidomastoid and trapezius muscles on both sides of the body. The strength of the trapezius muscle is assessed through a resisted shoulder shrug (figure 10.11), and the sternocleidomastoid muscle is assessed by resisting both turning and lifting of the chin. The presence of atrophy or weakness during resisted muscle movement suggests nerve injury.

Pathological Conditions

Pathological conditions discussed in this chapter are divided into sections as follows: brain and spinal cord disorders (SRC, stroke), paroxysmal disorders (head-aches, seizures), neuromuscular disorders (ALS), and pain disorders (CRPS).

The presentation and the diagnosis of many neurological conditions are based on a process of exclusion. To arrive at the correct diagnosis, the physician must exclude all other possible explanations for the patient's symptoms. Conditions such as ALS and CRPS have a rather insidious onset, and no single diagnostic test is available to confirm them. A thorough history is paramount in helping the clinician to arrive at the correct diagnosis. Patients often dismiss symptoms and attribute them to fatigue (vision problems, balance issues, or headaches), and a complete medical history should illuminate the symptoms specific to the neurological condition.

Brain and Spinal Cord Disorders

Sport-Related Concussion

This section on SRCs is contributed by Tamara C. Valovich McLeod.

SRC is a common injury in recreational activities and sports that may have possible short- and long-term sequelae. In collegiate sports, there are an estimated 10,560 concussions annually, representing approximately 6% of all collegiate sport-related injuries.[2] Data from children and adolescents suggest that between 1.1 and 1.9 million concussions are sustained annually.[3] It is also speculated that these numbers may be higher because of SRCs that are not recognized by the athlete and thus not reported.[1,4] Data from two national injury surveillance systems found that concussions represented 8.9% of all high school and 5.8% of all collegiate athletic injuries.[5]

The current definition of SRC, as outlined following the Fifth International Conference on Concussion in Sport and provided in the sidebar, Definition of a Sport-Related Concussion, is more comprehensive and describes the clinical, pathological, and biomechanical features of concussion that are important in identifying these injuries.[6] Immediate referral to the nearest emergency department is indicated for any athlete demonstrating any of the following signs and symptoms:

- Deterioration of neurological function
- Decreasing level of consciousness
- Decreasing or irregular respirations or pulse
- Unequal, unreactive, or dilated pupils
- Signs or symptoms of associated injuries
- Skull fracture (including CSF leaking from the nose or ears) or bleeding
- Decreasing mental status and seizures

CONDITION HIGHLIGHT

Definition of a Sport-Related Concussion

SRC is a traumatic brain injury induced by biomechanical forces. Several common features may be used in clinically defining the nature of a concussive head injury:

- SRC may be caused by a direct blow to the head, face, neck, or elsewhere on the body with an impulsive force transmitted to the head.

- SRC typically results in rapid onset of short-lived impairment of neurological function that resolves spontaneously. However, in some cases, signs and symptoms evolve over minutes to hours.

- SRC may result in neuropathological changes, but the acute clinical signs and symptoms largely reflect a functional disturbance rather than a structural injury and, as such, no abnormality is seen on standard structural neuroimaging studies.

- SRC results in a range of clinical signs and symptoms that may or may not involve loss of consciousness. Resolution of the clinical and cognitive features typically follows a sequential course. However, symptoms may be prolonged in some cases.

The clinical signs and symptoms of concussion cannot be explained by other injuries (e.g., cervical injuries, peripheral vestibular dysfunction, etc.), other comorbidities (e.g., psychological factors or coexisting medical conditions), or medication use, alcohol, or other substances.

Signs and Symptoms

The health care provider should be able to identify signs and symptoms associated with SRC. These signs and symptoms are often categorized as somatic (physical), emotional, cognitive, or sleep related.[7] Symptoms that warrant referral to a medical facility are listed in the physician referral guidelines. Each athlete may present differently, with respect to symptom severity and duration. In the National Collegiate Athletics Association (NCAA) Concussion Assessment, Research and Education (CARE) Consortium study, researchers noted an increase in reported symptoms immediately after concussion, followed by a gradual decrease in symptom complaints throughout the first week.[8] The average duration of symptom resolution was 8.83 ± 18.75 d, with more than 41% of patients taking longer than 7 d to report as asymptomatic.[8] Among pediatric patients, symptom resolution tends to take longer, with symptom resolution averaging approximately 17 d and just over one-fourth of patients taking longer than 4 wk to achieve symptom resolution.[9] Headache is the most common symptom reported and tends to last the longest.

Differential Diagnosis and Referral

As part of the initial assessment of SRC, the health care provider should try to rule out more severe head injuries such as skull fracture, cerebral contusion, and epidural hematoma.[4,10,11] Assessment of these injuries may reveal acute localized swelling, deformity, prolonged loss of consciousness, intractable vomiting, and often multiple positive neurological examination findings such as cranial nerve abnormalities and motor or sensory weakness. Positive findings during an initial examination for loss of consciousness on the field, amnesia lasting longer than 15 min, deterioration of neurological function or consciousness, unequal or unreactive pupils, or other systemic declines should warrant immediate transfer to an emergency department capable of managing a neurosurgical emergency.[10] The clinician should continue to monitor the athlete for any signs of changing or deteriorating condition in the acute injury phase and throughout the first week postinjury that would increase suspicion of a subdural hematoma. Patients should be given a take-home instruction form that lists the warnings for immediate referral and other information about home care of the SRC (figure 10.12). Each athletic trainer should work in collaboration with their directing physician to determine the most appropriate language and recommendations pertinent to their patient population.

Clinical Tips

Diagnosing Concussions

Diagnostic imaging in the management of SRC is used to rule out a more severe structural injury (intracranial hemorrhage, epidural hematoma, or subdural hematoma) and should not be used to aid in determining the severity of an SRC or to make return-to-play decisions.

PATIENT INSTRUCTIONS FOR SPORT-RELATED CONCUSSIONS

I believe that _____ sustained a concussion on _____. To make sure he or she recovers, please follow the following important recommendations:

1. _____ must report to the athletic training facility on _____ at ____ _____ for a follow-up evaluation.

2. If any of the problems below develop before the follow-up visit, please call _____ at ____ _____ or contact the local emergency medical system or your family physician.

- Decreasing level of consciousness
- Increasing confusion
- Increasing irritability
- Loss of or fluctuating level of consciousness
- Numbness in the arms or legs
- Pupils becoming unequal in size
- Repeated vomiting
- Seizures
- Slurred speech or inability to speak
- Inability to recognize people or places
- Worsening headache

Otherwise, you can follow the instructions outlined below.

It is OK to
- Use acetaminophen (Tylenol) for headaches
- Use ice pack on head and neck as needed for comfort
- Eat a carbohydrate-rich diet
- Go to sleep
- Engage in an initial brief period of rest (24-48 h) where you limit physical activity
- Engage in activities of daily living at home, school, and work to a level that does not worsen symptoms

There is NO need to
- Check eyes with flashlight
- Wake up frequently (unless otherwise instructed)
- Test reflexes
- Stay in bed

Do NOT
- Drink alcohol
- Drive a car or operate machinery
- Return to sports activity until cleared by a health care provider

Other recommendations:

Recommendations provided to _____

Please feel free to contact me if you have any questions. I can be reached at _____.

Please follow up in the athletic training facility on _____ (date).

FIGURE 10.12   Take-home instructions for patients with a sport-related concussion.

Adapted from Broglio et al. (2014).

Physician referral is also indicated for athletes who are not experiencing a typical recovery, for those who may still be symptomatic in the weeks after their initial injury, and for those who demonstrate an increase in symptoms in the postacute phase. A typical recovery time is 10 to 14 d for adults and up to 28 d for children and adolescents.[6] At this time, referral to a specific specialty, based on concussion phenotype, may be necessary. For example, an athlete with sleep disturbances may benefit from referral to a neurologist, whereas a patient with cognitive difficulties may be best referred to a neuropsychologist.[10]

Diagnostic Tests

SRC is a functional injury and does not normally include structural injury to the brain. Therefore, most diagnostic tests will result in negative imaging findings, thus making neuroimaging of little value for most SRCs.[4,11-13] Suspicion of an intracranial hemorrhage or hematoma should result in immediate referral for a computed tomography (CT) scan, functional magnetic resonance imaging (MRI), or other imaging study. Moreover, the sudden presence or deterioration of symptoms that had previously resolved or remained stable necessitates neuroimaging for a subdural hematoma, which may not be noted on a CT scan or an MRI scan for 1 to 2 wk after the initial concussion.[10] However, a negative imaging finding does not rule out SRC, and it should not be used to prematurely return a patient to activity.

Assessment

The assessment of SRC should begin off-season or during preseason in conjunction with the preparticipation physical examination (PPE) to obtain an adequate concussion history and to assess baseline measures of symptom reports, postural stability, and neurocognition. The PPE should include a thorough neurological injury history, including a history of SRC and other concussive injuries (e.g., motor vehicle accidents, falls), past medical history, and history of mental health concerns.[21] The PPE should contain an adequate series of questions regarding concussion history, including queries about perceived previous concussions and those focusing on earlier concussion-related symptoms sustained during both sport and nonsport activity. Knowledge of an athlete's concussion history is important, as research has demonstrated a relationship between previous concussions and increased risk for later injury.[10,11,22] In addition, baseline measures of symptoms, neurocognitive function, and postural stability should be obtained from athletes when they are healthy for future comparison with postconcussion scores, although baseline assessments are not required for all athletes.[6,13]

After a concussion, the athlete should be assessed immediately for symptom reports, mental status, and postural stability. Serial assessments using tools such as the Graded Symptom Checklist (GSC) or the Post-Concussion Symptom Scale (PCSS) take place at planned intervals (postgame and 24, 48, and 72 h postinjury) to assess the athlete's recovery. The GSC asks patients to relay symptoms, such as blurred vision, dizziness, feeling "in a fog," headache, nausea, irritability, and so on. The athletic trainer notes changes in symptom severity, the number of symptoms reported, or if new symptoms arise. Once the athlete reports symptom resolution, more complex neurocognitive assessments may be administered to determine whether cognitive recovery has occurred as well. Scores on all assessment tools should meet or improve to baseline or normative scores and the clinical examination should be normal before a return-to-play progression is begun.

Concussion Legislation and Policy

Health care providers need to be aware of laws and policies regarding SRC. In 2009, the first SRC law was passed in Washington State; since that time, all 50 states and the District of Columbia have passed concussion laws. All 51 laws apply to high school student-athletes, with 50 laws also applying to middle school students and 42 applicable to youth athletes.[1] The language in most laws differs, but most include three common components: (1) concussion education and informed consent, (2) removal from play, and (3) return-to-play guidelines.[14] The laws differ in the areas of required coach or health care provider training, liability waivers, designation of qualified medical providers, and the delivery mode for concussion education. A few studies have begun to evaluate the effects of these laws and have found an increase in coach knowledge[15,16] and health care utilization[17-19] after their implementation. Health care providers should understand the concussion laws in the states in which they practice to be sure they comply with all aspects.

In addition to state laws, many sport organizations, school districts, and schools have their own concussion policies. Most states have an interscholastic athletic association that oversees all sports and activities in its state, and most of these associations have concussion policies, which may be similar to or more conservative than the state law. Other organizations, such as Pop Warner Football[20] and USA Soccer, have developed concussion policies as well.

Self-Report Symptoms Assessment

Athletic trainers typically use instruments, such as the PCSS, to identify postconcussion signs and symptoms. There are several variations of PCSS tools, including both symptom checklists and graded symptom scales (GSSs), that differ in the number of symptoms they list and whether symptoms are grouped into the factors mentioned previously.[10,23] A PCSS checklist comprises a list of commonly noted concussion symptoms to which athletes simply provide a yes-or-no response as to whether they are experiencing each symptom. A GSS is a more objective measure that provides detailed information about concussion severity or duration. Using a Likert scale, athletes note the extent to which they are experiencing each symptom. The summative score can then be calculated. The first score is the sum of Likert scale responses and represents a "total symptom score." The second score is the total number of symptoms for which the athlete indicated a severity or duration score greater than zero.[10] In addition to these stand-alone PCSS tools, some computerized neurocognitive tests and Sport Concussion Assessment Tool (SCAT) iterations include symptom inventories.[24]

These symptom checklists and scales serve as an initial screen of the patient's symptom reports. Clinicians should ask follow-up questions for any symptom present to better understand its quality, frequency, duration, and other characteristics. For example, a patient who reports dizziness should be asked follow-up questions that address the quality of dizziness (e.g., patient's description of vertigo, lightheadedness, or unsteadiness), timing and duration of dizziness, triggers, and other associated symptoms. Patients reporting a headache should be asked about onset, location, duration, characteristics, and aggravating and alleviating factors. These follow-up questions provide the clinician with more detailed information about reported symptoms to help inform treatment and management plans of care.

In a meta-analysis investigating the degree to which concussion affected self-reported symptoms, neurocognitive ability, and postural stability, researchers found a significant increase in self-reported symptoms in the

Clinical Tips

Mobile Concussion Assessment Tools

Most concussion sideline assessment tools have an app one can load onto a mobile phone or tablet device. The responses collected can then be sent directly to a physician or medical file from the device.

immediate postinjury phase and during follow-up examinations within the first 14 d postinjury.[25] This finding further highlights the need for clinicians to use some tool to assess PCSS in all athletes with a suspected concussion.[25] Clinicians should ensure that the checklist or scale chosen is appropriate for their patients, as children and adolescents must be assessed with appropriate symptom inventories.[10,23]

Mental Status Assessment

Mental status assessments are often used on the sideline or in the acute postinjury phase to determine the presence of cognitive deficits in an athlete with a suspected concussion. These assessments differ from the computerized neurocognitive tests, in that they are simple cognitive screening tools and are most sensitive to deficits in cognition within the first 48 h postinjury.[26] These assessments may be more informal and can include questions regarding orientation and memory (Maddocks' questions),[27] repeating digits backward or forward, serial subtraction of threes or sevens,[28] or repeating days of the week or months of the year in reverse order. In addition, several more formal mental status assessments have been used in the evaluation of SRC, including the Standardized Assessment of Concussion (SAC)[26] and SCAT tools.[24]

The SAC has adequate reliability, validity, and sensitivity to change subsequent to SRC[26,29-31] and has been evaluated as an assessment tool in collegiate,[32,33] high school,[30,34] and youth sports athletes.[35] The SAC was found to indicate the largest negative effect (decrease in cognition) of all cognitive tests studied, including pencil-and-paper and computerized batteries, during the immediate postinjury assessment.[25] This finding supports single studies that evaluated the SAC and found it to be the most sensitive in detecting cognitive deficits in the first 48 h after concussion.[33]

Neurocognitive Assessment

Although mental status evaluation is important on the sideline and in the immediate postinjury phase, those assessments are not sensitive enough to determine the extent of more complex cognitive deficits. Nor are they useful in making return-to-play decisions during the later stages of recovery. Pencil-and-paper neurocognitive batteries or, more commonly, computerized neurocognitive concussion programs are used once an athlete is asymptomatic to determine whether cognitive deficits still exist. Clinicians using neurocognitive assessments should be aware of factors that might affect test performance and score interpretation, including demographic variables (age, race, ethnicity, native language, education level), medical conditions (learning disabilities, attention-deficit disorder, anxiety, sleep disorders, concussion history), preinjury cognitive function, and previous exposure to neurocognitive testing (learning effects).[36]

Pencil-and-paper batteries are typically developed by neuropsychologists trained to administer and interpret these types of assessments. A baseline battery may last up to 30 min, with postinjury assessments being slightly shorter, and is composed of several different neurocognitive tests that assess domains sensitive to impairment after SRC. These include attention, concentration, processing speed, learning, memory, and executive functioning.[26] Computerized neurocognitive assessments are also available from different companies in laptop, tablet, and mobile phone formats using a variety of applications.

Significant deficits in neurocognitive function have been noted during both initial assessment and subsequent follow-up evaluations, with the effect of concussion on neurocognition resulting in a smaller but still significant negative effect during the first 14 d postinjury.[25] The largest negative effect on cognition reported at the follow-up assessment was found with pencil-and-paper batteries, indicating that they were more sensitive to detecting cognitive deficits. Mild to moderate negative effects in cognitive function immediately after concussion and little effect, indicating full neurocognitive recovery, by 7 to 10 d postinjury were also reported in a prior meta-analysis of concussion and neurocognitive function.[37] Although both of these meta-analyses observed a lesser effect with computerized neurocognitive programs, these programs may be more cost-effective, time efficient, and clinician friendly in the assessment of SRC.

Postural Control Assessment

Assessment of postural control or postural stability has become another central component of concussion evaluation plans. Computerized force plate systems,[38] such as the NeuroCom Sensory Organization Test, and clinical balance measures,[39] such as the Balance Error Scoring System (BESS), have been advocated as means to assess postural stability. Both have been shown to be sensitive to deficits in postural stability until about 5 d postinjury.[38] In addition, large negative effects were found in postural control measures both immediately after SRC and during follow-up assessments.[25]

The BESS has several clinical advantages compared with force plate measures of postural stability, including cost-effectiveness (requiring only a stopwatch and a foam pad), efficiency (taking only 5 min to administer), and portability (the foam pad is transported easily). The BESS consists of six separate 20 s balance tests completed in three different stances on both firm and foam surfaces (figure 10.13): *(a)* double leg stance, *(b)* tandem leg stance (nondominant leg placed behind dominant leg), *(c)* single leg stance (standing on nondominant leg), *(d)* double leg stance on foam, *(e)* tandem leg stance on foam, and *(f)* single leg stance on foam.[39] During each test

condition, error scores are recorded when the athlete compensates to aid balance. Errors include each instance of opening the eyes; lifting the hands off the hips; stepping, falling, or lifting a foot or heel; remaining out of position more than 5 s; or maintaining the hip in more than 30° of abduction or flexion. Another clinical balance assessment called the *tandem gait task* was included in the SCAT-5 and has shown promising results as an inexpensive tool in the office setting. The inclusion of dual tasking, in which patients complete the tandem gait task with the addition of cognitive tasks, is also useful for increasing assessment difficulty.[40] Advancements in mobile technology have also led to the development of several applications for balance assessment using smartphones and tablets.

Oculomotor Testing

Oculomotor function is another dimension of vestibular function that should be assessed following a concussion. The cranial nerve assessment included as part of the neurologic evaluation should enable the clinician to evaluate visual acuity, saccades, smooth pursuits, eye motion, and vergence (convergence and divergence).[41,42] Two clinical assessments have been introduced that can supplement the clinical examination and provide objective measures of oculomotor function: the Vestibular Ocular Motor Screening (VOMS) and the King-Devick test. The VOMS is a clinical examination that evaluates smooth pursuits, horizontal and vertical saccades, convergence, horizontal vestibular–ocular reflex testing, and visual motor sensitivity, along with self-reported symptom assessment following each test to determine the presence of headache, dizziness, nausea, and fogginess.[42] The King-Devick test evaluates horizontal saccadic eye movement, processing speed, and attention.[43] In this timed, rapid number reading assessment, difficulty increases as the patient progresses through the three test cards. The test is scored as the total time required to read the three test cards, and the examiner also records the number of errors made during the testing time.[43,44]

Multifaceted Assessment

Although each of the previously described assessment categories is important, a multifaceted approach to concussion assessment has been advocated by several consensus and position statements[13,45] and supported by research.[18] These multifaceted concussion plans have been shown to increase diagnostic accuracy compared with individual tests of neurocognition, postural stability, or self-reported symptoms.[25,33,46] McCrea and colleagues reported increased sensitivity up to 93% with a protocol consisting of a GSS, the SAC, and the BESS compared with the sensitivity of each individual tool (89%, 80%, and 34%, respectively).[33] Similarly, PCSS sensitivity increased from 64% to 83% with the addition of the

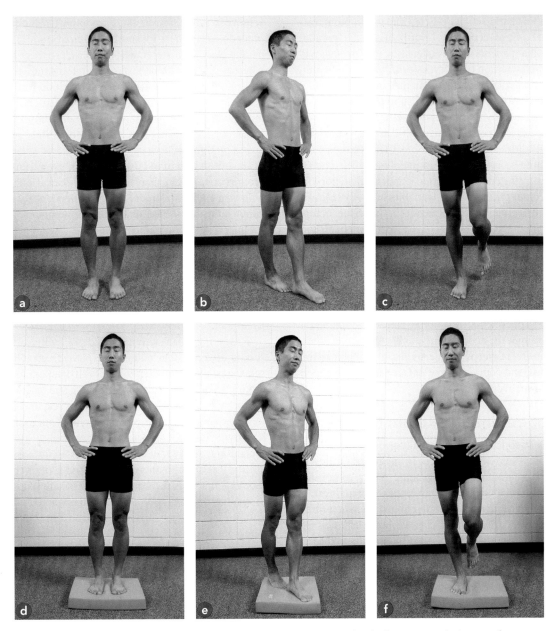

FIGURE 10.13   The Balance Error Scoring System (BESS) is one method of assessing balance after concussion.

ImPACT computerized concussion assessment tool.[46] Finally, higher sensitivity was found with the addition of postural stability measures and a GSS to ImPACT use (91.7%), the HeadMinder Concussion Resolution Index (89.3%), and pencil-and-paper neurocognitive batteries (95.7%).[47] Data from the NCAA CARE Consortium noted that a multimodal assessment that included symptom evaluation, postural control on the firm surface (e.g., BESS), and neurocognitive screening (e.g., SAC) resulted in the most optimal quantification of acute dysfunction following concussion.[12]

Clinicians may benefit the most by using a multifaceted assessment paradigm that includes a PCSS, the SAC, and a measure of postural stability during their initial assessment within the first 48 h postinjury. Once the athlete is asymptomatic, the clinician can then follow up using a PCSS, a postural stability measure, and a pencil-and-paper or computerized neurocognitive battery, which may provide more useful information for decision-making regarding concussion treatment and return to activity.

Concussion Treatment

Previous recommendations suggested that patients refrain from all physical and cognitive activities until symptom resolution, at which time initiating a return-to-school or return-to-play protocol is advised. However, evidence suggests that early activity is beneficial to symptom resolution and time to recovery.[48,49] Furthermore, the literature suggests that patients with a concussion may present with different concussion phenotypes or subtypes, indicating that different courses of treatment may be appropriate.[7,50] Classification into a concussion subtype is done based on the patient's symptom reports, clinical examination findings, and adjunct assessment results. The Concussion Clinical Profiles Screening (CP Screen) may be helpful in determining a patient's concussion phenotype.[7] The CP Screen is a 29-item self-reported symptom inventory for patients older than age 12 yr, and it includes five clinical profiles (affective, cognitive, headache-migraine, ocular, vestibular) and two modifiers (sleep, cervical). Each item is scored as none, mild, moderate, or severe, with a total score ranging from 0 to 87 and individual profiles scored on average from 0 to 3.[7]

Several taxonomies classify concussion into subtypes or phenotypes. An example is provided in table 10.1. Regardless of concussion subtype, current recommendations highlight the need for early subsymptom threshold aerobic exercise, sleep hygiene, monitoring of preexisting conditions, and counseling patients regarding the expectations of recovery.[51]

Management and Return to Activity

To manage concussion, an initial period of 24 to 48 h for physical and cognitive rest is suggested, followed by active treatments and a gradual return-to-activity progression.[6,11] During this time, patients should refrain from sport participation and other unrestricted activities, such as physical education classes; however, they are encouraged to engage in supervised subsymptom threshold aerobic exercise and other concussion treatments as indicated by the treating provider. In the acute phase, patients may also be prescribed a period of cognitive rest that may include academic adjustments in the classroom during the initial course of recovery.

Cognitive rest involves avoiding or limiting activities that produce mental exertion that could result in neurometabolic processes and stressors that may delay recovery.[52] Many concussion-related symptoms may follow cognitive activity, and patients should reduce mental challenges to levels that are tolerable during the first 24 to 48 h following SRC.[52] Cognitive rest may include a reduction in activities of daily living, scholastic stressors, time spent using technology, and school attendance and activities. However, bed rest or strict rest from all cognitive activities may worsen symptoms and result in a longer recovery.[53] Clinicians need to balance rest with light subsymptom threshold activity and progressively increase mental demands as the patient's symptoms resolve.

The progression of cognitive activities is also termed the *return-to-learn progression*, and it helps the patient achieve a full return to the classroom,[54] which should precede any return to sport participation.[6,10,54] Every patient will be different. Some may progress rapidly, whereas others with persisting symptoms may require a more gradual progression that may include formal academic accommodations, such as a 504 plan or academic modifications (e.g., Individualized Education Plan).[55,56] It has been suggested that patients should not return to even a modified school day until they can concentrate for at least 30 min without an increase in symptoms.[57] The progression should then move from partial attendance with academic adjustments, to full attendance with academic adjustments, to full attendance without additional support.[58] Academic adjustments are determined based on the types of symptoms the patient is experiencing, the clinical examination findings, and specifics related to individual coursework. Successful return-to-learn progressions require collaboration and communication between the patient's health care providers and school personnel.

Regarding other activities of daily living, clinicians should also consider counseling patients on when it is safe to resume driving. Driving is skill that requires multitasking, vision, coordination, attention, and reaction time. Furthermore, drivers must be able to respond quickly to any changes in the environment. Concussion can lead to dysfunction in oculomotor control, visual motor processing, and reaction time, which can impair driving ability.[59] Although there are limited evidence-based recommendations regarding when it is safe for a patient to resume driving, several studies have noted cognitive deficits and slowed driving reaction time, even after symptom resolution.[60-63] Based on the limited evidence, recommendations to restrict driving in the first 24 to 48 h following concussion may be prudent, although there is insufficient evidence for specific recommendations after the 48 h window.[64] Clinicians should use the information obtained in their clinical examination and adjunct testing to provide individualized recommendations regarding when it is safe for patients to resume driving.

Similarly, return-to-play guidelines follow a specific progression that begins with light subsymptom threshold exercise initiated as part of concussion treatment.[6] A stepwise progression calls for a 24 h symptom-free period between steps.[6,10,58] The progression allows the patient to begin performing exercises of increasing intensity, beginning with a subexertional exercise protocol of 10 to 15 min (e.g., stationary bike intervals) to determine whether symptoms return with exercise onset and the associated increase in heart rate and blood pressure. The patient can then participate in sport-specific exercises for a set duration of 20 to 30 min, followed by on-field practice with no contact, on-field practice with body contact, and then return to full competition. Many recommendation and consensus statements suggest that in the absence of

TABLE 10.1   **Concussion Phenotypes, Examination Findings, and Treatments**

Phenotype	Symptoms	Risk factors	Examination findings	Treatment options
Affective	• Anxiety, depression, worry, difficulty turning off thoughts, focus on symptoms, panic attacks • Sadness, limited social interactions, loss of interest	• Personal or family psychiatric history or medications • Comorbid migraine and sleep issues • Presence of significant life stressors	• Elevated scores above cutoff on mood or anxiety questionnaires • Otherwise normal physical examination	• Psychotherapy approaches (CBT, behavioral activation, exposure therapy) • Psychotropic medication
Cognitive	• Feeling in a fog, difficulty concentrating, memory problems, feeling slowed down • Fatigue or low energy • Symptoms worsen throughout the day	• Personal history of ADHD, learning disability	• Neurocognitive deficits • Multiple domains often affected	• Academic supports • Behavioral regulation • Medication with stimulants (if needed)
Fatigue	• Fatigue or low energy • Drowsiness • Trouble falling asleep • Difficulty concentrating • Feeling slowed down	• Preinjury sleep difficulties	• Normal physical examination • Tired or subdued appearance • Decreased arousal	• CBT • Graded exertional tolerance training
Headache-migraine	• Intermittent, moderate to intense headache, often present on waking • Headache with nausea and/or phonosensitivity, photosensitivity, or both • Visual aura including flashing or shimmering lights, zigzagging lines, or stars • Pulsating quality • Motion sickness and sleep problems common	• Personal or family history of migraine • Personal history of motion sickness • Comorbid anxiety disorder or sleep problems • Female	Neurocognitive deficits across domains	• Referral to headache specialist • Behavioral regulation
Ocular	• Blurry vision, diplopia, eye strain, difficulty focusing • Difficulty reading (e.g., skipping lines, reading comprehension) • Headache and fatigue triggered specifically by visual activity	• Personal or family history of eye muscle surgery, strabismus, amblyopia, or other ocular diplopia	• Abnormal near point convergence measurements • Tracking, saccadic deficits • Neurocognitive deficits typical, especially reaction time	• Vision therapy • Exposure/recovery approach when engaging in visually demanding tasks
Vestibular	• Slow, wavy dizziness with movement or change of positions • Dizziness, nausea, mental fogginess, and anxiety in busy environments • Balance problems • Motion sensitivity • Vertigo when lying down, looking up, or rolling over	• Personal history of motion sickness or sensitivity • Personal history of vestibular disorder • Comorbid migraine • Comorbid anxiety disorder	• Abnormal vestibular screening • Symptom provocation with vestibular–ocular reflex testing	• Vestibular rehabilitation • Dynamic exertion therapy • Exposure and/or recovery approach in day-to-day activity

Note: ADHD = attention-deficit/hyperactivity disorder; CBT = cognitive–behavioral therapy.

Data from Kontos (2019); Lumba-Brown (2020); Harmon (2019).

objective balance or neurocognitive assessments, a 7 d waiting period should be observed before beginning the stepladder return-to-play progression once the athlete reports being symptom free. In this progression, a level is not begun until the athlete is symptom free for 24 h after completing the previous step.[10,45] The progression outlined in current consensus and position statements lends itself best to contact and collision sports like football and soccer. For other noncontact sports, the clinician may need to modify the steps and should include sport-specific activities. For example, in swimming, considerations should be made regarding the appropriate time to initiate each stroke, flip turns, and diving from the blocks.[65] The literature is beginning to describe other sport-specific return-to-activity protocols.[66] Figure 10.14 is specific to adolescents and includes both return-to-activity and return-to-school protocols.

Prognosis

The prognosis for most patients after SRC is good. In general, adult patients recover in about 10 to 14 d and children and adolescents recover within 28 d.[6] However, some evidence suggests that athletes with certain modifying factors may be at risk of persisting symptoms or require a more conservative return-to-play progression.[6,22,67]

These modifying factors include age younger than 18 yr or history of migraine, depression or other mental health disorders, attention-deficit hyperactivity disorder, learning disabilities, or sleep disorders. Furthermore, patients with a prior concussion history, especially those with past injuries that occurred close together or that took longer for symptoms to resolve, should be treated more conservatively.[6,68] Several other injury-related characteristics are reported to have prognostic capabilities for persisting symptoms following concussion, including initial symptom burden and time to medical care.[69-71]

The Predicting and Preventing Postconcussive Problems in Pediatrics (5P) clinical risk score has been validated for pediatric patients presenting acutely following concussion. The clinical risk score uses nine commonly evaluated variables—age, sex, prior concussion history, migraine history, answering questions slowly, headache, fatigue, sensitivity to noise, and balance impairments—to determine a patient's risk for persisting symptoms. Each variable is scored, and the clinical risk score ranges from 0 (low risk) to 12 (high risk). The 5P clinical risk score is shown to predict persisting symptoms in patients presenting to the emergency department and to an outpatient sports medicine clinic.[72-74]

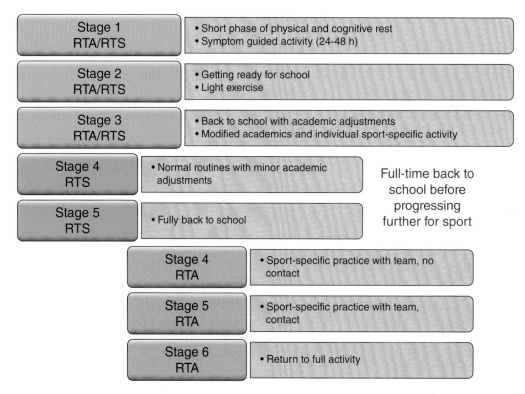

FIGURE 10.14 Concussion return-to-activity (RTA) and return-to-school (RTS) protocols.

Reprinted by permission from C.A. DeMatteo, S. Randall, C.A. Lin, and E.A. Claridge. "What Comes First: Return to School or Return to Activity for Youth After Concussion? Maybe We Don't Have to Choose," *Frontiers in Neurology* 10, no. 792 (2019), https://doi: 10.3389/fneur.2019.00792. Distributed under the terms of the Creative Commons Attribution 4.0 International License (http://creativecommons.org/licenses/by/4.0/).

Prevention

There is currently no evidence that helmets or headgear can effectively reduce SRC incidence or severity.[10,75-77] Mouthguard use has been shown to reduce concussion risk between 57% and 64% among NCAA and youth ice hockey athletes.[78,79] Some evidence suggests that contact restrictions and rule changes, specifically regarding body checking in ice hockey, can reduce the risk of head impacts and concussion.[80-83]

Awareness and education currently serve as the best means of prevention by informing athletes, coaches, parents, and health care providers about SRC signs and symptoms so these injuries can be reported appropriately. Several educational programs have been advocated, including the Centers for Disease Control and Prevention (CDC) concussion tool kits[84] and Canada's ThinkFirst program.[84,85]

Stroke

Stroke, also called a **cerebrovascular accident (CVA)**, is caused by a lack of oxygen to the brain and may lead to reversible or irreversible paralysis and other neurological damage. Such damage to a group of nerve cells in the brain is often caused by interrupted blood flow from a blood clot or aneurysm in which the blood vessel bursts. Depending on the area of the brain that is damaged, stroke can cause coma, paralysis, speech problems, dementia, or death. An often-overlooked category of stroke is the transient ischemic attack (TIA). Because the episode is momentary and often lasts only a few minutes, TIA does not permanently damage the brain; however, this does not diminish the gravity of the event. The cause, presentation, and risk factors are the same for TIA and stroke. Any damage is less noticeable because the blockage is temporary. Nonetheless, a TIA is a warning that full blood flow to the brain is not occurring. As with a stroke, the TIA is a medical emergency.

In a previous study, the American Heart Association stated that Black and Hispanic women older than age 70 yr had a higher risk of stroke compared with White women.[86] This increased risk was not demonstrated in older Black or Hispanic men compared with White men.[86] In the United States, the regions with the highest mortality from stroke are the Midwest through southeastern states.[86] The main risk factors for stroke are dyslipidemia (38%), smoking (34%), hypertension (20%), and diabetes mellitus (11%).[87] Other risk factors include obesity, high cholesterol (total cholesterol >200 mg/dl), family history of stroke or cardiovascular disease, and vitamin D deficiency.

Although rare, the incidence of ischemic stroke has been trending upward since 1990 among working-age adults.[88] A 22-year-old football player sustained a stroke secondary to an on-field whiplash injury,[89] a 15-year-old was misdiagnosed with migraine,[90] and a 27-year-old girl's basketball coach thought he had a dizzy spell,[91] but all were eventually diagnosed with stroke, and all recovered. A review article found 39 cases of stroke in athletes, and the authors reported that headache along with head trauma, neck trauma, or both were the most cited precursors to the stroke diagnosis.[92] In athletes, head injury may be a primary cause of stroke. Head injury often causes intracranial bleeding, with common sites including intracerebral areas, especially the inferior frontal and temporal lobes, and the subarachnoid, subdural, and epidural spaces (see figure 10.2). Another cause of stroke associated with intracerebral hemorrhage in young adults is drug abuse, specifically of designer drugs such as amphetamine, cocaine, and ecstasy.[87] In such cases, evaluation may be hindered when a cause is not readily apparent. A thorough clinical history obtained from the athlete or especially close friends and acquaintances is vital.

Signs and Symptoms

Health care providers working with physically active people must recognize the signs and symptoms of a possible stroke, and they should not rule it out simply because of the patient's age or fitness level. Speedy identification and access to medical care improve stroke recovery. The American Heart Association has a simple mnemonic for quickly recognizing a suspected stroke.[86,93] The mnemonic is Act FAST, but other organizations have added to the mnemonic with **BE-FAST**:[93]

B Balance: Assess for sudden balance loss.

E Eyes: Ask about sudden vision loss (may be unilateral).

F Face: Ask the person to smile. Does one side of the face droop?

A Arms: Ask the person to raise both arms. Does one arm drift downward?

S Speech: Ask the person to repeat a phrase. Is their speech slurred or strange?

T Time: Time is of the essence. If any of these signs are observed, call the emergency medical service (9-1-1).

Knowledge of the cranial nerves and their functions is also helpful in determining the extent of neurological involvement. Awareness of Brodmann's areas of the brain is very helpful in diagnosing where a problem may lie (see figure 10.4).

In the athletic setting, a differential diagnosis for stroke may include epileptic seizure with postictal Todd's

RED FLAGS FOR STROKE

Signs and symptoms of a possible stroke include sudden occurrence of the following:

- Numbness or weakness of the face, arm, or leg, especially on one side of the body
- Confusion, trouble speaking or understanding
- Vision difficulties in one or both eyes
- Problem with speaking, slurred speech
- Trouble walking, dizziness, loss of balance or coordination
- Severe headache with no known cause

paresis, a focal weakness after generalized or focal motor seizures that is uncommon in persistence for more than a few hours. Other differential diagnoses include tumor, migraine, metabolic encephalopathy caused by fever or infection, hyperglycemia, or hypercalcemia.[94] In addition, drug interactions, overdose, or substance abuse should not be overlooked.

Referral and Diagnostic Tests

A stroke is a medical emergency. Emergency treatment is crucial because every minute lost between symptom onset and emergency contact limits the window of opportunity for intervention. Many patients do not go to the emergency department until 24 h or more after symptom onset. The longer the delay, the greater the damage and loss of potential for recovery.

Diagnosis requires a complete medical history, physical and neurological examinations, complete blood count (CBC) including electrolyte levels, and a battery of specific diagnostic tests. These tests fall into four categories: (1) imaging tests, including CT and MRI scans; (2) **electroencephalogram (EEG)** and evoked potentials testing to record electrical activity and sensory response patterns; (3) Doppler blood flow studies to reveal the patency of the arteries at the base of the skull or in the neck; and (4) arteriography, in which dye is injected into the vessels, combined with radiography to reveal blood flow through the vessels in the brain and to show the size and location of any blockages.[95]

Treatment and Return to Participation

Acute treatment is designed to reverse or lessen the amount of tissue death. The goal is to stabilize the patient, perform imaging, and complete laboratory studies within 60 min of stroke onset.[96] Doing so involves medical support to optimize tissue perfusion and to prevent complications such as infection, deep vein thrombosis, and pulmonary embolism. Administration of pharmaceutical agents through intravenous or intraarterial lines may be combined with anticoagulant and antiplatelet agents, heparin or aspirin, and possibly hypothermia to mitigate cell destruction secondary to ischemia.[96]

Poststroke rehabilitation starts in the hospital as soon as possible. Stable patients can begin rehabilitation within 2 d after the stroke has occurred and continue as necessary after hospital discharge. The choice of rehabilitation options after stroke depends on tissue damage and severity and includes the following:

- Rehabilitation unit in the hospital
- Subacute care unit
- Rehabilitation hospital
- Home therapy
- Home with outpatient therapy
- Occupational therapy
- Speech–language therapy

The goal of rehabilitation is to improve function so that the stroke survivor can continue an independent lifestyle. Such training must be accomplished in a way that preserves dignity and motivates the patient to relearn basic skills for the activities of daily living that may have been lost, including communicating, eating, dressing, and walking.

It is not fully understood how the brain compensates for the damage caused by stroke. A slight interruption in the flow of oxygenated blood may damage a few brain cells temporarily that later resume functioning. In some cases, because different areas of the brain overlap in function, the brain can reorganize, with one area taking over for the area damaged by the stroke. Because of this organ fluidity, stroke survivors sometimes experience a remarkable and unanticipated recovery.

For the athlete, return to full athletic participation after stroke depends primarily on recovery level and residual impairment as well as the type of sport (i.e., contact or collision sports versus noncontact sports). An athlete who has incurred a stroke as a result of a head injury may be ruled medically ineligible to participate even when recovery is complete. Any athlete who has sustained a stroke related to a medical issue that could be exacerbated by activity should refrain from dangerous activity in the future. Further, the risk of additional injury may be too great to continue participation in sports such as hockey, football, or lacrosse.

Regarding participation in physical activity and exercise, studies have documented the positive effects of physical training on the recovery and rehabilitation process after stroke. In addition to the obvious physical benefits of a training and reconditioning program, a return to physical activity may also boost the athlete's psychological recovery. Activity intensity, duration, and volume are best chosen with guidance from the medical team and the athletic trainer supervising the athlete's recovery. A systematic review reported that stroke survivors expend more energy during walking than healthy people.[97] The take-home message is that typical low-intensity exercises may become moderate-level exercises after stroke, and the focus should be on patient efforts.[97,98] Recovery is generally slow and tedious and may take many months.

Prevention

Stroke prevention has two major components: lifestyle risk factors and trauma prevention factors. Lifestyle risk factors such as obesity, diabetes, hypertension, and smoking may not be issues for physically active people, but athletes should understand their significance for cerebrovascular disease later in life. In 2022, the CDC reported that stroke is the fifth leading cause of fatalities in the United States, following heart disease, cancer, COVID-19, and accidents.[99]

Hypertension in the athlete cannot be underestimated as a risk factor for stroke. Athletes who are hypertensive during the PPE should have serial blood pressures taken before and after exercise for several weeks to see whether the high readings continue. If blood pressures continue to be hypertensive, the athlete needs to be referred to a physician for further evaluation and possible medications.

Trauma protection is key in stroke prevention for athletes involved in collision sports, and this may include proper helmet fitting and compliance. Stroke caused by intracranial hemorrhage from head trauma is considered one of the most severe sequelae.

The American Heart Association suggests stroke prevention strategies such as increasing physical activity and consuming a diet high in fruits, vegetables, and whole grains and low in saturated fat. Moderate consumption of alcohol (e.g., one or two glasses of red wine a day) may lower stroke risk, but the negative effects of alcohol may negate the positive. The once-popular daily dose of aspirin to thin the blood also has negative consequences for the gastrointestinal system.[100]

Paroxysmal Disorders

Paroxysmal disorders are neurological conditions that have symptoms that come and go and are episodic in nature. Typically, these conditions go away on their own, only to return without warning. Examples of paroxysmal disorders discussed here are headaches, seizures, and vertigo.

Headaches

The International Classification of Headache Disorders identifies more than 150 varieties of headache divided into two categories: primary and secondary. Primary headaches are unconnected to any other underlying medical condition.[101] Examples of primary headaches are migraine, cluster, and tension headaches. Secondary headaches are symptoms of underlying sequelae, such as fever, hypoglycemia, hyperglycemia, stress, infection, allergy, hypertension, head trauma, tumors, emotional distress, sinus infection, and nerve disorders.[101] In general, headaches can serve as indicators of potentially critical underlying conditions. A migraine complex is a recurrent neurological disorder that is often associated with a trigger that predisposes the individual to migraine (see the Precipitating Factors for Migraine sidebar).[102] The disorder presents with an increasingly moderate to severe headache and can be accompanied by sensory manifestations.[103]

Migraine onset usually occurs during puberty or in the second to third decade of life (i.e., age 10-40 yr), with a familial occurrence of 50%.[104] Women tend to experience migraine more often than men, and migraine may partially or completely remit after age 50 yr. For many women, symptoms worsen with the use of oral contraceptives or vasodilatory medications, and they improve in both frequency and intensity after menopause. Symptoms also appear to worsen during the spring months, when pollen is higher.

Approximately 5% of children experience migraine during the grade school years, and this rate increases to 20% of adolescents during high school.[105] A strong female predominance is also evident in this age group. Onset of migraine with aura usually occurs around age 5 yr in boys and between ages 12 and 13 yr in girls; onset of migraine without aura peaks at ages 10 to 11 yr in boys and between ages 14 to 17 yr in girls.[102] A study conducted with nearly 800 NCAA Division I basketball athletes concluded that although women had an increased prevalence of migraine, these athletes in general had a lower incidence of migraine than did the general population.[103,106] A systematic review of 40 publications related to university students (n = 19,162) and migraine presence demonstrated that migraine incidence in university students is increasing and has associated negative consequences, including missed academic time.[103]

Some preventive strategies for younger athletes include eating regularly, avoiding skipping meals, getting adequate sleep by keeping a regular sleep schedule, and being aware of potential triggers such as particular foods. Other contributing factors are excessive exercise or physical activity, specific exercise regimens, physical or emotional stress, screen time (television, phone, or tablet), and an erratic or hectic schedule.

Signs and Symptoms

Secondary headaches attributable to underlying conditions usually have a rapid onset and present with unilateral throbbing pain in the frontal or temporal area. The headaches may occur in an episodic pattern and often last for hours as opposed to days. Conversely, migraines tend to start in the morning, peak about 2 h later, and resolve after 1 d, although they can recur daily. Cluster headaches, so named because they present as groups of headaches, are usually unilateral and on the face (orbital, supraorbital, temporal), last 15 min to 2.5 h, and can occur up to eight times a day.[107] Cluster headaches have been attributed to pathologies of the face, conjunctivitis, nasal congestion, ptosis, face edema, and rhinorrhea.[107] Another common secondary headache is the tension headache, named after the episodic condition, often triggered by stress.[107] This headache is bilateral, self-limiting, and most often attributed to continuous contraction of the scalp and neck muscles. Figure 10.15 demonstrates the typical anatomical location of pain related to specific types of headaches.

A migraine diagnosis is based largely on presenting symptoms. The classic migraine begins with an aura and is accompanied by extreme sensitivity to sound and light.[101,102] The aura may consist of visual disturbances, usually unilateral, such as scotomas (areas of darkness in the visual field), flashes of light, and bright-colored or white objects. These phenomena commonly last for 20 min and usually resolve before any pain or intense throbbing begins. Migraines generally last for days as opposed to hours, with associated symptoms including nausea, vomiting, diarrhea, weight gain, dizziness, and a prodromal period of endocrine dysfunction resulting in fluid retention. In addition, photophobia often accompanies these headaches.

Other types of migraine are associated with neurological deficits, such as the basilar artery migraine and the hemiplegic or ophthalmoplegic migraine. The basilar artery migraine is common in young women, occurring before their menstrual period. Symptoms last for minutes to hours and may include facial or finger paresthesias, vertigo, ataxia, dysarthria, and tinnitus. The hemiplegic or ophthalmoplegic migraine is more common in young adults and can present in two ways. One condition involves extraocular muscle palsies (CN III) and ptosis, which may become permanent in recurrent cases. The other involves hemiplegia and hemiparesis that can persist even after the headache resolves.

There are several differential diagnoses for migraine, including headache associated with a head injury; facial pain, such as temporomandibular joint pain, sinus headache, cluster headache, or trigeminal neuralgia; systemic conditions, including hypertension or infection whether viral, sinus, or influenza; side effects from medications, such as mood-altering substances, antidepressants, analgesics, antibiotics, antihypertensives, caffeine (or lack thereof if used habitually), steroids, or nicotine; and environmental factors, including high altitude, hypercapnia, and hyperthermia. Headaches associated with hunger are also possible in the athlete who comes to practice without adequate caloric intake.

Sinus	**Cluster**	**Tension**	**Migraine**
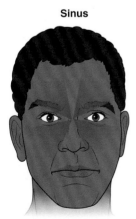	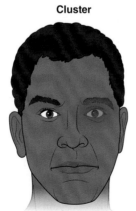	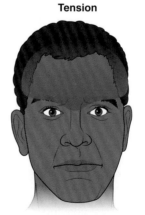	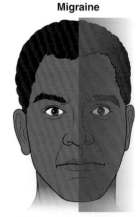
Pain is usually behind the forehead or cheekbones	Pain is in and around one eye	Pain is like a band squeezing the head	Pain, nausea, and visual changes are typical of classic form

FIGURE 10.15 Location of pain in the head for certain types of headaches.

Precipitating Factors for Migraine

Endocrine changes

    Premenstrual

    Menstrual

    Oral contraceptive pills

    Pregnancy

    Puberty

    Menopause

    Hyperthyroidism

Metabolic changes

    Fever

    Anemia

Rhinitis

Change in temperature or altitude

Change in activity

Alcohol, especially red wine

Foods

    Chocolate

    Cheese

    Hot dogs

    Nuts

Drugs

    Nitroglycerin

    Nitrates

    Indomethacin

Blood pressure changes

Sleep, too much or too little

Referral and Diagnostic Tests

A detailed and thorough clinical history helps to differentiate migraine from other types of headache. Merely recognizing the key presenting symptoms of vascular headaches can help to exclude tension headaches. The location of pain may also indicate the headache type (see figure 10.15).

Physical examination assesses commonly affected cranial nerves by testing visual acuity and visual fields, pupil reaction, extraocular muscle movements, and facial symmetry. A physician may also order a CBC, a biochemistry profile, skull and cervical spine radiographs, a CT scan or an MRI scan of the brain, an EEG, or a lumbar puncture. In addition, treatment responses can help pinpoint the diagnosis.[102,105,108] For instance, tension headaches caused by muscle contraction tend to respond positively to traditional nonsteroidal anti-inflammatory drugs (NSAIDs), whereas migraines generally do not.

It is important to distinguish whether a patient's headache is associated with exercise. These types of headaches include exercise-induced migraine, benign exertional headache (also referred to as *weightlifter's cephalgia*), and vascular headache resulting from prolonged exercise. All three of these headaches are classified as vascular but have definite distinguishing factors.

An effort- or exercise-induced migraine is a unilateral retroorbital headache that presents with a visual aura and is more prominent at the end of activity. The symptoms are more likely in hot weather and accompany dehydration. In benign exertional headache, the symptoms are bilateral, have rapid onset and short duration, and occur at the beginning of activity. They are often associated with the increased intrathecal pressure associated with

lifting weights with a closed glottis. Exertional headaches generally decrease in frequency over time. It is critically important that a physician evaluate patients with this type of headache because 10% will have associated intracranial pathology, such as arteriovenous malformation, Arnold-Chiari malformation, subdural hematoma, brain tumor, aneurysm, or basilar impression.[108] The vascular headache with prolonged activity presents true to its name and may last for up to 24 h after exercise. It may also have associated transient or persistent neurological deficits depending on the presence and severity of cerebral ischemia.[108]

The health care provider also needs to recognize the features of headaches associated with intracranial hemorrhage and head trauma for on-the-field evaluation of the athlete. Headaches associated with intracranial hemorrhage usually present with more severe neurological signs, especially involving altered levels of consciousness, than those associated with exertion or dehydration.

After head trauma, two headaches of special concern include posttraumatic migraine and **dysautonomic cephalgia**. Posttraumatic migraine is common in soccer players secondary to heading a ball. This headache presents as a classic migraine with prominent visual symptoms and usually has a cervical muscle–associated headache component. Dysautonomic cephalgia occurs with trauma to the anterior triangle of the neck and causes injury to the sympathetic nerve fibers near the carotid artery. Sympathetic nerve injury results in autonomic dysfunction presenting as Horner's syndrome, often with ptosis, hyperhidrosis, and a unilateral headache.

In addition, athletes with headache should always be referred for medical evaluation if there is a history of head trauma or loss of consciousness, signs of a postconcussion syndrome, or an exertional headache.[108,109] General headache symptoms that warrant further evaluation by a physician are the following:

- New or unusual headache
- Sudden onset of severe headache
- Change in the pattern of a headache
- Chronic headache with localized pain
- Headache that interrupts sleep during the night or in the early morning
- Headache that worsens over days
- Headache with severe nausea and vomiting leading to dehydration
- Visual disturbances
- Numbness, paralysis, or weakness of one side of the face or body
- Headache with associated stiff neck or meningeal signs
- Systemic symptoms, such as fever or weight loss
- Neurological symptoms
- Local extracranial symptoms

Treatment and Return to Participation

Treatment for migraine includes identifying the cause and appropriately treating the mechanism. The U.S. Food and Drug Administration (FDA) has approved a preventive medication, erenumab (Aimovig), for adults that works by blocking one peptide responsible for migraine. Another FDA-approved medication, lasmiditan (Reyvow), has been effective for short-term treatment. Some medications used to treat other conditions, such as epilepsy, depression, and hypertension, have demonstrated effectiveness for migraine as well.[105] Coenzyme Q_{10}, magnesium, riboflavin, and vitamin B_{12} are also being investigated as possible treatments.[105] Health care providers need to help the athlete learn to recognize the precursors of an episode and how to avoid them.

People with migraines may be discouraged from specific athletic activities, such as scuba diving, where the diving environment itself can induce migraines that are often of increased severity. Typical stresses experienced in the diving environment include anxiety, associated sinus barotrauma, cold exposure, and possible saltwater aspiration.

Prevention

The key prevention strategy for headaches is to identify and avoid precipitating factors, such as stress, smoking, sleep deprivation, red wine, chocolate, and tyramine-containing cheeses.[94,102,104] In addition, it is important to maintain good control of blood pressure and monitor medication side effects. Supportive psychotherapy can also assist in headache prevention by teaching techniques to reduce and relieve stress and tension. Regular exercise, healthy diet, adequate hydration, and quality sleep are all important for the athletic population and are also known prohibitors for migraine.[105]

Two preventive treatment protocols are specific to exercise-related headaches. Exercise-induced migraines brought on because of effort may be prevented by a graded warm-up period before exercise, which primes the sympathetic nervous system. In addition, avoiding training in hot weather and ensuring adequate hydration may also reduce the occurrence of these migraines. Rarely, in cases of severe unrelenting headache, the offending activity must be significantly reduced or discontinued.[110] Benign exertional headache is generally successfully treated with NSAIDs, neck massage, and hydration, and it may be prevented by the administration of acetaminophen or ibuprofen before exercise.[105,108,111]

Simple treatment options for migraine include placing the patient in a quiet, dark room and encouraging sleep, which will often neutralize the headache. Pharmacological treatment is often necessary. Medical therapy for migraine consists of two classes of drugs: abortive and preventive medications.

Seizure Disorder and Epilepsy

A seizure is caused by abnormal discharges of electrical activity in the brain, and it may arise from several pathologies. The outward manifestation of a seizure is altered awareness and, often, involuntary movements and convulsions. Seizures may occur because of brain injury or insult, heatstroke, hypoglycemia (low blood sugar), hyponatremia (too little salt in the blood as a result of overhydration), alcohol consumption, drug withdrawal, meningitis, encephalitis, drug interaction, or fever. Febrile seizures can occur in children younger than age 6 yr with a body temperature greater than 39 °C (102.2 °F). Complex febrile seizures last longer than 15 min or occur in a series; these require medical attention. There can be a relationship between childhood febrile seizures and epilepsy. Risk factors for epilepsy increase with family history, developmental delay, complex seizures, and neurological abnormalities.[112] The most common chronic seizure disorder is epilepsy, which is discussed next.

Although an estimated 10% to 30% of people will have a seizure at some point, epilepsy is a chronic condition that consists of unprovoked, randomly recurring seizures and occurs in approximately 3% of the population.[112] The diagnosis of epilepsy is based on the occurrence of more than two seizures; therefore, single-seizure episodes during a person's lifetime, including infantile febrile seizures, do not meet the clinical definition. The International League Against Epilepsy (ILAE) has classified epileptic seizures as (1) *focal-onset seizures* (the current term for the once called *partial seizure*) and (2) *generalized-onset seizures*, with the former originating in the focal area of the cerebral cortex and the latter in both cerebral hemispheres.[112]

As stated previously, a seizure is abnormal electrical activity in the brain that can cause involuntary systemic convulsions, depending on the area of brain involvement. There are many underlying causes of seizures, although more than one-half of cases are idiopathic.[113] The etiology is presumed to be some form of inherited neuronal abnormality. In general, most idiopathic seizures develop between the ages of 2 and 14 yr. Other seizures occurring in children younger than 2 yr are usually related to developmental defects, birth trauma, or metabolic diseases of the brain. In people older than age 25 yr, the etiology is usually identified.[112] In addition to those listed previously, some identifiable causes of seizure include recent or old brain injury, brain tumor, stroke, infection, metabolic disturbances, inherited disorders, sleep deprivation, and extreme emotional and physical stress.

Absence seizures (also termed *petit mal seizures*) are another type of generalized seizure, and they are characterized by brief episodes of loss of attention or awareness lasting between 3 and 15 s without aura or a postictal state. They are most common in children and are not usually a lifelong condition, but they tend to be genetically linked with family members with epilepsy.[114] Associated automatisms may include chewing, lip smacking, swallowing, or facial twitching. As many as 15 other types of generalized seizures occur, including myoclonic seizures and febrile seizures.

Exercise-induced seizures occur very infrequently and present during or immediately after exercise. In sports of prolonged activity, such as marathons and triathlons, the underlying cause may be metabolic imbalance (e.g., hyponatremia), as opposed to the exercise itself, or may be attributable to the exercise as in exertional heat-stroke.[115] Outside of the history and physical examination, an EEG performed during exercise is the best diagnostic approach for seizures that occur during or immediately after activity.

Signs and Symptoms

Seizures result in activity that can affect the level of consciousness and/or manifest as motor activity, sensory phenomena, psychic disturbances, or inappropriate behavior.

Generalized seizures involve electrical activity in both cerebral hemispheres. These types of seizures may have bilateral cerebral hemisphere involvement from the onset, or they may evolve from a focal seizure to involve both cerebral hemispheres. Generalized seizures are further classified as **tonic–clonic seizures**, such as those seen in intermittent or status epilepticus, absence seizures, or any of a variety of less common seizures. Intermittent tonic–clonic seizures are among the most common types. They are associated with the following: an aura of smells or sounds that alert the person to impending seizure; tongue biting caused by uncontrolled muscle contraction; incontinence; and a postictal state of disorientation, confusion, exhaustion, or lethargy. The postictal state is a 5 to 30 min period of altered consciousness resulting from an epileptic seizure.[95] These seizures are generally of short duration and are self-limited, at times requiring no medication. Continuous tonic–clonic seizures are called *status epilepticus* and are medical emergencies. These are defined as continuous tonic–clonic convulsions lasting more than 30 min or recurrent tonic–clonic convulsions without regaining consciousness between attacks. These seizures require immediate intervention with monitoring and support of the airway, breathing, and circulation and prompt administration of medications to abort the continued pattern.

A focal seizure starts with a localized presentation of a motor, sensory, autonomic, or psychic disturbance that manifests based on the area of its origin in one cerebral hemisphere. Examples of these disturbances include the following:

- Involuntary motor activity of the face, limbs, or head
- Somatosensory symptoms of tingling, numbness, or pins and needles
- Special sensory phenomena, such as visual, auditory, olfactory, or **gustatory hallucinations**
- Autonomic dysfunction, including diaphoresis (sweating) and flushing
- Psychic phenomena, such as feelings of **déjà vu, jamais vu**, paranoia, or fear

In simple focal seizures, consciousness is not impaired, and the manifestations are usually restricted to one anatomical area on only one side of the body. In complex focal seizures, consciousness is impaired, and this impairment may occur alone or in association with integrated purposeful movements or experiences such as automatisms or psychic disturbances. Automatisms may be simple, such as chewing, lip smacking, and swallowing, or complex, such as walking into a room or getting dressed. Both types of focal seizures can evolve into generalized seizures. There are also obvious focal seizures that cannot be further differentiated as simple or complex, and these account for approximately 7% of all seizures.[112]

Clinical Tips

The Fencing Response

Since the early 2000s, a visible sign following SRC has been widely documented via social media and news outlets. The *fencing response* is an acute seizure-like event that is manifested by a tonic extension of one arm and flexion of the contralateral arm. This posturing is initiated on impact to the head and is sustained for several seconds. Athletes who are hit in the head and exhibit the fencing response require medical attention, as this sign is indicative of a moderate brain injury with involvement of the brainstem.[148,149]

Convulsive activity caused by seizures must be differentiated from that prompted by other disorders, such as concussive convulsions and convulsive syncope. Concussive convulsions are brief periods of tonic posturing that are expressions of the concussion event. They are benign and require no specific treatment outside of that for the underlying concussion.[116] Convulsive syncope involves generalized convulsive movements, tongue biting, and incontinence during a syncopal or fainting event. Both entities involve convulsive movements related to reflex phenomena rather than abnormal cerebral electrical activity.

Referral and Diagnostic Tests

Any patient who experiences a seizure, whether of new or established onset, needs to be referred for neurological assessment to ensure appropriate diagnosis and management in new cases and to review medical management for effective control in established cases. Also, any athlete with a syncopal event needs to be referred for medical examination.

General evaluation of a patient with a seizure disorder involves a detailed medical history, including occurrences and precipitating factors, and a physical examination thoroughly reviewing the neurological system. Laboratory tests include a CBC, chemistry panel, and urinalysis. Prolactin levels are determined immediately after the event to determine the etiology (epileptic versus nonepileptic). Neurological testing may include an EEG, an MRI scan, or a CT of the brain as well as lumbar puncture in cases of suspected infection and possibly a positron emission tomography scan. CSF is evaluated if meningitis or encephalitis is suspected.[112]

Treatment and Return to Participation

Acute management includes protecting the patient from further harm by ensuring that all dangerous objects are out of the way during the seizure. This includes moving desks, chairs, and anything the patient may hit while seizing. It is neither necessary nor indicated to restrain someone undergoing a seizure. After a seizure, the patient is placed in the recovery position, on their left side with their head resting on their left arm (figure 10.16).

Although it has been reported that 25% to 30% of patients with seizure activity do not respond to anticonvulsant medications, they are still the best option for seizure management.[117,118] There are no pharmaceuticals that can cure epilepsy, but management of symptoms is possible. Medical control of epilepsy follows some general guidelines. Initially, a single medication is used to control the seizures. A second agent is added only when the maximal dosage of the first is attained, when side effects or toxicity limit further dosage increases, or

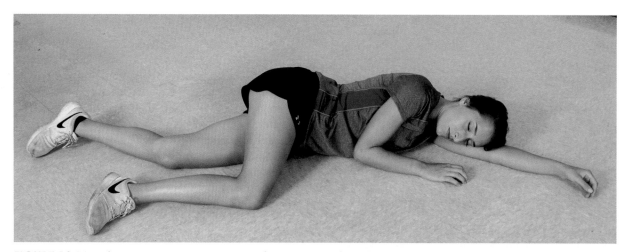

FIGURE 10.16   The correct recovery position for a person after a seizure.

when adequate seizure control is not attained with a single agent. Most medications prescribed for treating seizure activity have adverse effects. Additionally, two robust studies determined that only 64% of newly diagnosed patients with epilepsy are seizure free following a year of medication use.[112] The practitioner and the patient must weigh the benefits of a medication against its potential negative effects. It is important to monitor the serum levels of medications and the blood chemistry they may affect. Another consideration for treatment of epilepsy is the management of the disorder in older adults. Typically, senior adults have concomitant diseases and are prescribed medications for other afflictions. Antiepileptic agents tend to metabolize other drugs; therefore, patients must work closely with their physicians and pharmacists to ensure that no drug interactions will interfere with the seizure medications.[119]

Other medical treatments include implantable neurostimulation for patients with drug-resistant epilepsy and surgical intervention to the area of the brain most affected. Epilepsy surgery has shown promise but depends on the patient, type of epilepsy, and response to pharmacological treatment.[112]

The health care provider must also assess and treat underlying complications that can occur during seizures, such as fractures, dislocations, and head and neck injuries.

For patients with epilepsy, participation in sports or physical activity depends on the type of sport, risk of injury, and presence of preexisting neurological injury or dysfunction. The following criteria must be carefully considered before an athlete with epilepsy returns to participation:

- Sport type: collision, contact, or noncontact
- Risk of severe injury or death if seizure occurs during the activity
- Preexisting brain injury and neurological dysfunction
- Risk of traumatic brain injury from athletic participation
- Seizure control: frequency, association with exercise, medications
- Effects of medications on performance: sedation and impaired judgment

The ILAE seeks to create common classifications and language to effectively communicate about epilepsy's many facets. The ILAE Task Force on Sports and Epilepsy offers guidance in sports participation by dividing sports into three categories:[120]

- Group 1: sports with no significant additional risk. Examples include bowling, wrestling, judo, baseball, basketball, football, volleyball, and cross country.

- Group 2: sports with moderate risk to the person with epilepsy, but with no risk to bystanders. Examples include alpine skiing, pole vaulting, boxing, karate, cycling, gymnastics, horse show jumping, ice hockey, skateboarding, and snowboarding.

- Group 3: sports with major risks. Examples include aviation, climbing, diving, motor sports, parachuting, rodeo, scuba diving, and other such activities.

Each group has criteria regarding seizure activity that must be met for an individual to "qualify" for the sport. High-risk sports, including platform or springboard diving, parachuting, rock climbing, scuba diving, rodeo, surfing, and motor sports, should be avoided.[120] The medical team supporting the athlete, including the physician responsible for monitoring and treating the patient's epilepsy, should use evidence and jointly decide the sport or sports in which the athlete may participate.[121,122]

Return-to-participation guidance is approached with caution and on an individual basis. One factor to consider is the athlete's ability to commute to practices and events; people with epilepsy commonly need to prove stable seizure management before they can obtain or reinstate a driver's license. A person with epilepsy must meet certain additional legal obligations when operating a motor vehicle. The athlete and, as appropriate, their parents are alerted to this requirement. It is reported that there are more than 700,000 licensed drivers with epilepsy, and that all U.S. states permit people with epilepsy to drive.[123] The actual reporting of epilepsy to an appropriate governing authority varies from state to state, and guidelines are available from the websites of the National Institutes of Health, the Epilepsy Foundation, and local driver's license centers. More stringent legal requirements exist for commercial licensing because the U.S. Department of Transportation has made it illegal to license anyone with a history of epilepsy for interstate trucking. Criteria for other professions, such as air traffic controllers, border patrol agents, Federal Bureau of Investigation agents, law enforcement officers, firefighters, pilots, U.S. Postal Service mail carriers, and medical personnel, are also addressed on the Epilepsy Foundation website.[124]

The main approach to preventing epileptic seizures is to avoid or promptly treat precipitating factors.

Vertigo

Vertigo is defined as a sensation of instability, loss of equilibrium, or rotation usually caused by a disturbance in the semicircular canals of the inner ear or vestibular nuclei of the brainstem.[125] Vertigo is described as either central or peripheral. *Central vertigo* arises when the cause of vertigo is a result of brain or spinal cord anomaly; *peripheral vertigo* is attributable to problems with the inner ear.[126] Vertigo associated with hearing loss is referred to as *sudden sensorineural hearing loss* and is uncommon. The most common variety of vertigo falls under the peripheral category because it is associated with ailments of the inner ear. It is termed *benign paroxysmal positional vertigo* (BPPV) and is the focus here. BPPV is a brief sensation of spinning accompanied by nystagmus. It usually lasts less than a minute, but it can continue episodically up to 4 wk.[95,126,127] Typically, in BPPV, hearing is not affected. Dizziness should not be confused with vertigo, as dizziness comprises lightheadedness or unsteadiness, whereas vertigo involves sensations of spinning.[125,127]

Signs and Symptoms

Clinically, *subjective vertigo* is when one feels the body is spinning in space; *objective vertigo* is when one feels everything is spinning about the body.[125] Both are common in BPPV. BPPV is precipitated by changes in head position with respect to gravity, tends to affect women more than men, and has a peak onset between ages 50 and 60 yr.[127] The motion sensation can be so severe that the patient is temporarily debilitated. Nausea, vomiting, dizziness, and nystagmus are not unusual. It should be noted that patients with BPPV do not typically feel vertigo all the time, and severe attacks are triggered by motion of the head. Persistent vertigo should be investigated as a pathophysiology other than BPPV.[127]

Differential diagnoses for vertigo are many and varied. Stroke, Ménière's disease, migraine, otitis media with effusion, vestibular neuritis, tumor, hypoglycemia, alcohol intoxication, fatigue, and dehydration can all present with dizziness, which some confuse with vertigo or true vertigo.[94] Vertebral artery insufficiency is also a known cause of vertigo.[127] Certain medications acting alone, or in combination with alcohol, can elicit vertigo-like sensations. Idiopathic pathology and ear diseases comprise 68% of cases.[127] A complete medical history is critical, including medication review. Acute head trauma can also present with vertigo symptoms.

Referral and Diagnostic Tests

Unrelenting or recurring vertigo should be referred to a neurologist or otolaryngologist for specialized evaluation to include ruling out BPPV. Research has failed to find a correlation with low vitamin D levels and BPPV but did find significant evidence that patients with recurrent episodes of BPPV had low vitamin D levels,[128] and osteopenia is related to residual dizziness of patients with BPPV.[129] Therefore, assessment of serum vitamin D and bone density may be indicated. A thorough neurological examination is performed, which should include assessment for uncontrollable lateral eye movement, or nystagmus.

An otoscope is used to evaluate the tympanic membrane for swelling or effusion. If hearing loss is suspected, an audiometry test may be ordered. Depending on the findings, the health care provider may perform a "roll" or a Dix-Hallpike test, which involves rapid repositioning of the patient to re-create symptoms or nystagmus.[126,27] An MRI scan or a CT scan may be ordered to rule out central causes of vertigo. Of patients presenting with vertigo, 39% have no known etiology.[127]

Treatment and Return to Participation

BPPV usually resolves spontaneously, but intermittent treatments can retard symptoms.[104] Several physical maneuvers mitigate the spinning sensation. The most well-known and widely used first-line treatment is the Epley or canalith (crystal)–repositioning maneuver, in which specific head movements are performed to loosen the canaliths in the semicircular canals of the inner ear; this is reported to be 90% effective.[127,130] Initially, these movements may worsen vertigo, and they should first be performed by an experienced health care provider, athletic trainer, or physical therapist.[130,131] Contraindications for the canalith-repositioning maneuver include cervical pathologies and recent retinal detachment. There are also many head and eye exercises that the patient can perform to decrease symptoms. Watchful waiting has also been utilized, as BPPV is benign and typically resolves untreated over time.[127] Medications, if prescribed, include antinausea agents and benzodiazepines such as diazepam (Valium). Both medication classes have side effects that include significant drowsiness, and they are not recommended if the athlete wishes to participate in sport.

Caution should be exercised when determining the patient's ability to operate machinery and to physically train. Sports with rotational components, such as swimming, diving, wrestling, gymnastics, and cheerleading, should be considered off-limits until the patient's symptoms are fully resolved. Sports that involve rotating head motions, such as volleyball and tennis, where the athlete is constantly moving and looking up to follow the ball at every play, can exacerbate BPPV symptoms. Patients who report vertigo to the point of falling should not be allowed to participate in activities where they can sustain more harm.

Neuromuscular Disorders

Neuromuscular disorders are conditions that affect voluntary muscle via the nerves that control them. Muscles that do not receive adequate nerve impulses atrophy and become useless. The neuromuscular condition discussed here is ALS; multiple sclerosis is discussed in chapter 13. Both conditions strike healthy people with little warning, and both have serious sequelae.

Amyotrophic Lateral Sclerosis

ALS is also known as *Lou Gehrig's disease*, named after the famous New York Yankee baseball player who developed the disease at age 36 yr and succumbed to it in 1941. This fatal, progressive neurological disease slowly attacks neurons responsible for voluntary muscular actions. Both upper and lower neurons are affected, as they progressively degenerate and die. Without input from neurons, muscles begin to atrophy, leading to complete loss of all voluntary muscular movement. ALS does not affect other senses (sight, smell, taste, or hearing) or cognitive thought. So, patients with ALS are aware of their surroundings but are eventually unable to communicate by voice or to move. As a result of disease progression, patients require a wheelchair for mobility. Neurons of the diaphragm eventually weaken, leading to the need for a respirator to maintain breathing.

Because ALS is not a reportable disease, it is not tracked. There are estimated 25,000 active cases in the United States.[132] ALS onset may occur between adolescence and the late 80s, with a mean age of onset of 65 y.[133] The disease has a heredity component, although it is small (5%-10%). Studies have shown that a mutated enzyme (superoxide dismutase 1, or SOD1) may account for the genetic tendency toward ALS.[134,135] Robust evidence suggests that long-term occupational exposure to lead has a strong association with ALS.[136,137]

Interestingly, an increased incidence of ALS has been observed among veterans of the Gulf War (1990-1991). Deployed veterans had both a greater postwar risk of ALS and significantly more rapid progression than did veterans with ALS who were not deployed to the Gulf War region.[138] Because past deployment to Vietnam was also related to more rapid progression, researchers suggest a war-related environmental trigger for ALS.

The typical patient with ALS survives 3 yr from onset of muscle weakness but approximately 15% survive 5 yr or longer, with an additional 5% surviving 10 yr or more.[133] Researchers are investigating medications and treatment combinations to extend quality of life for patients with ALS. Because no definitive cause of ALS has been identified, there are no prevention strategies available.

Signs and Symptoms

The earliest symptoms of ALS may be attributed to being tired or clumsy, as 75% to 80% of patients report increased stumbling, tripping, or difficulty with small motor functions (e.g., buttoning a shirt, turning a key).[133] Symptoms often begin in one limb—a hand or leg, for example—and patients complain of a gradual awkwardness in motor skills. Difficulty in swallowing (dysphagia) or with speech has also been noted. Because upper motor neurons are involved, spasticity or hyperreflexia and an exaggerated gag reflex may be present. Between 20% and 25% of patients report slurred speech, hoarseness, and choking during meals as initial complaints causing them to seek medical attention.[104,133] Patients report muscular twitching and weakness. Weight loss, fatigue, and difficulty controlling facial expressions or tongue movements are all additional indicators of ALS.[139]

As the disease progresses, muscular atrophy spreads throughout the body. A person's intelligence, memory, and personality are typically not impaired. There are some reports of a small percentage of patients who experience memory loss and difficulty with decision-making. Because most do not experience a loss of cognitive abilities, anxiety and depression are common.

Multiple sclerosis, human immunodeficiency virus (HIV), multifocal motor neuropathy, spinal disc insult, myasthenia gravis, progressive strokes, and certain vitamin deficiencies (e.g., vitamin B_{12}) may all be differential diagnoses of ALS.

Referral and Diagnostic Tests

There is no definitive diagnostic test for ALS. Patients must experience signs and symptoms in both upper and lower motor neurons that cannot be linked to any other cause (table 10.2). To rule out multiple sclerosis and other potential causes of symptoms, physicians may order a brain MRI scan, electromyography (EMG) and **nerve conduction velocity (NCV)** analysis, and blood work to determine whether other diseases or conditions are present. The EMG determines electrical activity in normal muscles; the NCV denotes the speed at which nerve impulses travel to a given muscle.[139] When all

TABLE 10.2 Signs and Symptoms of Upper Versus Lower Motor Neuron Disorders

Feature	Upper lesion	Lower lesion
Reflexes	Increased	Decreased or absent
Atrophy	Absent*	Present
Fasciculations	Absent	Present
Tone	Increased (spastic)	Decreased or absent (flaccid)

*May appear with prolonged limb disuse.

other organic explanations for the symptoms have been dismissed, ALS is considered the culprit.

Treatment and Return to Participation

There are no effective treatments that prevent, stop, or reverse ALS progression, but an FDA-approved drug, riluzole (Rilutke), extends life.[139] Another medication, edaravone (Radicava), is approved to slow functional decline.[133] Riluzole does not relieve symptoms. Although baclofen or diazepam are prescribed to control muscular spasms, trihexyphenidyl or amitriptyline can address dysphagia. Patients with ALS often receive a gastrostomy to facilitate nutritional intake without swallowing. The patient and family should be informed about risks with unproven treatments and clinical trials and whether they should participate in life-extending decisions, such as long-term ventilation or gastrostomy.

Several studies promote a multidisciplinary approach to the care of the patient with ALS.[133,139] Critical components include health care providers who can address both the physical and emotional symptoms of the disease, including end-of-life decisions and care.

Bell's Palsy

Unlike other conditions in this chapter, Bell's palsy typically affects one nerve—the facial cranial nerve (CN VII)—resulting in unilateral or bilateral facial weakness or paralysis. It has a rapid onset and almost always resolves spontaneously. Bell's palsy affects individuals of all ages and both sexes equally, and it occurs most often in people 10 to 45 years old. The etiology of Bell's palsy is most likely secondary to an immune reaction or inflammatory response. Herpes simplex is thought to be the most common trigger.[95] Patients have a quite visible presentation, as their face appears to be distorted and they cannot perform bilateral facial expressions (figure 10.17). Corticosteroids are the treatment of choice. Most patients recover completely within 1 to 8 wk, but some experience permanent contractures. Other complications are blindness, corneal ulcers, and impaired nutrition (e.g., from the inability to chew on one side). Other conditions that could present with facial neuropathies include stroke, Lyme disease, parotid tumor, HIV, syphilis, or trauma.[95]

Rabies

Rabies is a preventable infection of the CNS (a viral encephalitis) acquired from the saliva of infected bats and other mammals. Exposure to saliva from an infected mammal may be through a bite, scratch, mucosa, or contact with the eyes or mouth via aerosol (sprayed) saliva.[140] Although rabies is not common in the United

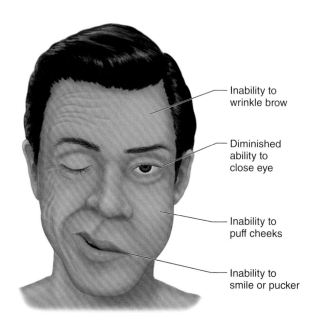

- Inability to wrinkle brow
- Diminished ability to close eye
- Inability to puff cheeks
- Inability to smile or pucker

FIGURE 10.17 Bell's palsy.

States, there are still approximately 15 deaths attributable to the infection annually.[140] The chief culprits are infected bats, raccoons, skunks, and foxes. However, rabies has been found in dogs, cats, ferrets, and several types of rodents, including gerbils, chipmunks, rabbits, groundhogs, and guinea pigs. Smaller rodents (rats, chipmunks, squirrels, mice, rabbits) tend to die of rabies before they can transmit it.[140] Death is almost always certain and occurs within 3 to 10 d after symptom onset. There is an incubation period of 20 to 90 d when the infected person is asymptomatic. After this is a period of 2 to 10 d when the virus enters the CNS and vague symptoms of malaise, headache, fever, anorexia, nausea, insomnia, and pharyngitis may present.[94] Patients who survive are identified early as possibly infected and receive immunoprophylaxis before developing symptoms. As the infection progresses, the patient experiences excessive salivation and encephalitis-related issues (hallucination, confusion, agitation, restlessness). It may be difficult to connect the injury (bite) to the symptoms, given the long incubation period of up to a year.

Pain Disorders

Complex Regional Pain Syndrome

CRPS involves overactivity of the sympathetic nervous system. CRPS can occur after minor injury as a result of trauma to a nerve or, more commonly, a condition of unknown etiology. CRPS type I was at one time termed *reflex sympathetic dystrophy*; it traditionally follows an injury, such as one in which soft tissue is damaged, crushed, or immobilized mechanically or pathologically (a too-tight cast or a frozen shoulder). *CRPS type II* is the current term for the condition causalgia, which is a documented injury to a nerve.[141] Both conditions present with sympathetic nervous system overactivity. The incidence of CRPS I is 21 per 100,000, and that of CRPS II is 4 per 100,000. The condition affects all races but is more common in women.[142] Strains or sprains are the most common cause of CRPS, followed by surgical wounds, fractures, and crush injuries. It is extremely unusual, but some cases have presented following lacerations, burns, electric shock, venipuncture, inflammatory processes, and spinal cord injuries.[143]

Both types of CRPS present with the hallmark symptom of pain out of proportion to the severity of injury. It generally appears posttraumatically with underlying ligament, bone, or nerve injury. The presentation in children is quite different from that in adults. For example, CRPS in adults has a higher incidence of upper extremity involvement, especially the shoulder, compared with a predominance of lower extremity involvement in children and adolescents, where ankle or foot sprains are the likely trigger. CRPS prognosis and treatment outcomes are generally better for children than for adults.

Signs and Symptoms

Patients report regional pain, not specific pinpoint pain or that which follows a dermatome. The onset of CRPS I can begin in a distal extremity in days or weeks following a seemingly benign injury. It is unusual to have an onset months after the original insult. Physical examination can be helpful in the accurate identification of CRPS and may even assist in determining its severity and chronic prognosis. Findings may reveal a warm, swollen joint with reduced and painful range of motion. The overlying skin may be sweaty and erythematous with dense hair growth and accelerated nail growth. These findings may change depending on the stage of CRPS at the time of presentation.[144] Over time, fat atrophy leads to thin, waxy, pale skin, muscle atrophy is prominent, nails become brittle and fractured, muscle spasms ensue, and extremity pain and stiffness progress. At the end stages of CRPS, irreversible changes to the extremity result in a nonfunctional atrophic extremity with joint contractures, lost mobility, and severe pain.

The signs and symptoms of CRPS could be attributed to disuse, owing to either immobilization or cognitive disuse, in which patients avoid using the injured area.[141] CRPS may progress through three distinct phases of deteriorating function: acute within less than 3 mo, dystrophic over 3 to 6 mo, and atrophic after more than 6 mo.[142]

Referral and Diagnostic Tests

In 2021, the International Association for the Study of Pain adapted diagnostic criteria for CRPS.[145]

1. The patient must meet each of the following four criteria:
   - The patient has continuing pain that is disproportionate to any inciting event.
   - The patient must report at least one symptom in three or more of the following categories.
   - The patient displays at least one sign in two or more of the following categories.
   - No other diagnosis can better explain the signs and symptoms.
2. Categories
   - Sensory: Complains of hyperesthesia and/or allodynia (light brush stroke, temperature sensation, deep pressure, and/or joint movement)
   - Vasomotor: Complains of temperature asymmetry, skin color changes, and/or skin color asymmetry
   - Submotor/edema: Complains of edema, sweating changes, and/or asymmetrical sweating
   - Motor/trophic: Complains of decreased range of motion, motor dysfunction (weakness, tremor, dystonia), and/or trophic changes (hair, nail, skin)

Following these criteria, a clinical diagnosis of CRPS has a sensitivity of 0.70 and a specificity of 0.94 for the condition.[144]

Often the best diagnostic tool for identifying and confirming CRPS is the clinical response to a coordinated comprehensive rehabilitation program. It is not uncommon for the therapeutic clinician to initially refer the patient to a physician for further evaluation. As the rehabilitation course progresses, slower recovery than expected is one of the first clues that CRPS may be developing. This finding alone may warrant rereferral to the physician for assessment as to whether early CRPS changes are occurring or whether there are other injuries that were not identified initially.

CRPS is primarily a clinical diagnosis that is made after a thorough medical history and examination and after other, more common conditions that prompt a high level of suspicion have been excluded. A CBC helps to rule out inflammatory pathologies, and EMG studies and/or bone scintigraphy can assist in differentiating CRPS from other pain syndromes, but they are not specific for the condition.[141] Diagnostic tests are generally nonspecific, and there is no one test to confirm the diagnosis

CONDITION HIGHLIGHT

Complex Regional Pain Syndrome

Patients with CRPS usually experience intense, unrelenting pain at a joint. The pain is generally worse with any weight bearing or loading of the affected extremity, and it is relieved by rest and joint immobilization in severe cases. This pain is accompanied by varying degrees of autonomic dysfunction, including vasomotor disturbances or dystrophic changes. In addition, the affected area may exhibit edema, sweating, nerve hypersensitivity (allodynia) in 90% of cases, and dermatographia.

Delayed recovery in the presence of pain disproportionate to the degree of injury, reduced joint motion, or hypersensitivity to touch and movement requires prompt rereferral to the physician for further evaluation for definite CRPS.

Diagnosis of CRPS is often made based on the exclusion of other probable medical conditions. It is vital to rule out other conditions that have a similar clinical presentation as well as underlying conditions that could cause the presenting CRPS. In the latter case, if these conditions are not identified and treated, the CRPS may never resolve or improve. Diagnoses to exclude include Raynaud's phenomenon, systemic lupus erythematosus, polymyositis, gout, myofascial pain syndrome, myositis ossification, compartment syndromes, and thrombophlebitis.[94] Demonstrated underlying causes of CRPS are peripheral nerve entrapment (e.g., carpal tunnel syndrome and tarsal tunnel syndrome), nerve injury caused by laceration or neuroma, ligament sprain or tear, and fracture.[146]

of CRPS. Radiographs taken early may be negative; however, within 2 to 3 mo, patchy juxtaarticular demineralization or osteoporosis may develop. Nuclear bone scans, although not very helpful, can also show changes of increased uptake in the juxtaarticular areas of bones, often involving joints distal to the actual site of injury. Yet again, the expected results will vary depending on the stage of the disorder, with these variations being much more common in children and adolescents.[147] Nerve conduction studies and electromyography are useful in determining only if a nerve is damaged, as it is in CRPS II; they are not helpful in diagnosing CRPS I.[143,147]

Another diagnostic approach tests the function of the sympathetic nervous system compared with the uninvolved side by skin wheal assessment, thermography, and sympathetic nerve blocks. Dermatographia is an abnormally prolonged wheal and erythematous response that can develop in CRPS after lightly scratching the skin of both extremities. An abnormal test result suggests sympathetic nervous system dysfunction. Thermography is often used in pain centers to assist in the diagnosis of CRPS. Because it also depends on the stage and severity of the condition, thermography is often inconsistent, nonspecific, and inconclusive.[95]

A plethora of medications have been used to relieve the pain of CRPS, with mixed reviews. One procedure that can be both therapeutic and diagnostic is a sympathetic anesthetic block. This block may be performed at the cervical level of C6 for upper extremity conditions, at the celiac plexus for upper abdominal area conditions, or at the lumbar level of L2 for lower extremity conditions. Ganglion nerve blocks and intravenous infusions have also been tried with varying responses.[141]

Treatment and Return to Participation

The mainstay in the treatment of CRPS is early motion and pain control. Prompt initiation of a physical rehabilitation program is critical. The goals of rehabilitation for CRPS are to do the following:

- Desensitize the extremity
- Increase joint and extremity range of motion
- Reduce pain
- Effect control of the extremity
- Restore strength and function

Desensitization techniques for hypersensitivity consist of challenging the area with increasingly abrasive

 RED FLAGS FOR COMPLEX REGIONAL PAIN SYNDROME

Signs and symptoms of CRPS include the following:

- Severe burning pain
- Hyperhidrosis
- Pain beyond what would be expected for the injury
- Local edema
- Pathological changes in skin
- Radiographic changes in bone
- Extreme sensitivity to pressure or touch

textured materials and stress loading the affected extremity. Range-of-motion activities are the central focus of rehabilitation, and they may be facilitated by use of ultrasound, transcutaneous electrical nerve stimulation, muscle stimulation, or hydrotherapy. Contrast baths and range-of-motion exercises (figure 10.18) may both help to reduce edema in the extremity. In addition, biofeedback may allow the patient to gain some control over the autonomic nervous system functions of sweating, skin temperature variations, and blood flow.[143,147] Supportive psychotherapy can offer these patients various skills to help them accept, cope with, and treat their pain. Some of these skills include relaxation training, biofeedback, and distraction techniques.[141,147]

A program of range-of-motion activities and stress-loading exercises for the affected joint or extremity amplifies the potential for a good response to treatment. Exercise provides a way to continue desensitizing the affected extremity. For example, in CRPS of the hand, a stress-loading protocol may consist of household chores that include scrubbing a 3 ft square area of floor for 20 min three times daily or lifting and carrying books several times each day. In some cases, the pain recurs during rehabilitation so intensely that a somatic block, such as an epidural block or brachial plexus block, may be necessary to calm the noxious stimuli coming from the muscles and joints in the affected extremity.

Prognosis in CRPS depends on the degree of severity and the progression of the condition. Most changes associated with CRPS are reversible in the early stages of the disease, within the first 4 to 6 mo, but they can become irreversible with time, often after 8 to 9 mo.[142] In most athletes, the condition is identified and treated early because of the limitations that it places on their performance. Athletes will seldom stay quiet for long when they cannot perform in sport. This propensity for early recognition and initiation of treatment in athletes is beneficial to both their recovery potential and their return to participation.

Given that recovery will vary depending on CRPS severity, the nature of the underlying injury, the extremity affected, and the athlete's sport, only general guidelines can be given for return-to-participation schedules. An athlete with CRPS can return to participation in sports when the following occur:

- Affected extremity and joint have full and pain-free range of motion
- Flexibility is symmetrical to that of the unaffected extremity
- Strength is at least 80% of that of the unaffected limb
- Coordinated firing patterns of the supporting muscles and muscular groups have been reestablished

The athlete must be able to perform challenging agility tasks that simulate sport activity with sound biomechanics and appropriate skill. The return to participation can be expedited if the affected extremity is not critical in the performance of the sport. In these cases, modification of the athletic activity may assist in the athlete's return, given adequate protection of the affected extremity.

Special Concerns in the Adolescent Athlete

A high level of suspicion for CRPS in active adolescents is always wise, because they often hide or downplay the symptom severity to return to play sooner or to avoid missing any activity. Precautions also need to be taken in prescribing medications for this age group. The physician and the athletic trainer must persist in encouraging compliance with therapy and maintenance programs in young athletes to ensure their recovery and to prevent chronic limitations, deformities, or disabilities.

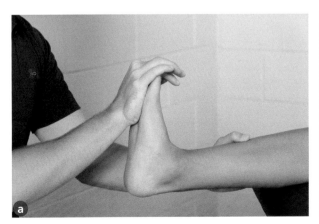
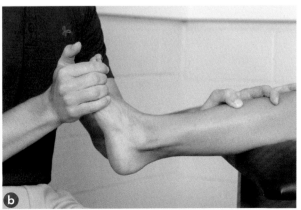

FIGURE 10.18   (a) Maintaining range of motion, shown here as passive dorsiflexion, and (b) training light resistance, shown here as eversion after an injury, are treatments for complex regional pain syndrome (CRPS).

Special Concerns in the Mature Athlete

The major concern with mature athletes is the tendency for stiffness to develop faster and to a greater degree than in younger people. Therefore, prompt initiation of joint and extremity mobilization in these athletes is critical.

Summary

Neurological disorders are alarming in the athletic population because they may be overlooked as symptoms of a benign condition. Without trauma, headaches are not typically a cause for concern in healthy people. This chapter describes conditions ranging from SRC to chronic disabling or fatal diseases, CRPS, epilepsy, and stroke that can all begin with a simple headache.

Two critical points in recognizing neurological disorders are (1) identifying symptoms that may seem benign, such as stumbling or chronic muscular twitching, and (2) understanding that strokes do occur in apparently healthy people. Rehabilitation of seemingly minor injuries that present with exaggerated pain should prompt the health care provider to consider CRPS. Having the knowledge to consider atypical neurological conditions in otherwise healthy athletes is critical to their future health.

Apply It!

Go to HK*Propel* to complete the case studies for this chapter.

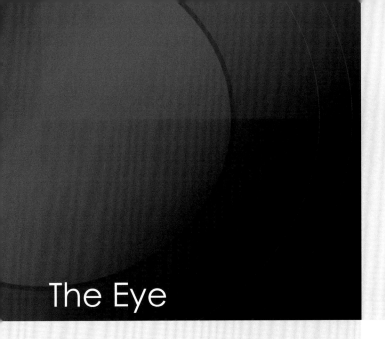

The Eye

OBJECTIVES

At the completion of this chapter the reader should be able to do the following:

1. Describe the basic anatomy and physiology of the eye.

2. Perform a basic eye examination.

3. Describe appropriate initial management of common conditions and injuries of the eye.

4. Recognize conditions of the eye that require referral.

5. Recognize conditions of the eye that may preclude the patient from participation in sport or physical activity.

Acute vision is vital to athletic success, and even minor eye disorders will sideline most individuals. An athletic trainer must understand the basic anatomy and physiology of the eye, be able to perform a basic eye examination, and know the common sport-related eye conditions and injuries for which referral to an eye care specialist is appropriate. This chapter discusses the structures of the eye, examination techniques for both healthy and injured eyes, and the pathological eye conditions that many athletic trainers might encounter.

Overview of Anatomy and Physiology

The anatomy of the eye consists of external and internal structures. All structures are contained within the bony eye socket. The eye socket, anatomically known as the bony orbit of the eye, comprises four walls made up of seven different facial bones of the skull, connective tissue, fat, blood vessels, and nerves (figure 11.1). Anteriorly, the orbit rim is created by the frontal, zygomatic, and maxillary bones (see figure 10.1). The sphenoid, lacrimal, ethmoid, and maxillary bones form the posterior and medial aspects of the orbit. The palatine, zygomatic, and maxillary bones create the floor of the orbit, and the zygomatic and sphenoid bones form the lateral aspect. The orbit provides protection for the eyeball (globe) and contains the lacrimal gland, which produces the tears that lubricate and rinse the surface of the eye. The bony orbit also provides anchorage for the six small extraocular muscles that move the eye. The optic nerve passes through the posterior aspect of the orbit. The visual cortex is located in the occipital lobe of the brain.

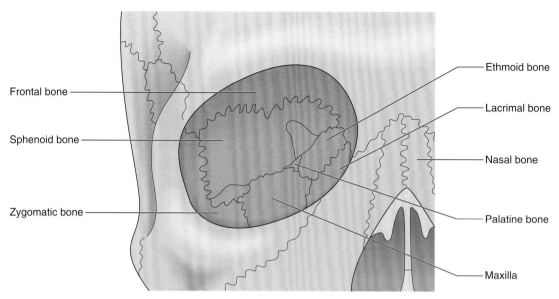

FIGURE 11.1 The eye socket, anatomically known as the bony orbit of the eye.

The external eye includes the eyelid, the conjunctiva, and the lacrimal gland (figure 11.2). These structures protect the eye from foreign objects and distribute tears evenly across the eye. The eyelids provide protection for the external surface of the eye. They help lubricate the ocular surface with their blinking action. The eyelid skin is the thinnest skin on the body. Within each eyelid is a relatively rigid tarsal plate containing meibomian glands, which secrete the oily component of the three-layered tear film. The conjunctiva is a thin, essentially transparent, highly vascular mucous membrane that covers the anterior sclera and the posterior surfaces of both the upper and lower eyelids.

The internal eye consists of many structures, including the sclera, cornea, iris, lens, retina, choroid, optic disk, and macula (figure 11.3). The sclera is the dense white connective tissue that makes up more than 90% of the outer layer of the globe and provides structure for the contents of the eyeball. The cornea serves as the barrier between the environment and the aqueous humor. The cornea is made up of several layers and is the clear window of the eye through which light passes. The iris creates the color of the eye. The pupil is the round, central opening in the iris that creates a pathway for light to reach the retina. This aperture dilates or constricts to regulate

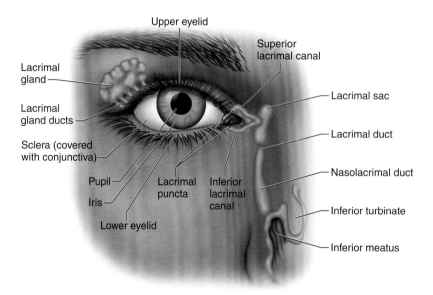

FIGURE 11.2 The external eye.

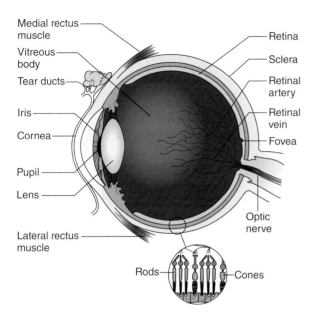

FIGURE 11.3   The internal eye.

the amount of light that enters the eye. Between the cornea and the iris is the anterior chamber. This space is filled with a clear fluid known as aqueous humor.

The crystalline lens is a round, transparent tissue located directly behind the iris. Tiny filaments called zonules, which are attached to the ciliary body, suspend the lens and control its thickness by contracting or relaxing it, allowing an image to be focused onto the retina. The ciliary body is responsible for production of the aqueous humor that fills the anterior chamber of the eye. The large space behind the lens is filled with the transparent gelatinous fluid of the eye known as the vitreous humor.[1]

The retina is the thin, transparent membrane lining the back of the eye that receives light and sends the initial visual signal through the optic nerve to the brain, where it is processed and interpreted. Between the retina and the sclera is the vascular tissue called the *choriocapillaris*. The choriocapillaris supplies blood and nourishment to the outer layers of the retina. The "red eye" seen in a photograph is caused by the reflection of the camera flash through a dilated pupil against the choriocapillaris. As the nerve fibers from the retina exit the eye through the optic nerve, they bunch together at the origin of the optic nerve to form the optic disk. The optic disk is the visible portion of the optic nerve that can be seen when examining the eye. The other structure that can be seen during examination with an ophthalmoscope is the macula and its center point, the fovea, which is considered the site of central vision and color perception of the eye. The majority of color receptors are found in the macula.[2]

Evaluation of the Eye

After taking a thorough history, the clinician will examine the anatomical structures of the eyes and surrounding areas and will also test visual acuity, pupillary responses, motility of the extraocular muscles, and peripheral vision. After the external structures are examined, the clinician may then examine the internal structures of the eye using an ophthalmoscope. The following sections describe a thorough examination of the eye.

Testing Visual Acuity

The most important part of an eye examination is the testing of visual acuity. The ability of the eye to focus clearly on distant or near objects is directly related to the structural integrity of all its parts. Visual acuity is assessed while the patient wears their glasses or contact lenses for distance vision. The Snellen chart is a quick and easy-to-use screening tool for far vision (figure 11.4a). The chart contains graduated sizes of letters with standardized acuity numbers at the end of each line. The patient is asked to read the lines of the chart while standing 20 ft away and covering one eye. The Snellen visual acuity is recorded as a fraction comparing the patient's performance with standard or normal performance. The first number, or numerator, represents the patient's distance from the eye chart, which should be 20 ft, and the second number, or denominator, represents the distance at which a normal person can read the same-size letter or letters on the same line of the chart. For example, if a patient can read down to the 20/40 line (from 20 ft away), this indicates that the patient can see a letter at 20 ft that a person with normal visual acuity can see at a distance of 40 ft, thus revealing that the patient has suboptimal acuity.[1] One must remember that this is a screening tool for distance vision only; it does not measure near vision or dynamic visual acuity. It may be necessary to refer a patient to an optometrist or ophthalmologist for a complete visual assessment. Each eye is tested independently while the other eye is covered with the palm of one hand or an opaque object. When testing acuity in children or nonreaders, an illiterate E or C or picture chart is used (figure 11.4b).

If a standard eye chart is not available, a near-vision card can be used to assess visual acuity (figure 11.5). These small cards can be easily added to a standard first-aid kit. If near vision is tested, then the patient should wear reading glasses or bifocals if they typically require corrective lenses to read. A common alcohol prep pad may be used in lieu of a near-vision card or Snellen eye chart when held at 14 in.

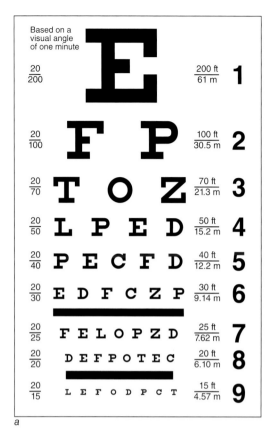 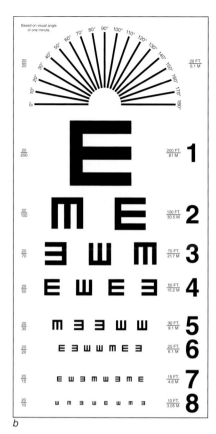

FIGURE 11.4 *(a)* The Snellen chart is used to test visual acuity. *(b)* When examining children or those who do not read, an illiterate E or C or picture chart may be used to test visual acuity.

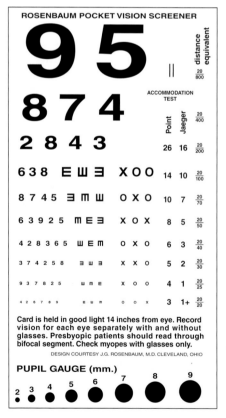

FIGURE 11.5 The Rosenbaum chart for testing near vision.

Visual Acuity

Normal visual acuity is 20/20. The top number indicates the distance at which a person is standing from the chart. The bottom number is the distance at which a normal eye can read that same line. The larger the denominator, the poorer the vision.

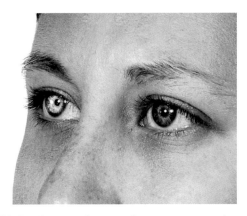

FIGURE 11.6   To test the pupillary response, the patient looks into the distance while a light is moved in toward the eye from the side and shone directly into the pupil. The speed of the pupillary constriction is compared with that of the other eye.

© Micki Cuppett

When a patient cannot see the largest letters of an eye chart, the clinician may hold up some of the fingers of one hand and ask the patient to count them at progressively closer distances to the eye. This is documented as "count fingers vision at [for example] 2 ft." If the patient cannot count the fingers, the examiner can wave a hand in front of the eye and ask if the patient can detect the motion. This is documented as *hand motion vision*. If the patient cannot detect hand motion, any bright light source (e.g., a penlight) can be used to determine the patient's ability to detect light. This is documented as *light perception vision*. Reduction of visual acuity in an injured eye is a serious ocular emergency. Immediate referral to an eye care specialist is warranted.

Testing Pupillary Responses

The pupil's ability to react to light is a basic feature of a normally functioning ocular system. Brisk pupil constriction in response to a bright light also suggests the presence of vision in the absence of any standard eye chart. While the patient is looking into the distance, a light is moved in toward the eye from the side and shone directly into the pupil (figure 11.6). The speed (briskness) of the pupillary constriction is noted. Each eye is examined separately and should be similar to the other.

After examining each eye for its light reactivity and responsiveness, the examiner performs a swinging light test by swinging a light from the normal eye to the injured one. This test is based on the fact that the same quantity of light (i.e., from the same light source) should constrict each pupil by the same amount. When internal ocular damage or optic nerve damage occurs in one eye, the pupil of the injured eye will appear to dilate when the light is moved from the normal eye to the injured eye, indicating that the same amount of light is not being transmitted through the optic nerve in the injured eye.[3] This is known as an **afferent pupillary defect** and represents a potentially severe ocular emergency. Immediate referral to an eye care specialist is warranted.

A pupil that is larger in the injured eye, that does not react to light (**traumatic mydriasis**), or that is no longer round (e.g., it is peaked or oval) may represent significant intraocular trauma (e.g., traumatic iritis). The patient should be immediately referred to an eye care specialist. The athletic trainer should know if the patient has a previously existing or congenitally larger pupil on one side, or **anisocoria**, because this may confuse the findings of the examination.

Testing Extraocular Muscle Motility

Part of the basic assessment of a patient's eye is the examination of ocular motility. The inability of one or both eyes to move into the cardinal fields of gaze (figure 11.7), especially after an eye injury, indicates a severe eye injury with possible eye socket pathology or entrapment of the extraocular muscles (figure 11.8). The examiner asks the patient to follow an object or a fingertip up, down, left, and right with both eyes together. The examiner assesses the patient for smooth, uninterrupted movements of both eyes in all fields of gaze. There should be no restriction of gaze in either eye; movements of the two eyes should be harmonious and parallel. Any change of extraocular movements after an injury may also represent a neurological condition, and it requires immediate medical attention.[4]

Testing Peripheral Vision

Although arguably not as crucial as central visual acuity, peripheral vision allows individuals to view the entire field of activity around them. For athletes, peripheral vision helps them see where their teammates or competitors might be while they focus their vision centrally. Before any injury occurs, the range of an individual's peripheral vision should be known from preparticipation vision testing.

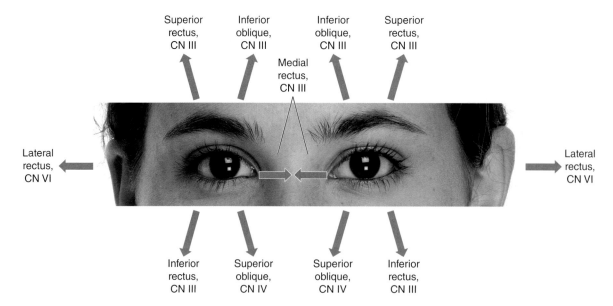

FIGURE 11.7   Eye motility should be tested in all cardinal fields of gaze. CN = cranial nerve.

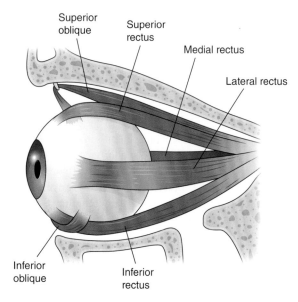

FIGURE 11.8   Extraocular muscles of the eye.

The method most often used to grossly test peripheral vision is called *confrontation visual field testing* (figure 11.9). The examiner tests the patient's peripheral vision one eye at a time. To test the right eye, the examiner stands approximately 3 ft directly in front of the patient. The patient, left hand over left eye, focuses only on the examiner's left eye. The examiner's right eye is closed. This allows the examiner to watch their own open hands during the examination while fixating on the patient's right eye.

The examiner holds up one, two, or three fingers, equidistant between the examiner and the patient and equidistant on either side of the direct line of sight between the patient's right eye and the examiner's left eye. Examiners must be able to see their own fingers during this kind of examination. The patient is asked to add the total number of fingers seen while fixating only on the examiner's left eye and without looking at the examiner's fingers. The examiner will be able to detect whether the patient looked away from the examiner's left eye. It is best not to hold up the same number of fingers on each hand at the same time. This will allow the examiner to know exactly which field of vision is defective. Next, the other eye is examined in a similar fashion. All the cardinal fields of vision—right, left, above, below, above and to the right, above and to the left, below and to the right, and below and to the left—need to be tested. Any finding of the patient's inability to see in a particular field of vision should be referred to an eye care specialist before participation.

Examining the Anatomical Structures of the Injured Eye

A good assessment of the eye can usually be made by simply having the patient open their eyes and examining them directly. On occasion, the eyelids may have to be held apart by either the patient or the examiner. Eyelid swelling is a common consequence of direct trauma to the eye. Therefore, the eye must be examined as soon as possible before swelling of the eyelid makes direct assessment impossible.

The examiner can use room lighting or a directed source of light (e.g., a flashlight or penlight) to assess the anterior portion of the eye. Inspection of the lids and palpation of the bony orbital rim can reveal serious trauma after a blunt injury. If there is any suspicion that the trauma was severe

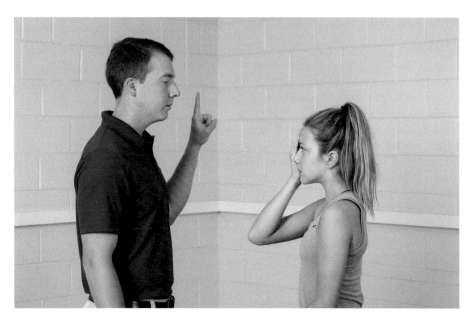

FIGURE 11.9 To test peripheral vision, confrontation visual field testing is used.

enough to penetrate or rupture the eyeball, then no external pressure should ever be placed on the eye or eyelids.

A light is directed toward the patient's opened eye; the patient is asked to look up while the examiner retracts the lower lid (figure 11.10*a*) and to look down while the examiner retracts the upper lid (figure 11.10*b*). This facilitates examination of the entire anterior aspect of the globe, including the conjunctiva, sclera, cornea, and iris. Foreign bodies are commonly found in the conjunctival fornices.[5] The **fornices** are the most posterior portions of the upper and lower portions of the conjunctiva, where the conjunctiva overlying the sclera (**bulbar conjunctiva**) and the conjunctiva lining the eyelids (**palpebral conjunctiva**) join together.

Obscuration of the structures behind the cornea, such as the iris or lens, because of a cloudy anterior chamber is an ominous sign of potential blood in the anterior chamber (hyphema). This can often be detected with a penlight, and it indicates a very serious eye injury. If the eye is anatomically distorted or bleeding, discontinue any further palpation or examination and seek emergency medical attention and ophthalmological referral.

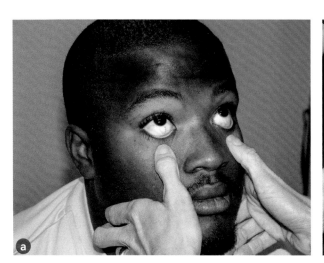
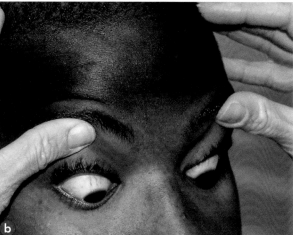

FIGURE 11.10 *(a)* Examining the anterior aspect of the globe with the lower lid retracted. *(b)* Examining the anterior aspect of the globe with the upper lid retracted.

Examining the Eye With the Ophthalmoscope

The ophthalmoscope (figure 11.11) is an instrument used to view the internal structures of the eye. The head of the instrument contains a light source that allows the examiner to visualize the inner eye through a series of lenses and apertures to allow for near or far focusing. The most commonly used aperture projects a large, round beam. Other apertures include the small aperture, the slit-lamp aperture to examine the anterior eye, the red-free filter aperture that shines a green beam to check the optic disk, and the grid aperture used to estimate the size of fundal lesions.[6]

The diopter of the ophthalmoscope—that is, the magnifying power of the lens—may be changed by turning the lens selector disk to the desired magnification.[1,2] The black numbers indicate positive magnification, and the red numbers indicate negative. Turning the wheel clockwise selects positive lenses, and rotating it counterclockwise selects negative lenses. Lens numbers range in magnification power from ±20 to ±140. The range of plus and minus lenses can compensate for myopia or hyperopia in both the examiner and the patient.[6] The diopter is

set at zero (clear glass) when both the patient's and the examiner's eyes are normal. The globe in a hyperopic eye is shorter than normal. The black numbers (convex lens) on the ophthalmoscope lens selector wheel are used to place the focal point on the retina. In the nearsighted person, the globe is longer than in the normal eye, so the lens selector wheel is moved to the red numbers (concave lens) to adjust for myopia in either the patient or the examiner.

The heads of both the ophthalmoscope and the otoscope (used to view the ear and nose) typically share a common handle containing a rechargeable battery. The heads are interchangeable so one can easily convert from one instrument to the other. To change from an otoscope head to an ophthalmoscope head, the examiner pushes down on the head that is currently on the handle while turning to unlock the attachment, inserts the other head, and fastens it to the handle in the same manner.

Both instruments are turned on in the same way: namely, by pushing the on/off switch while turning the black rheostat clockwise to the desired light intensity.

To examine a patient's eye with the ophthalmoscope, the athletic trainer turns on the ophthalmoscope and selects the large aperture. This should project a large, round light on the examiner's hand or the wall. Next the room is darkened. The examiner holds the handle of the ophthalmoscope in the right hand (to examine the patient's right eye) with the index or middle finger on the lens selector wheel. To examine the left eye, the left hand is used. The ophthalmoscope is held firmly against the bony orbit of the examiner's eye (right eye for examining the patient's right eye and left eye for the patient's left eye) with the handle tilted laterally. This will prevent the athletic trainer and the patient from bumping noses during the examination.

The patient is instructed to look up over the shoulder of the athletic trainer. The examiner should start about 15 in. away from the patient, shining the light into the eye to visualize the reddish orange glow (red reflex) from the light reflecting off the highly vascularized retina of the eye. The athletic trainer should approach the patient from the side at about a 15° angle. Shining the light directly into the patient's eye must be avoided because it will cause the

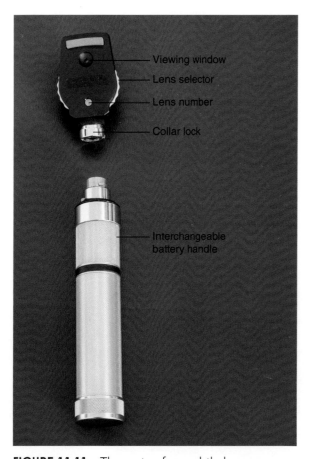

FIGURE 11.11 The parts of an ophthalmoscope.

Viewing window
Lens selector
Lens number
Collar lock
Interchangeable battery handle

pupil to constrict, making it more difficult to visualize the internal eye through an undilated pupil. While keeping the light focused on the red reflex, the athletic trainer moves in close to the eye, almost touching the patient's eyelashes. Absence of a red reflex is often the result of an improperly positioned ophthalmoscope.

To view the internal structures of the eye, such as the optic disk, arteries, veins, and retina, the athletic trainer may need to turn the lens selector wheel to focus on various structures. The fundus or retina will appear as a yellow or pink background with blood vessels branching away from the optic disk (figure 11.12). It is often easier to find the blood vessels and follow them back to the optic disk than to try to locate the optic disk by itself. The arterioles are smaller than the venules and reflect brighter light. The vessels should be followed as far as possible in each of the four quadrants of the eye (superior, inferior, nasal, and temporal) as they go away from the optic disk. When the optic disk is visualized, it should appear yellow to creamy pink, but it may be darker in

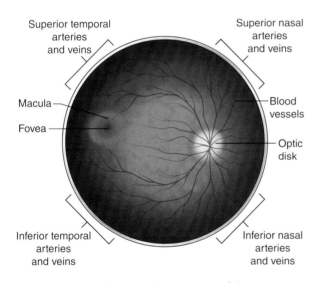

FIGURE 11.12   The retinal structures of the eye.

Clinical Tips
Retinal Vessels
The eye is the only place in the body where the blood vessels may be viewed directly. Many systemic diseases that affect the vascular system may show signs in the retinal vessels.

dark-skinned people.[6] The borders of the disk should be sharp and well defined. Moving in a temporal direction from the optic disk, the macula (fovea centralis) may be visualized. To bring the fovea into the field of vision, the examiner asks the patient to look directly at the light of the ophthalmoscope. It will appear as a yellow dot surrounded by a deep pink periphery and will not have any blood vessels running through it.[2] Considerable practice is needed to visualize the macula, and it may be impossible to view without the pupil being dilated.

Refractive Error

For clear vision, both near and distant images must be sharply focused onto the retina, which lines the back of the eyeball. The ability of the eye to focus these images is directly related to the length of the eye, the curvature of the cornea, the clarity of the ocular media, and the flexibility of the crystalline lens (figure 11.13). The first two parameters, length of eye and curvature of cornea, determine the refractive error of an eye.[7]

- **Myopia**, or nearsightedness, is produced by a longer-than-normal eye. A distant object is focused in front of the retina instead of on it.
- **Hyperopia**, or farsightedness, is produced by a shorter-than-normal eye. A distant object is out of focus when it reaches the retina and, theoretically, focuses behind the retina.

Common Misconceptions About Vision and the Eye

The following statements are often passed along as advice, but all are false.
- Reading in the dark is harmful to the eyes.
- Children will outgrow crossed eyes.
- A cataract is a film growing over the surface of the eye.
- One should avoid reading to save eyesight when vision is failing.
- Children must be cautioned not to sit too close to the television.
- Wearing someone else's glasses may damage one's eyes.
- Misuse of the eyes in childhood results in the need for glasses later in life.
- Emotional stress increases intraocular pressure.

The shape of the cornea is typically spherical (just like a tennis ball) on its anterior curvature. When this curvature is not spherical and has multiple curvatures (e.g., an egg or football), the eye is considered astigmatic. After age 40 yr, the crystalline lens inside the eye begins to lose its flexibility and thus its ability to focus on nearby objects. This is known as **presbyopia**. Patients with presbyopia eventually require reading glasses for near vision.

Signs and Symptoms

Mild degrees of refractive errors can remain undetected for years until very clear distance vision is needed, such as when an adolescent first begins an athletic season. In other cases, patients may complain of slowly declining visual acuity. Impaired visual acuity may be confirmed by testing with a Snellen chart. The vision should improve with pinhole testing, which is used to distinguish a refractive error (correctable with lenses) from organic eye disease. Pinhole testing is performed by punching several pinholes in a card. The patient looks through a pinhole in the card one eye at a time. If vision improves, the condition is refractory. A web-based distance visual acuity instrument (DigiVis) has been used to test patient's distance visual acuity and has shown good validity and reliability while allowing ophthalmic examination or consultation via telehealth.[8]

Referral and Diagnostic Tests

Patients who complain of poor vision, either at a distance or close up, need to be referred to an eye care practitioner who will determine the refraction of their eyes and perform other ocular tests. The refraction determines the refractive error of an eye. The refractive error will change over time as the shape and length of the eye change up to ages 23 to 25 yr. After that, the refractive error tends to stabilize.

Treatment and Return to Participation

The refractive error can be corrected with glasses or contact lenses. Refractive surgery, such as laser-assisted in situ keratomileusis (LASIK), is also an option for treatment. LASIK is performed to correct myopia, hyperopia, or astigmatism. In LASIK, a small, partial-thickness flap is made from the top of the cornea. A laser is used to reshape the corneal tissue under the flap and remove any refractive error present. The corneal flap is repositioned

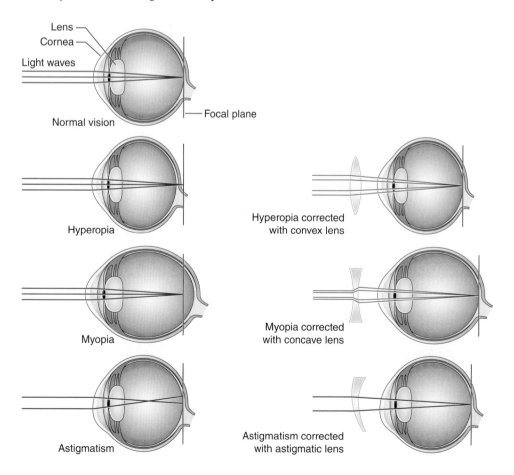

FIGURE 11.13   Common refractive disorders and their corrections.

onto the lasered cornea surface. This procedure takes approximately 15 to 30 min, with many patients capable of seeing an immediate improvement in their vision. Not everyone is eligible for LASIK. The success of the operation depends on the degree of initial refractive error and on the thickness of the cornea.[9] In one study, 36.4% of patients interviewed cited the desire to pursue sports and leisure activities as one of their main reasons for having LASIK.[10] Many active people consider having LASIK to avoid wearing glasses or contact lenses while playing sports. There have been no studies to date showing any improvement in the performance of players who have had LASIK. Although generally viewed as a safe procedure, there have been multiple case reports of dislodged flaps as a result of sport-related eye trauma.[10] LASIK should not be performed until the refraction has been stable for at least 2 yr, especially in the adolescent or young adult.[11]

The prognosis for the majority of refractive errors is excellent. Return to participation can be immediate after the patient has received correction for the refractive error.

Conjunctivitis

Conjunctivitis is a general term for an inflammation of the conjunctiva, the transparent vascular tissue covering the anterior sclera and the posterior surface of the eyelids. It is commonly caused by bacteria, viruses, allergies, or dry eye or occurs in response to a corneal injury or irritation.

Signs and Symptoms

The symptoms of conjunctivitis, sometimes called pink eye, are not specific to the causative agent and can include all or some of the following: redness, burning, itching, tearing, irritation, and foreign body sensation. Allergic conjunctivitis is classically characterized by itching. Viral conjunctivitis is often associated with recent cold or flu symptoms or recent contact with someone with a red eye.[12] The most obvious signs of conjunctivitis are redness or vascular engorgement (figure 11.14). There may be a discharge, ranging from watery to mucoid to frank purulence (pus). Redness of the conjunctiva in the space between the eyelids associated with a burning sensation is common after exposure to sun, wind, or dusty conditions, which are all common to outdoor athletics.

A few basic features can help differentiate bacterial, viral, and allergic conjunctivitis, especially if a **slit-lamp** biomicroscope is available. A watery or mucous discharge can be seen in both allergic and viral conjunctivitis.[12] Typically, the discharge in bacterial conjunctivitis is purulent (figure 11.15). Patients with allergic conjunctivitis typically complain that their eyes itch. Viral conjunctivitis often involves the cornea, which is difficult to visualize without high magnification. Viral conjunctivitis often presents with **preauricular lymphadenopathy**, a small, tender lymph node located just in front of the tragus of the ear.

Referral and Diagnostic Tests

Viral conjunctivitis is highly contagious. Therefore, referral to an eye care practitioner for diagnosis is important in most cases of conjunctivitis. Without the benefit of a slit-lamp biomicroscope used by the ophthalmologist or optometrist, determining the exact cause of conjunctivitis may be difficult. Follow these steps to assess the need for referral of a patient with red eye:

1. Check the patient's visual acuity.
2. Inspect for a pattern of redness. A diffuse pink color is quite different from a deep localized redness.

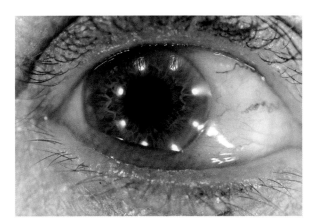

FIGURE 11.14   This photograph of allergic conjunctivitis shows the redundant conjunctiva rising over the edge of the lower lid margin in addition to redness and vascular engorgement of the sclera.

Photo courtesy of Charles B. Slonim.

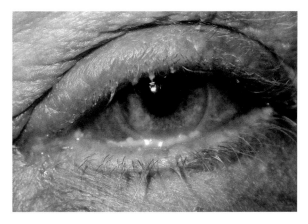

FIGURE 11.15   The discharge in bacterial conjunctivitis is typically purulent when compared with the watery discharge seen in allergic conjunctivitis in figure 11.14.

Photo courtesy of Charles B. Slonim.

3. Observe for the presence of discharge.

4. Use a fluorescein stain and blue cobalt light to observe for corneal defects if an abrasion is suspected.

5. Use an ophthalmoscope to observe the inner structures of the eye for irregularities.

6. Refer a patient with any abrasions, foreign bodies, hyphemas, or irregularities in the shape of the pupil to an eye care specialist immediately.

Treatment and Return to Participation

Standard treatment for mild acute bacterial conjunctivitis includes topical antibiotic eyedrops or ointments, such as fluoroquinolone ophthalmic drops (e.g., ofloxacin, ciprofloxacin, levofloxacin, moxifloxacin, gatifloxacin, besifloxacin), aminoglycoside ophthalmic drops (e.g., gentamicin, tobramycin), or erythromycin or bacitracin ophthalmic ointments. Viral conjunctivitis usually resolves spontaneously within 2 wk and cannot be treated effectively with topical antibiotics.[12] Typically, the worst signs and symptoms occur on the third to fifth days. Because antiviral therapies are not effective in treating viral conjunctivitis, treatment is directed at relieving symptoms such as redness and burning. This may involve the use of over-the-counter vasoconstrictors (i.e., whiteners), topical antiallergy drops (e.g., ketotifen), or simply artificial tears to lubricate the ocular surface. Allergic conjunctivitis is often self-treated with a variety of over-the-counter topical ophthalmic antihistamine or decongestant products. There are also prescription antiallergy ophthalmic products that can be prescribed by the eye care practitioner. These include topical ophthalmic antihistamines (e.g., emedastine), mast cell stabilizers (e.g., cromolyn sodium), mast cell stabilizer and antihistamine combinations (e.g., olopatadine, azelastine, epinastine), nonsteroidal anti-inflammatories (e.g., ketorolac), and steroids (e.g., loteprednol, fluorometholone).[13]

Viral conjunctivitis is highly contagious. Therefore, any patient with acute watery conjunctivitis should not be in close contact with others until the condition is resolved. Persistent or worsening conjunctivitis may be secondary to more aggressive bacteria or a moderately severe allergy. In such a case, the patient should receive an ophthalmic assessment. After 2 or 3 d, the patient can return to participation. Some extremely virulent strains of viral conjunctivitis can cause corneal clouding that can persist for weeks to months. This can adversely affect the patient's vision. Bacterial conjunctivitis, although contagious, is not as easily spread from one person to another as is viral conjunctivitis. After 1 or 2 d of topical antibiotic therapy, the patient can return to participation.[14]

Spread of viral conjunctivitis can be prevented by maintaining appropriate hygiene, handwashing, and isolating the patient with a red eye until it is properly diagnosed. Individuals are advised not to share cosmetics or other products used around their eyes.

Clinical Tip

The Cause of Red Eye

Many patients present with a chief complaint of a red eye. An engorgement of the conjunctival vessels causes the eye to be red. It may be associated with a subconjunctival hemorrhage that requires no treatment, or it may be a manifestation of a serious eye disorder that requires immediate attention. Common disorders involving red eye include the following:

- conjunctivitis—Bacterial, viral, allergic, and irritative
- herpes simplex keratitis—Inflammation of the cornea caused by herpesvirus
- scleritis—Inflammation of the sclera
- subconjunctival hemorrhage—Accumulation of blood in the potential space between the conjunctiva and the sclera
- abrasions and foreign bodies—Hyperemic response

Corneal Abrasions

A corneal abrasion results from a scratch to the surface of the cornea that causes a defect in the most superficial layer of cells, called the *epithelium*.[4,15] The most common cause of a corneal abrasion is direct trauma with a foreign object.

Signs and Symptoms

The most common symptom of a corneal abrasion is the sensation of having something in the eye, referred to as a foreign body sensation. Other symptoms include decreased vision, tearing, sensitivity to light, **blepharospasm** (abnormal blinking), and reactive conjunctivitis.[4]

Some corneal infections can have a similar presentation to a corneal abrasion, and it is important to distinguish between them by staining and magnification. Often a corneal abrasion is caused by an embedded foreign body that remains stuck to the ocular surface or possibly stuck onto the surface of the conjunctiva under the eyelids. Persistence of a foreign body sensation in the absence of an abrasion requires looking for a retained foreign body somewhere on the eye.

Referral and Diagnostic Tests

Most corneal abrasions should be referred to an eye care specialist in order to rule out an injury that might be deeper into the cornea than just the epithelial surface. A corneal abrasion can be difficult to see in a penlight examination. It is best visualized by a special ophthalmic vital dye staining technique. This technique involves placing a water-soluble orange dye, called fluorescein, on the ocular surface. Fluorescein dye is commercially available as individually wrapped, sterile paper strips that have been impregnated with the orange fluorescein dye.[16] To administer a fluorescein dye test, the clinician follows these steps:

1. Wet the tip of a fluorescein strip with sterile saline or eye wash.
2. Pull the lower lid down and away from the eye.
3. Touch the tip of the strip to the lower lid conjunctival cul-de-sac; do not place the strip directly on the eye.
4. Ask the patient to close their eye for a few seconds in order to spread the dye.
5. Darken the room.
6. Use a cobalt blue light to illuminate the eye.
7. Observe the eye; the dye fluoresces as a bright yellowish green color under the cobalt blue light and pinpoints abrasions (figure 11.16).

Treatment and Return to Participation

Initial treatment of any eye trauma is pain control, removal of contact lenses (if applicable), and protection of the eye to prevent further trauma. The treatment of a simple corneal abrasion is lubrication with artificial

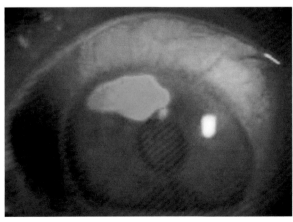

FIGURE 11.16 A corneal abrasion stained with fluorescein dye and "excited" with a cobalt blue filter.
Photo courtesy of Charles B. Slonim.

tears and occasionally a topical antibiotic drop (e.g., fluoroquinolone or aminoglycoside) or ointment (e.g., bacitracin or erythromycin) if the potential for a corneal infection exists. The antibiotic preparation should be administered as directed, and follow-up should be with the eye care practitioner as prescribed. Pain management is obtainable with topical, oral, intramuscular, or intravenous medications. The most common pain management medication is topical tetracaine.[17] Routine patching of small corneal abrasions is not recommended.[17]

Instead of a gauze patch, a soft contact lens with no refractive power, referred to as a *bandage contact lens*, can be placed over the corneal abrasion, which not only serves as a protective barrier to the movements of the eyelid but also aids in reepithelialization. In a previous study, patients treated with soft bandage contact lenses along with a nonsteroidal anti-inflammatory drop were able to return to normal activity much more quickly than those who were patched.[18] The addition of the anti-inflammatory drop significantly decreased the pain associated with the abrasion. Contact lenses should not be worn until the eye care specialist decides it is appropriate.

Simple noninfected corneal abrasions usually resolve clinically within 24 to 72 h.[4] After healing (reepithelialization) of the uncomplicated corneal abrasion, the area where it occurred is typically undetectable during future examinations, and it will not pose future problems for the patient. The patient can return to participation as soon as the foreign body sensation is gone. Larger abrasions may require more time for reepithelialization and symptom resolution.

Corneal or Scleral Lacerations

One of the most serious traumatic eye injuries is a corneal or corneal–scleral laceration, also known as an **open globe**.[4,19] An open globe is an eyeball that has been ruptured after blunt or sharp trauma or injury with a projectile foreign body (figure 11.17). Lacerations allow leakage of intraocular fluid or extrusion of intraocular tissues and contents. They also allow the introduction of infectious pathogens from the environment into the intraocular spaces.

Signs and Symptoms

The symptoms of an open globe are decreased vision and pain after trauma. The patient often has a hyphema, dense subconjunctival hemorrhage, decreased eye movements, or bloody tears. An open globe should be considered after any ocular trauma. Corneal lacerations can be penetrating, identified as open globe lacerations, or nonpenetrating.[19] Some penetrating or perforating injuries may or may not have an extrusion of intraocular contents. The differential diagnosis is left to the eye care specialist.

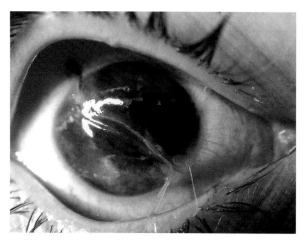

FIGURE 11.17 A corneal laceration (open globe) caused by a paintball injury.

Photo courtesy of Charles B. Slonim.

Referral and Diagnostic Tests

If a rupture is suspected, it is imperative that the eye not be touched and that the patient be immediately transported to the nearest emergency room.

Treatment and Return to Participation

A lacerated eye is treated with prompt surgical repair, often followed by several days of intravenous and topical antibiotics. Infection of the eye after an open globe can be catastrophic and can cause loss of vision or even loss of the eye.

Visual rehabilitation of an eye with a corneal laceration is prolonged. Even after prompt diagnosis and appropriate treatments, the eye may still develop a cataract or permanent scarring of the cornea. Scar tissue inside the eye often requires several eye surgeries to restore vision. Often the level of pretrauma vision cannot be regained, even after the most heroic efforts to restore the normal eye structure.

Corneal and Conjunctival Foreign Bodies

Any object embedded in or adhering to the conjunctiva or cornea is defined as an ocular foreign body (figure 11.18). The patient may or may not recall getting something in the eye. Most ocular bodies are washed off the surface of the eye by the rinsing lubrication of the tear film or brushed off by the blinking action of the eyelids. Foreign bodies that remain on the eye can cause the patient significant discomfort.

Signs and Symptoms

The symptoms of a foreign body are typically immediate. The patient may complain of a sensation of "something in the eye" or of "scratchiness." There is often associated reflex tearing as the eye reacts to the foreign body and tries to relieve the eye by lubricating it. The foreign body may not be visible to the examiner depending on its size, shape, and color.

A corneal or conjunctival abrasion without a foreign body can mimic the symptoms of a foreign body as the blinking eyelids continue to rub over the abraded surface. Frequently, the patient will feel as if the foreign body is under the upper eyelid even if the foreign body or abrasion is in the middle or lower part of the eye.

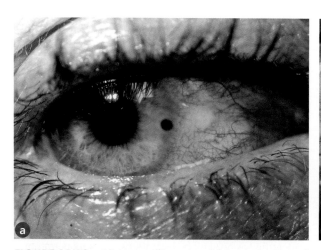
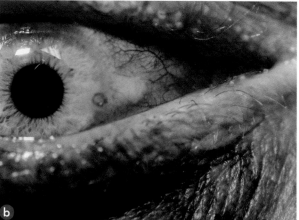

FIGURE 11.18 (a) A metallic corneal foreign body in the eye. (b) The same eye with a residual rust ring after the foreign body was removed.

Photos courtesy of Charles B. Slonim.

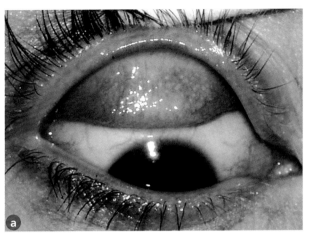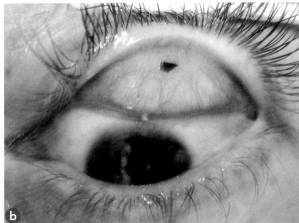

FIGURE 11.19   (a) The upper eyelid is everted with a cotton-tipped applicator. (b) A foreign body (plastic) on the upper eyelid.

Photos courtesy of Charles B. Slonim.

Referral and Diagnostic Tests

Most foreign bodies lodged on the less sensitive conjunctival surface can be removed on-site. Those on the extremely sensitive corneal surface may require referral to an eye care specialist if they cannot be removed with a few simple maneuvers.[17]

Treatment and Return to Participation

A loose foreign body on the ocular surface can often be rinsed off the eye with additional lubrication, such as an eye rinse or just a few drops of an artificial tear supplement. A contact lens in the affected eye should be removed before treatment. It is appropriate to wash an eye with a foreign body at an eye wash station if available. If the foreign body sensation persists after irrigation, the upper eyelid can be gently pulled away from the eyeball by grasping the upper lid eyelashes and pulling the upper eyelid down over the lower eyelid lashes. The lower eyelid lashes will then act as a "brush" against the back (conjunctival) side of the upper lid and potentially dislodge a loose foreign body from under the upper eyelid.

If the foreign body sensation persists after the brushing maneuver, the upper lid can be everted to allow a direct inspection of its conjunctival surface.[6] The examiner can pull the upper lid away from the eye by gently grasping the upper lid lashes and having the patient look down. When a small cotton-tipped applicator is placed against the upper eyelid crease (found approximately 1/2 in. above the margin of the eyelid), the eyelid can be rotated around the applicator (figure 11.19a). The examiner's finger can keep the lid everted by pressing the lashes against the brow. If the foreign body is located, the same applicator can be used to gently lift the foreign body off the surface of the conjunctiva.

The cornea should never be touched. No attempt to remove a foreign body from the cornea should be made, because inadvertent pressure on a sharp corneal foreign body could potentially push it deeper or even perforate the thin cornea. If the foreign body cannot be removed and remains embedded on the conjunctival or corneal surface, the patient needs to be referred to an eye care specialist.

Topical antibiotics (e.g., fluoroquinolone, aminoglycosides, erythromycin) are sometimes prescribed to prevent infection. Residual foreign body sensation, such as that caused by an abrasion from the foreign material, can be treated with artificial tears.

The prognosis for simple conjunctival foreign bodies is excellent. The patient can typically return to participation immediately after the foreign body has been removed. Sometimes the maneuvers to remove the foreign body may create an additional ocular surface abrasion. Although the foreign body is gone, the foreign body sensation may remain for another 24 h. The prognosis for removing corneal foreign bodies depends on their depth and size. The recovery time is usually a little longer and may require 24 to 48 h for the symptoms to completely resolve.

Hyphema

Blood in the anterior chamber of the eye is known as a **hyphema**, and it is a common complication of blunt trauma to the eyeball (figure 11.20). It is often associated with other types of orbital or ocular damage, such as corneal abrasions, orbital fractures, eyelid contusions, and open globe injuries.[20] The blood often comes from a damaged blood vessel in the iris or ciliary body. The appearance of blood in the anterior chamber of the eye begins as a crescent shape inferiorly and may progress until the entire anterior chamber is filled with blood.

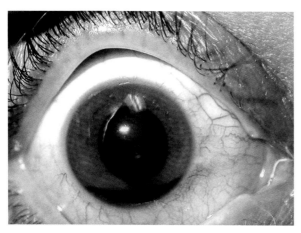

FIGURE 11.20   A hyphema most often is caused by trauma to the eye, as in this racquetball player's injury. This injury points out why it is important always to wear eye protection.

Photo courtesy of Charles B. Slonim.

Spontaneous hyphemas in the absence of trauma are rare and are associated with a variety of rare ocular syndromes.

Signs and Symptoms

The two main symptoms of a hyphema are pain and blurred vision. The pain is associated with both the initial trauma and the inflammatory effect that the blood has on the anterior structures of the eye. The blurred vision is associated with the interruption of the clear aqueous humor in the anterior chamber by the opaque blood. The blood can often be seen by close examination with an external light source. With a vertical head position, the blood will form a layer in the anterior chamber with the heavier blood settling to the bottom and the lighter aqueous humor rising to the top.[21] On occasion, the blood creates a very thin, microscopic layer at the bottom of the anterior chamber. This may be imperceptible to the naked eye of the examiner.

In the presence of trauma, blood in the anterior chamber can represent only a hyphema. On occasion, the source of the bleeding can be visualized. Hyphemas are associated with several other sight-threatening conditions and complications. The differential diagnoses are aimed at looking for other potential ocular damage that may have occurred in association with the hyphema. These conditions include a ruptured globe, corneal abrasion, dislocated lens, traumatic **cataract**, bleeding in the vitreous cavity, increased intraocular pressure (e.g., secondary glaucoma), and retinal tear or detachment.[21] The presence of a hyphema may make it difficult to examine the more posterior structures of the eye, such as the retina.

Referral and Diagnostic Tests

A hyphema represents a serious, sight-threatening condition that requires immediate referral to an eye care specialist. During transport, the patient should keep the head elevated in order to allow the blood to settle to the bottom of the anterior chamber. This will give the eye care specialist a better opportunity to visualize the rest of the ocular structures.

Treatment and Return to Participation

Protective eyewear can prevent the majority of hyphemas caused by direct trauma to an eye. The patient must wear protective eyewear after sustaining a hyphema to prevent a recurrence. An uncomplicated hyphema is typically managed with bed rest and the administration of topical steroids (e.g., prednisolone, loteprednol, dexamethasone), pupil-dilating drops known as mydriatics (e.g., **atropine**, **homatropine**), and, if required, eye pressure-lowering (antiglaucoma) agents.[22] The patient should sleep with the head of the bed slightly elevated. A significant late risk of hyphema is a rebleed that typically occurs between the third and fifth day after the initial injury. This rebleed can completely fill the anterior chamber with blood. This is commonly referred to as an *eight-ball hyphema*.[23] This can produce elevated intraocular pressure and permanent blood-staining of the inside of the cornea. Both conditions are sight-threatening. On occasion, systemic medication may be needed to control the bleeding and the high intraocular pressure. In cases of very high intraocular pressure or severe bleeding in the front of the eye, the patient may require hospitalization or surgical evacuation of the blood.

The prognosis for an uncomplicated hyphema is excellent. Depending on the size of the hyphema and the intraocular pressure measurement, daily follow-up by an eye care specialist may be needed until the blood starts to resorb. The patient can return to participation 2 to 3 wk after the blood has completely resolved.[22] Less frequent examinations by the eye care specialist over the following months may be required to rule out late complications such as secondary glaucoma. Undetected high intraocular pressures can cause irreversible damage to the optic nerve. Blood-staining of the cornea may require months to resolve.

Subconjunctival Hemorrhage

Bright-red blood appearing acutely in a sector of the eye under the clear conjunctiva and in front of the white sclera is termed a **subconjunctival hemorrhage** (figure 11.21). Although striking in appearance, this condition is benign. It represents a broken blood vessel under the conjunctiva and is analogous to a subcutaneous hematoma.

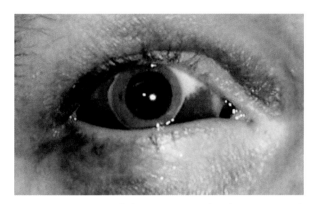

FIGURE 11.21   Eyelid contusion with subconjunctival hemorrhage.

Photo courtesy of Charles B. Slonim.

Signs and Symptoms

Subconjunctival hemorrhages can be caused by trauma, coughing or straining, high blood pressure, breath-holding or the Valsalva maneuver, bleeding disorders, and ingestion of blood thinners. They can occur spontaneously without a known cause and are usually without symptoms; however, other people observing the eye can easily detect the blood. Rarely, more serious conditions such as conjunctival tumors can emulate a subconjunctival hemorrhage.

Referral and Diagnostic Tests

Unless there has been blunt trauma, subconjunctival hemorrhage does not require ophthalmic evaluation as long as no other signs or symptoms are present and vision is unaffected.

Treatment and Return to Participation

Because of the nature of its pathophysiology, except for direct trauma, there is no way to prevent a subconjunctival hemorrhage. Protective eyewear should prevent subconjunctival hemorrhage caused by direct trauma to the conjunctival surface. For mild irritation, artificial tears can be given. A simple subconjunctival hemorrhage usually clears within 2 or 3 wk; it may change color as the blood resolves, similar to a bruise.

Prognosis is excellent. Athletic participation is not restricted because of subconjunctival hemorrhage. If there are recurrent bleeding episodes, visual symptoms, pain, or persistence of blood, an ophthalmic referral should be sought.

Eyelid Lacerations

The eyelids and periorbital skin are very susceptible to both blunt and sharp trauma. The eyelid skin is the thinnest skin on the body. The thicker periorbital skin overlies a relatively solid orbital rim. These tissues are readily vulnerable to direct trauma.

Signs and Symptoms

In the presence of trauma, eyelid lacerations present as an open wound of the eyelids or surrounding tissues. As with any tissue laceration, the presence of a foreign body needs to be ruled out. An examination for other evidence of ocular damage must be performed.

Referral and Diagnostic Tests

Lacerations that are not amenable to adhesive strip bandages and require suturing need to be referred to the appropriate oculofacial surgeon or ophthalmologist. Complete examination of the eyeball remains the highest priority before closure of the wounds.

Treatment and Return to Participation

Although the eyelids are not amenable to adhesive strips for closure of lacerations, for small wounds around the periorbital area, such as to the eyebrows, adhesive strips usually work well. Tissue adhesives (e.g., Dermabond) can be used to close small eyelid or periorbital wounds. Suturing is the most effective way to close an eyelid wound. During wound cleaning and antisepsis, care must be taken to avoid getting nonophthalmic antiseptic solutions, rinses, and ointments in the eye.

Most eyelid and periorbital lacerations heal nicely and uneventfully. Most athletes without visual complaints or increasing or persistent pain can return to participation as long as the swelling of the eyelid or periorbital tissue does not compromise their vision.

Orbital Fracture

Among the seven bones that make up the walls of the bony orbit are some of the thinnest bones of the body. When there is a blunt injury to the eye, the forces against the orbit create a sudden increase in pressure within the orbit. The orbital contents, including the eyeball, are displaced posteriorly, toward the back of the orbit. This pressure can break the thin orbital walls, causing an orbital wall fracture that is often referred to as a *blowout fracture*. Often the nearby orbital contents, such as the extraocular muscles and orbital fat, can be forced through the fracture site and become incarcerated in the space behind the fractured wall. The two orbital walls that most commonly fracture during blunt trauma are the inferior wall (orbital floor) and the medial wall. The spaces behind these two walls are the maxillary and ethmoid sinuses, respectively.

Signs and Symptoms

Depending on the severity of the injury and fracture, the symptoms of an orbital fracture can include pain with attempted eye movement, double vision (**diplopia**) when orbital contents are trapped in the fracture site, and numbness, or hypesthesia, in the distribution of the infraorbital nerve, which gives sensation to the cheek, upper lip, and upper teeth.[24,25] The double vision resolves when the patient covers one eye. The patient may show signs of restricted eye movements in up- or down-gaze (figure 11.22), decreased sensation in the cheek or upper lip on the same side as the injury, misalignment of the orbital rim on palpation along with point tenderness, and sometimes a "crunchy" sensation under the skin of the orbit.[25] This latter condition, called **orbital emphysema**, is a result of air from the sinus that has become trapped beneath the skin. Eyelid ecchymoses are often seen.

Blunt head trauma can damage certain cranial nerves associated with extraocular movements (e.g., cranial nerves III, IV, and VI), and the patient can present with diplopia.[26] Localized swelling over the infraorbital nerve can cause temporary hypesthesia along its sensory distribution. Retrobulbar (behind the globe) hematomas can cause irreversible optic nerve damage.

Referral and Diagnostic Tests

A patient with a suspected orbital fracture requires orbital imaging studies. The most important diagnostic test is a computed tomography (CT) scan of the orbit with both coronal and axial views. It is also important to examine the eye for potential intraocular injuries (e.g., retinal detachment, hyphema, open globe injury, foreign body).

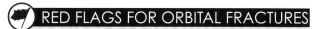

RED FLAGS FOR ORBITAL FRACTURES

An orbital fracture often causes the patient's eye on the affected side to have restricted upward movement as a result of trapping of the inferior rectus muscle through the orbital floor. Any patient with unilateral restricted eye movement must be referred for further examination.

Treatment and Return to Participation

Not all orbital fractures require surgical repair. Depending on the size, location, and whether there is tissue entrapment, an orbital fracture may be monitored to determine whether the patient's signs and symptoms spontaneously resolve with time. An orbital fracture technically represents an open fracture because the normally closed orbital space can allow sinus air to enter through the fracture site. For this reason, systemic antibiotics are administered. Ice compresses for the first 24 to 48 h can help reduce the periorbital swelling. No compresses are used until the eyeball has been cleared of any injuries. Patients with suspected orbital fractures are instructed not to blow their nose because this can force bacteria-laden air from the paranasal sinuses under the eyelids or into the orbit and cause a secondary infection.[25] For large fractures or persistent diplopia in primary or down-gaze, surgical repair of the fracture is often required. The patient may be observed for up to 2 wk before any surgical intervention to determine whether the signs and symptoms resolve spontaneously. Ophthalmologists, otolaryngologists, plastic surgeons, and maxillofacial surgeons perform this surgery.

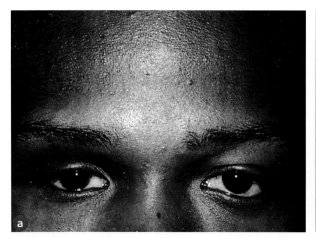
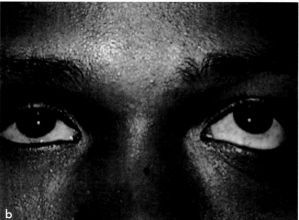

FIGURE 11.22 This right orbital floor fracture injury seen in a basketball player is assessed by (a) having the patient look straight ahead, and (b) noting the restricted upward gaze of the right eye, which is on the reader's left.
Photos courtesy of Charles B. Slonim.

The prognosis for complete resolution of the signs and symptoms of an orbital fracture depends on the spontaneous resolution of symptoms or the success of the surgical outcome. Persistent diplopia may require further extraocular muscle surgery. Shrinkage of the orbital fat after orbital trauma may cause delayed **enophthalmos** (movement of the eyeball deeper into the orbit). Infraorbital nerve hypesthesia may be transient or permanent, depending on the extent of injury to that nerve. Athletes may return to participation in approximately 2 to 4 wk, with facial and eyewear protection for approximately 4 to 6 mo.[27]

Retinal Tear and Detachment

The retina is the delicate transparent tissue lining the back of the eye. Light-sensitive retinal fibers receive images projected through the lens and send them to the brain through the optic nerve for interpretation as a visualized image. When the retina is damaged, transmission of the images is distorted or absent. Retinal tears and retinal detachments (figure 11.23) may occur through illness, injury, or heredity or as the result of normal aging. These conditions are most typically found in people who are nearsighted or have undergone previous eye surgery, have experienced eye trauma, or have a family history of retinal detachment. Middle-aged and older people are at higher risk than the younger population. Retinal tears and detachments are also likely to recur in patients with a history of a previous retinal tear or detachment. Patients with risk factors associated with retinal tears or detachments should avoid contact sports in which head or eye trauma is possible. Protective eyewear can prevent direct trauma to the eye that can cause retinal tears or detachments; however, blunt head trauma without direct eye trauma can also cause these conditions.

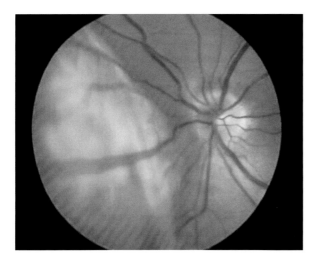

FIGURE 11.23 Retinal detachment.

Photo courtesy of Charles B. Slonim.

Retinal detachment typically begins with one or more small holes or tears in the retina. These holes are caused by shrinkage (e.g., during the aging process) or sudden movement (e.g., in trauma) of the vitreous humor that is intimately attached to the retina. Once a tear has occurred, more liquid vitreous humor may flow through the hole or tear, causing the retina to elevate and detach.

Signs and Symptoms

A retinal tear or detachment typically occurs in only one eye. The most common symptoms of a tear in the retina are brief flashes of light (**photopsia**) in the peripheral visual field or an abrupt increase in vitreous floaters. *Floaters* are the perception of images caused by opacity in the vitreous; they are common but typically few, and they only appear occasionally. The most common symptoms of a retinal detachment are the same as for a retinal tear, plus a curtain or shadow moving over the field of vision. Sometimes central visual acuity may be lost. A retinal tear or detachment may be identified through the direct visualization of the elevated or torn retina.

As people age, the vitreous begins to liquefy. Eventually, it becomes so liquid that it collapses into itself and peels away from the retina. This phenomenon is called **posterior vitreous detachment (PVD)** or posterior vitreous separation. People who have had a PVD often notice floaters in their vision caused by small opacities in the vitreous that cast shadows on the retina. They may also experience a split-second flash of light in the corner of their vision. These symptoms are similar to those of a retinal tear.

Referral and Diagnostic Tests

Patients with a new onset of flashes or floaters, or what appears to be a curtain moving over their vision, especially after trauma, must be immediately referred to an eye care professional. These patients are often referred to retina specialists. Proper examination requires pharmacological dilation of the pupil, along with a detailed examination of the retinal periphery with specialized ophthalmic instruments.

Treatment and Return to Participation

Retinal detachments caused by traumatic breaks or tears to the retina are treated surgically. Ophthalmologists use lasers or cryoprobes to create adhesions between the detached retina and the back surface of the eye.[28] Silicone oil, filtered air, or special gases are sometimes injected into the vitreous cavity to push the retina against the back of the eye during the healing process.

The prognosis for a retinal tear or detachment is based on the number of tears or holes or the size and location of the detachment. Early diagnosis and treatment are critical factors in successful surgical outcomes. If the central retina (macula), which is responsible for central 20/20 acuity, is not detached, successful surgery can preserve excellent central vision. However, complications of surgery, infection, redetachment, or a primary detachment of the central part of the retina can drastically decrease vision. Once a patient has had retinal surgery, the eye requires several weeks to heal. The risk of redetachment is higher in a patient with a previous history of one.[29] Return to participation depends on the extent of the retinal injury and the success of the repair. It also depends on the sport involved (e.g., contact versus noncontact). Lengthy discussions between the athlete and the retina specialist are necessary to determine the athlete's safety and the risk of future visual loss when returning to sports.

Dislocated Contact Lens

More than 30 million Americans wear contact lenses as a substitute for glasses to correct refractive errors and to improve their visual acuity. Contact lenses are categorized by the flexibility of the plastic material from which they are manufactured.

- Soft contact lenses are relatively large, soft, and pliable. They are designed to cover the entire corneal surface and extend approximately 1 to 2 mm beyond the cornea onto the conjunctiva and sclera.

- Rigid contact lenses are relatively small, are less flexible, and are designed to fit only on the corneal surface. Rigid contact lenses are made of durable plastic material (typically silicone), are gas permeable, and may be a better choice when the patient has an irregular cornea, high prescription, or dry eye.[30]

Contact lenses can be moved from their normal central location over the cornea when the eye is subjected to a shearing force, such as a tangential trauma from a ball or a hand. Studies have indicated that soft contact lenses may have a protective effect for corneal abrasions.[31] Protective eyewear or visors for helmets can prevent shearing forces from displacing contact lenses. The use of prescription safety goggles eliminates the risks associated with contact lenses and simultaneously protects the eyes from other trauma but generally is not as appealing to the athlete.

Signs and Symptoms

The symptoms of a displaced contact lens include loss of visual acuity and the presence of a foreign body sensation. Most currently available contact lenses have a visible tint for easy handling. This makes it easier for the examiner to identify a dislocated lens against the background of the white sclera. Nontinted lenses may be more difficult to see. Soft lenses may become rolled up and lodged in the upper limits of the conjunctiva under the upper eyelid.

Other acute conditions associated with contact lens wear can present with decreased acuity and a foreign body sensation, including corneal abrasions, corneal foreign bodies, some corneal infections, an inside-out contact lens, and hypersensitivity to a new or overused contact lens cleaning solution.

Referral and Diagnostic Tests

If the dislocated lens is located but cannot be removed by either the patient or the athletic trainer, then referral to an eye care specialist may be necessary. If no lens is found but a foreign body sensation remains, the patient may need the services of an eye specialist to rule out a possible corneal or conjunctival abrasion and to further examine the eye for the dislocated lens. If a patient believes that a contact lens has become dislocated, the athletic trainer should help find it. Often the patient can manipulate the lens and reposition it.

Treatment and Return to Participation

Pulling the upper and lower lids away from the eye to inspect the conjunctiva will often reveal the dislocated contact lens.

Before a displaced contact lens is removed, the eye should be lubricated with saline eye wash, an artificial tear solution, or contact lens rewetting solution. If the contact lens is dislodged under the upper lid, the lid must be everted. Once the lens is located, the eyelid is allowed to assume its normal position by simply asking the patient to look up. The lens can be moved to the lower portion of the eye by applying gentle, direct pressure through the eyelid. The athletic trainer must avoid excessive pressure on the contact lens. If the contact lens is dislodged under the lower lid, the conjunctiva is exposed by pulling the lower eyelid away from the eye. The lens can be repositioned by gentle finger pressure through the eyelid or removed from the eye. Applying a small contact lens suction cup, which should be included in the athletic trainer's kit, to a rigid lens can assist in lifting the lens out. The suction cup technique is not effective with soft contact lenses, and the suction cup should never be placed on the cornea.

A rigid lens may be reinserted on the cornea, if necessary. A soft lens should not be reinserted until it has been disinfected. Once good acuity is achieved, either through replacement contact lenses or corrective glasses, the patient may return to participation.

Chemical Burns

Any chemical substance that comes into contact with the ocular surface has the potential to cause a serious chemical burn. Common chemicals that can produce serious, vision-threatening conditions and that are found in athletic training facilities include cleaning solutions or solvents, detergents, and aerosol hygiene products. Chemical compounds typically found around an athletic facility should be well labeled and kept away from areas where accidental spills and splashes can occur. Protective eyewear can prevent some splash injuries.

Signs and Symptoms

The symptoms of a chemical burn are the rapid onset of pain, a foreign body sensation, and frequently, loss of vision after contact with a chemical substance. The signs of a chemical burn of the ocular surface range from defects on the corneal surface to corneal opacification with pronounced swelling and blanching of the cornea or conjunctiva (figure 11.24).[32] Burns to the surrounding skin of the face may also occur where the substance touches it.

A radiation burn to the cornea can present with symptoms similar to those of a chemical burn. The differential diagnosis is based on the presence or absence of a history of contact with a noxious substance.

Referral and Diagnostic Tests

Any chemical burn to the eye should be evaluated by an eye care professional. Treatment must be initiated before

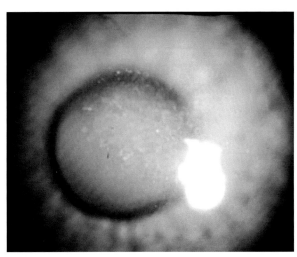

FIGURE 11.24   A chemical burn to the cornea; note the tiny white dots, which are irregularities on the corneal surface. Each dot represents a tiny corneal abrasion.

Photo courtesy of Charles B. Slonim.

transporting the patient to the nearest emergency facility. Evaluation of the eye with a chemical burn requires biomicroscopic (slit-lamp) examination, occasional assessment of the pH of the eye with test strips, and fluorescein staining of the cornea.[33]

Treatment and Return to Participation

The most important treatment for a chemical burn to the ocular surface is immediate irrigation of the eye with copious amounts of any available clean fluid or liquid. These include saline eye wash, sink or shower water, a very low-pressure water fountain or hose, or noncarbonated sports beverages. Irrigation should be performed from the nasal corner of the eye to the temporal (lateral) side of the eye whenever possible to avoid flushing the chemical into the other eye. Irrigation should continue until the eye can be assessed at an emergency facility. A cooperative patient should have the conjunctival pockets under the upper and lower eyelids swept with a moistened cotton swab and have the upper eyelid everted and irrigated. Irrigation is continued at the emergency facility until the pH of the eye has returned to normal. The patient should then be treated by aggressive lubrication with an ointment, possibly one containing a topical steroid (e.g., prednisolone, loteprednol, or fluorometholone), if significant inflammation is present.[33] Topical antibiotics should be considered if an abrasion is present. Associated complications, such as corneal damage or opacification and elevated intraocular pressure, may require further treatment.

Prognoses for chemical burns to the eye can vary widely depending on the severity of the burn and the type of chemical causing the injury. Alkali burns tend to create more serious ocular injuries than do acid burns. Most chemical burns create large corneal or conjunctival abrasions. A rapid resolution, with a rehabilitation course similar to that for a corneal abrasion, is common when irrigation is promptly initiated. However, if irrigation is delayed, vision-threatening ocular surface damage can result. Return to participation depends on the severity of the chemical burn.

Clinical Tips

Chemical Burns

A chemically injured eye must be immediately irrigated with copious amounts of clean water or saline solution. Irrigate from the nasal side to the temporal side of the eye whenever possible to avoid flushing the chemical into the nonaffected eye.

Periorbital Contusion

Direct trauma to periorbital structures (e.g., eyebrows, eyelids, cheeks) can result in localized swelling and subcutaneous hemorrhages. Periorbital contusion is commonly referred to as a *black eye*. The dark purple, or "black and blue," appearance beneath the skin of the tissues around the eye is attributable to damaged blood vessels in the skin and muscles (ecchymoses) of the eyelids and face. These hemorrhages may extend to the subconjunctival space. The collection of blood and fluid produces the discoloration as well as the swelling within the surrounding ocular tissues.

Signs and Symptoms

Anyone who suffers a periorbital contusion can present with localized pain from the initial traumatic event. Diplopia may occur. The swelling and hemorrhages can be so severe that the eyelids may be swollen shut and may prevent access to the eyeball for an appropriate examination (figure 11.25). The external signs of a periorbital contusion with hemorrhage are usually obvious to the examiner. They include facial and eyelid ecchymoses with or without tissue edema and swelling.[4] Extraocular muscle motility may be reduced as a result of severe periorbital swelling that prevents the eye from moving in all fields of gaze. An increase in the pressure around the eye or inside the anterior orbit may give the appearance that the eyeball is being pushed forward (proptosis).

The typical appearance of a black eye with bruising and swelling often worsens within 1 to 2 d after blunt periorbital trauma. Prolonged increased pressure within the orbit can damage both the optic nerve and extraocular muscle functions.

Any orbital or ocular injury resulting from blunt trauma may present with mild to severe periorbital contusions. Therefore, all potential orbital or ocular injuries (e.g., open globe, hyphema, orbital fracture) must be ruled out.

Referral and Diagnostic Tests

In the absence of any intraocular or visual damage, periorbital contusions can be treated without referral to an eye care specialist. If there are any visual symptoms or evidence of intraocular injury, the patient is referred to an eye care specialist for a complete ophthalmic examination.

Treatment and Return to Participation

In the absence of intraocular or visual damage, conservative therapy, consisting of ice compresses for the first 48 h followed by warm compresses until the ecchymoses have resolved, typically results in resolution within 1 to 2 wk. Pain can usually be controlled with non–aspirin-containing analgesics.

Most periorbital contusions resolve spontaneously and uneventfully. Most patients without visual complaints or increasing or persistent pain can return to participation in sports or work as long as the swelling of the periorbital tissue does not compromise their vision.

Traumatic Iritis

Traumatic iritis refers to an inflammation of the iris secondary to blunt traumatic injury to the eye. This term is

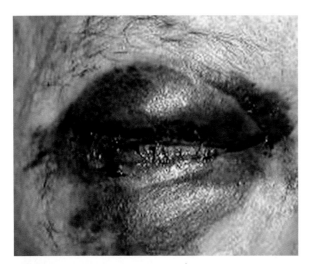

FIGURE 11.25 A severe periorbital contusion. An examiner would not be able to do an appropriate examination of the eye because the eyelids are swollen shut.

Photo courtesy of Charles B. Slonim.

 RED FLAGS FOR CONDITIONS FOR IMMEDIATE REFERRAL

- Persistent blurred vision
- Diplopia
- Restricted eye movement
- Hyphema
- Distorted pupil
- Unilateral pupil dilation or constriction
- Foreign body protruding into the eye
- Large lacerations of the eyelids
- Lacerations that involve the margins of the eyelid
- Persistent floaters

often used to refer to an inflammation within the anterior chamber of the eye. The many nontraumatic causes of iritis are related to various medical and ocular conditions.

Signs and Symptoms

Inflammation of the iris or anterior chamber of the eye is associated with a dull, deep, aching pain when either the iris or pupil moves. The most common symptom of traumatic iritis is **photophobia** or pain when light is shone into the eye. This results from the constriction and movement of the pupil and iris when stimulated by a direct light source. Traumatic iritis can occur 1 to 7 d after the initial trauma.[34] In addition to a mild to marked sensitivity to light, the patient may also complain of decreased vision, different-sized pupils (traumatic mydriasis), or a red eye with the redness forming a ring just outside the edge of the cornea. A definitive diagnosis is difficult without a slit-lamp biomicroscope.

In the presence of blunt ocular trauma, light sensitivity is caused by traumatic iritis until proven otherwise. Other ocular injuries associated with blunt trauma (e.g., corneal abrasion, hyphema, retinal detachment) need to be ruled out through a complete ophthalmic examination.[4]

Referral and Diagnostic Tests

An eye care specialist must evaluate for suspected traumatic iritis. The diagnosis of iritis can only be made under the high magnification of a slit-lamp biomicroscope. In iritis, microscopic inflammatory white cells can be seen floating in the aqueous humor within the anterior chamber of the eye. These cells can plug the outflow tract of the aqueous humor, causing the intraocular pressure to rise (secondary glaucoma).

Treatment and Return to Participation

The treatment of traumatic iritis involves preventing the iris from moving and reducing the internal ocular inflammation. Dilation and temporary paralysis of the pupil with mydriatic drops (e.g., cyclopentolate) will typically alleviate the photophobia. Topical ophthalmic steroid drops, such as prednisolone and loteprednol, are used to reduce the anterior chamber inflammation. Depending on the severity of the inflammation, the treatment may last 2 to 4 wk. The topical steroid must be tapered to prevent a rebound of the inflammatory response. On occasion, additional drops (e.g., brimonidine, timolol) to treat secondary glaucoma may be necessary.[15]

The prognosis for traumatic iritis is excellent. Improvement of symptoms begins as soon as the pupil is dilated. Reduction of the internal inflammation often occurs within 5 to 7 d. Eyedrops are discontinued once the inflammation is resolved. The patient should receive a thorough eye examination within 1 mo of symptom resolution to check for other, subtle signs of anatomical damage from the blunt trauma. Patients can return to participation once the inflammation has subsided.

Proptosis

Direct trauma to the orbit can result in deep orbital swelling and hemorrhages. Swelling that occurs behind the eye can push the eyeball forward, causing a bulging of the eye from between the eyelids (figure 11.26). This is called **proptosis**, or **exophthalmos**. Swelling and hemorrhages behind the eyeball can cause direct damage to the optic nerve by compromising its blood supply. This same swelling can put pressure on the outside of the eyeball, which can subsequently increase the pressure inside the eye (secondary **glaucoma**).[34] The hemorrhages may extend to the subconjunctival space.

Signs and Symptoms

Patients who suffer from traumatic proptosis often present with a bulging eye. The patient may complain of diplopia. Often the patient also complains of pain and possibly nausea. Extraocular movements may be significantly reduced or absent. The eyelids may not close all the way (**lagophthalmos**), or there may be a severe subconjunctival hemorrhage that protrudes between the eyelids. Eyelid ecchymoses are not uncommon. These may not be evident for a day or two after the injury. Prolonged increased pressure within the orbit can damage both the optic nerve and extraocular muscle functions.

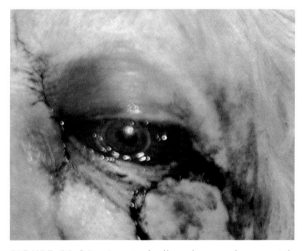

FIGURE 11.26   A retrobulbar hemorrhage with proptosis.

Photo courtesy of Charles B. Slonim.

In the presence of blunt trauma, proptosis may also be caused by significant orbital ecchymoses originating from a sinus as a result of an orbital fracture. All potential orbital or ocular injuries, including open globe, hyphema, and orbital fracture, must be ruled out.

Referral and Diagnostic Tests

Protrusion of the eye after blunt trauma must be referred immediately to an eye care specialist. A patient with a suspected orbital hemorrhage requires orbital imaging studies. Either a CT or magnetic resonance imaging scan of the orbit with both coronal and axial views should be performed. It is also important to examine the eye for potential intraocular injuries, such as retinal detachment, hyphema, and open globe injury.

Treatment and Return to Participation

In the absence of any intraocular or visual damage, conservative therapy consisting of ice pack application for the first 24 to 48 h, ocular lubricants to protect the cornea from drying out, and careful observation may be all that is required. Pain can usually be controlled with non–aspirin-containing analgesics. In the presence of any intraocular or visual damage, orbital decompression surgery may be required to preserve vision.[23,35] Systemic (e.g., acetazolamide) and topical medications (e.g., brimonidine, timolol) to reduce intraocular pressure may be needed.

Traumatic proptosis has a guarded prognosis depending on the severity of the proptosis and damage to the ocular structures. Many cases resolve spontaneously and uneventfully, whereas others require surgical intervention. Most patients without visual complaints or increasing or persistent pain can return to participation after proptosis has completely subsided.

Protective Eyewear

Nearly 30,000 sports-related eye injuries are treated in U.S. emergency rooms each year, and the majority of such injuries occur in athletes younger than age 25 yr.[36] Basketball is the leading cause of sports-related eye injuries in the United States, followed by baseball, softball, airsoft rifles, pellet guns, racquetball, and hockey.[36] Many eye injuries sustained in athletics are permanent and are associated with serious vision loss. Appropriate eye protection reduces the risk of eye injuries by at least 90% during any sport.[37] For sports use, polycarbonate lenses must be used with protectors that meet or exceed the current sport-specific requirements of ASTM International (American Society for Testing and Materials), a global standards development organization.[38] Polycarbonate lenses are the most impact resistant, are thinner and lighter than plastic, are shatterproof, and provide ultraviolet (UV) protection. Most sports have an ASTM standard that is directed to the specific risks likely to be encountered in that sport. Look for the appropriate ASTM standard on the product and/or its packaging before making a purchase.[38]

The American Academy of Ophthalmology and Prevent Blindness both recommend specific protective eye guards or goggles with the ASTM rating listed.

- Basketball and soccer: The recommendation is F803-19.[36] When tested, both the frame and lenses must withstand projectiles sized from 40 to 65.1 mm fired at a rate of 90 mph to receive the F3164 rating. This requirement replaced the old F803 rating.
- Football: A polycarbonate visor shield can be attached to the helmet. Collegiate football players are not allowed to wear tinted shields, while National Football League players can only wear a tinted shield if there is a specific league-approved medical reason for the tint.

Clinical Tips

Choosing Protective Eye Guards

- Fit an athlete who wears prescription glasses with prescription eye guards.
- Purchase nonprescription eye guards at sport specialty stores or optical stores.
- Only "lensed" protectors are recommended for sports use.
- Fogging of lenses can be a problem for an active athlete. Some eye guards are available with antifog coating; others have side vents for additional ventilation. Antifog lens wipes can be beneficial in decreasing the amount of lens fogging.
- Look for an indication on the eye guard's packaging that it has been tested and approved for the athlete's sport. Polycarbonate eye guards are the most impact resistant.
- Make sure the eye guard is padded or cushioned along the brow and bridge of the nose. Padding will prevent the eye guard from cutting the athlete's skin during rugged sport activity.
- Adjust the eye guard straps to be secure on the face but not so tight that the eye guard is uncomfortable.

CONDITION HIGHLIGHT

Cataract

Although not as common in young athletic patients, cataracts are very common in the middle-aged and older population, and the athletic trainer may encounter a patient with a cataract or a family history of the condition. Early-onset cataracts are attributable to chronic inhaled steroids (typically used for sinus or allergy treatment) or systemic steroid use. A cataract is a clouding of the lens of the eye; it is the leading cause of blindness among people older than 55 yr. Cataracts are generally painless and usually start out as a small opaque spot or a complaint of inability to see at night because of glare. Vision is not usually affected until a larger area of the lens becomes opaque. Other symptoms include blurred vision, impaired night vision, light sensitivity, or changes in eyewear prescription. The diagnosis is determined by slit-lamp examination and retinal examination. Surgery is the only cure for cataracts, although some never need treatment. The surgical procedure involves removing the clouded lens and replacing it with a lens implant.[40]

- Hockey: A wire or a polycarbonate visor or shield is attached to the helmet. Types B1/B2 (full-face protector) and C (visor) are to be worn by persons other than goaltenders. All hockey eye and face protectors should bear the Hockey Equipment Certification Council (HECC) label.
- Field hockey: Eye guards should be approved to ASTM F2713-18.
- Racket sports (including pickleball): The recommendation is F3164-19.[38]

For patients who are functionally monocular, such as those with a history of **amblyopia** (*lazy eye*) or a history of a prior eye injury, wearing protective eyewear should be mandatory at all times during any sport participation.[37] Patients with functional vision in only one eye should consider sports other than contact sports and should not participate in sports involving high-velocity projectiles such as ball sports and hockey. Contact lenses offer no protection from eye injuries, and protective eyewear without a refractive correction should be worn over contact lenses for the best protection.

Because athletes (and coaches) spend considerable time in the sun, special consideration should be given to wearing sunglasses to decrease the effects of UV rays on the eyes. Prolonged UV exposure can contribute to cataracts, macular degeneration, and growths on the eyes. Ophthalmologists recommend wearing 99% (and higher)

UV-absorbent sunglasses and a brimmed hat when in the sun for prolonged periods of time. Just as chapter 16 discusses the importance of applying sunscreen, protecting the eyes with sunglasses is equally important.[39] The color and darkness of the lenses do not indicate their ability to block UV light. Even clear lenses can be coated to block UV. Wraparound frames are shaped to keep light from entering the eyes from the side, and sunglasses with such frames seem to be most effective in reducing the amount of UV light reaching the eyes.[39]

Summary

Athletic trainers must recognize eye conditions that require immediate attention and referral to an eye care practitioner. This chapter describes how to perform a basic examination of the eye, including tests for visual acuity and eye motility. If blurred vision is prolonged or eye motility is hindered, the patient should be referred. The patient who presents with an abnormally shaped pupil or diplopia also must be referred immediately. The athletic trainer should be skilled in the basic visualization of the internal structures of the eye and should be able to recognize abnormal conditions. The skilled use of an ophthalmoscope is necessary to visualize the internal structures of the eye. Protective eyewear is the patient's best defense against periorbital and ocular trauma.

 Apply It!

Go to HK*Propel* to complete the case studies for this chapter.

Ear, Nose, Mouth, and Throat

12

This chapter covers nontraumatic conditions of the ear, nose, mouth, and throat. Many of these conditions are common occurrences in physically active people, and the athletic trainer may have ample opportunity to see them. Clinicians must understand the anatomy and physiology discussed in this chapter and feel comfortable performing an examination of the patient. Diagnosis of these conditions can usually be made based on patient history, signs and symptoms, and caregiver observations.

Overview of Anatomy and Physiology

This section provides an overview of the anatomy and physiology of the ear, nose, throat, and mouth. Each body part is discussed independently, but the clinician must be aware of the interaction among the ears, nose, mouth, and throat, and the history and examination must address all of these areas.

Ear

The ear serves two main functions: (1) to identify, locate, and interpret sound and (2) to maintain equilibrium. It consists of three distinct parts: external, middle, and inner (figure 12.1). The external ear consists of the pinna (or auricle), the external auditory canal, and the lateral surface of the tympanic membrane. The pinna has a cartilage framework that is covered in skin, whereas the earlobe is fat covered in skin. The shape of the pinna is designed to gather or channel sound into the canal. The canal is approximately 2.5 cm long and is lined with epithelial cells, hairs, sebaceous glands, and ceruminous glands.[1] The ceruminous glands produce **cerumen**, or earwax, which lubricates the ear canal and tympanic membrane

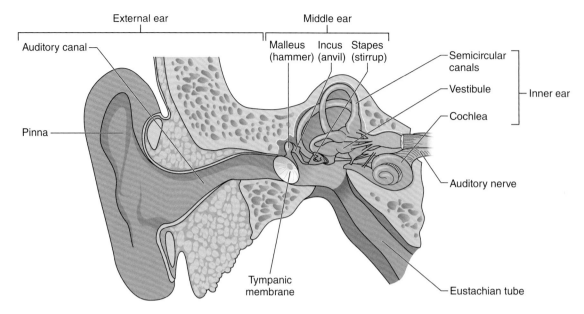

FIGURE 12.1 Anatomy of the ear.

while serving as a protective barrier against foreign matter and bacteria. The outer third of the canal is flexible where it attaches to the pinna but is rigid for the last two-thirds as it enters the skull.

The external ear and the middle ear are separated by the tympanic membrane. The translucent tympanic membrane permits visualization of the middle ear, which is an air-filled cavity in the temporal bone that contains the ossicles: the malleus, incus, and stapes. These bones transmit vibrations from the tympanic membrane mechanically to the inner ear, where the mechanical vibrations are changed to electrical signals. The middle ear is connected to the **nasopharynx** by the **eustachian tube**. This passage opens briefly to equalize pressure in the inner ear when that pressure changes with swallowing, sneezing, or yawning.[2,3]

The inner ear consists of the vestibule, semicircular canals, and cochlea. The cochlea encodes the mechanical vibrations as electrical impulses that are then sent to the eighth cranial (vestibulocochlear) nerve. The vestibule is directly responsible for balance, as the fluid in the semicircular canals shifts with head movement. Feedback from this movement is provided to the brain, helping to maintain upright posture and balance.[2]

Hearing is an interpretation of sound waves received through an air conduction path. The most efficient and normal hearing pathway is through the air conduction pathway, which produces sound from the tympanic membrane to the stapes to the basilar membrane of the cochlea. Bone also conducts sound by transmitting the vibrations of the skull directly to the inner ear and the vestibulocochlear nerve (figure 12.2).

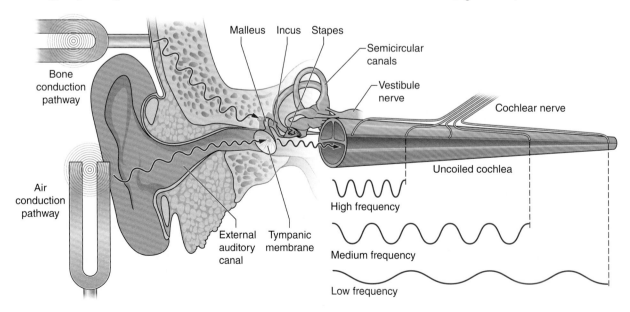

FIGURE 12.2 Pathways of hearing.

Nose and Nasopharynx

The external nose consists of bone in the proximal third of the nose and cartilage in the lower two-thirds covered by skin. The nasal bones arise from extensions of the frontal and maxillary bones, forming the nasal bridge. The hard and soft palates form the floor of the nose, and the frontal and sphenoid bones form the roof. The external nose humidifies, filters, and warms inspired air and serves as a passageway for expired air.[1]

The internal nose is divided into two anterior cavities, or vestibules, by the septum (figure 12.3). Air enters the nose through the nostrils and passes posteriorly to the nasopharynx through one of the **choanae**, separated by one of three turbinate bones. The **cribriform plate** that is part of the ethmoid bone on the roof of the nose houses the sensory endings of the olfactory nerve (cranial nerve I). A group of small, fragile arteries and veins is located on the anterior superior portion of the septum. This group of arteries and veins is called **Kiesselbach's plexus** and is often responsible for epistaxis. The **adenoids** lie on the posterior wall of the nasopharynx.

Three turbinate bones form the lateral walls of the nose. Covered by vascular mucous membrane, the turbinates separate the nose into a superior meatus, medial meatus, and inferior meatus. The turbinates help to increase the surface area for warming, filtering, and humidifying air.

The paranasal sinuses are a group of four paired air-filled spaces within the cranium.[3] They are generally named for their location in relationship to the eyes:

- Maxillary sinuses are under the eyes.
- Ethmoid sinuses are between the eyes.
- Frontal sinuses are above the eyes.
- Sphenoidal sinuses are behind the eyes.

The sinuses drain into their respective nasal cavities. The sinuses lighten the weight of the skull bones and serve as resonators for sound production. They also produce mucus from the membranes that line the sinus cavities, and this mucus drains into the nasal cavity. Because the sinus openings are narrow and occlude easily, they are a common site for inflammation.

Mouth, Oropharynx, and Throat

The oral cavity consists of the lips, cheeks, tongue, teeth, and salivary glands (figure 12.4). It functions in several capacities, including serving as a passage for food as well as the initiation of digestion by mastication and salivary secretion. The mouth and oropharynx also emit air for vocalization and expiration.

The oral cavity may be divided into the mouth and vestibule. The vestibule is the area between the buccal mucosa and the outer surface of the teeth and gums.[1] The roof of the mouth, which is formed by the hard and soft palates, separates the oral cavity from the nasal cavity. The soft palate is muscular tissue covered by mucous membrane that plays an active role in swallowing and vocal resonance. The soft palate, tonsillar pillars, tonsils, base of the tongue, and posterior pharyngeal walls make up the oropharynx. The tongue is a skeletal muscle cov-

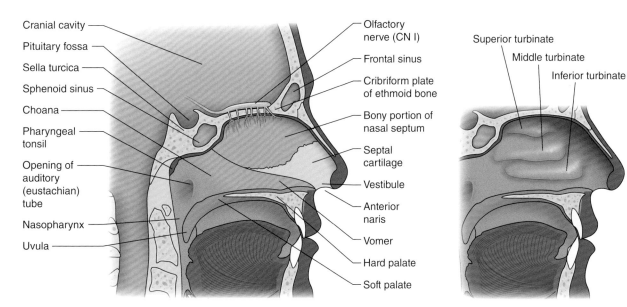

FIGURE 12.3   The nose and nasal septum.

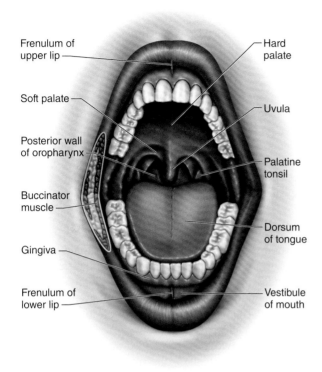

FIGURE 12.4 The anatomical structures of the oral cavity.

ered by mucous membrane, which helps to form the floor of the mouth, and is anchored to the floor of the mouth by the frenulum (figure 12.5). Papillae cover the surface of the tongue to assist in the movement of food. Taste buds are contained within the papillae, and they allow people to taste what they are consuming.

Three pairs of salivary glands are located in the mouth. The parotid, submandibular, and sublingual glands secrete saliva to moisten and lubricate food and to begin the digestive process (figure 12.6). A parotid gland lies within each cheek, just anterior to the ear; for each gland, a duct, known as *Stensen's duct*, extends to an opening on the buccal mucosa opposite the second molar. The submandibular glands lie beneath the left and right mandibles at the angle of the jaw. For each, a duct runs to the floor of the mouth, with the opening on either side of the frenulum. The sublingual glands are the smallest of the three pairs and are located under the tongue.

The teeth are embedded in the alveolar ridges and are protected by **gingivae** that cover the neck and roots of each tooth. The teeth and gums are inspected during any evaluation of the mouth. Adults typically have 32 permanent teeth that are divided into upper and lower rows (figure 12.7). Each tooth consists of enamel, dentin, and pulp (figure 12.8). The enamel is an extremely hard surface that covers the dentin. The periodontal ligament that surrounds the root of the tooth helps keep the tooth

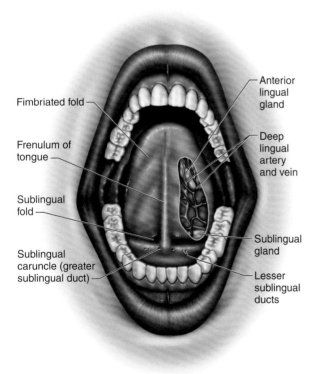

FIGURE 12.5 The ventral surface of the tongue showing anatomical landmarks.

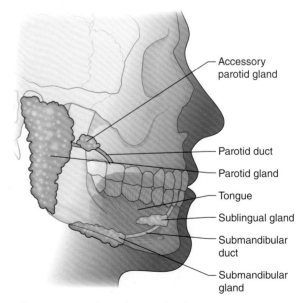

FIGURE 12.6 The salivary glands.

stable. The pulp chamber contains the pulp, nerves, and blood vessels.[1]

The pharynx consists of the combined upper parts of the respiratory and digestive tracts: the nasopharynx, oropharynx, and laryngopharynx (see figure 6.1). The larynx functions in respiration, prevents food and saliva from entering the respiratory tract, and produces sound.

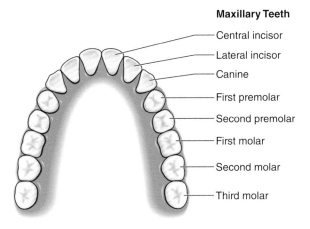

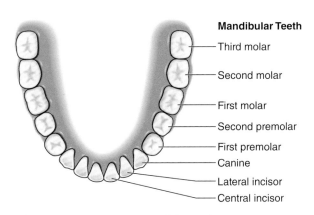

FIGURE 12.7   Permanent adult teeth.

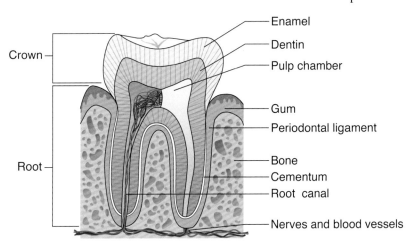

FIGURE 12.8   Anatomy of a tooth.

It is protected anteriorly by the thyroid cartilage and inferiorly by the cricoid cartilage.[2]

Evaluation of the Ear, Nose, Mouth, and Throat

Evaluation of the ear, nose, mouth, and throat is most commonly completed as a single examination because many conditions affect more than one anatomical area. For example, sinusitis may affect not only the sinuses but also the nose, ears, and throat. Often patients with sinusitis will complain of pain in their teeth. Examination of each anatomical area may reveal important signs and symptoms from which to determine a diagnosis.

Examination of the Ear

When examining the ears, the examiner begins with a general inspection of the auricle, or pinna, noting its general size, shape, and symmetry. The clinician notes any deformities or discoloration that may indicate trauma to the external ear. The examiner also looks for lesions or nodules. The ear examination includes an inspection of the external auditory canal for obvious discharge or odor. Straw-colored fluid draining from the ear after a head injury could be cerebrospinal fluid (CSF), which is indicative of a brain injury. The auricles and mastoid areas are palpated for point tenderness, swelling, and nonvisible nodules. The auricle should be firm and mobile without nodules.

The clinician conducts a gross determination of hearing when hearing loss is suspected. The patient's response to questions or directions may give a good indication of gross hearing ability. To distinguish between sensorineural and conductive hearing loss, the Weber and Rinne tests may be used (see the corresponding sidebar).

An otoscope with a disposal speculum is used to inspect the ear canal. Specula come in different sizes to conform to different-sized ears. The largest speculum that can be comfortably fit into the ear is used to allow the best view of the canal and the tympanic membrane. The otoscope is turned on by rotating the dial on top of the handle. The examiner asks the patient to tip the head slightly toward the opposite shoulder and to avoid moving during the examination.

Because the canal slopes inferiorly and forward toward the eye, the external auditory canal must be "straightened" from its S shape by pulling up and back on the pinna (figure 12.9). Otitis externa is suspected if the patient experiences

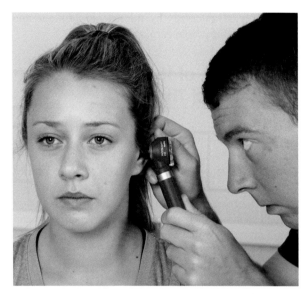

FIGURE 12.9   To view the inner structure of the ear with an otoscope, the ear canal must be straightened by pulling the pinna up and back.

pain while the examiner is pulling on the pinna. The speculum is inserted gently and slightly down and forward approximately 1/2 in. into the ear canal. The examiner places a finger or side of the hand against the cheek to guard against inserting the speculum too far into the ear.

The canal lining is lubricated with cerumen that is secreted by the sebaceous glands in the distal one-third of the canal. Cerumen often builds up in the external canal; impacted cerumen may be a cause of **otalgia** or hearing loss, and it makes examination of the tympanic membrane difficult. The skin in the external auditory canal is examined; it should be smooth and somewhat pink or "flesh" colored. The examiner looks for and notes any scaling or increased redness in the canal as well as any discharge, lesions, or foreign bodies. A reddened canal with discharge signifies inflammation or infection.

Clinical Tips

Ear Examination

- Use the largest speculum that can comfortably fit in the ear.
- Pull the pinna up and back to straighten the canal.
- Do not insert the speculum too deep.
- Expect the normal ear canal to look pink, without scaling or discharge.
- Expect the normal tympanic membrane to be pearly gray, with no perforations, bulging, or redness.

To visualize the tympanic membrane, the otoscope must be slowly moved in a circular direction, as if looking at a large area through a small window. The tympanic membrane appears translucent and pearly gray in color (figure 12.10). The translucent nature of a healthy tympanic membrane allows visualization of the middle ear cavity, including the malleus. The tympanic membrane is concave because it is pulled in at the center, or umbo, by the malleus, allowing a light reflex to be visible when it is inspected with an otoscope. The light reflex occurs as a result of the otoscope's light beam reflecting off the semitransparent tympanic membrane. It can be seen as a wedge-shaped bright spot originating from the umbo. The tympanic membrane should be free from holes or breaks and should not be bulging or bloody. These signs may indicate a tympanic membrane puncture. Abnormal findings of the tympanic membrane and their possible indications are as follows:

- Pink or red, bulging: inflammation of the tympanic membrane
- Bluish or dark color: blood behind the tympanic membrane
- White color: pus behind the tympanic membrane
- Perforations or scarring: current or previous tympanic membrane rupture

A pneumatic otoscope (which can deliver a small puff of air to the tympanic membrane) may be used to confirm the flexibility of the tympanic membrane. A tympanic membrane that is bulging because of inflammation or infection is not flaccid; rather, it is rigid when the puff of air strikes it. This is indicative of otitis media.

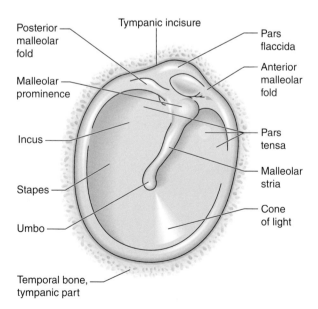

FIGURE 12.10   Anatomic landmarks of the tympanic membrane.

Weber Test and Rinne Test to Distinguish Between Sensorineural and Conductive Hearing Loss

Weber Test for Lateralization of Sound

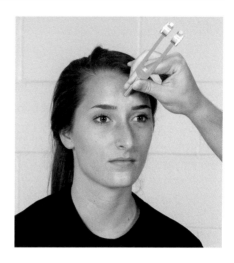

1. Hold the tuning fork at its base and tap it lightly against the palm of the hand to start its vibrations.
2. Place the tuning fork at the vertex of the patient's head.
3. Ask the patient if the sound is heard better in one ear or equally in both.

Results

- Normal finding: sound heard equally in both ears
- Conduction hearing loss: sound heard best in impaired ear
- Unilateral sensorineural hearing loss: sound identified only in normal ear

Rinne Test

1. Hold the tuning fork at its base and tap it lightly against the palm of the hand to start its vibrations.
2. Place the stem of the tuning fork against the patient's mastoid process *(a)*.
3. Ask the patient to say when the sound is no longer heard. Count the seconds until the sound is no longer heard (by bone conduction) and note the number of seconds.
4. Quickly, place the still-vibrating tines 1/2 to 1 in. from the ear canal *(b)*.
5. Ask the patient to say when the sound is no longer heard. Count the seconds until the sound is no longer heard (by air conduction) and note the number of seconds.
6. Compare the number of seconds the sound is heard through the air and when in contact with the bone.

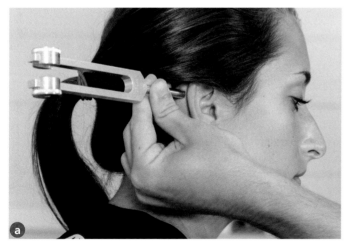
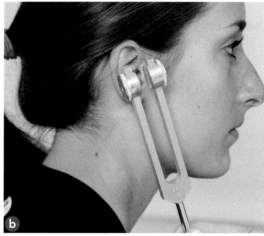

Results

- Normal finding: air-conducted sound heard twice as long as bone-conducted sound
- Conduction hearing loss: bone-conducted sound can be heard longer
- Sensorineural hearing loss: sound reduced and heard longer through the air

Clinical Tips

Nose Examination

- Use universal precautions when bleeding or discharge is present.
- Stop the epistaxis before performing an examination.
- Look for deformity of the external nose.
- Compare the sizes of the **nares** bilaterally.
- Determine the characteristics of any discharge.
- Determine the nature of any obstruction: unilateral or bilateral.
- Use a short speculum to examine the septum and nasal cavity.

Examination of the Nose and Nasopharynx

Nasal disorders may present with local symptoms, or they may result from disorders of other structures such as the paranasal sinuses. The major nontraumatic problems related to the nose are nasal obstruction, drainage, facial pain or headache, epistaxis, and change in smell or taste. A thorough history of symptoms will help the examiner to determine the nature of the nasal disorder.

The examiner asks the patient about the onset and duration of symptoms. In the case of nasal obstruction, it is important to determine whether trauma was involved or whether the onset was insidious. It is also important to determine whether the obstruction is bilateral or unilateral and whether it is constant or intermittent. Assessment of inspiratory and expiratory airflow is done by occluding one nostril at a time while the patient inspires (figure 12.11).

Unilateral obstruction may indicate an anatomical problem, such as a deviated septum or polyp, whereas bilateral obstruction could arise from a simple cold.[4] If drainage is present, it is helpful to determine its characteristics. Is it unilateral or bilateral? Is it clear or discolored? Clear drainage suggests **rhinitis**, either

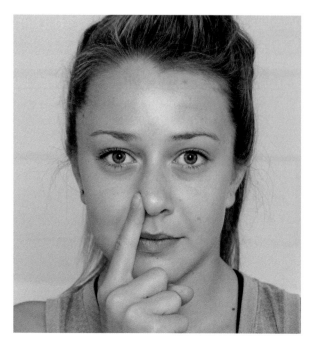

FIGURE 12.11 Determining whether an obstruction is unilateral or bilateral may be done by occluding one nostril at a time during inspiration and expiration.

allergic or nonallergic, whereas yellow, green, or brown drainage suggests bacterial or viral infection (table 12.1). Straw-colored drainage occurring after a head injury could be CSF and an indicator of possible brain injury. If discharge is present, the examiner should wear gloves for the examination.

The patient may also experience facial pain and headache. Many nasal or sinus disorders will present with headaches, but these should be differentiated from headache or face pain caused by migraine, tension headache, or temporomandibular joint (TMJ) pain. Dental disorders may also cause diffuse facial pain. When pain and swelling occur over the sinuses accompanied by purulent drainage, sinusitis may be suspected.

During or after the history, the clinician visually examines the external nose, noting its shape, size, and color. The patient is asked whether there are subtle changes in shape. Sometimes standing behind the patient and looking

TABLE 12.1 Differential Diagnoses of Nasal Conditions With Drainage

Drainage characteristics	Typical other symptoms	Conditions
Watery discharge	Sneezing, watery eyes, sore throat, facial pain, itchiness, lower airway symptoms, congestion	Allergic or nonallergic rhinitis
Purulent yellowish or greenish discharge	Sinus or upper respiratory infection	Sinusitis (bacterial or viral)
Bloody discharge	Traumatic or dry nasal mucosa	Epistaxis

down the nose while the patient is sitting allows better visualization of whether the nose is straight. Next, the nares are examined for discharge as well as any unilateral flaring or narrowing.

Palpation may reveal swelling, tenderness, or masses as well as any displacement of bone or cartilage. The patency of the nares is evaluated by gently squeezing them together. Unilateral variations may indicate a deviated septum or polyp in the nose. One must remember that recent trauma may cause ecchymosis and edema of the nose and surrounding areas as well as localized tenderness.

The examiner palpates the facial bones and the sinuses to determine any areas of tenderness, swelling, or deformity. The facial areas over the frontal sinuses are palpated by pressing upward beneath the patient's supraorbital ridge (figure 12.12*a*). The maxillary sinuses are palpated by pressing with thumbs up under the zygomatic process (figure 12.12*b*). Healthy sinuses are not generally tender to the touch, and pain with palpation of the facial bones over the sinuses often indicates inflammation from infection or allergy.

Transillumination

The sinuses also may be transilluminated. Transillumination is often performed by the physician, but the athletic trainer may want to try the technique. Transillumination is done in a darkened room, using a penlight or an otoscope.

The frontal sinus may be transilluminated by placing a light against the medial aspect of each supraorbital rim while looking for a slight red glow of light just above the eyebrow.[1] The absence of a glow in the sinus indicates that the sinus contains secretions. Likewise, the maxillary sinus may be illuminated by placing the light lateral to the patient's nose beneath the medial aspect of the eye while asking the patient to open the mouth. If the sinus is clear, the hard palate will be illuminated.

Speculum Examination

To view the septum and turbinates, the examiner tips the patient's head slightly backward. The nares may be dilated and viewed using a speculum and a light, or the speculum on an otoscope may be used. The speculum is held in one hand while the other guides the patient's head.

The septum may be visualized by tipping the speculum toward the midline (figure 12.13). The septum is normally pink and glistening, and it should be thicker anteriorly. The examiner checks for any discoloration, perforations, bleeding, or crusting and notes differences such as polyps, holes, swelling, or abnormal coloring.[3] The septum should be straight and positioned close to the midline. To determine the position of the septum, it is best to compare sides bilaterally, ensuring that the space between the lateral wall of the nose and the septum is the same in both nostrils.

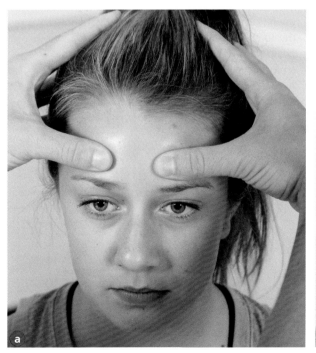

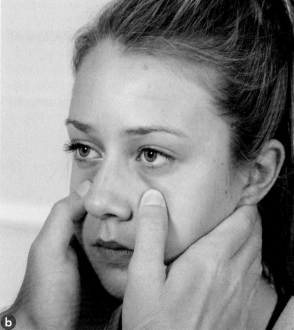

FIGURE 12.12   Palpation. *(a)* Frontal sinuses. *(b)* Maxillary sinuses.

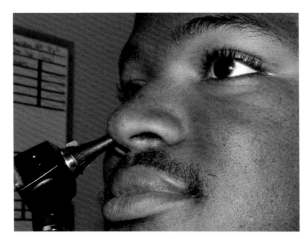

FIGURE 12.13 The septum is examined with an otoscope equipped with a nasal speculum.
© Micki Cuppett

After the integrity of the septum is determined, the vestibule and the turbinates can be visualized with the patient's head erect. The examiner tilts the patient's head backward to see the middle meatus and middle turbinates (figure 12.14). The turbinates should be pink, moist, and free of any lesions or discolorations.

Examination of the Mouth and Throat

The assessment of the mouth and oropharynx starts with an inspection of the face, head, and neck. The face, ears, and neck are observed, noting any asymmetry or changes on the skin. The neck is palpated, with the examiner paying special attention to the hyoid bone, thyroid cartilage, cricoid cartilage, and the thyroid gland. Special attention should be paid to the size of the various glands in the face and neck, including the parotid glands in the cheeks over the mandible, the submandibular glands that lie beneath the mandible at the "angle" of the jaw, and the thyroid gland. During palpation, the examiner should also note swelling or tenderness of the lymph nodes in the neck and along the jaw. Examination continues with evaluation of the lips with the mouth both open and closed, noting the texture, color, and any surface abnormalities (figure 12.15a).

The examiner asks the patient to open the mouth and visually examines the labial mucosa and the maxillary and mandibular vestibules, noting the color and texture as well as any swelling of the mucosa or gingivae. The buccal mucosa is examined, extending from the labial commissure back to the anterior tonsillar pillar. A tongue depressor or gloved finger may be used to pull the buccal mucosa away from the teeth (figure 12.15b). The examiner notes pigmentation, color, texture, mobility, and other abnormalities of the mucosa.

The examiner inspects the buccal and labial aspects of the gingivae and alveolar ridges (processes) by starting with the right maxillary posterior gingivae and alveolar ridge and then moving around the arch to the left posterior area.[3] The inspection continues with the left mandibular posterior gingivae and alveolar ridge and moves around the arch to the right posterior area. The examiner looks for any abnormal lesions, especially white or dark pigmented areas. Stensen's duct, the opening of the parotid gland, will look like a small dimple opposite the upper second molar.[1]

With the patient's tongue at rest and the mouth partially open, the dorsum of the tongue is inspected for any swelling, ulceration, coating, or variation in size, color, or texture. The examiner visualizes the papillary pattern on the surface of the tongue, asks the patient to stick out the tongue, and notes any abnormality of mobility or positioning. Then the tip of the tongue is grasped with a piece of gauze to assist in its full protrusion and to aid in the examination of the more posterior aspects of the tongue's lateral borders. The ventral surface of the tongue is examined along with the floor of the mouth.

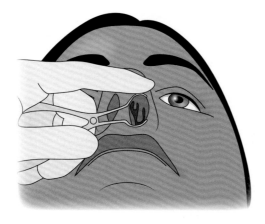
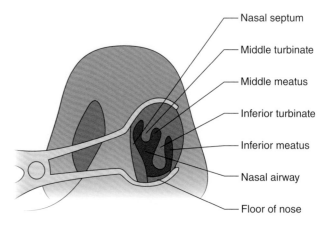

Nasal septum
Middle turbinate
Middle meatus
Inferior turbinate
Inferior meatus
Nasal airway
Floor of nose

FIGURE 12.14 The patient's head is tilted backward in order to view the nasal mucosa and middle turbinate through a nasal speculum.

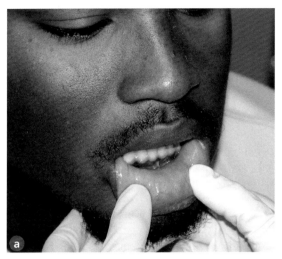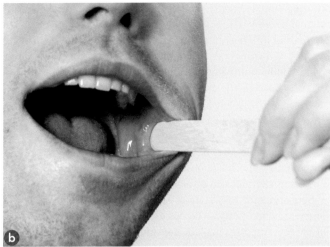

FIGURE 12.15   Inspection. *(a)* Inner oral mucosa. *(b)* Retraction of the buccal mucosa.

(a) © Micki Cuppett

The examiner is looking for changes in color, texture, swelling, or other surface abnormalities. With the mouth wide open and the patient's head tilted back, the base of the tongue is gently depressed with a tongue blade. The hard palate is examined, followed by the soft palate and oropharyngeal tissues. Movement of the soft palate may be evaluated by asking the patient to say "ah." This also tests cranial nerves IX and X, the glossopharyngeal and vagus nerves, respectively.

Clinical Tips

Mouth and Throat Examination

- Inspect the lips, noting color and lesions.
- Note any cracking of the lips that may indicate dehydration.
- Note the condition of the teeth and gums as an overall indicator of general health.
- Inspect the tongue and buccal mucosa for color, lesions, and presence of white plaque.
- Inspect the sides of the tongue for lesions.
- Use a tongue depressor to hold down the tongue to visualize the tonsils, uvula, and pharynx; redness, swelling, exudates, or spots indicate inflammation or infection.
- Palpate the mouth when indicated, being sure to wear gloves.
- Palpate the cervical lymph nodes for swelling.

Next, the oropharynx is inspected while keeping the tongue depressed with a tongue blade. The tonsillar pillars should be pink and should blend in with the integrity of the retropharyngeal wall. Hypertrophied or reddened tonsils that may be covered in exudates indicate a viral or bacterial infection. The posterior wall is normally pink and smooth, although some irregular spots of lymphatic tissue may be present. A yellowish film may indicate postnasal drip. The examiner may elicit the gag reflex at this point in the examination, which also tests the glossopharyngeal and vagus nerves.

Pathological Conditions of the Ear

Hearing Loss

Hearing loss may include the inability to hear a specific pitch or the inability to detect any sound. In 2019, Global Burden of Disease study investigators estimated that more than 1.57 billion people have some form of hearing loss. Hearing loss affects approximately one-third of adults ages 61 to 70 yr and 80% of those older than age 85 yr.[5] It is estimated that 10% to 15% of the population younger than age 60 yr has some degree of hearing impairment. However, globally only 17% of people who need hearing aids make use of them.[6] Hearing loss is not just a concern for older patients. It is estimated that the prevalence of hearing loss in children may be as high as 18% by age 18 yr.[7] The inability to detect any sound is referred to as *deafness*.

The most efficient and normal hearing pathway is through air conduction; however, bone also conducts sound. In bone conduction, the vibrations of the skull are transmitted directly to the vestibulocochlear nerve (cranial nerve VIII).[2]

Hearing loss may be divided into two types: conductive and sensorineural. In conductive hearing loss, the sound conduction pathway is blocked, and sound does not pass through the external and middle ear to reach the inner ear. It is considered a mechanical dysfunction because the person can hear if the sound is amplified enough. A buildup of impacted wax, injury, foreign body, or infection in the external ear can cause conductive loss. Otitis media, sinus infections, small or blocked eustachian tubes, and allergies can also cause conductive loss.[7]

Sensorineural loss is more serious and involves the inner ear, where sensory receptors convert sound waves into neural impulses that are transmitted to the brain for translation. Most people who are born Deaf have this type of loss. Causes of sensorineural loss are generally idiopathic. Other identified causes include hereditary factors, meningitis, measles, scarlet fever, mumps, and encephalitis. Hearing loss caused by gradual nerve degeneration, known as **presbycusis**,[7] often occurs with aging and may cause the person to be unable to understand words. Simple amplification of sound will not increase the ability to hear in cases of sensorineural hearing loss. Balance problems may also accompany this type of loss. A patient who has hearing loss with additional symptoms of vertigo and tinnitus requires follow-up, as these symptoms may be indicative of a more serious condition such as Ménière's disease.[8] A combination of both conductive and sensorineural hearing loss in the same ear is called a *mixed hearing loss*. If hearing impairment is suspected, the patient should be referred as soon as possible for proper diagnosis and treatment. Treatment depends on the cause of the hearing loss.

Signs and Symptoms

Patients with hearing loss have trouble hearing in either general or specific situations. Often patients complain of hearing loss after bathing or swimming; they may also note hearing loss associated with upper respiratory infection. It should be noted whether the patient has any pain, dizziness, vertigo, or **tinnitus**.

Referral and Diagnostic Tests

Quick tests for hearing may be performed while taking the patient's history. These include observing the responses to questions spoken at different intensities. Comparing the patient's ability to hear sounds with whispering, normal conversational intensity, and shouting gives rough estimates of the amount of hearing loss. Additional tests include the Rinne test and the Weber test to differentiate between conductive and sensorineural hearing loss.[1] Audiometry may be performed by an audiologist to determine the extent of the hearing deficit.

Treatment and Return to Participation

Prognosis and return to participation after hearing loss are usually determined by the cause of the hearing deficit. Treatment of the condition responsible for the hearing loss may return the hearing to normal.

Prevention of hearing loss largely depends on preventing exposure to situations that may cause damage to the ear: sharp objects in the ear that may perforate the tympanic membrane, extremely loud noises, blows to the ear, and excessive buildup of cerumen. Because some hearing loss is congenital or occurs with age, there is no definitive method of prevention.

Otitis Externa

Otitis externa is an inflammation or infection of the external auditory canal and tympanic membrane (figure 12.16). Subgroups include acute localized otitis externa (furunculosis), acute diffuse bacterial otitis externa (swimmer's ear), chronic otitis externa, eczematous otitis externa, fungal otitis externa (otomycosis), and, rarely, invasive or necrotizing otitis externa.[9] Otitis externa occurs in 4 of every 1,000 Americans each year, and this incidence is higher during the summer months. The condition is more prevalent in people with narrow inner ear canals or with ear canals that slope downward more than normal. Because prolonged water exposure causes tissue swelling and oozing, otitis externa is a common malady seen in swimmers and others involved in water sports. Eczema, seborrhea, or psoriasis may also be present. Excessive cleaning of the external auditory canal may also contribute to otitis externa by removing the canal's protective cerumen.[10] A normal acidic balance in the external canal maintains the level of *Pseudomonas aeruginosa* that is present in virtually all auditory canals. When the epidermal barrier is compromised, the

RED FLAGS FOR HEARING LOSS

- Blood or pus coming from the ear
- Sudden onset or rapidly progressive hearing loss
- An unexplained conductive hearing loss
- Evidence of traumatic deformity of the ear or ruptured tympanic membrane
- Dizziness or vertigo
- Tinnitus

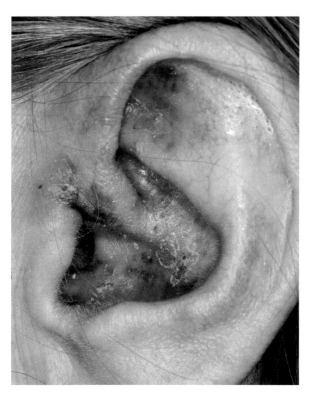

FIGURE 12.16   Otitis externa.

Dr P. Marazzi / Science Source

pH protection is lost, and the *Pseudomonas* organisms proliferate, causing serous exudates.[10]

Signs and Symptoms

Signs and symptoms of otitis externa include pain, itching, or burning with possible drainage. The external auditory canal will be edematous and erythematous, perhaps causing narrowing of the canal. Scaling or crusting of the canal's epithelial cells and an apparent absence of cerumen may be noted. Pulling on the pinna will increase pain in a person with otitis externa. The patient may present with inflammation outside the ear canal as well. This is typically cellulitis and not otitis externa. With otitis externa, the middle ear is generally not involved, and the patient will not have systemic symptoms, such as fever or chills. Acute otitis externa should be distinguished from acute otitis media, impacted cerumen, cellulitis, and ruptured tympanic membrane. The telltale symptom of otitis externa that is not present with middle ear problems is the pain the patient experiences when the pinna is pulled. Other conditions to consider are herpes zoster and foreign bodies in the ear.[9]

Referral and Diagnostic Tests

A thorough history and physical examination are typically the primary diagnostic tests. Cultures are gener-ally ordered only when the patient is not responding to treatment.

Treatment and Return to Participation

Treatment typically includes the application of ear drops, three or four times daily. The drops may contain an acidifying agent, such as aluminum acetate or vinegar, and a drying agent, which is often isopropyl alcohol. Many ear drops also contain broad-spectrum antibiotics or topical steroids. The efficacy of topical antibiotics and steroids in the treatment of otitis externa has been debated; however, oral antibiotics may be appropriate for swimming athletes.[10] Treatment with ear drops usually cures acute otitis externa in 1 to 2 d. Chronic conditions take much longer—that is, weeks or even months. Oral analgesics may be used for pain. Some physicians advocate application of a hot pack to the side of the face for its soothing properties.

Patients, other than those in water sports, may participate in vigorous activity and athletics as symptoms allow, provided the head stays dry. Aquatic athletes with otitis externa are kept out of the pool until they have completed at least 24 h of antibiotics. Persistent or recurrent otitis externa may require the swimming athlete to discontinue in-pool training for longer. When the patient is restricted from the pool, on-land exercises, such as weight training or conditioning, may be continued. Mild infections may be treated with rubbing alcohol or a mixture of alcohol and vinegar. Creating a more acidic atmosphere will prevent the growth of bacteria.[4]

Prevention

Although recurrent otitis externa is not completely preventable, several measures may help reduce its occurrence. Swimming in potentially contaminated waters, such as lakes or rivers, increases the incidence of otitis externa compared with swimming in a chlorinated pool. The ear canals should be emptied of water and dried carefully after swimming or bathing. Self-inflicted trauma to the ears, such as using cotton swabs or inserting objects into the canal, should be avoided. Frequent washing of the ears with soap may leave an alkaline residue in the ear canal, thereby reducing the normally acidic pH of the canal. Application of acidifying ear drops after swimming to help dry and acidify the ear is helpful for patients who are susceptible to recurrent otitis externa.

Otitis Media

Otitis media is the presence of fluid in the middle ear accompanied by signs and symptoms of infection (figure 12.17). It is the second most common childhood disease (following upper respiratory infection), with a peak incidence between 6 and 36 mo and between 4 and 6 yr. Otitis media often recurs, with more than one-third of children experiencing more than six episodes before age 7 yr.[11,12] The incidence of otitis media decreases dramatically with age, and it occurs infrequently in adults.

Otitis media often occurs simultaneously with an upper respiratory infection or other viral respiratory infection, such as severe acute respiratory syndrome coronavirus 2, and can be caused by a virus or bacteria. Common bacterial sources for otitis media are *Streptococcus pneumoniae* and *Haemophilus influenzae*.[9,13] Although otitis media is any inflammation of the middle ear without reference to pathology, the most important factor in recurrent otitis media is a dysfunctional eustachian tube.

Signs and Symptoms

Common signs and symptoms of otitis media include otalgia (earache), fever, a feeling of fullness in the ear, dizziness, tinnitus, headache, and diminished hearing. The diagnosis of acute otitis media can only be made when the following are simultaneously present: acute onset of otalgia, signs of tympanic membrane inflammation, and presence of middle ear effusion (MEE). Fever is reported in about 50% of patients with acute otitis media.[13] The young child will often pull or rub the affected ear, with the otalgia increasing when the child is lying down. Rubbing or pulling of the ear alone is not specific enough for a diagnosis of acute otitis media without the other presentations cited earlier.

The primary differential diagnoses for otalgia are otitis media, otitis externa, and TMJ dysfunction. People with TMJ problems typically do not have hearing difficulties,

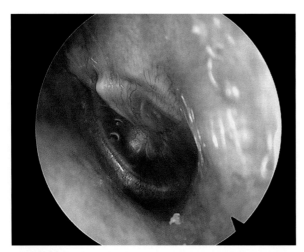

FIGURE 12.17   Otitis media.

Professor Tony Wright, Institute of Laryngology & Otology / Science Source

and physical examination should rule out otitis externa. As noted next, the location of patient-reported ear pain is a clue to its cause.

External Auditory Canal

- Otitis externa
- Auricular hematoma
- Foreign body in the ear
- Obstructive cerumen

Middle Ear

- Acute otitis media
- Chronic otitis media
- Ruptured tympanic membrane

Referred Pain

- Temporomandibular joint dysfunction
- Inflammation from the nasopharynx, larynx, or pharynx

Referral and Diagnostic Tests

Otitis media may be confirmed by physical examination with an otoscope. Visualization of the tympanic membrane may be difficult and painful in the otalgic ear, but the tympanic membrane will appear erythematous, bulging, and perhaps more opaque than normal. Pneumatic otoscopy will reveal less mobility in the tympanic membrane and is considered the standard examination technique for patients with suspected otitis media. Unfortunately, visualizing the entire tympanic membrane is difficult and requires a clean ear canal. Most children have considerable cerumen buildup in the external auditory canal, especially in the otalgic ear. Otomicroscopy has been used to increase the sensitivity and specificity of acute otitis media diagnosis. It shows an enlarged view and binocular viewing, which permits depth perception, complete evaluation of the tympanic membrane, and, when needed, easier cerumen removal.[13] A Weber test will confirm conductive hearing loss in the affected ear. The patient is referred to a physician for treatment as soon as possible.

Treatment and Return to Participation

The physician will often prescribe a broad-spectrum antibiotic, such as amoxicillin, for otitis media. However, because of growing concern regarding antibiotic-resistant strains of bacteria, the American Academy of Pediatrics currently recommends that the clinician treat the pain on the first visit and observe the condition to determine whether it meets criteria for acute otitis media before prescribing antibiotic therapy. If all three conditions for acute otitis media are present (acute onset, presence of MEE, and signs or symptoms of middle ear inflammation), then antibiotic therapy is recommended for any patient older than age 2 yr. Amoxicillin is still the most used antibiotic for acute otitis media, but a cephalosporin or erythromycin may be used for patients with penicillin allergy. There is a significant difference in revisits or recurrence of acute otitis media if patients are treated with antibiotics within the first 3 d.[14] Chapter 4 provides more information about antibiotics. Antihistamines and decongestants have not proven beneficial for managing otitis media.

After resolving the discomfort that accompanies otitis media, the patient who is afebrile may return to participation. Air travel should be avoided until the middle ear has returned to normal appearance and function, because of the increased risk of ruptured tympanic membrane from pressure changes on ascent and descent. If antibiotic treatment does not improve symptoms within 72 h, then high-dose antibiotics are indicated. Complications of acute otitis media are uncommon but are best recognized early and treated aggressively. These complications may include meningitis, facial nerve paralysis, and neck infection.[13]

Prevention

Avoidance of situations that introduce bacteria into the ear may help decrease the occurrence of otitis media. Aggressive treatment and prevention of upper respiratory infection may also reduce the risk, as seen during the COVID-19 pandemic when mitigation efforts were stressed to prevent infection. During that time, the incidence of acute otitis media decreased significantly.[13] The efficacy of prophylactic antibiotic treatment for upper respiratory infection for those who are susceptible to otitis media is debatable.

Ruptured Tympanic Membrane

A ruptured tympanic membrane, or tympanic membrane perforation (TMP), may occur when there is a sudden change in air pressure caused by blunt trauma or an infection that inhibits the ability to regulate inner ear pressure.[15] Infection is the principal cause of TMP. The increasing pressure in the middle ear often causes extreme pain before rupture. Sticking a sharp object, even a cotton swab, in the ear may also rupture the membrane, as can incorrect irrigation of the ear canal.

Signs and Symptoms

Signs and symptoms of TMP include audible whistling sounds and decreased hearing. Leaking of purulent fluid

or bleeding from the ear may be noted. TMP may be painless if not accompanied by infection, typically otitis media. The hearing loss is more severe if the ossicular chain is disrupted or the inner ear injured. Vertigo may be present if the inner ear is injured.

Other causes of hearing loss, otalgia, and **otorrhea** should be ruled out, including otitis media, impacted cerumen, otitis externa, or infectious myringitis. A TMP can usually be visualized with an otoscope, thus differentiating it from other ear conditions.

Referral and Diagnostic Tests

Radiography and magnetic resonance imaging are usually of no use in uncomplicated TMP and are typically not performed. TMP is usually diagnosed based on simple history, physical examination, and otoscopy. The presence of a hole or perforation in the tympanic membrane is often visible on examination (figure 12.18). In the absence of an obvious perforation, a **tympanogram** may be performed to determine tympanic membrane integrity. Audiometry is typically performed by the physician to determine the amount of hearing loss and is particularly relevant before any attempt at repair.

Treatment and Return to Participation

The tympanic membrane tends to heal itself, and even eardrums that have been perforated multiple times often remain intact. Larger perforations may take 3 to 6 mo to heal. Patients with a small perforation tend to heal quickly, but the injury must be protected from water and debris.[15] Over-the-counter analgesics may be needed during the initial healing stages if the patient is in pain. If the TMP was caused by an infection, the physician will generally prescribe drying agent drops as well as topical and oral antibiotics.

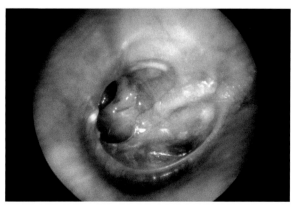

FIGURE 12.18   View of a large tympanic membrane perforation.

Professor Tony Wright, Institute of Laryngology & Otology / Science Source

Larger or complicated ruptures may require surgery by an **otolaryngologist** and involve a graft of surgical paper, fat, muscle, or other material.[15] These procedures are usually done in the office with the patient under local anesthesia.

The prognosis for small, uncomplicated perforations of the tympanic membrane is good and should result in minimal time lost, especially in the nonswimming athlete. Larger or multiple perforations may cause scarring of the tympanic membrane and some resultant hearing loss.[16] Divers may be held out of activity longer than swimmers because of the combination of water and pressure changes associated with the sport. Patients with TMP are more susceptible to middle ear infections, and they must take special care to keep the ear dry until it heals.

Prevention

Prevention of TMP includes keeping foreign objects out of the ear, such as sharp objects or cotton-tipped applicators that are inserted too deeply. Treating otitis media aggressively to reduce pressure on the tympanic membrane will also reduce the chances of TMP. The patient with otitis media also needs to avoid sudden altitude changes resulting in pressure from air or water. A TMP from a blow to the external ear may be unavoidable unless head or ear protection is worn.

Pathological Conditions of the Nose

Allergic Rhinitis

Allergic rhinitis is an immunoglobulin E–mediated response to nasally inhaled allergens that causes sneezing, **rhinorrhea**, nasal pruritus, and congestion.[17] This condition affects 10% to 20% of the U.S. population.[9] Seasonal allergic rhinitis occurs in the spring, summer, and fall and is triggered by pollen, ragweed, or grasses. Perennial rhinitis occurs daily and is typically triggered by dust, animal allergens, smoke, detergents, or soaps. Although allergic rhinitis is common, its effect on performance and daily activities should not be underestimated.

Signs and Symptoms

Allergic rhinitis presents with clear nasal discharge and sneezing, nasal congestion, cough, and a sensation of plugged ears, accompanied by itchy, watering eyes. The mucosa of the turbinates may appear pale from venous engorgement. The throat may appear erythematous from postnasal drip.[9]

Allergic rhinitis must be distinguished from viral, bacterial, or fungal rhinitis and from influenza. Septal obstruction must also be ruled out as a cause of nasal congestion. In addition, rhinitis medicamentosa from cocaine use or excessive nasal drop use should be considered.

Allergic rhinitis can be associated with several comorbid conditions, including asthma, atopic dermatitis, and nasal polyps. Uncontrolled allergic rhinitis can worsen the inflammation associated with these disorders.[18]

Referral and Diagnostic Tests

Diagnostic tests are often unnecessary; however, a detailed medical history is useful in identifying the irritating allergen. Temperature may be taken to confirm that the patient is afebrile. A patient with chronic symptoms that affect athletic or job performance should be referred to a physician, especially if over-the-counter medications have not been effective in the past.[9] If symptoms persist for more than 7 d, the patient should be referred to a physician. Some patients may benefit from allergy testing.

Treatment and Return to Participation

Optimal treatment includes allergen avoidance and pharmacotherapy. Second-generation antihistamines (loratadine, fexofenadine, or cetirizine) are readily available over the counter, generally control symptoms, and have fewer adverse effects than first-generation antihistamines. Fluticasone proprionate, an over-the-counter intranasal corticosteroid, may be used as a first-line treatment for allergic rhinitis with symptoms that affect patient quality of life. Targeted symptom control with immunotherapy should be considered for patients with moderate or severe persistent allergic rhinitis that does not respond to usual treatment. Chapter 4 provides a more complete description of antihistamines.

One must not underestimate the effectiveness of eliminating or reducing the allergen. Dust allergens may be the easiest to control, as several types of filters are readily available. Studies have not found any benefit to using mite-proof impermeable mattresses or pillow covers.[17] Most patients experience considerable relief by avoiding the allergens and properly using medications. Patients may participate in sports as they are able. Avoidance of the irritating allergens is the best form of prevention for patients with allergic rhinitis. Air conditioning, indoor humidity maintained below 50%, and air filter use may also be helpful.

Nonallergic Rhinitis

Nonallergic rhinitis is characterized by nasal congestion, rhinorrhea, sneezing, and/or posterior nasal drainage and can be either inflammatory or noninflammatory.

Inflammatory causes include postinfectious rhinitis and rhinitis associated with nasal polyps. Noninflammatory causes include vasomotor rhinitis, infection, or medication-induced rhinitis or may be occupational, hormone related (e.g., pregnancy), or systemic disease related.[19] Regardless of the cause, rhinitis causes excessive production of mucus, resulting in nasal congestion and mucous discharge. Infectious rhinitis is most commonly caused by rhinovirus, adenovirus, and parainfluenza virus. Vasomotor rhinitis symptoms are exacerbated by changes in temperature and humidity or exposure to hot and cold foods. Drug-induced rhinitis is termed *rhinitis medicamentosa* and results from cocaine use, excessive nasal drop use, or other medications. Patients may also experience rhinitis only at work; this is deemed *occupational rhinitis* and is caused by an inhaled irritant. Patients may also exhibit rhinitis only during hormonal changes, such as puberty, pregnancy, or the introduction of hormone therapy. Gustatory rhinitis occurs after eating, particularly with hot and spicy foods.

Signs and Symptoms

Nonallergic rhinitis is similar to perennial allergic rhinitis, with symptoms of nasal obstruction, clear rhinorrhea, sneezing, watery eyes, and pruritus of the nose, eyes, and palate, but it fails to show responses on allergy testing. Nonallergic rhinitis is differentiated from allergic rhinitis, sinusitis, nasal obstruction, nasal polyps, and noninflammatory rhinitis. Many nasal conditions result in rhinorrhea. Yellow or brown discharge accompanied by a fever indicates a bacterial condition and not rhinitis (see table 12.1). Rhinitis typically resolves in 7 to 10 d if viral.

Referral and Diagnostic Tests

The patient is referred to a physician for further evaluation if the symptoms persist for more than 7 d. The patient's temperature may be taken to rule out a fever. Allergy tests may be performed to rule out allergic rhinitis.

Treatment and Return to Participation

Rhinitis is usually treated symptomatically with over-the-counter medications. For patients participating in athletics or working in industrial settings, second-generation antihistamines should be used because of their nonsedating properties. Decongestants and intranasal steroid spray are also used for symptom management. Patients taking antihistamines should maintain adequate hydration because of the drying effects of these medications. Rhinitis is self-limiting, and typically patients can participate in sports with few limitations.

Sinusitis and Rhinosinusitis

Sinusitis is a common respiratory illness with more than 30 million diagnoses in the United States each year.[20] **Sinusitis** is an inflammation of the mucous membrane lining of the nasal cavity or one or more of the paranasal sinuses. It is almost always accompanied by inflammation of the nasal mucosa and thus may be more correctly termed *rhinosinusitis*. Sinusitis may be acute, subacute, recurrent, or chronic and occurs when mucus or other infectious material causes blockage within the passageways connecting the sinuses to the nasal cavity. Most cases of sinusitis are caused by bacterial infection. Acute viral infection may be preceded by infection with the common cold or influenza. This is typically followed by mucosal edema and sinus infection. The drainage of thick secretions is decreased, resulting in obstruction of the sinuses.[9] The decrease in sinus drainage results in the entrapment of bacteria in the sinuses, resulting in a secondary bacterial infection.

Signs and Symptoms

Patients with sinusitis typically present with a history of previous upper respiratory infection with postnasal drip lasting more than 7 to 10 d. Patients may experience purulent nasal discharge, facial tightness, nasal obstruction, and headache.[9] They may also complain of point tenderness over the infected sinus and toothache if the maxillary sinus is involved. On occasion, patients present with a cough that is worse at night.

Because of the facial pain associated with sinusitis, it should be differentiated from migraine headache and dental infection. Sinusitis should also be differentiated from viral or bacterial rhinitis and influenza.

Referral and Diagnostic Tests

Clinicians should refer patients with suspected sinusitis to a physician so that the diagnosis can be confirmed and pharmacological treatment started. Diagnosis is typically done through history and examination. Transillumination of the sinuses may help to confirm that the sinuses are indeed blocked. For chronic conditions that do not improve with medication, a radiological examination may be performed, but this is helpful only to rule out, not confirm, sinusitis.[21]

Treatment and Return to Participation

Symptomatic treatment can be initiated for patients with mild symptoms using analgesics, antipyretics, decongestants, or mucolytics. Saline nasal spray may help clear nasal crusts and thick mucus. The use of topical

---

CONDITION HIGHLIGHT

Sinusitis and Rhinosinusitis

Sinusitis and rhinosinusitis are very common in the United States, with more than 30 million cases diagnosed each year. The maxillary sinus is commonly involved, but the frontal sinus can also be involved in adults, whereas children tend to experience sinusitis in the ethmoid sinus. Sinusitis may be acute, subacute, chronic, or recurrent. Risk factors include allergens, smoke exposure, and air pollutants as well as anatomical anomalies, such as nasal polyps and septal deviation. Most sinusitis is viral and is called *rhinovirus* because it is mainly in the nasal passages. Other common viruses involved in sinusitis are influenza and adenovirus. Bacterial etiology includes *S. pneumoniae* and *H. influenzae*.[21] The clinician should watch for fever greater than 39 °C (102.2 °F) or visual complaints (diplopia) and severe facial or dental pain. These conditions require referral. The athletic trainer can assist with decreasing unnecessary antibiotic treatment of sinusitis and rhinosinusitis by suggesting that the patient try over-the-counter medications first and give the illness time to resolve, as opposed to sending the patient immediately to a physician.

---

decongestants, if necessary, should be short term only. Systemic decongestants may also be used to help dry up the sinuses. Because most cases of acute sinusitis have a viral etiology, they resolve within about 2 wk without pharmacological treatment. However, physicians in the United States prescribe antibiotics for this condition in 90% of patients, which contributes to the direct cost of management of this condition and recommendations that antibiotics only be used if signs and symptoms are persistent for more than 10 d or are severe for at least 3 to 4 d with fever and purulent nasal discharge.[20] Non-pharmacological treatments include air humidification, hydration, and application of hot compresses over the sinuses to help promote sinus drainage. An afebrile patient who feels well enough may be allowed to resume normal activities, including athletics. Chronic sinusitis represents a persistent low-grade infection involving the paranasal sinuses with persistent mucosal thickening and may be exacerbated by inappropriate frequent antibiotic use for sinus infections.[20] More aggressive treatment is often required for chronic sinusitis to prevent long-term complications, and surgical procedures may be needed to relieve the obstruction.

Prevention

Seventy percent of cases of acute sinusitis are caused by *S. pneumoniae* or *H. influenzae*.[21] Frequent handwashing is one of the best lines of defense when in contact with people known to have *S. pneumoniae* or *H. influenzae*, and it may drastically reduce the incidence of infection. Rapid treatment of upper respiratory tract infection may decrease the incidence of sinusitis. Not swimming in contaminated water will also reduce the incidence.

Deviated Septum

A deviated septum typically occurs from trauma, often a blow to the side of the nose. It may present with epistaxis and is often associated with nasal fracture. A deviated septum often is discovered well after the initial trauma has healed and may present with only a minor deformity or complaints of chronic nasal obstruction. Whereas figure 12.19*a* shows an obvious deviation, most septal deviations are less obvious (as in figure 12.19*b*), so the clinician needs to recognize the difference in the spacing of the nares.

Signs and Symptoms

The patient with a deviated septum typically presents with a history of trauma to the nose and initially has swelling and pain throughout the nose. There may be external nasal deformity. The patient may complain of a unilateral nasal obstruction, often confirmed on examination by visualization of the space between the septum and the lateral nasal wall on the affected and the nonaffected sides. The nasal passage will appear narrow on the side to which the septum is deviated.

Referral and Diagnostic Tests

A deviated septum may be diagnosed based on the history and physical examination. Visualization of the nasal passage will usually reveal the deviation; radiographs are inconsequential. When a deviated septum is suspected, both nasal fracture and septal hematoma should be ruled out. Other causes of unilateral nasal obstruction, such as polyps or a foreign body, must also be eliminated.

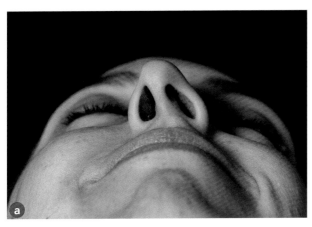 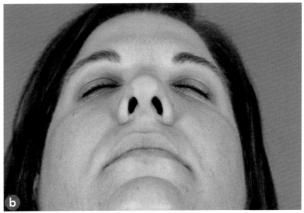

FIGURE 12.19 A septal deviation may be recognized by the difference between the spacing in the nares and the angulation of the septum. *(a)* Obvious septal deviation. *(b)* Less obvious septal deviation.

(a) JodiJacobson/E+/Getty Images

Treatment and Return to Participation

The acute treatment of nasal trauma involves stopping the epistaxis and minimizing the swelling. If considerable swelling occurs, it may be more difficult to correct the deviation by a minor surgical procedure. The patient must be seen quickly to prevent long-term complications from septal deviations.[22] Correction of a deviated septum is typically a minor elective surgical procedure that is performed with the patient under local anesthesia. If an external nasal deformity is also present, then a **rhinoplasty** may also be performed to improve both function and cosmetic appearance.

Early recognition and treatment of the deviated septum may prevent long-term complications, and the patient should be able to return to participation as soon as the septum has been reduced and healed. The physician may allow the patient to return sooner if the nose is adequately protected with a mask. If the septum is not treated expediently, the patient may have chronic unilateral nasal

RED FLAGS FOR NASAL CONDITIONS

- Unilateral blockage following trauma
- Visualization of polyps
- Visualization of deformity
- Loss of smell
- Unexplained epistaxis

obstruction later in life. The incidence of deviated septum by trauma is drastically reduced in athletes who wear facial protection. Many collision sports require facial protection; however, many traumatic nasal injuries occur in noncollision sports, in which the unprotected athlete is still at risk from contact with another athlete or with a ball, bat, or tennis racket.

Epistaxis

Epistaxis, commonly known as nosebleed, is a common occurrence among athletes and physically active individuals. It is typically associated with trauma to the nose but may occur without trauma. Epistaxis can be divided into anterior bleeds and posterior bleeds, depending on where the bleeding originates. More than 90% of all epistaxis occurs anteriorly, where Kiesselbach's plexus forms on the septum.[9] Epistaxis is often attributable to an erosion of the mucosa that causes the vessels to become exposed. Anterior bleeds from capillaries and veins provide a constant ooze rather than the profuse pumping of blood observed from an artery.

Posterior epistaxis is usually more profuse and often has an arterial origin. A posterior bleed is a more serious hemorrhage that presents a greater risk of airway obstruction and difficulty in controlling bleeding.

Signs and Symptoms

Epistaxis presents with blood coming from the nostrils. The patient generally complains of swallowing and spitting up blood. Epistaxis may result from local or systemic factors. Local causes generally occur in young children and are usually spontaneous events. Epistaxis resulting from local events is often related to nose picking, excessive blowing, sneezing, or rubbing of the nose. Recurrent bleeding may occur if a scab forms at the bleeding site and becomes dislodged. In adults, bleeding tends to be caused by external trauma to the nose,[23] or it may be caused by the previously mentioned local factors, especially in very dry or high climates, in which nasal membranes tend to dry.

Systemic epistaxis may be caused by intrinsic coagulopathies, such as hemophilia, or by acquired coagulopathies, such as blood thinner use or long-term aspirin use.[24] Hypertension is not a cause of epistaxis but may impede clotting.

It is important to determine the cause of the epistaxis. If it is caused by trauma, a deviated septum, nasal fracture, and septal hematoma must all be ruled out. If the epistaxis is recurrent, a thorough history may reveal information leading to its cause.

Referral and Diagnostic Tests

Typically, the diagnosis of epistaxis is made through the history and physical examination. A nasal speculum is used to visualize the site of bleeding once the active bleeding is slowed. Sinus radiographs are done only when tumors are suspected as the cause of the bleeding.

Treatment and Return to Participation

Management of epistaxis depends on the bleeding site, severity, and etiology. If the patient presents with active bleeding, necessary treatment may precede the normal history and palpation of a nasal examination. As in all cases in which the clinician is handling body fluids, universal precautions must be followed.

Most anterior epistaxes stop spontaneously with direct pressure applied to the nose. The patient should be encouraged to sit with the head elevated but not hyperextended, which may cause bleeding into the pharynx. Digital compression or pinching of the nose should be done for 4 to 5 min. In traumatic situations, ice should also be applied. A cotton or gauze plug may be inserted into the nose to absorb the blood.[25]

If direct pressure proves inadequate to treat an anterior bleed, gauze moistened with phenylephrine (Neo-Synephrine) or pseudoephedrine (Afrin) may be placed in the affected nostril to help promote vasoconstriction.[24,26]

For recurrent nosebleeds, conservative treatment, such as improving the humidity of inspired air, using saline nasal drops, and applying antibiotic ointments to the affected area, may be beneficial. Further evaluation by a physician should be sought to determine the etiology of the epistaxis.

Most cases of anterior epistaxis from Kiesselbach's plexus can be stopped by nasal compression and local vasoconstriction. If there is no indication of nasal fracture, septal deviation, or septal hematoma, the patient may return to participation once the nose has stopped bleeding. Because minimal aggravation can restart the bleeding, it is important to protect the patient from trauma to the nose. If possible, strenuous physical activity should be avoided when bleeding is active.

Prevention

The incidence of epistaxis may be decreased by ensuring proper humidity and hydration, especially for patients in dry environments or at high altitudes. Saline nasal drops may be helpful in reducing dryness in the nose. Additional humidification using humidifiers and vaporizers may be needed. Repeated trauma to the nose should be avoided, including foreign bodies, nose picking, and trauma in sports. Patients susceptible to epistaxis may need to wear facial protection during athletic participation.

Pathological Conditions of the Mouth and Throat

Pharyngitis and Tonsillitis

Pharyngitis is an inflammation of the pharynx and is commonly known as a *sore throat*. Tonsillitis is an inflammation of the tonsils. Both may be caused by bacteria or a virus. Pharyngitis is initially viral in most cases, but it may be followed by a bacterial infection (figure 12.20a). Tonsillitis is most caused by β-hemolytic *Streptococcus* (figure 12.20b). When caused by *Streptococcus*, pharyngitis is called *strep throat*.[27] Pharyngitis may be secondary to sinusitis, tonsillitis, smoking, or alcoholism. Because many of the symptoms are identical, pharyngitis and tonsillitis are discussed together here. Pharyngitis and tonsillitis occur equally in males and females, with peak incidence occurring in late winter to early spring.

Signs and Symptoms

Common signs and symptoms of pharyngitis and tonsillitis include sore throat, pain with swallowing, hoarseness, and possibly chills or fever. In both viral and bacterial pharyngitis, the mucous membranes may be inflamed mildly to more severely and may be covered with purulent exudates. If the pharyngitis is viral, it is usually accompanied by rhinorrhea, conjunctivitis, and cough. Bacterial infections normally present with a much higher fever and systemic signs of infection. Rapid antigen detection tests and throat cultures can be used with clinical findings to identify the inciting organism.[28] Tonsillitis (either viral

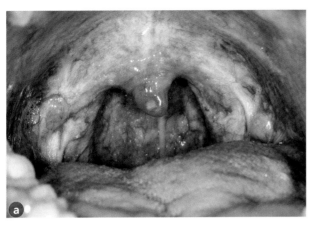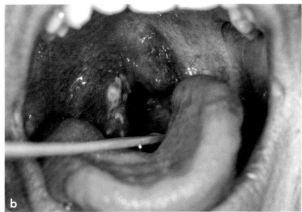

FIGURE 12.20   Examination of the mouth and throat may reveal *(a)* acute viral pharyngitis or *(b)* pharyngitis caused by *Streptococcus* (strep throat).

(a) Dr P. Marazzi / Science Source; *(b)* Scott Camazine / Science Source

or bacterial) will present with red and swollen tonsils, possibly covered in white exudates. Fever and swollen neck lymph nodes are common.

When diagnosing pharyngitis or tonsillitis, other conditions that cause throat pain and fever must be ruled out. These include upper respiratory infection, laryngitis, and influenza. Viral infections may present with rhinorrhea, conjunctivitis, and cough, whereas patients with bacterial infections will not have these symptoms.

Referral and Diagnostic Tests

The health care provider should monitor the patient's temperature. A patient with a fever or symptoms persisting for more than 5 d should be referred to a physician. If the tonsils or pharynx present with exudates on observation, the patient must be referred. It is difficult to tell from physical examination alone whether pharyngitis is viral or bacterial. A throat culture and rapid antigen tests can be conducted to determine whether the pharyngitis or tonsillitis is indeed caused by a *Streptococcus* strain.[28] A mononucleosis spot test (monospot test) may also be performed to rule out mononucleosis. Laboratory tests may also include a complete blood count with differential; a high leukocyte count supports the diagnosis of bacterial infection.

Treatment and Return to Participation

Historically, physicians have prescribed a course of antibiotics (usually penicillin or erythromycin) for 10 d to prevent complications from pharyngitis or tonsillitis. With increased use of diagnostic testing to determine the origin (bacterial or viral), unnecessary antibiotic use is decreased.[29] Nonpharmacological treatment includes consuming plenty of fluids and gargling with saltwater. Acetaminophen is often given to decrease discomfort and reduce fever. The patient should be afebrile and must be able to tolerate fluids before participating in vigorous athletic activities. Full recovery typically occurs in 7 to 14 d.[28,29] Several serious complications, such as rheumatic fever, can arise from untreated streptococcal infection.

Recurrent streptococcal infection is common and may represent reinfection from others in the living or working environment. As with other bacterial and viral conditions, frequent handwashing when in contact with people known to have the infection may drastically reduce spread and the incidence of recurrence.

Laryngitis

Inflammation of the larynx is termed **laryngitis**. It often occurs simultaneously with the common cold, bronchitis, pneumonia, or influenza, and it can be acute or chronic. Laryngitis may also be caused by direct trauma to the throat, gastroesophageal reflux disease (GERD), allergies, cigarette smoke, or excessive use of the voice. This condition is especially common in the athletic population and has been termed **cheerleader's nodules**.

Signs and Symptoms

The patient with laryngitis typically experiences a hoarse or weak voice and, in some cases, may be unable to speak. A constant urge to clear the throat or a tickling sensation may also occur. In more severe cases, fever, **dysphagia**, malaise, and throat pain may occur.[9] Edema of the larynx may cause dyspnea. Other conditions that can cause throat pain and dysphagia should be considered, including viral or bacterial pharyngitis, mononucleosis, or candidiasis. In chronic laryngitis, laryngeal tumors and papillomatosis must be ruled out.

Referral and Diagnostic Tests

The patient should be referred to a physician if symptoms do not resolve within 5 to 7 d. The physician may perform an indirect laryngoscopy that may disclose mild to marked erythema of the mucous membrane. Laryngeal cultures and biopsies may be performed if an etiology other than viral infection or irritation is suspected.

Treatment and Return to Participation

Voice rest and increased humidification through a vaporizer may help relieve symptoms. Alcohol and caffeine should be avoided because of their diuretic effect, and decongestants should be avoided because of their drying effect. Acetaminophen or other analgesics for pain may be helpful, as may other supporting treatments, such as throat lozenges or sprays. Guaifenesin may be useful as a mucolytic agent. Elimination or treatment of the irritating cause of chronic laryngitis (e.g., GERD, inhaled smoke) may decrease symptoms dramatically. Most cases of laryngitis are viral, and antibiotics are usually indicated only if a specific pathogen is isolated. Most symptoms of uncomplicated laryngitis usually resolve within a few days. Patients with laryngitis may participate in sports if they are afebrile and otherwise feel well. Chronic laryngitis is typically the result of overuse or exposure to irritants. The patient susceptible to chronic laryngitis caused by these irritants should try to avoid smoke, air pollution, and straining the voice as in cheerleading or singing.

Oral Mucosal Lesions

Lesions on the mouth and lips are common in athletics and may be caused by local trauma, infectious disease, autoimmune disorders, neoplastic disease, and toxic reactions. Identification of atraumatic oral lesions is especially important because it may allow early recognition and referral for oral cancer or infectious disease (table 12.2). Oral lesions are often the first clinical evidence of human immunodeficiency virus (HIV) infection and acquired immunodeficiency syndrome.

Oral lesions may be categorized and described based on clinical appearance, similar to skin disorders. They are often described as white or pigmented and as vesicular or ulcerated. Many oral lesions present as a white plaque and can be differentiated depending on their location. White lesions that are easily removed by wiping them off suggest candidiasis, whereas a defect that cannot be wiped away is consistent with precancerous leukoplakia or squamous cell carcinoma.

Brown- or black-pigmented macules on the oral mucosa may be caused by something as benign as localized melanin production, or they may be the sign of something much more significant, including malignant melanoma.

Oral Candidiasis

Oral candidiasis is caused by the yeast-like fungus *Candida albicans*. It is called *thrush* in infants and is the most common white lesion of the oral cavity (figure 12.21).

Signs and Symptoms

Oral candidiasis presents as a white, cheesy, curd-like patch on the tongue and buccal mucosa. It is seen most commonly in newborns, and it also may occur after antibiotic use, in immunosuppressed patients, and in association with corticosteroid treatment.

Referral and Diagnostic Tests

The white, curd-like patch characteristic of oral candidiasis can be scraped from the tongue or buccal mucosa with a tongue depressor and typically bleeds easily. If the plaque does not easily scrape off the surface, other oral lesions should be considered. In the adult with oral candidiasis, tests should be conducted for HIV infection.

Treatment and Return to Participation

Candidiasis is typically treated with an oral rinse of nystatin and oral antifungal medications. Antifungals such as fluconazole (Diflucan) are administered for 2 wk or until symptoms resolve.[9] Candidiasis can often be

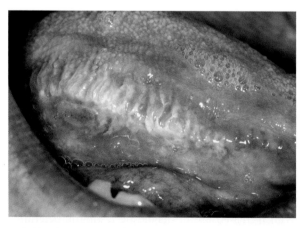

FIGURE 12.21 Candidiasis.

Dr P. Marazzi / Science Source

persistent, requiring treatment for several weeks. The patient with oral candidiasis who is otherwise in good health may participate in activities including athletics.

Oral Cancers

Oral cancer is a very serious condition and often involves the tongue, lips, and gums. This form of cancer is the sixth most common in the world and accounts for more than 400,000 new cases globally each year. Most oral cancers are oral squamous cell carcinomas (OSCCs). Although oral cancer has a poor prognosis, early diagnosis greatly increases recovery chances.[30] The many predisposing risk factors include any type of tobacco use, excessive alcohol use, poor oral hygiene, age older than 40 yr, and a family history of oral cancer. At least 75% of head and neck cancers are caused by tobacco and alcohol use.[31] Men have twice the risk of women. Smokeless tobacco use

TABLE 12.2 **Differential Diagnoses of Conditions Affecting the Oral Cavity**

Disease	Cause	Signs and symptoms	Appearance
Basal cell carcinoma of the lips	Prolonged exposure to sunlight	Lesion ulcerates, heals over, and then breaks down again; history of ultraviolet light exposure	Crusted ulcer with heaped or rolled borders
Candidiasis	*Candida albicans*	White to yellow lesions in the cheeks, at folds, and on tongue	Soft, white to yellow, slightly elevated plaques; milky curds
Gingival cyst	Developmental	Typically found on oral examination; presents as a bump	Painless nodule; normal in color; should be biopsied to rule out other lesions
Herpes simplex	Herpes simplex virus type 1	Itching, complaints of neuralgiform symptoms in prodrome, changing to pain when lesions form	Recurrent, episodic eruptions of yellowish, fluid-filled vesicles on upper or lower lip or nose
Herpes zoster infection (shingles)	Varicella-zoster virus	Extremely painful; burning pain, fever, and malaise; lesions may appear in the mouth, depending on which cranial nerve is affected	Unilateral vesicles on the buccal mucosa, tongue, uvula, pharynx, or larynx; erosions noted when vesicles rupture
Kaposi's sarcoma	HIV infection	Purplish, tender or painful nodules on mucous membranes	Purplish macules; can also be raised, nodular, or ulcerated
Leukoplakia	Multifactorial (tobacco use, trauma, lupus, irritative reactions)	Painless, white patch or plaque on surface of mucosa	White patch typically on lips, tongue, palate, floor of mouth, or buccal mucosa
Lymphoepithelial cyst	HIV infection	Presents as a parotid gland swelling	Small (<1 cm), well-circumscribed, yellow or white, soft-tissue nodule located in the floor of the mouth or ventral-lateral surface of the tongue
Squamous cell carcinoma; oral cavity, floor of mouth, or anterior tongue	Lack of specific etiology; tobacco smoking, alcohol use, and poor oral hygiene are implicated as contributors	Usually a painless ulcer unless nerves or periosteum are involved; fetid breath	Ulcerated lesion with raised borders
Thyroglossal tract cyst	Developmental	Mass or lump located at the midline of the neck	Nonpainful, movable, and fluctuant

⚑ RED FLAGS FOR EARLY SIGNS OF LIP AND ORAL CANCER

- A sore in the mouth that does not heal in 2 to 3 wk
- Any sores that are painful or bleed easily
- Any unusual lumps in the mouth
- Numbness or pain in the mouth and throat
- Persistent red or white patches on the oral mucosa
- A change in voice not associated with a cold or allergies
- Difficulty chewing or swallowing

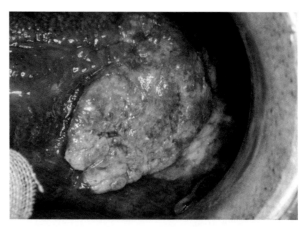

FIGURE 12.22 Oral leukoplakia on the lateral border of the tongue.

Clinical Photography, Central Manchester University Hospitals NHS Foundation Trust, UK / Science Source

increases the risk of oral leukoplakia to 5% for tobacco chewers and ranges from 29% to 63% for snuff users. The variation in the increased incidence is based on the amount used per day. The overall survival rate of patients with oral cancer is greater than 50%.[31]

Signs and Symptoms

Patients with oral cancer typically present with red or white lesions or other open wounds in the mouth. The lesions become opaquer with increased tobacco use. Patients may experience tongue swelling and dysphagia as well as abnormal taste sensation. Crusting lesions of the lips or ulcerated lesions within the mouth are prime suspects for oral cancer. Ninety percent of all oral cancer cells arise on the floor of the mouth, the ventrolateral aspect of the tongue, or the soft palate.[30] Treatment, prognosis, and return to athletic participation after oral cancer are discussed in general terms.

Leukoplakia (Keratosis)

Leukoplakia is a precancerous lesion of the mucosa and is usually found on the sides of the tongue (figure 12.22), the lower lip, and the floor of the mouth. It appears as a white patch that cannot be removed by scraping. The early keratosis caused by snuff is a ribbed, translucent white patch. The rate of occurrence of leukoplakia is approximately 1.5% to 12% in nonsmokers and more than 16% in smokers. Lesions can vary in appearance from a flat, almost translucent area to a raised, rough patch.[30] Lesions will often resolve when the user quits using tobacco or moves the tobacco to another part of the mouth. Several conditions may present as leukoplakia on the buccal mucosa, so any suspicious lesion should be

referred for biopsy. Leukoplakia, which is considered precancerous, can progress to OSCC if left untreated, with a progression rate of approximately 2% to 3% each year.[30] Treatment for leukoplakia is based on the nature of the lesion and varies depending on whether the lesion is benign or whether it exhibits malignant changes.

Oral Squamous Cell Carcinoma

OSCC is the most common type of malignant oral cancer, representing 90% of all oral cancers. It starts as a non-healing, painless, red ulceration that may grow rapidly. Light-skinned people who do not tan well are susceptible to squamous cell carcinomas on the lower lip because of prolonged exposure to the sun. Other factors associated with OSCC are as follows:

- Use of smoking tobacco
- Use of smokeless tobacco
- Infections
- Human papillomavirus (HPV) infection
- Epstein-Barr virus (EBV) infection
- Human immunodeficiency virus (HIV) infection
- *Candida albicans* infection
- Chronic irritation (e.g., dental caries, overuse of mouthwash)
- Prolonged sun exposure
- Alcohol consumption

Squamous cell carcinomas that are detected early and removed almost always have a good result. Otherwise, they may spread from the oral cavity to the cervical and submandibular lymph nodes.

Kaposi's Sarcoma

Unlike leukoplakia, **Kaposi's sarcoma** is a pigmented lesion that may be either flat or raised, and it is reddish to purple in color. It is found more often in males than females and is a common manifestation of HIV infection. Kaposi's sarcoma is initially asymptomatic, but it progresses to a painful lesion that interferes with eating and talking.

Referral and Diagnostic Tests

Other cancerous lesions, such as basal cell carcinoma and various melanomas, may also be found in and around the mouth. The reader is referred to chapter 16 for descriptions of these skin cancers. The health care provider should refer any patient with an unusual skin lesion in the mouth to a physician for biopsy. This includes any lesion that does not heal in a timely manner or that heals and then breaks down again.[32] One should be especially suspicious if multifactorial risk factors, such as alcohol use, excessive sunlight exposure, and tobacco use, are present. Judicious use of sunscreen on the lips and face must be emphasized with athletic teams, coaches, and support staff who are exposed to sunlight over a prolonged period.

Treatment and Return to Participation

Early cancers of the lips and oral cavity are highly curable by surgery or radiation therapy. The choice of treatment, as well as the prognosis, often depends on the location of the cancer, how early it is detected, and anticipated functional and cosmetic results of treatment. Treatment options include excision, curettage, cryosurgery, radiation, and some topical medications.

The extent to which the patient can participate in activity depends largely on the treatment and not necessarily on the disease itself, as often the disease goes undetected for a considerable time. For the patient being treated by radiation therapy or surgery, participation will be determined by the extent of treatment.

Dental Disease

Many conditions fall under the category of dental disease. For the purposes of this book, only gingivitis and periodontitis are discussed. **Gingivitis** is an inflammatory condition of the gums, caused by bacteria (figure 12.23). Bacteria, present in food and not removed because of inadequate brushing and flossing, produce plaque deposits, leading to gingivitis. **Periodontitis** may occur

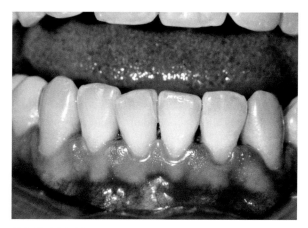
FIGURE 12.23   Gingivitis.
CNRI / Science Source

if gingivitis is left untreated. Periodontitis results in a receding gum line and loss of alveolar bone.

Signs and Symptoms

With gingivitis, the gums often appear red and swollen, and the patient will state that tooth brushing causes pain and bleeding gums.[33] The patient may also have bad breath or complain of a bad taste in the mouth. If the disease progresses to periodontitis, the patient will experience tooth sensitivity, red and swollen gums, pain and bleeding with brushing, and possibly loosening of the teeth. Gingivitis and periodontitis should be differentiated from other conditions that may cause oral pain or sensitivity to hot or cold, including gum lacerations, oral lesions, or tooth decay.

Referral and Diagnostic Tests

Patients with swollen or bleeding gums are referred to a dentist or periodontist for evaluation. Radiographs and observation of the gums will reveal the extent of the disease.

Treatment and Return to Participation

Treatment of gingivitis includes an aggressive oral hygiene program to stimulate the gingivae. This may include flossing and the use of dental picks and oral stimulators.[33] Advanced gingivitis may require treatment with antibiotics, tooth scaling, and removal of plaque below the gum line. The patient with periodontal disease may participate in sports as able. If advanced periodontitis results in loosening of teeth, the patient participating in contact sports must be cautious and use appropriate mouth guards.

Prevention

Dental disease continues to be a problem, and neglected dental hygiene may result in time lost from work or participation in athletics.[34] Prevention of periodontal disease includes frequent brushing and flossing as well as the use of antibacterial mouth rinses. Regular dental hygiene visits allow periodontal disease to be detected at an early, reversible stage.

Dental Caries

Although dental caries is a common condition, the patient will typically seek the advice and treatment of a dentist for all dental problems. Dental caries represents a multifaceted disease that involves interactions among the teeth, the normal microflora, saliva, and diet. Tooth decay occurs when bacteria in the mouth accumulate on the enamel surface to form plaque, which collects on the teeth both above and below the gum line. The plaque then produces acids that cause tooth decay. Decay starts at the enamel and may extend into the dentin and even the pulp of the tooth. If the decay is caught early, only the enamel is affected, and the condition is easily remedied. If the bacteria reach the pulp, the tooth will die, and an abscess may form near the root.[35]

Good dental hygiene and annual dental checkups will help catch dental decay in the early stages, when it can be easily treated. New dental treatments, such as early childhood fluoride and tooth-sealing treatments, have dramatically reduced the frequency of dental caries.

Signs and Symptoms

Decay will initially look white and chalky and later turn brown or black (figure 12.24). Clinically, dental caries can be classified as pit and fissure, smooth surface, cemental, or recurrent. Smooth surface caries is less common but appears as a white, "chalky" demineralization of the enamel.[35] The dental decay is often asymptomatic in the early stages; however, in advanced stages, the patient's teeth may be sensitive to hot or cold. Later stages of dental decay may also be accompanied by red, swollen gums. The patient may note a roughness on the tooth when feeling it with the tongue. If an abscess forms, the area around the tooth will be painful, and the tooth will be sensitive to heat. There will be a fluctuant mass on the buccal side of the tooth.

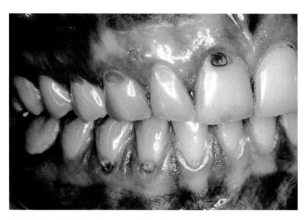

FIGURE 12.24 Teeth with decay.
CNRI / Science Source

Referral and Diagnostic Tests

All individuals need to practice good dental hygiene. A patient with poor dental hygiene should be educated about annual dental health visits and the importance of proper nutrition. A patient who presents with tooth decay can be referred to a dentist for treatment. Other conditions that may cause oral pain or sensitivity to hot or cold include gingivitis, periodontitis, fractured teeth, and oral lesions.

Treatment and Return to Participation

Treatment depends on the severity of decay. Cavities caused by mild tooth decay are repaired with fillings, whereas more severe tooth decay requires repair with a crown. If the pulp is involved, a root canal treatment may be needed; in extreme cases, the tooth may need to be extracted. The patient with dental caries has no restrictions, and participation in vigorous activity is self-limited.

Summary

The athletic trainer will commonly see injuries and conditions of the ears, nose, mouth, and throat because of athletic participation as well as from other causes. This chapter reviews the anatomy and evaluation of the ear, nose, mouth, and throat and highlights nontraumatic medical conditions common to these areas. The clinician must be able to recognize normal and abnormal conditions in the ear, nose, mouth, and throat and know when to refer the patient to a physician for more definitive diagnostic testing and treatment.

Apply It!

Go to HK*Propel* to complete the case studies for this chapter.

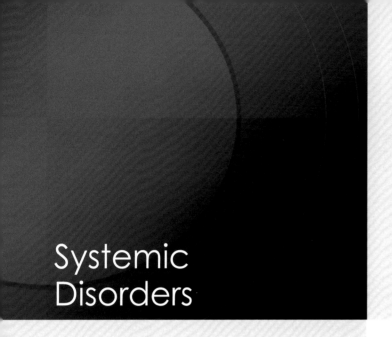

Systemic Disorders

At the completion of this chapter the reader should be able to do the following:

1. Appreciate the complexity of systemic disorders.

2. Recognize signs and symptoms of common systemic ailments.

3. Identify conditions that warrant referral to a physician.

4. Relate the warning signs of malignancies involving the lymphatic system and blood.

5. Contrast chronic or autoimmune disorders with common physical training fatigue.

6. Describe prevention strategies for vector-borne Lyme disease.

7. Recognize and refer arthritides conditions.

8. Differentiate inflammatory myopathies from typical muscle soreness.

Systemic disorders have shortened the careers of many athletes and affect many physically active patients. The athletic trainer serves as a gatekeeper to the health care system for patients: This critically important role cannot be overlooked, because early detection often can prevent permanent disability or deadly consequences. Many systemic conditions can affect a person's general health. These range from vector-borne infections to life-threatening malignancies. Typically, systemic disorders cross several body systems and present in multiple fashions.

Because the discussion of systemic conditions can apply to all body systems, the organization of this chapter differs slightly from the other chapters. The chapter begins with a review of the anatomy and physiology of the lymphatic system, followed by sections on malignancies, vector-borne conditions, chronic and autoimmune disorders, arthritides, and inflammatory myopathies. The anatomy and physiology of the respiratory, cardiovascular, gastrointestinal, genitourinary, gynecological, and neurological systems are discussed in earlier chapters, and the integumentary system is covered in chapter 16.

Most chronic systemic conditions are treatable, but they require special care both to ensure patients' safety and to optimize their quality of life and participation in activity. The conditions discussed here are typically not preventable; however, prevention is discussed when applicable.

Overview of Anatomy and Physiology of the Lymphatic System

The lymphatic system facilitates the spread of some pathological conditions, especially the lymphomas, so understanding of its anatomy and physiology is important. The role of this system is to maintain internal fluid balance and assist with immune functions in the body. It is a collection of vessels, ducts, nodes, organs, and tissue that transport fats, proteins, and lymphatic fluid throughout the body (figure 13.1). The system restores most of the fluid that filters out of the blood during normal homeostasis. It does this by collecting fluid that leaks from capillaries into surrounding tissues and returning it to the blood. The lymphatic system consists of lymph nodes, organs (spleen, thymus, and tonsils), and vessels that parallel veins. The lymph nodes are home to lymphocytes (T-cells and B-cells), the white blood cells that are largely responsible for producing antibodies to combat infections. A healthy node is typically round or kidney shaped and up to 1 in. (2.54 cm) in diameter. Nodes cluster in the cervical region, axilla, and groin. Infections in these regions produce swollen nodes, which become enlarged and tender to palpation as the macrophage cells fight invading cells. In addition to lymphatic system structures, many areas in the body support lymph tissue, such as bone marrow, the intestines, liver, skin, heart, and lungs.

The lymphatic system is not a closed circuit like the circulatory system, but it has access to all body organs and can facilitate disease spread throughout the body. Lymph is moved within this system through normal muscular movement and respiration. A malfunctioning lymphatic system can result in edema in the appendages.

The lymphatic system contains both lymph and interstitial fluid. Lymph is the clear fluid in the lymph vessels, whereas interstitial fluid is a by-product of lymph as it passes into surrounding cells. Lymph consists primarily of protein, salts, glucose, and urea. Lymph vessels collect interstitial fluid and return it to the circulatory system through the larger veins in the thorax. Compared with the cardiovascular system, lymphatic vessels are thinner and have more valves. Rarely are conditions of the lymphatic system preventable.

Malignancies

Cancer is another name for malignant entities, especially carcinomas and sarcomas. As a group, cancers represent the second leading cause of death in adults.[1] By their nature, malignant cells migrate to adjacent tissues, or they use the blood or lymph to transport cells to distant regions of the body. Once there, they infiltrate healthy cells and spread the cancer.

Because the cause of specific malignancies is largely unknown, cancer is difficult to prevent. Cancer occurs when a cell mutates and no longer performs the function for which it was intended. These cells are abnormal in appearance, function, and growth. As the malignant cells

divide and multiply, the cancer grows and potentially spreads. The lymphatic and circulatory systems are especially well suited to facilitate the spread of cancer throughout the body; thus, they are associated with the **metastasis** of lymphomas. Cancers discussed in this chapter have systemic ramifications because they present with vague symptoms and can have whole-body sequelae. Cancers of specific regions are discussed in the chapters devoted to those body regions. For example, lung cancer is discussed in the respiratory system chapter, colon cancer is covered in the gastrointestinal system chapter, and breast and testicular cancers are discussed in the genitourinary and gynecological systems chapter. The malignancies discussed here involve both the lymphatic system and blood. Both are similar in presentation: a swollen lymph node, fatigue, and vague symptoms that can present systemically.

Non-Hodgkin's Lymphoma

Non-Hodgkin's lymphoma (NHL) is a group of malignancies of the **lymphoreticular system**. This system is a collection of lymph nodes and lymphoid tissues formed by several types of immune system cells from both the lymph and reticuloendothelial systems that fight primarily against infection. Although NHL occurs in childhood (5% of adolescent cancer is NHL), the diagnosis increases with age, peaking in the third decade of life.[2] There are several types of NHL and several different classifications. In 2022, nearly 90,000 new cases of NHL were diagnosed in the United States, and about 21,000 patients died of the disease.[2] Some evidence links pesticide and herbicide exposure to a greater incidence of NHL.[3]

Signs and Symptoms

Because NHL is a group of lymphatic cancers, patients can present with a variety of symptoms depending on the site affected. The most common sites are the abdomen, mediastinum, and neck. If the abdomen is affected, the patient can experience nausea, vomiting, or diarrhea, usually accompanied by abdominal pain and weight loss. The patient may also have an enlarged spleen or liver or a palpable mass in the abdomen. Other general signs include excessive sweating, including night sweats, weight loss, fatigue, and unexplained fevers.[3] When the mediastinum is affected, the disease generally progresses more rapidly. Presenting symptoms can range from chest pain to severe shortness of breath on exertion. Neck masses and enlarged lymph nodes can also present as NHL. Figure 13.1*a* shows the location of specific cervical lymph nodes.

In patients with enlarged lymph nodes, the differential diagnoses are extensive. Hodgkin's disease, bacterial

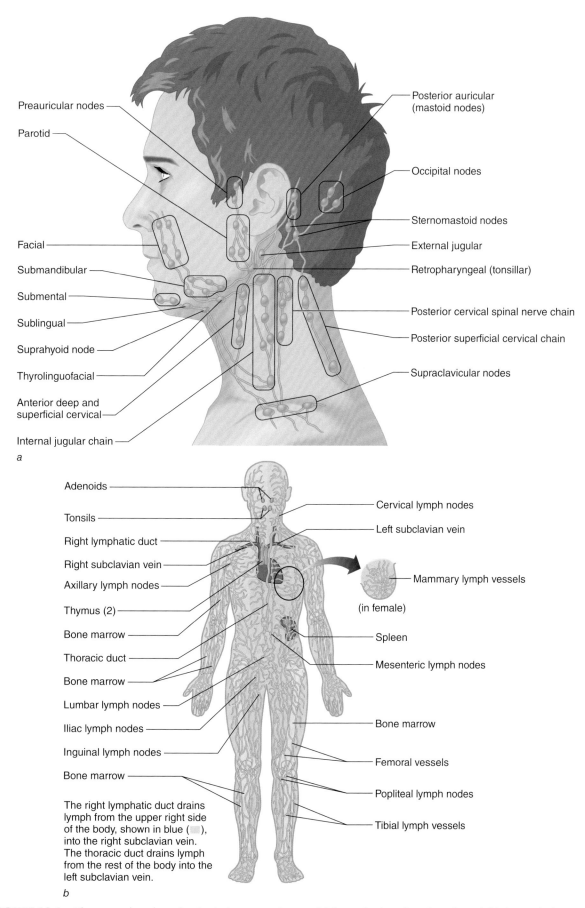

FIGURE 13.1 The complete lymphatic drainage pathways (a) from the head and neck and (b) through the trunk and extremities. The shaded area is drained through the right lymphatic duct, and lymph from the remainder of the body drains through the thoracic duct. The limbs have an extensive drainage system that follows venous return to the heart.

infections, human immunodeficiency virus (HIV), infectious mononucleosis, and sarcoidosis are just a few that need to be considered. Patients with chest pain or dyspnea would have differential diagnoses of hypertrophic cardiomyopathy, coronary artery disease, gastroesophageal reflux disease, asthma, or influenza.[3,4]

Referral and Diagnostic Tests

People who have enlarged lymph nodes without apparent cause, such as infection distal to the gland, inexplicable chest pain, or dyspnea, should be referred to a physician for further evaluation. When NHL is suspected, imaging by computed tomography (CT) or ultrasound can help confirm the presence and size of enlarged lymph nodes. The diagnosis is confirmed by sampling tissue from these lymph nodes by fine-needle biopsy or by removing them for pathological analysis. If the diagnosis is confirmed by biopsy, the patient should be referred to an oncologist for specific treatment.

Patients suspected of having NHL will undergo a complete history and physical examination followed by laboratory work. Initially, patients may present with mild anemia and elevated lactate dehydrogenase (LDH).[5] A battery of other blood tests is performed to help stage the disease, as are laparoscopic lymph node biopsy, bone marrow evaluation, positron emission tomography (PET) scan, and other more common laboratory evaluations. Lymphomas are staged according to the four stages of the Ann Arbor system (I-IV; see table 13.1). Stage I involves a single lymph node or localized organ, whereas stage IV comprises dissipated multifocal involvements of one or more extralymphatic sites.[3]

Treatment and Return to Participation

Treatment depends on the histological type and the stage of NHL. Radiation therapy, chemotherapy, or both can be implemented as treatment and are performed by oncologists.

Prognosis varies widely and depends on the stage, size, and histological type of the disease. The survival rate has steadily increased since the early 2000s with improvements in therapeutic treatments. Patients with high-grade or metastasized NHL tend to do better and may achieve a cure with aggressive chemotherapy. The five-year survival rate for patients with NHL is 72%.[3]

A decision to return to athletic competition must be made once treatment has ended. Because of the prognosis of NHL and risks associated with treatment, athletes with NHL should remain out of competition during treatment, and any return to competition must be made after consultation with physicians.

Hodgkin's Lymphoma

Hodgkin's lymphoma is a malignant condition of lymphoreticular origin, different from NHL because of the existence of **Reed-Sternberg cells** (multinucleated giant cells).[5] The incidence of the disease increases throughout childhood and into the late teenage years, but peaks from ages 15 to 34 yr and again after age 50 yr. It is less prevalent than NHL, with predictions of roughly 8,500 new cases and 950 deaths annually.[6] Hodgkin's lymphoma is more common among Caucasians, groups from higher socioeconomic backgrounds, and males; 80% of teens with Hodgkin's lymphoma are male. The five-year survival rate is steadily increasing, likely as a result of earlier and better detection.[6] There are five types of Hodgkin's lymphoma, but all present similarly and have similar initial signs and symptoms.

Signs and Symptoms

Although Hodgkin's lymphoma has several possible presenting signs, the most common initial sign is an enlarged lymph node, typically in the lower anterior neck region. The lymph node is usually nontender, discrete, firm, and rubbery, and it is not fixed to adjacent structures and can vary in size.[7] Patients with mediastinal chest involvement can present with shortness of breath, chest pain, or cough. On occasion, enlarged lymph nodes are present in the axillary or inguinal region. Splenomegaly or **hepatomegaly** is not uncommon. Figure 13.2 illustrates the

TABLE 13.1 **Lugano Staging for Lymphomas**

Stage	Classification
I	Cancer affects a single lymph node region (cervical, axillary, inguinal, etc.) or lymph gland
II	Cancer affects two or more lymph node regions or lymph tissue on the same side of the diaphragm
III	Cancer affects lymph node region(s) or lymphoid tissue(s) on both sides of the diaphragm
IV	Cancer cells are widespread and involve one or more extranodal tissue(s) or organ(s) outside of the lymph system

Adapted from PDQ Pediatric Treatment Editorial Board, "Childhood Hodgkin Lymphoma Treatment (PDQ®): Health Professional Version," *DQ Cancer Information Summaries* (Bethesda, MD: National Cancer Institute, 2002), Table 2, Lugano Classification for Hodgkin and Non-Hodgkin Lymphoma, https://www.ncbi.nlm.nih.gov/books/NBK66057/table/CDR0000062707__1075/; Adapted from Cheson et al. (2014).

common sites of Hodgkin's lymphoma. Intense itching and intermittent fevers associated with night sweats are classic symptoms. Other systemic signs and symptoms are fatigue, fever, weight loss, **pruritus**, and central nervous system (CNS) signs or symptoms.[7]

In patients who present with enlarged lymph nodes, the differential diagnoses are extensive. Non-Hodgkin's disease, bacterial infection, HIV, infectious mononucleosis, and sarcoidosis are just a few diagnoses that should be considered.

Referral and Diagnostic Tests

Individuals with persistent neck masses, any enlarged lymph node (figure 13.3), or constitutional symptoms, such as night sweats, intermittent fevers, and a weight loss greater than 10% of total body weight over 6 mo, should be evaluated by a physician. If the diagnosis is confirmed, the patient is referred to an oncologist for further treatment. Blood work is performed, including assessment of complete blood count (CBC), LDH, and erythrocyte sedimentation rate (ESR).

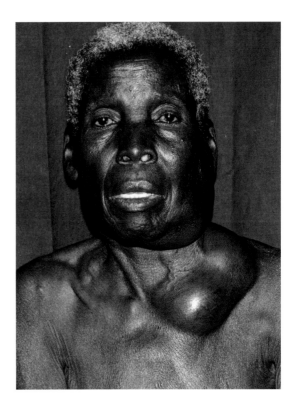

FIGURE 13.3 Sublingual swelling consistent with malignant Hodgkin's lymphoma.
Dr M.A. Ansary / Science Source

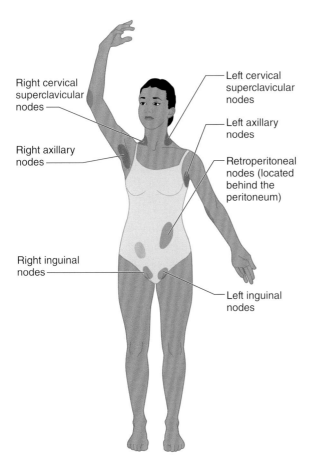

Right cervical superclavicular nodes

Right axillary nodes

Right inguinal nodes

Left cervical superclavicular nodes

Left axillary nodes

Retroperitoneal nodes (located behind the peritoneum)

Left inguinal nodes

FIGURE 13.2 Sites common to Hodgkin's lymphoma. Note that red areas represent common sites and blue areas represent uncommon sites.

If a patient presents with a persistent neck mass that does not respond to antibiotics or is not associated with an infection, an excisional or fine-needle lymph node biopsy is performed. This tissue can then be sent for histological diagnosis. If a persistent cough or other chest symptoms are found, a chest radiograph is taken. Imaging studies are vital for staging the disease and include CT scans of the chest, abdomen, and pelvis.[5,7]

Treatment and Return to Participation

Treatment revolves around histological diagnosis and staging, but Hodgkin's lymphoma generally requires radiation therapy and chemotherapy. With advances in treatment, Hodgkin's lymphoma can be cured in most patients with both localized and advanced disease. Surgery may be indicated if the disease is extensive.

The overall survival rate for Hodgkin's lymphoma is 86% at 5 yr, depending on the type and involvement, but this comes with significant sequelae.[7] Data indicate that late and long-term side effects of treatment for Hodgkin's lymphoma include a higher risk of secondary cancers, fertility issues, thyroid or cardiovascular issues, and challenges fighting off infections.[6] Return-to-participation decisions are made by the patient's physician. It is best to avoid competition during both acute illness and treatment, because the immune system response to the additional stress of competition may be detrimental to a timely recovery.

Leukemia

The several types of **leukemias** have different treatments and prognoses. In general, leukemias are characterized by uncontrolled proliferation of white blood cells in the bone marrow, which accumulate and replace normal blood cells in the marrow. They can then spread to different parts of the body, including the lymph nodes, liver, and spleen; occasionally the gonads, kidneys, and CNS can be affected.[8] As a group, there were more than 60,700 new diagnoses of leukemia in the United States in 2022 and about 24,400 deaths.[6]

Cancers that start from other places and then spread to the bone marrow are not leukemias. It was thought at one time that lymphomas arose only from the lymphatic system, and leukemias from bone marrow, and that these two malignancies were distinctly different. This is no longer supported, as the distinction between the two is often vague.

Leukemia is among the top eight types of cancer in adults but is the most common malignancy in children, comprising 30% of all childhood cancers.[9] Leukemia arises from bone marrow and is divided into four main groups based on both the cell type and speed of growth (acute versus chronic). In adults with leukemia, the most common types are chronic lymphocytic leukemia (CLL [33%]) and acute myeloid leukemia (AML [31%]). In individuals younger than age 19 yr with leukemia, acute lymphocytic leukemia (ALL) affects 75% and AML occurs in 17%.

The specific etiology of leukemia is unknown; however, several risk factors are associated with increased incidence. These include prior chemotherapy with certain agents, history of prior radiation therapy, viral infection (e.g., Epstein-Barr virus), genetic syndromes (e.g., Down syndrome), and family history of leukemia.[5,10,11]

 RED FLAGS FOR ENLARGED LYMPH NODES

The athletic trainer or health care provider should always be suspicious of any enlarged lymph gland. It could indicate a distal infection (e.g., an enlarged groin lymph gland may be attributable to an infected knee turf burn), but it could also be a warning sign of many cancers.

Signs and Symptoms

The diagnosis of leukemia is challenging because the initial symptoms can be nonspecific and can mimic a common viral infection. Approximately 25% to 50% of patients with chronic forms of leukemia may be asymptomatic.[12] Adults and children can present with generalized fatigue, loss of appetite, fever, enlarged lymph nodes, and weakness. Additional findings include pallor, **petechiae**, ecchymoses, frequent nosebleeds, and weight loss. An enlarged liver or spleen noted on physical examination can be the explanation for a patient's abdominal pain. If leukemia spreads to the CNS, it may cause seizures, blurred vision, headache, and loss of balance. Because leukemia is characterized by infiltration of malignant lymphocytic cells in bone marrow, bone pain, bruising, and pallor often occur.[5] Some patients are diagnosed based on abnormal findings on a routine CBC even though their symptoms may be very mild or absent. There are no screening tests for leukemia.[10,12]

In children and adults, the differential diagnoses are similar. This includes infectious mononucleosis caused by the Epstein-Barr virus, infiltrative diseases of the bone marrow, and aplastic anemia. The most significant among the differential diagnoses is leukemia in its various forms, which can usually be proven by bone marrow biopsy or a peripheral blood smear.

Referral and Diagnostic Tests

Individuals suspected of having leukemia should be referred to a hematologist or oncologist as quickly as possible to allow for initiation of treatment.

Several different findings evident on a CBC are helpful in the diagnosis of leukemia. Patients can have a very low (<5,000/mm^3) or very high (>100,000/mm^3) white blood cell count. See table 2.4 for normal blood values. The CBC may also reveal a low platelet count or anemia, which would explain easy bruising and fatigue, respectively. The key for identifying the type of leukemia is a peripheral blood smear or a bone marrow biopsy, which will show the type of abnormal white blood cells that predominate. Other abnormal laboratory findings include elevated LDH and uric acid levels. Chest radiographs are routinely performed to rule out mediastinal masses. CT, magnetic resonance imaging (MRI), or ultrasound of the abdomen is used to check for hepatomegaly or splenomegaly.

Treatment and Return to Participation

Treatment varies depending on the type of leukemia diagnosed. In general, treatments include radiation, chemotherapy, blood transfusions, platelet transfusions, and possibly bone marrow or stem cell transplantation. Prognosis depends on disease severity, health of the patient before diagnosis, and treatment. Adults with the more common CLL may experience a rapid decline and death within 2 to 3 yr of onset or a progressive decline over 5 to 10 yr and death.[12] Among adults with ALL, only 20% to 40% are cured with the treatments currently available.[10] In general, people with ALL are characterized by prognostic risk (good, intermediate, and poor) following treatments. The "good" criteria include age younger than 30 yr and complete remission within 4 wk, whereas the "poor" criteria include age older than 60 yr and failure to achieve complete remission within 4 wk.[10]

Avoidance of activity during treatment is essential, and return-to-participation decisions are made under oncologist supervision. Follow-up examinations, laboratory work, and CT and PET scans are essential in the years after treatment to check for disease recurrence.

Vector-Borne Disease

A vector-borne disease is one that is carried by an infected organism (e.g., a tick or mosquito) to a healthy person. This group of diseases is largely preventable by avoiding the habitats where these organisms live or by applying repellent. Here we discuss Lyme disease, a condition brought about by an infected tick bite. In chapter 14, we cover other vector-borne conditions from mosquitoes (West Nile and Zika viruses) that are infectious.

Lyme Disease

Lyme disease, the most common tick-borne illness in the United States, was first described in the late 1970s in Lyme, Connecticut. This multisystem disorder, when left untreated, can lead to serious arthritic and neurological symptoms that become increasingly difficult to treat because of permanent tissue damage.[13] The culprit responsible for Lyme disease is *Borrelia burgdorferi*. This spirochetal bacterium is transmitted to humans from infected ticks, usually the common blacklegged tick, also known as the deer tick (*Ixodes scapularis*), and by the western blacklegged tick (*Ixodes pacificus*).[13-15] These ticks reside in wooded areas and on the tips of grass, bushes, and shrubs. Athletes active in these areas, such as mountain bikers, hikers, and runners, are susceptible to infection from ticks.

People most affected by Lyme disease are those who spend a large amount of time outdoors and are bitten by ticks between May and September. In 2022, an estimated 476,000 people were treated for Lyme disease in the United States.[16,17] The environment is also a factor with infected ticks. In general, ticks thrive in areas that have milder winters, ample rainfall, and warmer temperatures, with the states of New Hampshire, Maine, Vermont, Delaware, and Connecticut leading the numbers of diagnoses annually.[68]

Signs and Symptoms

Lyme disease can be grouped into three different categories based on symptom longevity: early, early disseminated, and late. In 70% to 80% of patients, early localized Lyme disease begins as a red, circular rash called **erythema migrans** that enlarges over days (figure 13.4). This rash, which can stretch to 12 in. (30 cm), can appear anywhere from 3 to 30 d after a tick bite and generally occurs on the trunk.[13] The rash is usually accompanied by a viral-like illness, with symptoms that can include headache, muscle ache, fever, joint ache, fatigue, and, occasionally, neck stiffness.[18]

Disease not treated at rash onset can lead to early disseminated Lyme disease within weeks to months. Patients may present with Bell's palsy or even meningitis, carditis, or adenopathies.[18] Patients who develop lymphocytic meningitis generally have only neck pain and stiffness, but they may not have the typical findings associated with meningitis on physical examination, such as positive **Brudzinski's sign** and **Kernig's sign** (see figure 14.9).

Early disseminated Lyme disease can also present with cardiac manifestations occurring anywhere from 1 wk to 7 mo after the bite and peaking at 1 to 2 mo. Affected patients may have a variety of symptoms, including chest pain, palpitations, weakness, fatigue, or shortness of breath. These symptoms may result from a conduction abnormality in the heart, leading to irregular rhythms or abnormal findings on an electrocardiogram. The heart muscle may also become inflamed because of infection of the heart tissue.[14]

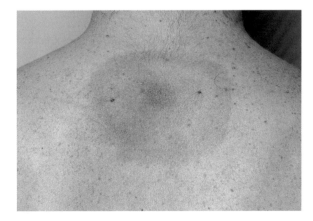

FIGURE 13.4   Erythema migrans rash consistent with Lyme disease.

Paul Whitten / Science Source

Late Lyme disease is characterized by manifestations involving the musculoskeletal system or CNS. Patients may experience intermittent attacks of brief joint swelling followed by chronic pain and arthritic changes. This can occur from weeks to years after the initial tick bite, and its incidence approaches 50% among those who were untreated at the time of infection.[18,19] *Tertiary neuroborreliosis* is the name given to a syndrome of progressively worsening cognitive function, which is thought to be caused by infection of the CNS by the spirochete that is passed on from the infected tick, *B. burgdorferi*.

Differential diagnoses for Lyme disease include depression, fibromyalgia, cellulitis, and chronic fatigue syndrome. In athletes with no trauma and a joint effusion, autoimmune, infectious, neoplastic, and other inflammatory processes must also be considered.[18,19]

Referral and Diagnostic Tests

Patients who have recently visited wooded areas and have a rash that looks like erythema migrans are referred to a primary care physician. Once signs and symptoms of Lyme disease are identified, the diagnosis can be confirmed definitively only by laboratory testing. A positive test result without symptoms does not support the diagnosis of Lyme disease because 3% to 5% of those tested can have false-positive results. Additionally, the blood tests detect antibodies, which can take weeks to develop.[19] The Centers for Disease Control and Prevention (CDC) recommends a two-step process: Blood tests routinely used include an enzyme-linked immunoassay (EIA or ELISA) to identify antibodies to *B. burgdorferi*. If the ELISA is positive, it must then be confirmed on the same blood sample by a Western blot test. These two sequential tests must both be positive for the diagnosis of Lyme disease to be affirmative.[16,18,19]

Despite this information, routine serological testing of individuals with erythema migrans is not recommended, because only one-third of those patients with a single lesion will have a positive test result. If several erythema migrans lesions are noted, the number of positive test results jumps to 90%. Persons with suspected Lyme disease without the rash should have samples taken immediately, with repeated sampling in 4 to 6 wk. Regardless of the laboratory outcomes, treatment should be initiated if the symptoms are consistent with Lyme disease. The diagnosis of Lyme disease that has spread to the CNS is confirmed by testing spinal fluid taken by means of a lumbar puncture.

If the patient has a clinical history of a tick bite and CNS manifestations or a swollen joint, fluid from the affected area should be taken for analysis. The clinician should remember that not all swollen joints are necessarily caused by trauma or injury; if suspicion is high, Lyme arthritis needs to be ruled out to ensure appropriate treatment.

Treatment and Return to Participation

Early treatment of Lyme disease usually prevents any of the aforementioned complications. For early disease, oral antibiotics, including doxycycline (100 mg twice a day), amoxicillin (500 mg three times a day), or cefuroxime axetil (500 mg twice a day), are used. For pregnant females, nursing mothers, or children younger than age 8 yr, amoxicillin or cefuroxime axetil is suggested.[18,19] Cases diagnosed later or that involve the CNS or cardiovascular system typically require intravenous antibiotics. Giving antibiotics to symptom-free people who have been bitten by ticks has not been proven to lessen Lyme incidence. The current recommendation is to monitor closely those bitten by ticks for findings of Lyme disease, including erythema migrans, and to treat those infected appropriately.

As with any acute illness, an individual assessment must be made to determine clearance to play. Most patients can return to participation when any aggravating symptoms have dissipated and proper treatment has been initiated. Transmission of Lyme disease from person to person cannot occur.

Clinical Tips

Tick Removal

It is important to remove a tick as soon as possible to prevent Lyme disease. Follow these steps:

1. Cleanse the area with a povidone–iodine solution or antibacterial soap.

2. Grasp the tick as close to the skin as possible, using tweezers, forceps, or even gloved fingers.

3. Pull the tick up and perpendicular to the skin without twisting or jerking; such movements can break off parts of the insect's mouth and leave them embedded in the skin.

4. Remove the tick, taking care not to crush, squeeze, or puncture its body while it is attached to the skin, as it may release infectious fluid into the body.

5. Cleanse the area again as described previously.

6. To dispose of the tick, place it in a sealed container, wrap it tightly in tape, or flush it down a toilet. Never use fingers to crush a tick.

Prevention

With appropriate and expeditious treatment of Lyme disease, major late sequelae can be prevented, including CNS manifestations, carditis, and recurrent arthritis.[18,19] Efforts to create a viable vaccine to prevent infection have yet to be successful and are ongoing.[18]

Primary prevention comprises the following: avoid ticks, wear proper clothing, including long pants tucked into socks, use insect repellent, and routinely inspect for ticks after possible exposure. Spraying skin and clothing with insect repellent containing the compound *N,N*-diethyl-3-methylbenzamide (DEET) has been shown to be especially helpful in deterring ticks.[16,20] Prompt and early tick removal is essential because transmission of *B. burgdorferi* is rare unless the tick has been attached to the human host for more than 24 h.[18] A joint publication by the Infectious Diseases Society of America, the American Academy of Neurology, and the American College of Rheumatology recommends prophylactic antibiotic therapy be provided to adults (not children) within 72 h of removal of an identified high-risk tick bite.[20] If the tick bite cannot be distinctly identified, a wait-and-watch period is advised.[20]

Chronic and Autoimmune Disorders

Raynaud's Disease

Raynaud's disease is characterized by vasospasm of the arteries, primarily in the hands, but it can also affect the feet, nose, and ears. The two presentations of Raynaud's disease are primary and secondary. Typically, the primary condition is referred to as *Raynaud's disease* if no other cause can be found beyond vasospasm. Secondary Raynaud's is caused by an underlying problem and is termed **Raynaud's phenomenon**. The many causes for Raynaud's phenomenon include medications (e.g., oral contraceptives), systemic lupus erythematosus (SLE), rheumatoid arthritis (RA), scleroderma, chemical exposure, smoking, arteriovascular disease, hyperthyroidism, pulmonary hypertension, and repetitive trauma from tools that cause vibration.[5] Stressors, including cold temperatures and emotional trauma, exacerbate the phenomenon.

Raynaud's phenomenon is found in 11% of women and 8% of men. Primary Raynaud's is more common than secondary Raynaud's and occurs more often in women and in people younger than age 40 yr.[21]

Signs and Symptoms

Patients typically present with a **triphasic** color response to cold exposure:

- *Pallor:* The skin, most often of the fingers, will become pale, or pallid, because of vasospasm (figure 13.5).

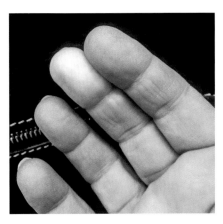

FIGURE 13.5   Raynaud's phenomenon, presenting initially as pallor of the digits when exposed to cold or stress.
© Katie Walsh Flanagan

- *Cyanosis:* The skin will then become blue because of the increase in venous, or deoxygenated, blood in the digits.
- *Erythema:* The skin turns red when the vasospasm resolves, and a rush of blood enters the digits, causing pain and numbness.

As noted previously, these symptoms can happen in the hands, feet, nose, and ears and usually occur bilaterally. The symptoms generally resolve over minutes but can lead to ulcerations, gangrene, and dead tissue if they persist.[21]

Differential diagnoses of Raynaud's phenomenon include the secondary causes listed previously as well as **CREST syndrome** (*c*alcinosis cutis, *R*aynaud's phenomenon, *e*sophageal dysfunction, *s*clerodactyly, *t*elangiectasia), scleroderma, carpal tunnel syndrome, thoracic outlet syndrome, peripheral vascular disease, and dermatomyositis (discussed later in this chapter).[4,21]

Referral and Diagnostic Tests

If Raynaud's phenomenon is suspected, the appropriate referral should be made to determine the underlying cause. A rheumatologist should be involved for cases with underlying autoimmune diseases. The most common association with Raynaud's phenomenon is **scleroderma** (90%) and SLE (85%).[21]

A history of the symptoms is usually enough to diagnose Raynaud's disease. Once the diagnosis is made, a thorough history and physical examination should help in ruling out secondary causes of Raynaud's disease. If a secondary cause is suggested, the physician will order appropriate blood work. On occasion, the diagnosis can be "seen" by having the patient expose the fingers to a cold environment, such as ice water, and monitoring the results. No blood tests assist in the diagnosis of Raynaud's, but a CBC, basic electrolytes, kidney function test, liver function test, ESR test, and urinalysis should be ordered to help differentiate it from other diseases.

Treatment and Return to Participation

The simplest treatment is to avoid the triggers that propagate Raynaud's. For example, avoid medications that may cause it, stay out of the cold, wear appropriate protective clothing, and avoid other triggers such as caffeine and tobacco.[21] For those with no relief from the nonpharmacological approach, medications can be used to decrease symptoms. Calcium-channel blockers, such as nifedipine, have proven to be the most effective treatment for Raynaud's disease. Other medications that have proven helpful include α-blockers and, to a lesser extent, aspirin and topical nitrates.

Patients with primary Raynaud's can usually control their symptoms with nonpharmacological treatments. Unfortunately, for those with secondary Raynaud's caused by CREST syndrome or scleroderma, symptoms may be so severe that the disease causes ulcerations, gangrene, and even autoamputations.[8]

Systemic Lupus Erythematosus

SLE is a chronic autoimmune disorder that potentially affects many parts of the body, including the musculoskeletal system, skin, kidneys, cardiac cells, and nervous system. In lupus erythematosus, the immune system makes autoantibodies (i.e., antibodies to the body's own proteins), which then form complexes that cause injury and pain. It tends to be an exacerbation–remission disorder with long-term consequences. Of the four main types of lupus, SLE is the most common and predominantly affects women. Black and Latina women of childbearing age (14-44 yr) are more commonly affected, and they are 2 to 3 times more likely than White women to not only develop lupus but also to have more severe progression.[22] Twenty percent of patients with lupus are children.[23]

The four main types of lupus are as follows:

- *Systemic lupus erythematosus:* Often simply called *lupus*, SLE can affect any part of the body.
- *Discoid lupus erythematosus:* This form can present as an acute, subacute, or chronic skin condition, can be localized or generalized, and can begin in childhood. It can occur independent of SLE or in conjunction with it.[24]
- *Drug-induced lupus erythematosus:* This is a form of SLE triggered by certain medications that abates once the drug therapy is terminated.[25]
- *Neonatal lupus erythematosus:* This rare form is passed in utero from mother to child. Infants with this form of lupus are born with a mild plaque rash that typically disappears within 6 mo.[26]

The exact cause of SLE is not known, but it may involve a genetic predisposition triggered by environmental factors. SLE is a chronic, progressive disorder that can affect several different systems at various times throughout the disease course. The effects of the condition range from mild to life-threatening, and there is no cure.

Signs and Symptoms

SLE is a multisystem disease process, so the patient often presents with multiple complaints. Fatigue, skin rash, fever, and hair loss are common. At some point during their disease course, 90% of patients with SLE will have musculoskeletal complaints. Typically, patients experience muscle aches and pains as well as arthritis or swelling of several joints.[8] As a result of long-term corticosteroid treatment, many patients with SLE have a much higher risk of osteoporosis and a high risk of avascular necrosis, typically presenting in the hip. Several large studies have reported that approximately 22% to 47% of patients with SLE will also present with fibromyalgia.[27,28]

The skin is often affected in patients with SLE. The hallmark sign is a red rash over the malar eminence of the face, with sparing of the nasolabial folds (the area between the nose and upper lip). It is called a *butterfly rash* because of its typical appearance (figure 13.6). Patients can also present with hair loss, red and scaly patches that turn to plaques, and oral ulcers as well as photophobic skin responses to sunlight.[29]

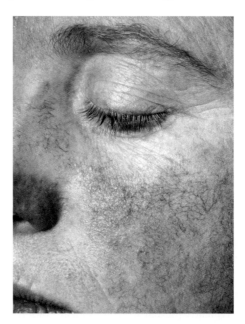

FIGURE 13.6 Butterfly rash of systemic lupus erythematosus.

BSIP / Science Source

Patients with SLE have a high risk of cardiovascular problems. There is a significant relationship between autoimmune diseases and increased atherosclerosis. In women, the risk of myocardial infarction is increased by 50% for patients with SLE compared with the same sex and age population. Blood clots forming in the circulatory system also occur in SLE because of the production of specialized **antiphospholipid antibodies**.[29]

In addition, the kidneys can be affected, with approximately one-half of patients with SLE developing lupus nephritis. Although the treatment for lupus nephritis can keep the kidneys functioning well, kidney problems are a major cause of morbidity and mortality among patients with SLE.

CNS effects of SLE are many and widely varied. Patients can present with seizures, psychosis, decreased cognitive function, stroke, or even coma.

Referral and Diagnostic Tests

Individuals who complain of unexplained joint pain and swelling, especially if accompanied by a butterfly rash, should consult a physician for further testing. Referrals depend on the disease severity and the organ systems involved. In addition to a primary care physician, patients with SLE need a rheumatologist to oversee their care. Nephrologists should be involved for patients with kidney disorders, hematologists for those with blood manifestations, and, if needed, orthopedic surgeons for those with avascular necrosis.

In 2019, the American College of Rheumatology (ACR) and the European Alliance of Associations for Rheumatology (EULAR; formerly the European League Against Rheumatism) updated previous criteria to aid in SLE diagnosis. Four of the 11 criteria must be met for a positive diagnosis.[30] In addition to the criteria, several blood tests can be performed to help in the diagnosis of SLE. For an SLE diagnosis, the presence of antinuclear antibody (ANA), of at least 1:80 on Hep-2 cells, or an equivalent positive test result at least once must be observed. Other laboratory examinations indicate the level of inflammation in the body, and a urinalysis is performed to determine whether protein or blood is present. Chest X-rays and electrocardiograms (ECGs) may be ordered to evaluate the level of possible lung and cardiac involvement.[31] Two charts are used to diagnose SLE: one is presented in table 13.2, and the other relates to three categories of antibodies or proteins.

TABLE 13.2 **EULAR and ACR Clinical Domains and Criteria for Systemic Lupus Erythematosus**

Patients must meet at least one clinical domain and 10 or more points to be diagnosed.

Domain	Criteria	Points
Constitutional	Fever	2
Hematologic	Leukopenia Thrombocytopenia Autoimmune hemolysis	3 4 4
Neuropsychiatric	Delirium Psychosis Seizure	2 3 5
Mucocutaneous	Nonscarring alopecia Oral ulcers Subacute cutaneous or discoid lupus Acute cutaneous lupus	2 2 4 6
Serosal	Pleural or pericardial effusion Acute pericarditis	5 6
Musculoskeletal	Joint involvement	6
Renal	Proteinuria >0.5 g/24 h Kidney biopsy class II or V lupus nephritis Kidney biopsy class III or IV lupus nephritis	4 8 10

Note: ACR = American College of Rheumatology; EULAR = European Alliance of Associations for Rheumatology (formerly the European League Against Rheumatism).

Adapted from Aringer et al. (2019).

Because SLE affects multiple systems, many other illnesses, including various infections and malignancies (e.g., lymphoma and leukemia), must be excluded in the differential diagnosis. Because of their musculoskeletal involvement, RA and mixed connective tissue disease (e.g., scleroderma, dermatomyositis) may also produce symptoms similar to those of SLE.

Treatment and Return to Participation

The goal of treatment is to reduce the acute symptoms while avoiding the progressive, damaging effects of SLE in the long term. Antimalarial drugs (e.g., hydroxychloroquine) are typically recommended for every patient diagnosed with SLE.[23,31] Photosensitivity for those with skin manifestations can be controlled with sunscreen use, protective hats and clothing, and avoidance of sunlight. Patients with musculoskeletal symptoms can benefit from nonsteroidal anti-inflammatory drugs (NSAIDs) or steroids. Corticosteroids have been the mainstay of treatment for SLE symptoms affecting the renal, nervous, and hematological systems. Although corticosteroid treatment is extremely beneficial for patients with SLE, its many side effects complicate the disease itself. Patients taking long-term corticosteroids have a higher likelihood of infections, osteoporosis, avascular necrosis, steroid-induced diabetes, and several skin ramifications (see chapter 4). All of these side effects need to be monitored and treated appropriately while the patient continues to take corticosteroids. The key is to have the patient take the lowest dose that controls the disease while limiting the side effects. Two additional treatments were approved by the U.S. Food and Drug Administration (FDA) in 2021. Voclosporin (Lupkynis) was approved to treat lupus nephritis in adults. Anifrolumab-fnia (Saphnelo) is delivered via venous puncture and has been a successful secondary targeted treatment for SLE.[23]

Because patients with SLE tend to experience remissions and exacerbations, the prognosis is often complicated. Infection resulting from immunosuppression, owing to not only the disease but also chronic corticosteroid treatment, is the leading cause of death in patients with SLE. Other causes of death in patients with SLE include renal and neurological diseases. Systematic reviews of patients with SLE determine that they show less cardiovascular response to exercise than others without the disease.[32,33] Therefore, patients with SLE who are returned to activity must be monitored for exacerbations and new disease complications while balancing the potential side effects of treatment.

Fibromyalgia

Fibromyalgia is a chronic, noninflammatory, diffuse pain syndrome characterized by multiple areas of musculoskeletal pain, sleep disturbances, fatigue, and depression.[36] Women tend to lead men in the diagnosis of fibromyalgia, but this depends on how it is diagnosed. It can occur at any age, even in childhood, but the predominant age range at diagnosis is between 20 and 50 yr.[34] The overall prevalence of fibromyalgia in the United States is 2% to 4%.[36] People with an autoimmune disease (e.g., SLE, RA, or **Sjogren's syndrome**) are at higher risk of fibromyalgia.[28]

The cause of fibromyalgia remains unknown, but genetics and environmental factors have been identified to predispose one to it.[5] Although how this process is set in motion in some people and not others is unknown, it is thought that a precipitating event, such as injury, surgery, infection, or emotional trauma, is often involved.[35,36] Research has discovered that patients with fibromyalgia have an abnormal and exaggerated response to pain in the neuroreceptors in the brain.[36,37]

Signs and Symptoms

Patients with fibromyalgia typically experience severe and diffuse musculoskeletal pain that is unrelated to a clearly defined anatomical lesion. The pain is located mostly in the neck and lower back, but it can also affect the extremities. This pain syndrome will wax and wane not only in severity but also in location, and it may be exacerbated by any stress or emotional or physical trauma.[4] If a patient has any findings consistent with another disease process or injury, such as a swollen joint, warmth or redness over the affected site, or abnormal X-ray findings, a diagnosis other than fibromyalgia should be investigated thoroughly. Complaints of fatigue, ineffective sleep (the ACR terms this *waking unrefreshed*), or impaired cognition, inability to concentrate, and memory challenges are also used to determine the presence of fibromyalgia.[36-38]

The differential diagnoses of fibromyalgia include many diseases with similar signs and symptoms. These include depression, chronic fatigue syndrome, myofascial pain syndrome, hypothyroidism, RA, and SLE.[8,29]

Referral and Diagnostic Tests

Health care providers should watch for patients whose symptoms last longer than usual for a given injury or illness. If a patient has symptoms for 3 mo or longer that are thought to be consistent with fibromyalgia, referral to a primary care physician is appropriate to help with the diagnosis. The patient can be referred to a rheumatologist, psychiatrist, physical therapist, or a specialist in fibromyalgia as needed.

The diagnosis of fibromyalgia rests on a thorough history, physical examination, and set of criteria established in 2010 by the ACR (see the Diagnostic Criteria for Fibromyalgia sidebar). These criteria include widespread, bilateral pain located above and below the waist and pain involving the axial skeleton that has been present for at least 3 mo. To meet the diagnosis of fibromyalgia, the patient must also have pain at 7 of 19 sites when the examiner applies pressure and must have fatigue, cognitive issues, unrefreshed awakening, and no other health issue that would explain the symptoms.[29,36] Physicians evaluate patients on two scales: the widespread pain index (WPI), which is the number of places the patient has pain, and symptom severity, which relates the level of severity to fatigue, sleep, and cognitive symptoms. In 2011, a patient self-report form was included in the diagnostic criteria; in 2018, an international group proffered diagnostic criteria that would also include other chronic pain disorders, but the 2010 criteria are the most used.[36] Basic laboratory evaluations, including assessment of CBC, creatinine kinase, thyroid-stimulating hormone, iron levels, vitamin B_{12} levels, and ESR, are performed to differentiate fibromyalgia from other diseases that have overlapping symptoms.[34]

Treatment and Return to Participation

Treatment for fibromyalgia usually incorporates a variety of disciplines. The key element is patient education and management of flare-ups. Counseling is also an important part of treating fibromyalgia, especially for patients with manifestations of depression or poor coping skills.[29] Exercise has proven to be beneficial because deconditioning plays a large role in fibromyalgia.[39,40] Good sleep habits and mild exercise have a positive effect on mood disorders and depression (see chapter 17).[34] Cardiovascular exercise and muscle strengthening seem to provide more benefit than stretching and flexibility exercises, although these work for some patients. After a 3 mo program, some patients can see benefits that last for up to a year. Water aerobics, swimming, biking, yoga, and other nonimpact exercises are appropriate. A 9 yr study of patients with fibromyalgia and healthy individuals concluded that regular, moderate-intensive activity had a positive effect on long-term fitness, decreased pain, and effects of fibromyalgia symptoms.[41] Exercise compliance can be difficult because some patients perceive exercise to cause their pain and fatigue. However, counseling the patient to start out slowly and at a low intensity, gradually increasing their exercise tolerance, has been helpful.[37]

The patient with fibromyalgia may also benefit from pharmacological treatment. Antidepressants, especially

---

Diagnostic Criteria for Fibromyalgia

The following criteria have been established by the American College of Rheumatology:[38]

- History of widespread pain over the four quadrants of the body, lasting more than 3 mo
- Presence of specific widespread pain points (WPI). The ACR has identified the following 19 specific areas; 7 areas must be represented for fibromyalgia to be considered:

    Shoulder girdle (R/L)   Jaw (R/L)
    Upper arm (R/L)   Upper back
    Lower arm (R/L)   Lower back
    Hip (buttock, greater trochanter) (R/L)   Chest
    Upper leg (R/L)   Abdomen
    Lower leg (R/L)   Neck

- Symptom severity (SS)

    Fatigue
    Waking unrefreshed
    Cognitive symptoms

    L = left; R = right; WPI = widespread pain.

tricyclic antidepressants, such as amitriptyline (Elavil) at low doses, have been shown to help. Not only do antidepressants aid in addressing the possible underlying depression, but their sedative effect helps improve sleep, especially when taken before bedtime. The FDA has approved the following drugs in the treatment of fibromyalgia: pregabalin (Lyrica), duloxetine (Cymbalta), and milnacipran (Savella).[34] These medications are effective in altering the chemicals (serotonin and norepinephrine) that process pain perception, improving sleep, and reducing depression. Muscle relaxants such as cyclobenzaprine (Flexeril) have shown merit in helping patients with fibromyalgia, and they also have a sedating effect. Selective serotonin reuptake inhibitors, such as fluoxetine (Prozac), paroxetine (Paxil), and sertraline (Zoloft), also have proven beneficial, but they should be monitored because of their potential for abuse.[34] NSAIDs have not proven to be beneficial for patients with fibromyalgia. It is important to note that all of these medications have side effects that may make them detrimental in specific cases.

Other treatments that may help patients with fibromyalgia include hypnosis, chiropractic treatments, acupuncture, and herbal medications. These modalities need to be further studied to determine their true effectiveness. A study of 400 women with fibromyalgia showed that only a small percentage (16%) were engaged in the 10,000 minimum step recommendations compared to the same number of healthy women in the same age range.[39] The authors suggested that engaging in more activity—at least minimum daily standards—might be a helpful treatment for those with fibromyalgia.[34]

The prognosis for patients with fibromyalgia is uncertain because the symptoms commonly come and go over the disease course. Although patients can show improvement, there is no known cure. An aggressive, multifaceted, organized approach to treatment will help lead to a substantial improvement in and ideally remission of symptoms. Participation in athletics is determined on an individual basis. Most patients can function if their symptoms are well controlled.

Chronic Fatigue Syndrome

Chronic fatigue syndrome (CFS), also termed *myalgic encephalomyelitis* (ME), is often a disabling illness. The primary symptom is severe fatigue that is exacerbated with exertion, persisting for 6 mo or longer.[42] This is often accompanied by several other symptoms, most often cognitive difficulties, but the musculoskeletal, immunological, and neurological systems can be affected. Up to 2.5 million people of all races and ages have CFS, but it is two to four times more prevalent in women.[43,44] CFS has an average age of onset of 33 yr but has been documented in people age 10 to 70 yr.[42]

There is no known cause of CFS, and no specific diagnostic tests are available.[43,44] CFS is likely a spectrum of illnesses sharing a common pathogenesis with varying degrees of fatigue and associated symptoms. Some studies indicate that certain infectious diseases, Epstein-Barr virus, pneumonia, infection (e.g., upper respiratory infection), or diarrhea may be the culprit in CFS, but the research is not definitive.[42]

Signs and Symptoms

There are three primary core symptoms for CFS and one of two additional symptoms are required for diagnosis. (See the Primary Symptoms for CFS and ME Diagnosis sidebar.) Symptoms must continue for 6 mo or longer and accompany cognitive difficulties. Several other symptoms can be present as well; however, these vary widely and are used mainly to differentiate CFS from other causes of persistent fatigue. Other symptoms are listed next in the CDC criteria for diagnosis.

Referral and Diagnostic Tests

The diagnosis of CFS is one of exclusion. Because symptoms of CFS overlap with several other diseases, including depression, fibromyalgia, and infectious mononucleosis, several criteria must be met in order to achieve a CFS diagnosis. A complete history and physical examination are mandatory to help exclude other disease processes. The CDC has determined that other common symptoms are as follows:[45]

- Muscle aches and pains, weakness
- Joint pain absent swelling or redness
- Headache (new type, pattern, or severity)
- Frequent or recurring sore throat
- Tender lymph nodes
- Digestive issues
- Chills and night sweats
- Allergies and sensitivities to foods, odors, chemicals, light, or noise
- Shortness of breath
- Irregular heartbeat

Laboratory tests include a standard CBC, thyroid function, ESR, and liver function tests, but other tests are ordered depending on the patient's symptoms.[42] Patients are often referred to infectious disease specialists because of elevated immunoglobulin levels. In CFS, the results of laboratory examinations are within normal limits. A host of diseases must be excluded before allowing the diagnosis of CFS, including the following:

Primary Symptoms for CFS and ME Diagnosis

The following are the three core symptoms for CFS:

- Dramatically lowered ability to do activities that were previously not taxing: A decline in activity levels, combined with fatigue, must last longer than 6 mo.

- Declining CFS and ME symptoms after exertion or mental activity (postexertional malaise): This can be accompanied by problems sleeping, sore throat, headache, dizziness, or severe tiredness, which is often described as a "crash" from which it can take days, weeks, or longer for the patient to recover.

- Sleep challenges: Patients will describe they do not feel better or rested after a full night's sleep, or have difficulty getting to or remaining asleep.

In addition to the core symptoms, one of the following is required for diagnosis:

- Difficulty with cognition and memory: Patients complain of "brain fog" or difficulty thinking quickly, remembering, or having attention to details.

- Worsening symptoms with standing or sitting upright (orthostatic intolerance): Symptoms include dizziness, weakness, blurry vision, or near-syncopal episodes.

Adapted from "Symptoms of ME/CFS," Center for Disease Control and Prevention, last modified January 27, 2021, https://www.cdc.gov/me-cfs/symptoms-diagnosis/symptoms.html.

- Anemia
- Chronic hepatitis B or C
- Depression
- Diabetes mellitus
- Fibromyalgia
- Human immunodeficiency virus
- Hypopituitarism
- Hypothyroidism
- Leukemia
- Lyme disease
- Medication reaction
- Mononucleosis
- Multiple sclerosis
- Myasthenia gravis
- Narcolepsy
- Pregnancy
- Rheumatoid arthritis
- Sleep apnea
- Systemic lupus erythematosus
- Thyroiditis
- Tuberculosis

Treatment and Return to Participation

Optimal treatment of CFS includes a multifactorial approach aimed at managing the disease and its manifestations. There are no FDA-approved medications to treat CFS. Because there is no definitive cure and it may be related to a viral infection, treatment needs to be tailored to the individual. The basic treatment in current use seems to have a beneficial effect in managing the disease. Most medications and vitamins have proven ineffective, as have antidepressants.[42] Suggested management includes supportive treatment, including a graded exercise program, proper nutrition, and improved sleep.

Counseling is important in the athletic setting because CFS can hamper a person's performance substantially, making return to competition at any level challenging.

Treatment of any other coexisting disorders, such as depression, fibromyalgia, panic disorders, and irritable bowel syndrome, is also important in the overall approach to patients with CFS.

The prognosis for people with CFS is unknown because there is no definitive cure for the disease. The hope is that, with a multidisciplinary approach, the athlete will be able to return to the previous level of competition; however, this may take months to years to accomplish.

Multiple Sclerosis

Multiple sclerosis (MS) is a neurodegenerative, lifelong, chronic disease diagnosed primarily in young adults. It is characterized by the gradual accumulation of focal plaques of demyelination in the brain. Peripheral nerves are not affected. The pathophysiology of MS involves myelinated cells being destroyed and replaced by hard sclerotic tissue. The result may be permanent disability in the affected nerves. In Western societies, MS is second only to trauma as a cause of neurological disability arising in early to middle adulthood.[46]

Current evidence indicates that MS is an autoimmune disease. The precise cause of MS remains unknown, but several epidemiological facts have been clearly established. MS develops in genetically susceptible individuals who reside in certain permissive environments. It affects approximately 400,000 Americans and 2.3 million people worldwide and is approximately two to three times as common in females as in males.[47,48] In both sexes, the incidence rises steadily from adolescence to age 35 yr and declines gradually thereafter. About two-thirds of cases have an onset between ages 20 and 40 yr, and research has linked the risk factor for MS to genetics. MS can be found in most racial groups but is more common in Caucasians. Factors such as vitamin D deficiency have been linked, and there is growing evidence that individuals with obesity and smokers have a higher incidence of MS. Epstein-Barr virus contracted after childhood has been associated with increased risk.[46,48] In contrast, vaccines, stress, allergies, exposure to metals, and traumatic events have shown no evidence of increased risk of MS.[48] The presence of MS is increasing globally, as is the prevalence of women diagnosed with the condition.[47]

There are four distinct forms of MS that differ in their presentation but are similar in signs, symptoms, and treatment:[48,49]

Relapsing–Remitting MS (RRMS)

- Cyclic episodes of worsening neurological function, followed by complete recovery periods (remissions). Attacks are termed *relapses*, *flare-ups*, or *exacerbations*.
- Eighty-five percent of people with MS have this form of the disease.

Primary–Progressive MS (PPMS)

- Gradually worsening neurological function without distinct remission.
- Ten percent of people with MS have this form of the disease.

Secondary–Progressive MS (SPMS)

- After a period of relapsing–remitting MS, these patients develop a secondary progressive decline in neurological function.

Progressive–Relapsing MS (PRMS)

- Progressive worsening of neurological function occurs, punctuated by occasional attacks of accelerated deterioration; no remission occurs.
- Only five percent of people have this rare form of MS.

Manifestations of MS vary from a benign illness to a rapidly evolving and incapacitating disease requiring profound adjustments in lifestyle and goals for patients and their families. Complications from MS affect multiple body systems.[5,8]

Signs and Symptoms

Often, the first indicator of MS or relapse is a squeezing feeling about the torso, similar to a sphygmomanometer tightening for a blood pressure reading. This condition is termed *dysesthesia* but is referred to as a "MS hug."[48]

The following are common signs and symptoms of MS:[48]

- MS hug (dysesthesia)
- Problems with balance and coordination
- Challenges with normal gait
- Spasticity
- Fatigue
- Visual problems
- Dizziness or vertigo
- Pain and itching
- Numbness or tingling
- Bladder or bowel dysfunction
- Emotional behavior changes
- Cognitive function changes

Symptoms of MS may be mild or severe, may be of long or short duration, and may appear in various combinations. Most frequently, the disease is relapsing and remitting, with symptoms that may come and go over time. Weakness or numbness in one or more extremities is the initial symptom in about one-half of patients. The initial presentation in about 25% of all patients with MS is an episode of optic neuritis.[50] Optic neuritis is a syndrome in which partial or total loss of vision, usually in one eye, evolves rapidly over several hours to days. Some patients may experience pain within the orbit that may be made worse with eye movement or palpation of the globe 1 or 2 d before visual loss. Other visual symptoms may include blurred vision, double vision, or red-green color distortion. About one-third of patients with optic neuritis recover completely, and others generally improve significantly even when the initial visual loss was profound.

Systemic fatigue is also a common complaint associated with MS. Sixty percent of patients with MS judge fatigue to be their worst symptom.[5,50] This symptom makes diagnosis challenging in the active population, in whom fatigue is common.

Heat is a culprit for the worsening of many MS symptoms, and active patients with this disorder should be monitored carefully during warmer days.[48]

Several other diseases produce symptoms like those seen in MS. The possibility of an alternative diagnosis must be considered and eventually ruled out. Initially MS may mimic stroke, lupus, progressive myelopathy, migraine, spinal cord tumor, arteriovenous disorders, Lyme disease, arthritis, Guillain-Barré syndrome (GBS), vitamin D deficiency, autoimmune conditions, and syphilis, among other conditions.[4,50]

Referral and Diagnostic Tests

The symptoms of MS are often vague, insidious, and nonspecific. However, patients who experience fatigue, numbness and tingling (in the arms, legs, or elsewhere in the body), or vision irregularities must be referred to a physician. These are among the early indications of MS. Often the symptoms will be unilateral and will occur without trauma. Static tremors may be present, and a physician will determine whether a neurological condition, such as MS, may be the cause.

Physicians perform a neurological examination and take a medical history when they suspect MS. Imaging technologies include MRI, which provides an anatomical picture of lesions, and magnetic resonance spectroscopy, which yields information about the biochemistry of the brain. Other tests include a spinal tap to obtain a cerebrospinal fluid (CSF) sample to study the immunoglobulin G antibody, an EEG, sensory evoked potential studies, and an electromyogram.[48,50] Evoked potential tests record the nervous system's electrical response to stimulation (e.g., visual, auditory). People with MS have slower response times than do individuals without the condition. No single test unequivocally detects MS.

Other tests performed to diagnose MS include testing deep tendon reflexes, which are generally increased in the disease. Many times, the challenge is to rule out other conditions, resulting in a diagnosis of MS. There are three criteria for diagnosing MS, according to the National Multiple Sclerosis Society: (1) the presence of damage in at least two separate areas of the CNS, (2) evidence that the damage took place at different points in time, and (3) exclusion of all other conditions.[48] Diagnostic criteria were further delineated in the revised McDonald criteria in 2017 to include CSF analysis.[51] These additional tests can confirm the diagnosis after only one attack.

Treatment and Return to Participation

There is no cure for MS. Approximately 85% of patients have the relapsing–remitting form of the disease, in which they experience acute exacerbations or relapses with near or complete recovery.[48] Treatment is divided into two categories: (1) immunomodulatory therapy (*disease-modifying agents*) to treat the underlying immune disorder and (2) symptom management. Several agents have been successful for immunomodulatory therapy, including interferon and monoclonal antibodies, among others showing promise. Recent and remarkable advances in treatment options for MS have been made in the disease-modifying category. Ten such treatments have significantly changed the short- and intermediate-term natural progression of the disease.[46,49] Clinicians referring patients would be wise to align with progressive physicians who are informed of current and emerging MS therapies that are effective and have few side effects.

MS may also be progressive. Medications to relieve symptoms in progressive MS include corticosteroids, muscle relaxants, and medications to reduce fatigue. Many medications are used for the muscle stiffness, depression, pain, and bladder control problems often associated with MS. Drugs for arthritis and medications that suppress the immune system may slow MS in some cases.

In addition to medications, other treatments may relieve MS symptoms. These include physical and occupational therapy, with the goal of preserving independence by performing flexibility, strengthening, and proprioceptive exercises and using assistive devices to ease daily tasks.

Counseling for individuals or in group therapy sessions may help both the patient and family cope with MS and relieve emotional stress.[48-50] Exercise is an excellent treatment for patients with MS when performed in moderation; the benefits of mild to moderate exercise for MS patients include the following:

- Decreases fatigue
- Allows more independent functioning
- Helps overcome depression
- Improves the following:

  Stamina

  Strength

  Muscle tone

  Balance

  Coordination

  Overall mood

  Sense of well-being

Exercise may also have some adverse effects, particularly if prolonged or practiced in hot environments. These adverse effects include increased fatigue, weakness, pain, and spasticity. MS or medications used to control some symptoms can alter the body's ability to dissipate heat. Overheating increases MS symptoms. In addition, muscle weakness around the joints can leave patients with MS unstable and vulnerable to injury, which causes pain that makes spasticity worse and promotes more weakness.

Because the exact cause of MS remains unknown, the clinical course and prognosis are as variable as the symptoms. Whereas one patient may present with the disease and have a virtually benign course, another may rapidly progress to wheelchair use and catheters for voiding.

Most people with MS have a normal, if not slightly shorter, life expectancy. The remission–exacerbation components of the disease make it challenging to predict future disability. Untreated, 30% of patients experience significant physical disability, and males with primary–progressive MS have the worst prognosis.[50] Patients with a disease course that is progressive from the start are more likely to experience progression of disability. In the worst cases, MS can render a person unable to write, speak, or walk.

A young athlete who develops this chronic, debilitating disease can be particularly devastated. One of the first questions may be, "Can I continue to exercise or train?" The answer is, "Yes, but..." Research has shown that although exercise does not change impairment, physical exercise helps the patient feel better, both mentally and physically. The good news is that much work is being done: Congress passed a bill for fiscal year 2023 that includes funding for MS, with $20 million dedicated specifically to MS research as well as funding for policies and programs that benefit people living with MS.[48]

Because MS affects people in different ways, some athletes who have completely or almost completely recovered from an exacerbation may be able to run 5 or 10 mi or bicycle 75 mi per day. Others may experience severe disability and require use of a powered wheelchair. Finding the optimal exercise management program requires a team effort among the physician, the athletic trainer, the physical therapist, and the patient. The best program combines elements of cardiovascular training, strength, flexibility, balance, coordination, and appropriate functional exercises and is designed with independence and quality of life in mind.

Guillain-Barré Syndrome

GBS is an acute, diffuse demyelinating disorder of the spinal roots and peripheral nerves. Physiologically, there are specific lymphocytes thought to produce antibodies against components of the myelin sheath and may contribute to the destruction of myelin. As noted previously, without myelin, nerve conduction is interrupted and the nerve is ineffective. GBS has several subtypes, but all are similar in development and symptoms.[52] The GBS polyneuropathy is an autoimmune syndrome that is sudden, often severe, and rapidly progressive.[5] GBS has a 2% to 12% mortality rate. It can be rapidly regressive, such as tetraplegia within 24 h, and incomplete recovery within 18 mo.[52] Typically, GBS peaks in 10 to 14 d, with ambulatory and respiratory challenges, but recovery within weeks. However, the usual experience is days on a ventilator (without treatment) to assist breathing. Eighty percent of patients can walk without assistance at 6 mo,

and more than half regain full motor strength within 12 mo. Unfortunately, 5% to 10% of patients with GBS have extended illness, with months of ventilator dependence and incomplete recovery.[52]

Approximately 3,000 to 6,000 cases of GBS are diagnosed annually in North America. The condition may occur in either sex but favors males over females (1.5:1). GBS is uncommon in early childhood but has two age-related peaks: age 15 to 35 yr and 50 to 75 yr. Race is not a factor. The incidence increases with age, and about two-thirds of patients with GBS experience symptoms of viral respiratory or gastrointestinal infection 1 to 3 wk before the onset of neurological symptoms.[53] There have been small increases in GBS following some vaccines, but the studies reporting these are not replicated under more robust research.[66,67] Although the trend is to blame vaccines for the illness, there are no confirmed data since 2021 that support this claim.[53,65] In a study of 147 cases of GBS onset related to SARS-CoV-2 (COVID-19) infection, it was suggested that COVID-19 could trigger GBS, but more studies are necessary for a definitive correlation.[54] GBS is not contagious.

The health care provider must be able to recognize the symptoms of rapid onset of bilateral muscle weakness in the lower extremities with the absence of fever or other systemic symptoms and refer the patient immediately to the appropriate medical facility, usually the hospital emergency department.

Signs and Symptoms

The major clinical symptom of GBS is distal muscle weakness and loss of deep tendon reflexes that occurs bilaterally. The pattern is typically an ascending paralysis initially noted in the legs. The weakness evolves quickly over several hours or days and may be accompanied by tingling and dysesthesias in all extremities. The trunk, intercostals, neck, and cranial muscles may be involved later. Weakness may progress to total motor paralysis with death from respiratory failure within a few days. Frequently, early symptoms will also include paresthesias and numbness. A varying degree of sensory loss occurs in the first days and in a few days is barely detectable. When sensory deficits are present, deep sensations such as touch, pressure, and vibration are likely to be more affected than superficial sensations to pain or temperature. Complaints of pain and an aching discomfort, especially in muscles of the hips, thighs, and back, occur in 50% or more of the patients.[4,52] Patients with GBS may also present with a facial droop like Bell's palsy, diplopia, and difficulty with speech or swallowing.

Differential diagnoses for GBS include metabolic myopathies, poliomyelitis, spinal cord compression, heavy metal intoxication, botulism, tick paralysis, and basilar artery occlusion.[52]

Referral and Diagnostic Tests

A patient who experiences bilateral, rapidly evolving muscle weakness with absence of fever or other systemic symptoms and has a history of a recent viral upper respiratory infection or gastrointestinal illness must be referred to a physician immediately. GBS in its most severe form is a medical emergency. Most patients require hospitalization, and almost 30% require breathing assistance at some time during the illness. Severe GBS may result in total paralysis and the inability to breathe without the help of a ventilator. Thirty percent of patients complain of residual weakness 3 yr after recovery.[52,53,55]

In addition to deficient deep tendon reflexes, key diagnostic and laboratory tests include an electromyologram (EMG) and CSF analysis via a lumbar puncture. An EMG records and measures the electrical activity produced by a specific skeletal muscle. The test is performed by applying surface electrodes or by inserting small needle electrodes into a muscle. This test is performed to determine whether there is any defect in the nerve associated with the muscle or whether the nerve is not responding normally because of disease or impingement. CSF findings are distinctive but conclusive only after the first week. They include an elevated CSF protein level (100-1,000 mg/dL) without an accompanying increase in cells. When symptoms have been present for less than 48 h, the CSF is often normal. Nearly 75% of patients diagnosed with GBS reach their lowest point of clinical function within 1 wk, and the remainder reach it within 1 mo.[4,55]

Nerve conduction velocity (NCV) has also proven to be diagnostic, as the rate at which the nerve impulse travels to the muscle is often slower in a limb affected with GBS. The principal EMG findings are a reduction in the amplitudes of muscle action potentials, slowed conduction velocity, and conduction block in motor nerves.[52] GBS is described as a syndrome and not a disease because there is no specific disease-causing agent.

RED FLAGS FOR GUILLAIN-BARRÉ SYNDROME

Signs and symptoms of Guillain-Barré syndrome include the following:

- Progressive weakness beginning distally and moving proximally
- Areflexia
- Afebrile state
- Pain with slightest movement of affected area
- Nocturnal muscular cramps

Diagnosis is made by a physician carefully evaluating the patient's symptoms and recognizing the pattern of rapidly evolving signs of paralysis, diminished or absent reflexes, lack of fever or other systemic symptoms, and the results of laboratory tests, EMG, NCV, and CSF analysis. If the diagnosis is strongly suspected, treatment is initiated without waiting for the occurrence of characteristic EMG and CSF findings.

Treatment and Return to Participation

Treatment is initiated as soon after diagnosis as possible. There is no cure for GBS. Although patients do get better, they rarely recover completely. Therapies are aimed at lessening symptom severity, accelerating the rate of recovery in most patients, and managing GBS complications such as fluctuations in blood pressure and heart rate, inability to breathe without respiratory assistance, and inability to chew and swallow. Plasmapheresis and high-dose immunoglobulin therapy have been demonstrated to be effective.[52]

Rehabilitation involves being prudent with respect to possible thrombophlebitis, urine retention, and airway management for the sickest of patients. Skin conditions such as bedsores and contractures can occur. These can be circumvented with diligent skin care and inspection and range-of-motion exercises.

Most people reach the stage of greatest weakness within the first week after symptoms appear, and by the third week of the illness, 90% of all patients are at their weakest.[53] The recovery period may be as short as a few weeks or several years. Approximately 85% of patients with GBS recover completely or nearly completely, with mild motor deficits in the feet or legs. About 3% may suffer a relapse of muscle weakness and tingling sensations many years after the initial attack.[53] Evidence of widespread axonal damage, as well as early and prolonged mechanical ventilatory assistance, occur in those with the most severe and rapidly progressing form of the disease. EMG findings are consistent predictors of residual weakness.

Return to participation will be determined by the level of symptom resolution and clearance by the medical team. It may take 1 yr or more for symptoms to resolve.

Arthritides

Gout

Gout is one of the more painful of the rheumatic arthritides. The ancient Greeks first described it in the fifth century BC. Gout is usually acute in onset and is associated with pain, erythema, and warmth in one joint (monoarticular). It is a potentially disabling form of arthritis that results from the deposition of uric acid crystals within a joint, in the connective tissues surrounding a joint as deposits called *tophi*, or a combination of the two. Gout is increasing in the United States, owing in part to increasing population age and obesity prevalence, and is more common in males.[56,57]

Pseudogout is sometimes confused with gout because it produces similar symptoms of inflammation. However, in pseudogout, also called *chondrocalcinosis*, deposits are made up of calcium pyrophosphate dihydrate (CPPD) crystals, not uric acid.[56] Pseudogout typically affects the knee, whereas gout most commonly affects the great toe but may affect any joint.

Uric acid is a nitrogen-based substance that is the product of purine metabolism. Uric acid is primarily excreted through the kidneys and eliminated in the urine and gastrointestinal tract. **Hyperuricemia** results from either the increased production of uric acid or the decreased elimination of uric acid by the kidneys. Hyperuricemia itself is not a disease and does not cause symptoms. However, if excess uric acid crystals form because of hyperuricemia, the clinical presentation of gout may develop. The presence of uric acid crystals in the joint activates several inflammatory pathways. Clinical gout presents if uric acid crystals from hyperuricemia are formed and deposited within the joint cavity, inducing several inflammatory responses.

Gout may be considered a continuum ranging from asymptomatic hyperuricemia to the acute gouty flare-up to formation of tophi (deposits of uric acid crystals in soft tissue). Hyperuricemia occurs when an individual has elevated levels of uric acid in the blood but no other symptoms. Acute gout, or acute gouty arthropathy, occurs when the hyperuricemia has caused the deposition of uric acid crystals into the joint space. This leads to a sudden onset of pain and localized swelling in the joint. The joint is also usually very warm, red, and tender. Acute gouty arthropathy often occurs at night and may be triggered by several risk factors. (See the Gout Risk Factors sidebar.) Flare-ups usually subside within 5 to 10 d, even without

treatment, and subsequent episodes may not occur for months or even years.[5]

Interval or intercritical gout is the period between acute flare-ups. During this time, the individual is usually asymptomatic. Prophylactic medications may be used to prevent flare-ups.

Chronic tophaceous gout is the most disabling stage and usually develops over several years of recurrent flares. *Tophi* is a term used to describe the deposition of uric acid crystals in soft tissue, typically found in the pinnae of the ears, around the interphalangeal (IP) joints, Achilles tendon, and olecranon bursa. The disease may cause permanent damage to the affected joints and sometimes to the kidneys. With proper treatment, most people with gout do not progress to this advanced stage.[4]

Signs and Symptoms

The patient usually presents with the sudden onset of a severe, painful, swollen joint (figure 13.7). Physical examination confirms the extremely tender, erythematous, inflamed joint. The pain is often worsened with motion or direct pressure. Motion is often restricted because of the swelling.[56]

Initial onset of gout may be confused with other orthopedic conditions that cause sudden onset of a painful swollen joint. Gout is atraumatic, which can differentiate

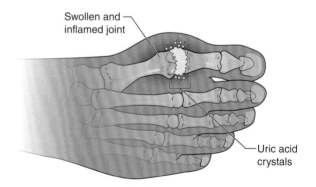

FIGURE 13.7 Gout of the great toe presents with an inflamed, painful first metatarsophalangeal joint.

Gout Risk Factors

- Foods high in purines (red meat, shellfish)
- Medications, such as diuretics, salicylates, niacin, cyclosporine, levodopa
- Family history, for males, postmenopausal females, and African Americans
- Medical conditions, such as diabetes, kidney disease, obesity, hypertension, hyperlipidemia, or sickle cell anemia
- Other factors, such as dehydration, trauma, surgery, or alcoholism

it from joint sprains or fractures. Other conditions that may present with similar signs and symptoms are pseudogout, septic arthritis, cellulitis, acute rheumatic fever, juvenile RA, tenosynovitis, bursitis, and palindromic rheumatism.[56]

Referral and Diagnostic Tests

The active patient with atraumatic, sudden onset of pain and swelling in a joint, especially the great toe, is referred for diagnostic tests to confirm the presence of gout. A definitive diagnosis is made by joint aspiration and evidence of uric acid crystals in the joint fluid. The fluid is usually evaluated for evidence of infection, since this could be an additional cause of joint pain and swelling. Blood uric acid levels may be elevated but this is often transient. Radiographs are often normal in acute flare-ups but may show characteristic findings of joint erosion or tophaceous deposits in chronic cases of gout.

Treatment and Return to Participation

Treatment consists of trying to decrease pain and inflammation while restoring normal uric acid levels to avoid formation of tophi and kidney stones. NSAIDs are very beneficial, and analgesics are sometimes needed as well. An acute flare-up of gout can be treated with NSAIDs, corticosteroids, or colchicine. Colchicine is very effective, especially if it is started within the first 12 to 24 h of an attack; however, it has frequent side effects and is often not well tolerated. Corticosteroids can be given orally or by injection during joint aspiration.

For patients who have had multiple episodes, therapy should be directed at normalizing uric acid levels in the blood as a prophylactic measure. Uricosuric agents (probenecid, febuxostat) lower the serum concentration of uric acid by increasing excretion. Drugs such as allopurinol help slow the production of uric acid and may be used alone or in combination with a uricosuric agent.[56]

Patients whose gout-associated symptoms are adequately controlled with diet and oral medications have a very good prognosis, and no restrictions on activity are necessary. Patients who continue to have flare-ups despite medications and lifestyle changes, however, may need to modify their activities. The athletic trainer can counsel the individual with gout about lifestyle issues that may be contributing to the flare-ups, including discussion of avoiding fad diets, maintaining a healthy weight, and monitoring consumption of foods high in purines, alcohol use, and certain medications. Maintaining adequate hydration, especially in times of increased exercise, can also help limit flare-ups.[57]

Pseudogout

Pseudogout refers to a condition that closely resembles gout, except the crystals are composed of CPPD. Patients present in a similar fashion to gout. However, aspiration reveals CPPD deposits as opposed to uric acid crystals in the joint. The term *chondrocalcinosis* is used to describe the calcium-containing deposits that are found in cartilage and are usually visible on joint radiographs (figure 13.8).

The etiology of pseudogout is unknown. There may be a familial predisposition or an association with thyroid or parathyroid gland disorders. NSAIDs, corticosteroid injections, and colchicine are successful in shortening the course of flare-ups and may be effective in preventing attacks. No treatments are available to dissolve the crystal deposits. Controlling inflammation helps to halt the progression of joint degeneration that often accompanies pseudogout.[5,56]

Rheumatoid Arthritis

RA is a systemic autoimmune inflammatory disease that typically causes symmetrical joint pain, swelling, and stiffness and eventually results in loss of motion and decreased function. Morning joint stiffness that may last for hours is a hallmark of the disease. Although RA may affect any joint, it most commonly presents in the wrists and carpometacarpal (CMC) and IP joints. Patients with RA may also experience systemic symptoms, including

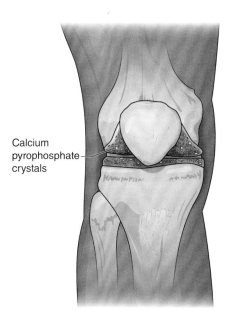

Calcium pyrophosphate crystals

FIGURE 13.8 Pseudogout presents with intermittent flare-ups of pain and inflammation, creating a cumulative joint degeneration over time.

generalized fatigue, malaise, and fever. Other systemic effects may include ocular dryness, skin ulcerations, **neutropenia**, or **splenomegaly**. These systemic symptoms associated with RA are also called Felty's syndrome. RA can affect individuals transiently or in cycles with periods of remission and flare-ups that progressively worsen over time. RA affects women more commonly than men and occurs in all racial and ethnic groups. RA typically begins in middle age and occurs with increased frequency in older people.[58]

An identical disease that occurs in children is known as juvenile chronic arthritis (juvenile RA). Juvenile RA can interfere with growth and lead to joint deformities because of chronic joint inflammation. Another common progression of juvenile RA is the inflammation of the iris in the eye that can lead to permanent eye damage.[59]

The cartilage damage seen in RA is thought to be a result of lymphocytic infiltration of the neutrophils in synovial fluid, chondrocytes, and hypertrophic synovium, which destroy articular cartilage.[58] The exact mechanism for the initiation of these processes is not clear.

Signs and Symptoms

Physical examination usually reveals symmetrical, tender, warm, swollen joints. Range of motion begins to be limited as the disease progresses. Eventually, joint deformities may develop, including ulnar drifting of the metacarpophalangeal (MCP) joints and boutonnière and swan neck deformity of the IP joints (figure 13.9). Rheumatoid nodules may also develop on the extensor surface of the digits and upper extremities. Rheumatoid nodules are small subcutaneous areas of fibrous necrosis

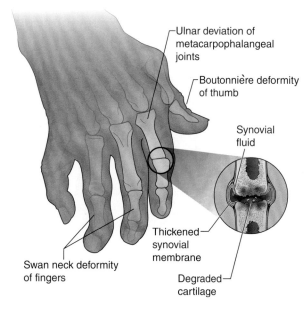

Ulnar deviation of metacarpophalangeal joints

Boutonnière deformity of thumb

Synovial fluid

Thickened synovial membrane

Swan neck deformity of fingers

Degraded cartilage

FIGURE 13.9 Rheumatoid arthritis presents with painful, stiff joints, and awkwardly twisted fingers.

surrounded by epithelial cells. In rare cases, these nodules may also be found systemically within the heart or lungs.

RA should be differentiated from other orthopedic presentations, such as osteoarthritis (OA), psoriatic arthritis, gout, Lyme disease, and fibromyalgia.

Referral and Diagnostic Tests

Patients with oligo- or polyarticular symptoms raise special concern for systemic evolvement. Laboratory tests typically reveal elevated levels of rheumatoid factors (immunoglobulin M) and ANAs. RA frequently causes chronic anemia, the severity of which often parallels the disease course. ESR and C-reactive protein are usually elevated because of the systemic inflammatory response.

Radiographs typically reveal osteoporosis and soft-tissue swelling in the early stages. As the disease progresses, joint space narrowing and eventually erosion of the articular surfaces of the joint will be evident on radiographs. Radiographs of the wrists, hands, and feet are usually the most dramatic.[58,59]

Treatment and Return to Participation

There is no known cure for RA, so treatment focuses on reducing pain, restoring joint motion, and improving overall function to allow the individual to lead a normal life. The most important aspect of management is to educate the patient about the condition and to begin a regular exercise program with appropriate periods of rest. Exercise helps to maintain muscle strength, joint mobility, and function and prevent osteoporosis. Medications may be used for pain relief and to reduce inflammation. NSAIDs, corticosteroids, and disease-modifying agents are classes of medications used to treat RA. Newer medications may be used to attempt to modify the disease itself. Most individuals do very well with a combination of treatments. Some individuals will continue to have a certain level of symptoms despite aggressive therapy. These individuals must rest their joints during flare-ups and maintain a regular, nonimpact exercise program.

Surgery is available to patients with severe joint damage. As with other treatments, the goals of surgery are to reduce pain, improve function of the affected joint, and restore the patient's ability to perform daily activities. Surgery is usually not performed on a pain-free functional joint regardless of the cosmetic deformity.[58,59]

Osteoarthritis

OA is the most common of the rheumatologic disorders and affects 32 million people, primarily older individuals, in the United States.[60] Although it is commonly known by the term *degenerative joint disease*, OA is a complicated process that involves damage to the underlying collagen structure and increasing water content in the articular cartilage (figure 13.10). There is an increase in chondrocytes, which results in an increase in degradative enzymes that shift the homeostasis of the joint from a status of repair to one of breakdown. This process has a greater effect on the articular surface than mechanical degeneration. Several factors have been shown to hasten this degradative process, including trauma, anterior cruciate ligament deficiency, and joint malalignment.[5]

Other risk factors include obesity, a positive family history, and performing heavy labor for a living. Interestingly, long-distance runners show no increased risk of developing OA. OA is seen primarily in the IP and first CMC joints of the hand, cervical and lower lumbar spine, hips, knees, and the first metatarsophalangeal joint but may affect any joint.[4,59]

Signs and Symptoms

The most common presenting complaint is pain that typically is worse with activity and resolves with rest. However, pain at night and following prolonged immobilization is also common. The symptoms are usually monoarticular or localized to one joint but may affect any number of joints. Joint stiffness in the morning and after rest or inactivity are common but usually resolve quickly in OA unlike in RA, in which stiffness may last for several hours. Patients often experience soreness associated with changes in the weather, especially with barometric changes and cold temperatures.[8,60]

Physical examination of the knee usually reveals joint crepitus, tenderness, and enlargement of bony promi-

nences because of osteophyte formation. Knee pain may also be noted in the proximal tibia.[60] Examination of the hands reveals enlargements around the IP joints, which are known as Heberden's nodes when distal and Bouchard's nodes when proximal. As osteophytes progress, joint stiffness and mechanical loss of motion begin to occur. OA in the hip typically presents as groin pain but may also present as buttock, thigh, or even knee pain. Internal rotation of the hip usually reproduces symptoms. Lower lumbar OA typically produces buttock or thigh pain. Cervical OA usually produces pain that radiates into the shoulder and arm. In the cervical and lumbar regions, the radiated pain is a result of nerve root impingement.[60]

OA should be differentiated from other orthopedic conditions, such as RA, psoriatic arthritis, gout, Lyme disease, and fibromyalgia.

Referral and Diagnostic Tests

Radiographs confirm the diagnosis of OA, although in early cases these films may show very minimal joint destruction. Eventually, loss of joint space and osteophyte formation occur (figure 13.11). Weight-bearing films are recommended to get a true sense of joint height. Subchondral bone cysts and irregularities in the intraarticular joint surface begin to appear in the later stages of the disease. Laboratory tests are usually normal.

Treatment and Return to Participation

No treatments are available that reverse OA, but many modalities, including pharmacological and surgical

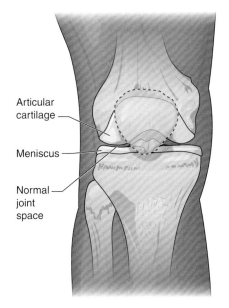
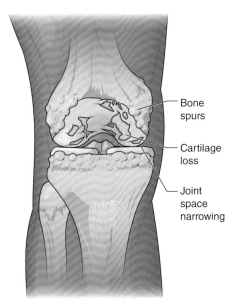

Articular cartilage

Meniscus

Normal joint space

Bone spurs

Cartilage loss

Joint space narrowing

FIGURE 13.10   Osteoarthritis of the knee joint showing a gradual breakdown of hyaline cartilage and narrowing joint space.

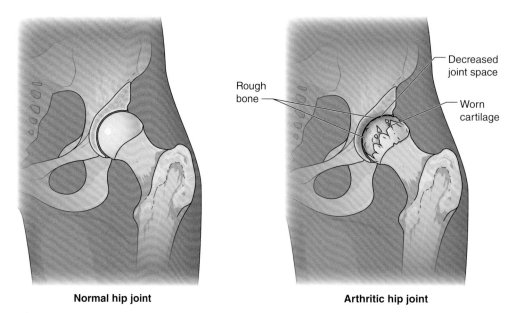

Normal hip joint   **Arthritic hip joint**

FIGURE 13.11 Osteoarthritis of the head of the femur. The image on the left is a normal smooth femoral-pelvis articulation, and the image on the right shows the effect of OA on the joint.

interventions, can be helpful in decreasing joint pain and preserving joint mobility and function (table 13.3). Exercise and lifestyle changes to maintain and improve joint range of motion and muscular strength should be initiated. At the same time, limiting impact-loading activities can decrease stress on the affected joints.

Pharmacological treatment follows a path from least to most invasive by beginning with acetaminophen, progressing to NSAIDs, then to corticosteroid injections. Other over-the-counter treatments, such as topical ointments, may provide superficial pain relief. Supplements such as glucosamine and chondroitin sulfate have shown some promise in treating OA symptoms in some individuals. In addition, analgesics are used for pain in patients whose symptoms are not controlled with other means.[4]

More invasive treatments such as corticosteroid injections have a beneficial effect on most arthritic joints, especially during flare-up of symptoms. Corticosteroid injections may safely be performed two or three times per year in any joint. Injectable hyaluronic acid has been used as a series of weekly injections that may help decrease symptoms for as long as 6 to 12 mo. When conservative measures are not successful in alleviating a patient's symptoms, more aggressive interventions are appropriate. These may include arthroscopic debridement and **lavage** for intraarticular pathology, such as meniscal tears, loose bodies, and articular cartilage flaps. Simply lavaging the joint and removing degenerative particles may also have a temporary benefit.[4,60]

A more aggressive procedure is an arthroplasty to replace or resurface the joint. Arthroplasty ranges from arthroscopic resurfacing of the joint to a complete replacement of the damaged joint via the commonly called *joint replacement* (figure 13.12). A joint replacement may provide a better chance of long-term relief from symptoms. More recently, a less invasive procedure that involves placing a small metal disk in the affected joint space of the knee has shown some promise in younger patients or patients with OA isolated to one side of the joint.

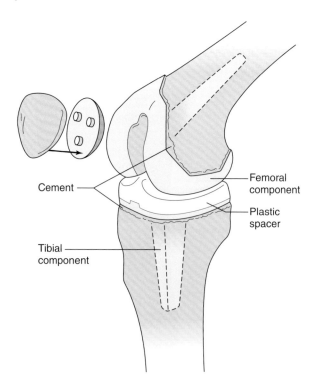

FIGURE 13.12 Knee arthroplasty. Replacing the joint surfaces is the final step in treatment of osteoarthritis.

TABLE 13.3   **Nonsurgical Treatment Options for Osteoarthritis**

Treatment	Benefits and possible adverse effects
Exercise	Decreased pain and stiffness; improved daily function and activity level. Some types of exercise will aggravate symptoms in some patients
Oral analgesics	
Acetaminophen (Tylenol)	Mild to moderate pain relief; appropriate for those taking anticoagulants
NSAIDs	Useful when analgesics no longer provide relief. This entire category has possible increased risk of gastrointestinal distress and is associated with increased risk of cardiovascular disease
COX-2–selective anti-inflammatory drugs, such as celecoxib (Celebrex)	Lower incidence of gastrointestinal challenges compared with other NSAIDs
Non–COX-2–selective anti-inflammatory drugs, such as ibuprofen (Advil, Motrin IB, Caldolor, Neo-Profen)	Widely available, inexpensive
Diclofenac (Voltaren XR, Cataflam, Cambia, Zipsor)	Has an enteric-coated, delayed-release option. Low risk of gastrointestinal bleeding. Monitor liver enzymes first 8 wk of treatment
Naproxen (Aleve, Anaprox, Anaprox DS, Naprelan, Naprosyn)	Primarily for mild to moderate pain
Topical analgesics	
Capsaicin (Qutenza)	This is the preferred topical analgesic for OA. May need 14 d to reach full skin and/or joint insensitivity
Narcotics (opioids)	Used for acute pain. Potential for abuse
Tramadol (Ultram, UltramER, ConZip)	Alters and inhibits pain pathways
Oxycodone (OxyContin, Roxicodone)	OA initial drug of choice, but short acting
Intraarticular injections	
Corticosteroids, such as triamcinolone acetonide ER (Zilretta)	Intended as single intraarticular injection
Betamethasone (Celestone), triamcinolone (Kenalog), or dexamethasone	Decreases inflammation by various physiological mechanisms
Hyaluronic acid (Hyalgan, Supartz), Hylan G-F 20 (Synvisc-One), or high-molecular weight hyaluronan (Orthovisc)	Primarily for OA of the knee: Varies from single injection, to up to five at weekly intervals. Avoid strenuous activity 48 h postinjection
Braces	
Elastic or neoprene knee sleeve	Added support for ADLs; control inflammation
Unloader brace	Reduces stresses placed on knee with normal weight-bearing activities

Note: ADL = activity of daily living; COX-2 = cyclooxygenase-2; NSAID = nonsteroidal anti-inflammatory drug; OA = osteoarthritis.

Adapted from Lozada (2022); "Hyaluronic Acid and Derivatives (Rx)," Medscape, https://reference.medscape.com/drug/orthovisc-synvisc-hyaluronic-acid-and-derivatives-999526.

As with all the degenerative arthropathies, the long-term prognosis for OA is not good. However, most patients do very well with some combination of therapies and are able to lead a healthy and active, if somewhat restricted, lifestyle. Specific restrictions are based on a patient's pain and disease progression.

Osteomyelitis

Osteomyelitis is an infection caused by a bacterium that affects the bone. This bacterium often is *Staphylococcus aureus*, but it could be any causative organism.[62] Osteomyelitis occurs in both acute and chronic forms. It can occur in any age group but is most seen in young children, older adults, and people with an underlying disease that leaves them immunocompromised.[61]

When a bone becomes infected, the marrow may swell and press against cortical bone. This causes the blood vessels in the marrow to be compromised, thus cutting off the blood supply to the bone and causing extreme pain. Bone requires this blood supply to survive and will break down without it. The infection may also break through the cortical bone, forming abscesses in surrounding muscle or other soft tissues.

Osteomyelitis is typically caused by one of several routes. The hematogenous route carries the infection through the bloodstream. Other routes include direct invasion from a penetrating trauma or retained metal implants or via infection in adjacent bone or soft tissues, such as soft-tissue ulcerations.[8] Individuals with artificial joints or metal attached to bone should use prophylactic antibiotics before any type of dental work and most surgeries, because these procedures have the potential to release bacteria into the bloodstream.

Signs and Symptoms

Osteomyelitis can present in many ways, but typically an individual has pain in the infected bone and may experience fever. The area around the infection may be painful to touch, erythematous, edematous, warm, and painful with movement. General signs of infection, such as malaise and fatigue, are common.[4]

Chronic osteomyelitis may develop if the initial bone infection is not treated adequately. This persistent infection can be very difficult to eliminate. It may be dormant for extended periods or, more commonly, cause recurrent infections in the soft tissue surrounding the bone with recurrent drainage of **purulent** fluid through a sinus tract in the skin.[61]

Other orthopedic conditions, such as gout and stress fracture, need to be ruled out. Systemic conditions also must be considered, such as reactive bone marrow edema, cellulitis, deep vein thrombosis, emboli, or carcinoma.[62]

Referral and Diagnostic Tests

Blood tests usually reveal an elevated level of white blood cells, ESR, and C-reactive protein. White blood cells are elevated as a response to infection, whereas ESR and C-reactive protein are elevated as a response to inflammation. Radiographs may not register any bone changes until the infection has progressed for several weeks (figure 13.13). Osteomyelitis is reliably diagnosed via PET, MRI, and single-photon emission CT scans, but MRI does not expose the patient to X-rays and is used more often.[62] Aspiration of the affected area may be required to confirm the diagnosis. This is typically done in the operating room, with preparations made for possibly surgically opening the area for thorough cleaning and debridement.[61,62]

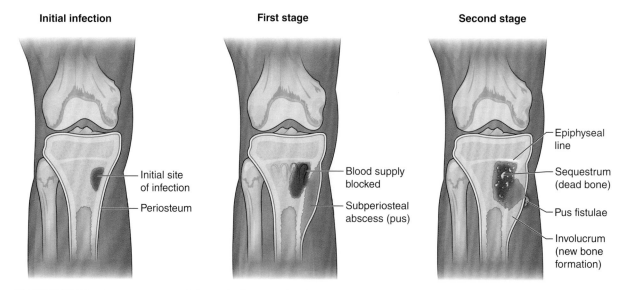

FIGURE 13.13 Anterior view of the right knee with advancing degrees of an osteomyelitis infection.

Treatment and Return to Participation

Appropriate antibiotic therapy based on the organism suspected is the basis for treatment. *S. aureus* is the most seen organism, but others may include mycobacteria, fungal infections, and even viruses. Additionally, methicillin-resistant *S. aureus* (MRSA) may be a culprit and may be more challenging to adequately treat.[62] Empirical treatment is often initiated before a specific organism is identified. Intravenous antibiotics are usually begun and subsequently switched to oral medications after a period depending on the organism, the patient's response to antibiotics, and the patient's overall health.[4] Antibiotics are typically continued for 4 to 8 wk, although they may be continued for several months in some cases (see chapter 3).

If osteomyelitis is detected early and treated appropriately, the prognosis is usually very good. When chronic osteomyelitis occurs, treatment may have to be cycled intermittently for several years.

Inflammatory Myopathies

The inflammatory myopathies are a group of diseases characterized by inflammation of muscle and other connective tissues (i.e., skin). Inflammatory myopathies may occur because of bacterial, fungal, or parasitic infections or toxic exposures or other known causes of muscle damage, such as myositis ossificans. The most common inflammatory myopathies are polymyositis and dermatomyositis.

Polymyositis and Dermatomyositis

Both polymyositis and dermatomyositis are connective tissue disorders, and as such, collagen associated with muscles, ligaments, and tendons are affected. The two conditions have many similarities, but polymyositis primarily affects muscles, whereas dermatomyositis also relates to skin manifestations. Both conditions are similar in that they have no specific cause, although immune reactions and viruses are among the more likely culprits.

Signs and Symptoms

Both polymyositis and dermatomyositis present more often in females than in males. Whereas polymyositis is uncommon in children, dermatomyositis is found in both children (onset age 5-15 yr) and adults (40-50 yr).[63,64] Polymyositis may present acutely or over the course of weeks to months. It is characterized by the insidious onset of proximal muscle weakness in which individuals notice the inability to rise from a chair, climb stairs, and reach overhead. It later may involve distal or pharyngeal muscles. Polymyositis is usually painless, but those affected often describe fatigue, general soreness, and cramping.[64]

Dermatomyositis is like polymyositis, with insidious onset of muscle weakness, often accompanied by other systemic symptoms, including fever, malaise, arthralgias, stomach ulcerations, and cutaneous lesions that result from inflammatory changes in the skin. Additional signs and symptoms of dermatomyositis are the characteristic scaling of the skin on the face and dorsal IP joints.[63] Gottron's papules, which are erythematous plaques usually seen over extensor surfaces of the MCP joints, and the **heliotrope rash**, a purplish discoloration around the upper eyelids (figure 13.14), are pathognomonic for the disease. Other cutaneous manifestations may include scaly rashes on other areas of the body, cuticle overgrowth, dryness and cracking of the palmar surfaces of the fingers, and erythema in the V of the neck.

Other conditions that may present in a similar fashion to polymyositis include Cushing's syndrome, fibromyalgia, thyroid disease, polymyalgia rheumatica, sarcoidosis, SLE, amyotrophic lateral sclerosis, infectious myositis, limb-girdle muscular dystrophy, and myasthenia gravis.[5,63,64]

Referral and Diagnostic Tests

When polymyositis is suspected, a CBC may show leukocytosis (present in 50% of patients) or thrombocytosis. An elevated ESR is present in 50% of patients with polymyositis. In both polymyositis and dermatomyositis, assessment of the muscle enzymes and creatine kinase (CK) levels is key to diagnosis; additionally, specific antibodies are investigated to confirm diagnosis.[5]

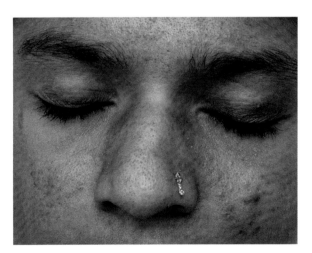

FIGURE 13.14 Dermatomyositis. One sign of the condition is the heliotrope rash surrounding the eyes and eyelids.

Science Photo Library / Science Source

Screening for both conditions includes tests for myoglobinuria and autoantibodies. Positive rheumatoid factors are performed to assist in diagnosis. Chest and abdominal CT scans and MRI tests are preformed, depending on presentation. EMG analysis is helpful to distinguish myopathy from neuropathy and is usually abnormal, with various motor unit potential changes and evidence of denervation or reinnervation in chronic cases. Diagnosis is also dependent on clinical signs, a pulmonary function test, and ECG. An echocardiogram and/or swallow study would be part of the battery of evaluative tests performed.[63,64] Depending on results of other examinations, a muscle biopsy may be collected. Muscle biopsy is performed to confirm the diagnosis and rule out other potential causes of muscle inflammation. Radiographs are generally not helpful.

Treatment and Return to Participation

Initial treatment for polymyositis includes prednisone for 1 to 2 mo until CK levels return to normal. Immunosuppressive medications may be introduced if steroids alone do not improve the patient's condition.[64] For dermatomyositis, skin, muscular, and other systemic challenges must be addressed. Typical treatment plans include avoiding the sun with both sunscreen and photoprotective clothing and using topical corticosteroid agents. People with muscular presentations are treated with corticosteroids and immunosuppressive medications. Oral corticosteroids are helpful in decreasing muscle inflammation, and immunosuppressive drugs are sometimes used when symptoms do not respond to conventional treatments. Other common medications include immunomodulatory medications (methotrexate, mycophenolate mofetil, or intravenous immunoglobulin).[63] Patients taking corticosteroids must be monitored for adverse side effects, such as hypertension, diabetes mellitus, osteopenia, and steroid myopathy.[5,63,64]

Patients should be encouraged to begin supervised activity as soon as possible and early in the disease. Activity includes passive range of motion, stretching, and flexibility exercises to prevent joint contractures. As the disease course subsides, a gradual increase to active and isometric exercise is permitted, progressing to isotonic exercises with light resistance. Aerobic exercise can begin once the disease is inactive.[64]

Prognosis for polymyositis and dermatomyositis is extremely variable. Most patients have a good response to therapies and can return to moderate levels of activity, although some patients do not achieve any response to therapies and experience significant disability. Mortality is rare but may occur in patients with severe disease who develop progressive muscle weakness and eventually dysphagia, malnutrition, pneumonia, or respiratory failure.

Summary

Systemic disorders are not uncommon in the general population and are often accompanied by general maladies, such as body aches and fatigue. The challenge with active people is to distinguish exercise-related body aches from something more ominous. Persistent fatigue, body aches, weight loss, or slower-than-typical healing must alert the athletic trainer to conditions that may warrant referral to a physician. Many systemic disorders, once correctly diagnosed, can be effectively treated, allowing the active patient to continue participation in sports.

Apply It!   Go to HK*Propel* to complete the case studies for this chapter.

Infectious Diseases

14

At the completion of this chapter the reader should be able to do the following:

1. Explain how infections are commonly transmitted and how to prevent transmission.

2. Justify the importance of maintaining immunity against those diseases for which vaccine is available.

3. Describe the reporting rationales for communicable diseases.

4. List the signs and symptoms of common infectious diseases.

5. Recognize common childhood diseases and explain how to prevent them.

6. Demonstrate universal precautions for the prevention and transmission of infectious diseases.

Nearly every chapter in this text addresses an infectious condition. For example, pneumonia is addressed in chapter 6 on the respiratory system, urinary tract infection in chapter 9 on the genitourinary and gynecological systems, and sinusitis in chapter 12 on the ear, nose, mouth, and throat. This chapter provides an overview of the infectious disease process, including common transmission mechanisms and routes, and discusses preventive measures to stop the infection cycle and protect people and the population at large. The conditions discussed in this chapter include many common childhood diseases, in addition to hepatitis, streptococcal, staphylococcal, and neurological infections. Sexually transmitted infections (STIs) are discussed in chapter 9.

This chapter is critical for learning how to recognize and refer infectious conditions. Because the signs and symptoms of many infections cross several body systems, this chapter builds on the previous ones to help the reader discern infections from other differential diagnoses previously discussed, in addition to transmittable conditions introduced here. All illnesses in this chapter can be passed to another individual or group of people. With knowledge gained in the previous chapters, readers will think outside a specific body system, ask better questions, and be able to consider system-crossing ailments, including infectious diseases. This chapter begins with a discussion of basic disease transmission prevention, including bloodborne pathogens (BBPs) and barriers to disease transmission.

Prevention of Disease Transmission

Everyone who works in health care appreciates the need to prevent disease transmission. Protection from infection and maintaining a sanitary environment are two critical elements in caring for patients with illnesses. Another prevention technique is immunization from specific diseases by vaccine. This chapter discusses vaccination as well as established standards for preventing the spread of disease and illnesses.

There are federal mandates that address disease prevention and spread. States and institutions may also impose restrictions for safety, and health care providers must know the policies and regulations for their own workplaces. Intercollegiate sports medicine guidelines require that all necessary materials, such as barriers, bleach, waste receptacles, and wound coverings, comply with universal precautions and be available to all health care providers.[1]

The Occupational Safety and Health Administration (OSHA) sets standards to protect health care workers and their patients. OSHA standards apply only to established relationships between employers and employees and do not extend federal protections to students.[2] However, students such as those in the health care field, who could be exposed to hazardous waste in facilities where they practice or observe, should follow the safety standards set forth by OSHA, receive training, and have ready access to precautionary materials, such as barriers and proper disposal containers.

OSHA can inspect any facility under its auspices without prior notification, and it has the power to suspend or shut down a facility as well as to impose hefty fines for noncompliance with standards.[2] The most familiar OSHA requirement affecting athletic medical care concerns the BBP standard. Athletic trainers must be intimately familiar with this standard because athletes often receive open wounds during their activities, with the consequent risk of infection.

Bloodborne Pathogens

The OSHA BBP standard is intended to safeguard health care workers against hazards resulting from exposure to infectious body fluids, and it covers anyone who could reasonably anticipate having occupational exposure to infectious waste (e.g., blood). Included in this standard is a description of how to formulate an individualized institutional or setting exposure control plan. A written document outlines steps to take and specific people to call in the event of an exposure to infectious waste. An exposure may range from a needlestick to blood spilled onto intact skin. All health care workers must have an operating knowledge of their employer's plan, access to personal protective equipment, BBP training, and knowledge about whom to contact should an exposure occur.[2] Typically, these instructions are visibly posted throughout the facility.

The BBP standard uses the phrase *universal precautions* to emphasize that all human waste should be treated as if it were infectious and that health care workers and patients must be protected in every situation in which they might be exposed to body fluid, including contact with blood, genital secretions, or mucous membranes in the eyes, mouth, or nose. Any sharp object that may be contaminated with infectious waste, such as needles, scalpels, or broken glass, is also considered potentially hazardous material.[2]

The National Collegiate Athletics Association (NCAA) and the National Federation of State High School Associations (NFHS) have explicit regulations that address infection control and bleeding athletes or those with blood on their uniform.[1,4] These regulations require that a bleeding athlete be removed from activ-

---

Clinical Tips

Handling Infectious Waste

- All infectious waste must be placed in a closeable, leakproof-approved container for storage, transporting, or shipping.
- An OSHA-approved plan for proper disposal of infectious waste bags and sharps units must be on hand and followed.
- Gloves must be worn when personnel handle infectious laundry.
- Laundry contaminated with infectious waste must be separated from other materials to be cleaned.
- Personal protective equipment (gowns, masks, gloves) shall be properly disposed of before leaving the treatment room or on contamination.
- While wearing gloves, personnel may clean bloodstains on material (uniforms, towels) with hydrogen peroxide in cold water and immediately rinse.
- Only red hazardous waste bags should be used to dispose of infectious materials.
- In the absence of antibacterial soap and running water, personnel should use antibacterial wipes or gels to sanitize hands often.
- Personnel should avoid putting ungloved hands to face (eyes, nose, mouth) when around ill patients or when working with infectious waste.

Data from Parson (2014); United States Department of Labor (2022).

ity until the bleeding has been stopped and the wound covered with a dressing sturdy enough to withstand the demands of activity. Soiled uniforms must be cleaned or changed before resumption of activity.[1] Again, the requirements of storing and disposing of infectious waste are intended to protect both the athlete and the health care provider and prevent them from transmitting diseases.

Barriers to Disease Transmission

Barriers are devices worn to protect both the health care worker and the patient against disease spread. The traditionally accepted barrier is latex gloves, but OSHA also requires access to face and eye protection, gowns, and mouthpieces for resuscitation.[1-3] Health care workers with a latex allergy must be provided with an alternative material suitable as a barrier against the BBP transmission.

All health care workers must have ready access to barriers that fit properly to retard infection from hazardous materials. Washing with soap and water is the best way to clean hands before and after glove use. If soap and water are not readily available, commercial disinfectant gels or single-use wipes can sanitize hands.

Workers should remove and properly dispose of soiled barriers before leaving the treatment area. Brightly labeled red infectious waste bags are the most common means of storing such waste until it can be disposed of

Clinical Tips
Correct Glove Use

1. Thoroughly wash all aspects of both hands and fingers, with liberal use of an antibacterial soap and plenty of water.
2. Dry hands with a disposable single-use hand towel.
3. Apply gloves without touching the external surfaces of the gloves.

When the procedure requiring gloves is complete, do the following:

1. Use the gloved index finger and thumb of one hand; gently pinch the glove at the wrist and pull toward fingertips.
2. Invert the glove and remove all but the index finger and thumb.
3. Repeat the procedure with the second hand, inverting the glove as it is removed.
4. Fold the gloves inside out and dispose of them in a red (OSHA-approved) bag.
5. Thoroughly wash and dry the hands as described previously.

per OSHA protocol. These bags must be contained in a sturdy, leakproof container with a lid and located in an easily accessible area for all to use.

Sharps Containers

Sharps containers are specifically built, self-contained units that have one-way valves (figure 14.1) and are used to accommodate sharp instruments, such as needles and scalpels, that may have infectious materials on them. Some sharps containers are locked to a wall so that only an OSHA-approved provider can remove them for proper disposal. These containers should never be opened or overstuffed. Typically, institutions that have sharps containers have a service that maintains them, including scheduled emptying and inspection for safety.

Disinfection

Another component in the prevention of infection spread is disinfection of surfaces used for examination, and treatment and disinfection of soiled materials, including uniforms and clothing. Disinfection is a critical aspect of every athletic training facility because of its potential to stop disease spread. The simple acts of sterilizing treatment tables after use and washing hands often can diminish disease transmission considerably. Many infections, such as hepatitis B virus (HBV), are quite hardy and can live outside the body if not obliterated properly.

The Environmental Protection Agency (EPA) registers all disinfectants in the United States. The EPA has prior approval on all test methods that companies use to determine whether their product is effective against a particular organism.[5] The product labels of EPA-approved disinfectants include a registration number and a list of

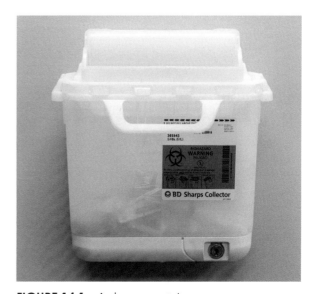

FIGURE 14.1 A sharps container.

organisms targeted. To be labeled as "hospital strength," a disinfectant must eradicate 100% of all organisms listed on the label. Household chlorine bleach contains 5.25% active sodium hypochlorite and 94.75% water. Although chlorine bleach is extremely effective against *Staphylococcus* and *Streptococcus* bacteria, *Salmonella* species, *Escherichia coli*, certain fungi, and influenza types A and B, it is not a cleaner. The EPA and U.S. Department of Agriculture have deemed chlorine bleach safe for use in food preparation and as a disinfectant. It is registered with the EPA for appropriate use as a hospital disinfectant, and the Centers for Disease Control and Prevention (CDC) has written guidelines for its use in health care facilities.[5]

The difference between a disinfectant and a disinfectant-cleaner is that a disinfectant merely kills microorganisms, whereas a combination cleaner removes soils and disinfects in one step. Regulations governing how these cleaners and disinfectants are dispersed include the following: If the material is removed from its original container, it must have all the product information transferred to the second receptacle, including a notation that the cleaner was moved, for example, from a gallon container to a spray bottle.[2,3] When sanitizing surfaces soiled with possible BBPs, OSHA recommends properly using barriers, cleaning all blood from the surface, properly

---

Clinical Tips

OSHA Mandates on Disinfectant Agents

- Contaminated surfaces must be sprayed to saturation with the disinfectant.
- Human immunodeficiency virus type 1 (HIV-1) disinfection requires 30 s of saturation.
- Hepatitis B virus disinfection requires 10 min of saturation.

From United States Department of Labor (2022).

Clinical Tips

Nosocomial Infections

A **nosocomial infection** is acquired in the athletic training facility or medical facility and is unrelated to the athlete's or patient's purpose for the visit. Many infections and illnesses discussed in this text can be acquired in the athletic training setting from other athletes or personnel. These include influenza, sinusitis, conjunctivitis, and certain staphylococcal and streptococcal infections.

---

disposing of the waste, and then disinfecting the area.[2]

The *2014-15 NCAA Sports Medicine Handbook* suggests using a 1:100 ratio of freshly prepared bleach-to-water solution for disinfecting surfaces.[1] The NFHS calls for a more proactive approach to disinfecting surfaces, and it recommends cleaning equipment and pads weekly with this bleach solution.[4]

Transmission

Most infections arise from one of four transmission routes:

- Airborne
- Direct contact
- Bloodborne
- Waterborne and foodborne

Sick people can spread infectious organisms by these pathways, so sanitary precautions are the most important line of defense in preventing illness. Healthy humans live in harmony with microbial flora that protect against the invasion of disease-causing microorganisms.[7] These flora reside in specific organs of the body, such as the skin, respiratory system, and gastrointestinal tract, and they help to protect the natural environments of these organs. Certain medications can disrupt this balance, as can repeated exposure to infectious organisms in an overtrained athlete. Many flora that protect humans can also invade their hosts under certain conditions. Disease transmission routes are discussed with each disorder.

Prevention

Increased infection prevention is achieved through vaccination and attention to personal hygiene. There are many vaccines available that are dependable, effective, and have minimal, if any, side effects. There are no robust, data-driven published studies that tie vaccines to lifelong sequelae, and unvaccinated individuals are at risk of developing the condition the immunization is intended to prevent. Sometimes, well-meaning parents mitigate vaccine effectiveness by providing infants and children with acetaminophen (Tylenol) or a similar medication to alleviate side effects. Some evidence suggests that follow-up booster vaccinations may be required in certain circumstances.

Good personal hygiene is also critical in preventing the spread of disease. Often the simple practice of handwashing with soap and water can deter infection or disease spread. Finally, proper nutrition and rest help the body resist opportunistic infection owing to a weakened immune system.

Vaccination

Practicing universal precautions and sanitation measures can prevent the transmission of most infectious diseases. In addition, immunization, such as for measles, mumps, and rubella (MMR), has deterred the spread of many adult and childhood diseases.

Researchers continue to provide new vaccines in the hope of preventing infectious diseases. Vaccines have been approved and distributed to prevent meningitis, human papillomavirus (HPV), and varicella (chicken pox). Colleges often require proof of meningitis vaccination before admission, and pediatricians are encouraging girls ages 12 to 15 yr to receive a three-shot series that may prevent future cervical cancer attributable to HPV. A varicella vaccine was approved in 1995. Studies indicate that a two-dose series is warranted for the vaccine to truly be effective, and the recommendation that all children receive the two-dose immunization for full immunity was made in 1996.[7-9] Adults are not exempt from immunizations. In addition to pneumonia vaccine for those older than age 65 yr and annual influenza protection, the Food and Drug Administration (FDA) recommended in 2008 that adults older than age 60 yr be vaccinated to prevent varicella-zoster virus (shingles).[7,8]

Some adults missed the window of opportunity for certain immunizations because they were born before they became available. For example, an effective vaccine for HBV was not established until 1982. Immunization against HPV is also an example, as females ages 13 to 26 yr are encouraged to complete the series if they missed their window of opportunity.[8] Adults who were not immunized as children and have no history of a particular disease should be vaccinated as adults, especially if they work in areas where they would be susceptible to the disease. Figures 14.2 and 14.3 provide the recommended schedules for vaccination for children and adults.

Children are no longer routinely vaccinated for small-pox because this disease has not been found in humans for more than a generation. Other communicable diseases, such as typhus, botulism, *E. coli*, polio, and anthrax, are not common but are extremely dangerous if contracted.[89] The danger with rare and dormant diseases is that they do still live in some laboratories, and terrorist attacks have made many people aware that releasing these organisms could initiate global germ warfare. Because few people are currently vaccinated against these dormant, yet deadly, diseases, their rapid spread is plausible.[7] The same is true with vaccine-preventable diseases. Individuals who choose to forgo available immunizations put themselves at risk should the disease reoccur.

Because of the threat of germ warfare, vaccines exist for typhoid and yellow fever but they are not widely used. These are typically available for persons traveling to countries where the contagion is more common than

> ## Clinical Tips
>
> ### Records of Immunization
>
> Immunization records with proof of vaccination against communicable diseases are required for entrance into most public schools and colleges. Some colleges now require proof of vaccination against meningococcal infections, which tend to affect college students living in dormitories.

in the United States, and there are significant side effects, especially for certain populations. The smallpox vaccine is another with many contraindications and tedious instructions for the weeks following immunization.[10]

U.S. public health officials established a goal through the Healthy People 2010 program to eliminate diphtheria, HBV, measles, mumps, polio, rubella, varicella, and tetanus by the year 2010. However, data show that little improvement has been made since the goal was established, and it remains a goal for Healthy People 2030.[11] Immunity after vaccination is not always guaranteed. In a 2006 outbreak, 6,584 people contracted mumps; 77% to 97% of the college students who acquired the illness had received the required two-dose MMR vaccine.[12] The updated Healthy People 2030 program continues to promote healthier behaviors, including immunization and other more current issues.[11]

With prevention being paramount, health histories typically include immunization records. However, in a study of the immune status of first-year medical students in New South Wales, Australia, immunity corresponded poorly with the self-reported histories. Tests were performed to determine students' antibody titers to certain vaccine-preventable diseases. The results showed that students' antibody titers were inadequate to protect them from future infection. Other studies have provided evidence for what many parents already know: Giving an infant acetaminophen to reduce fever caused by immunization actually reduces the effect of the vaccine.[10] This research may shed light on why so many previously immunized people have had less than the desired benefit of the vaccine later in life.

Although there may be little debate among health care providers over recommended vaccines, not all agencies have adopted minimal standards for immunization, leaving it to institutional autonomy or state authority. Even the Commission on Accreditation of Athletic Training Education standards only call for the institution to provide public access to requirements of the program, including "documentation of immunizations requirements" (Standard 24J) and "immunization requirements" (Standard 26F) for athletic training students; they do not articulate from what diseases the students should be immune.[13]

Table 1 Recommended Child and Adolescent Immunization Schedule for ages 18 years or younger, United States, 2023

These recommendations must be read with the notes that follow. For those who fall behind or start late, provide catch-up vaccination at the earliest opportunity as indicated by the green bars. To determine minimum intervals between doses, see the catch-up schedule (Table 2).

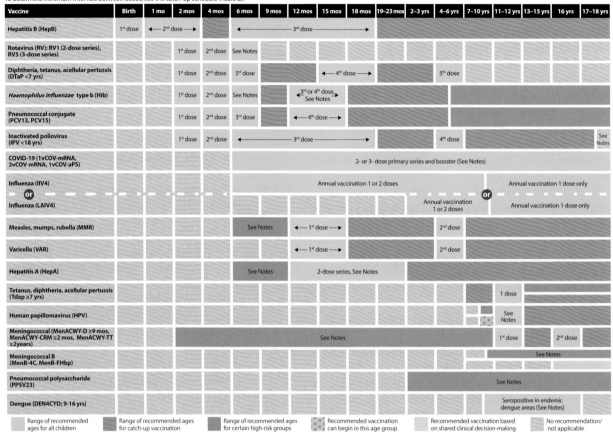

Vaccine	Birth	1 mo	2 mos	4 mos	6 mos	9 mos	12 mos	15 mos	18 mos	19–23 mos	2–3 yrs	4–6 yrs	7–10 yrs	11–12 yrs	13–15 yrs	16 yrs	17–18 yrs
Hepatitis B (HepB)	1st dose	◀---- 2nd dose ----▶			◀-------------------- 3rd dose --------------------▶												
Rotavirus (RV): RV1 (2-dose series), RV5 (3-dose series)			1st dose	2nd dose	See Notes												
Diphtheria, tetanus, acellular pertussis (DTaP <7 yrs)			1st dose	2nd dose	3rd dose			◀---- 4th dose ----▶				5th dose					
Haemophilus influenzae type b (Hib)			1st dose	2nd dose	See Notes		3rd or 4th dose, See Notes										
Pneumococcal conjugate (PCV13, PCV15)			1st dose	2nd dose	3rd dose		◀---- 4th dose ----▶										
Inactivated poliovirus (IPV <18 yrs)			1st dose	2nd dose	◀-------------------- 3rd dose --------------------▶							4th dose					See Notes
COVID-19 (1vCOV-mRNA, 2vCOV-mRNA, 1vCOV-aPS)					2- or 3- dose primary series and booster (See Notes)												
Influenza (IIV4) **or** **Influenza (LAIV4)**							Annual vaccination 1 or 2 doses				Annual vaccination 1 or 2 doses			**or**	Annual vaccination 1 dose only	Annual vaccination 1 dose only	
Measles, mumps, rubella (MMR)					See Notes		◀---- 1st dose ----▶					2nd dose					
Varicella (VAR)							◀---- 1st dose ----▶					2nd dose					
Hepatitis A (HepA)					See Notes		2-dose series, See Notes										
Tetanus, diphtheria, acellular pertussis (Tdap ≥7 yrs)														1 dose			
Human papillomavirus (HPV)														See Notes			
Meningococcal (MenACWY-D ≥9 mos, MenACWY-CRM ≥2 mos, MenACWY-TT ≥2years)							See Notes							1st dose		2nd dose	
Meningococcal B (MenB-4C, MenB-FHbp)															See Notes		
Pneumococcal polysaccharide (PPSV23)														See Notes			
Dengue (DEN4CYD; 9-16 yrs)														Seropositive in endemic dengue areas (See Notes)			

░ Range of recommended ages for all children	▓ Range of recommended ages for catch-up vaccination	▓ Range of recommended ages for certain high-risk groups	▒ Recommended vaccination can begin in this age group
░ Recommended vaccination based on shared clinical decision-making	▞ No recommendation/ not applicable		

FIGURE 14.2 Child and adolescent immunization schedule.

Reprinted from "Child and Adolescent Immunization Schedule by Age," Centers for Disease Control and Prevention, https://www.cdc.gov/vaccines/schedules/hcp/imz/child-adolescent.html.

Interestingly, according to the CDC, only 60% of health care workers in the United States have completed the three-series HBV vaccine.[14] In a 2017 study in Tanzania on health care workers, 57% had received one of the three HBV vaccination shots, whereas only 33.6% had completed the series.[15] In a 2021 study involving researchers working with biological samples in India, only 26% of students, faculty, and staff were fully immunized against HBV.[16]

Annual Immunization

An annual influenza shot for health care workers, older adults, children, and those with a weakened immune system has become an important health care benchmark each fall.[17] The seasonal influenza shot is usually targeted for a specific type of influenza; it does not provide global immunity against all types of influenza. Typically, influenza types A and B cause seasonal epidemics in the winter

months in the United States.[17] Each influenza type has subtypes and a slightly different physiological makeup. Vaccines are created annually to deter the viruses, but these illnesses have been known to alter themselves genetically to better fit a host. When this occurs, the vaccine becomes ineffective against the new strain. The two most common influenza vaccines are the inactivated influenza vaccine (IIV) and the live attenuated influenza vaccine (LAIV). IIV is administered via an intramuscular injection, whereas LAIV is a nasal spray that provides a small amount of live virus. The FluMist nasal spray has some contraindications. Those with chronic respiratory conditions or sinusitis must receive the injectable version because of potential complications from inhalation of the live virus. The live virus usually creates some flu-like symptoms within a few days of administration, whereas the injected variety does not. Because seasonal influenza most often strikes in the winter months (typically between October and March), it is recommended that patients

Table 1 Recommended Adult Immunization Schedule by Age Group, United States, 2023

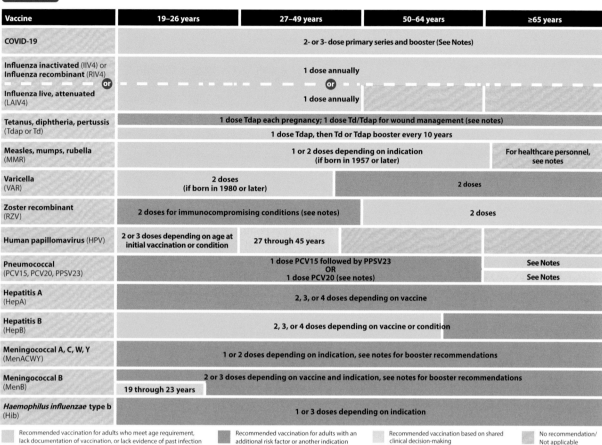

Vaccine	19–26 years	27–49 years	50–64 years	≥65 years
COVID-19	2- or 3- dose primary series and booster (See Notes)			
Influenza inactivated (IIV4) or Influenza recombinant (RIV4)	1 dose annually			
Influenza live, attenuated (LAIV4)	1 dose annually			
Tetanus, diphtheria, pertussis (Tdap or Td)	1 dose Tdap each pregnancy; 1 dose Td/Tdap for wound management (see notes)			
	1 dose Tdap, then Td or Tdap booster every 10 years			
Measles, mumps, rubella (MMR)	1 or 2 doses depending on indication (if born in 1957 or later)			For healthcare personnel, see notes
Varicella (VAR)	2 doses (if born in 1980 or later)		2 doses	
Zoster recombinant (RZV)	2 doses for immunocompromising conditions (see notes)		2 doses	
Human papillomavirus (HPV)	2 or 3 doses depending on age at initial vaccination or condition	27 through 45 years		
Pneumococcal (PCV15, PCV20, PPSV23)	1 dose PCV15 followed by PPSV23 OR 1 dose PCV20 (see notes)			See Notes / See Notes
Hepatitis A (HepA)	2, 3, or 4 doses depending on vaccine			
Hepatitis B (HepB)	2, 3, or 4 doses depending on vaccine or condition			
Meningococcal A, C, W, Y (MenACWY)	1 or 2 doses depending on indication, see notes for booster recommendations			
Meningococcal B (MenB)	2 or 3 doses depending on vaccine and indication, see notes for booster recommendations			
	19 through 23 years			
Haemophilus influenzae type b (Hib)	1 or 3 doses depending on indication			

Recommended vaccination for adults who meet age requirement, lack documentation of vaccination, or lack evidence of past infection

Recommended vaccination for adults with an additional risk factor or another indication

Recommended vaccination based on shared clinical decision-making

No recommendation/ Not applicable

FIGURE 14.3 Adult immunization schedule.

Reprinted from "Adult Immunization Schedule by Age," Centers for Disease Control and Prevention, https://www.cdc.gov/vaccines/schedules/hcp/imz/adult.html; www.cdc.gov/vaccines/schedules/downloads/adult/adult-schedule-easy-read.pdf

receive their annual dose in October to provide full-season coverage that lasts through mid-spring.[17,18]

As mentioned previously, airborne transmission and direct contact are two ways to infect others with communicable diseases. In sports, the close surroundings of athletic huddles, time-outs, locker rooms, and team buses present many opportunities to spread infections among team members.[19,86] However, common-sense precautions can help prevent infection transmission. The basic practices of personal hygiene are underappreciated in the fight against disease spread. Simple habits such as frequent handwashing, covering one's mouth or nose when coughing or sneezing, showering with quality antibacterial soap, and protecting the skin, including good foot care, are all examples of personal responsibility in hygiene that can be practiced in all walks of life.[20] Athletes with infections are isolated while they are contagious, and any equipment or clothing that they have worn is sanitized before the next use.

Methods of protection against disease that could affect the whole team include safeguarding the water source and containers and sanitizing surfaces that athletes have contact with, such as treatment tables, mats, and rehabilitation equipment. Certain states have regulations about the type of hose that may be used to draw potable (drinkable) water. These regulations may be found on state health department and OSHA websites. When sanitizing equipment, surfaces, and water containers, such as coolers, ice containers, and water bottles, a solution of 1:100 ratio of bleach to water is effective as a germicide.[19,86]

It is not difficult to prevent the spread of many of the infectious diseases discussed in this chapter. Compliance with preventive immunization programs when available can be followed up with good hygiene, sanitation, and the practice of universal precautions.

Reporting Communicable Diseases

The health care provider has a legal obligation to report certain medical conditions, such as some STIs or tuberculosis, to the public health authorities. The rationale behind reporting these conditions is to protect the public from an outbreak. Courts have ruled that for certain medical conditions, the risks of exposure outweigh the patient's right to privacy. Local, state, and national agencies review the lists of reportable diseases and report them to the proper authority when diagnosed by physicians or in laboratories.[21]

In the United States, the National Notifiable Diseases Surveillance System (NNDSS) is used to report communicable diseases from all public health agencies. When a physician has confirmed a certain infectious disease, the disease, but not the patient, is reported to the appropriate agency.[21,22] The NNDSS works in collaboration with agencies to monitor, control, and prevent communicable disease spread. On rare occasions, such as with an STI, the infectious person is identified and any partners who may have been infected are contacted.

The purpose of reporting communicable diseases is twofold:

1. To isolate a given disease and retard its spread
2. To generate data about current disease trends so they may be prevented in the future

Our discussion of the reporting system will focus on the local level. Basic reporting involves both individual cases and epidemics.

Local health officials, in conjunction with state and federal agencies, decide which individual cases are to be routinely reported and develop policies for collecting, documenting, and reporting the information. Physicians and other health care workers with knowledge of a reportable illness are required by law to report it. Hospitals generally have a specific officer who handles such reports; smaller medical clinics often have similar protocols, policies, and procedures for reporting communicable diseases. Minimal data for these reports include the patient's name, address, diagnosis, age, sex, and date

---

Clinical Tips

Comparing an Epidemic to a Pandemic

An *epidemic* is a (usually sudden) increase in the number of cases of a disease or condition beyond what is expected in a given region. A *pandemic* is an epidemic that has spread to a multitude of countries or continents.[23]

---

of report. The right to privacy is paramount, but so is the right of the community to prevent communicable disease spread and to protect unsuspecting people. Collective reports can simply list the number of cases for a given disease in a specific time frame. Diseases and conditions that are considered reportable vary by state, and state public health organizations are encouraged to enter cases into the NNDSS.[22]

Pandemic

The term *pandemic* refers to an illness that affects an exceptionally high proportion of the population in a wide geographic area. Pandemics in modern history include coronavirus disease 2019 (COVID-19), human immunodeficiency virus (HIV), and H1N1 influenza (swine flu). Pandemics are infectious diseases that cross continents; seasonal influenzas are not included. Historically significant pandemics include cholera, typhus, smallpox, measles, tuberculosis, leprosy, malaria, and yellow fever. A disease must meet three criteria to be called a pandemic by the World Health Organization (WHO):[23]

- Nearly simultaneous transmission occurs worldwide or is rapidly spread worldwide.
- It infects humans, causing serious illness.
- It is easily spread and sustained among humans.

The reason some illnesses (e.g., avian flu or bird flu) are not pandemics is that they do not have easily sustainable human-to-human transmission.

Influenza

In the United States during fall 2022 through spring 2023, there were an estimated 19,000 to 58,000 deaths and 290,000 to 650,000 hospitalizations from seasonal influenza. Ninety percent of the deaths and 60% of the hospitalizations were among adults older than age 65 yr.[87] In 2022, approximately 83% of the U.S. population met the criteria to undergo vaccination to prevent the common forms of influenza, yet only 54% to 74% of the eligible population received the influenza vaccine.[88] Illnesses and deaths owing to seasonal influenza decreased from 2020 to 2022, which is attributed to behaviors used to prevent COVID-19 spread. Infectious respiratory conditions were mitigated when there were no large gatherings of people and entire populations wore masks, maintained social distance, and washed hands often.

The two main human influenza viruses that cause epidemics each year are types A and B, but influenza A is further broken down into subcategories. Influenza A is labeled for two proteins, hemagglutinin (H) and neuraminidase (N). Within each protein are subtypes that generate viruses named H1 though H18 and N1 through

SARS-CoV-2

Severe acute respiratory syndrome (SARS) is not new, having first appeared in China in 2002. The virus was rapidly contained and has not been diagnosed since 2004. Severe acute respiratory syndrome coronavirus 2 (SARS-CoV-2) causes COVID-19,[24] which spreads through release of respiratory droplets into the air. The COVID-19 pandemic led to the worldwide practice of wearing surgical-grade medical masks, maintaining a six-foot distance between people, and renewing campaigns for frequent handwashing.

COVID-19 invades via the spike protein on its cell membrane that binds with angiotensin-converting enzyme 2 (ACE2) receptors to invade and interfere with the function of other cells. ACE2 receptors are found most often in human lungs, heart, liver, kidney, and gastrointestinal system, which is why signs and symptoms of COVID-19 relate to the system most affected.[25,26] The most common presentation is flu-like symptoms.

Johns Hopkins University managed a resource page that tracked illnesses and deaths, globally and regionally, giving up-to-date information throughout the COVID-19 pandemic.[27] According to their site, 3 yr after the virus was discovered, COVID-19 was the source of nearly 97 million cases of the virus and over 1 million deaths in the United States.[27] Globally, there were over 627 million cases of the disease and nearly 7 million deaths worldwide in the 3 yr since its onset in late 2019.[27]

N11. Influenza B is not subdivided. The CDC adheres to internationally approved methods for naming influenza viruses.[17] The name depends on the following:

- Antigen type (e.g., A, B)
- Host of origin (e.g., swine, bird, equine)
- Geographic origin (e.g., Taiwan, Denver)
- Year of isolation (e.g., 2009, 2014)
- Protein type for influenza A (e.g., H1N1, H3N2)[17]

One popular influenza variant that has re-emerged globally is swine flu. Originally detected in 1976, swine flu was transmitted from pigs to humans. In 2009, another outbreak occurred, this time attributed to the H1N1 influenza virus. The WHO designated H1N1 as a pandemic in June 2009; by July that year, there were more than 94,000 confirmed cases in more than 100 countries.[28] H1N1 differs from the 1976 strain of swine flu, such that those vaccinated in 1976 were most likely not immune to the 2009 strain.[17]

Avian influenza (bird flu) was first discovered in 1997 in Hong Kong, and outbreaks in humans occurred in China in 2003. There are three main varietals categorized with nine subtypes in each influenza A: H5, H7, and H9. Each is represented with H5N1 to H5N9, with the first number changing to represent varietal 7 or 9, as the proteins have changed slightly and create different strains. Bird flu is not easily transmitted between humans and therefore does not pose a pandemic threat. The purpose of identifying the strains of influenza is to determine which vaccine to create to protect against the projected virus for the coming season. Each February, the WHO collaborates with more than 100 countries to review the influenza viruses reported for the preceding year. From these data, laboratories create a vaccine to prevent the most common influenza strains identified. In 2016, a vaccine was created to protect against influenza A H1N1, H3N2, and influenza B/Phuket, but this vaccine may not be effective after that year because of the changes in influenza strains.[17]

Signs and Symptoms

Signs and symptoms of influenza include fever, cough, sore throat, body ache, headache, stuffy nose, chills, and fatigue. People are contagious from 1 d before symptom onset until up to 7 d after they realize they are sick. For referral and diagnostic tests and treatment and return-to-participation guidelines for influenza, please see chapter 6.

Infectious Mononucleosis

Infectious **mononucleosis (mono)** has also been called the *kissing disease* because it is easily transmitted by oropharyngeal contact. Caused by the Epstein-Barr virus (EBV), mononucleosis is a common occurrence in the college-aged population, but 50% of children have also shown serologic evidence of the infection by age 5 yr.[29] There is some speculation that chronic fatigue syndrome is associated with chronic EBV infection, but little evidence supports this theory.[7]

EBV is a herpesvirus that attacks lymphocytes and nasopharyngeal cells. It is found in oropharyngeal saliva secretions of up to 25% of healthy, nonsymptomatic adults. Despite its reputation as the kissing disease, mononucleosis is not particularly contagious, as only 5% of patients have a recent history of contact with an

⚑ **RED FLAGS FOR SPLENOMEGALY**

Splenomegaly is a possible side effect of mononucleosis, which causes the spleen to enlarge and protrude out from under the normal protection of the lower-left ribs. Unprotected, the spleen is susceptible to injury and rupture from athletic activity. An unrecognized ruptured spleen is life-threatening.

infected person.[7] For reported direct exposure, the incubation period is 10 to 50 d. Nevertheless, individuals are warned to avoid sharing drinking cups and putting their mouth on common water bottle spouts.

Signs and Symptoms

The chief signs and symptoms of infectious mononucleosis are fatigue, pharyngitis, fever, and **lymphadenopathy**, but not all signs and symptoms are present in every patient. Often, the first complaint is of overwhelming fatigue and the inability to get enough sleep. The patient will feel run down or will experience a sore throat. Other manifestations include tonsillitis, hepatomegaly, jaundice, and a **maculopapular rash**.[29]

Splenomegaly (figure 14.4) is present in 50% of mononucleosis cases and is most prevalent in the second and third weeks of the disease.[7] A blow to the left ribs of a patient with splenomegaly can rupture the spleen, causing a life-threatening emergency if the injury is not quickly recognized and treated.

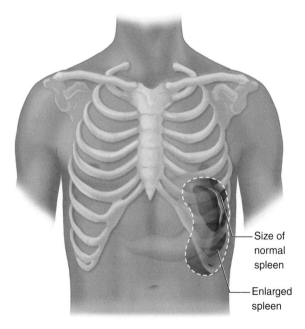

Size of normal spleen

Enlarged spleen

FIGURE 14.4 Splenomegaly, an enlargement of the spleen, is sometimes associated with acute infections such as mononucleosis.

Although 10% to 30% of patients experience hepatomegaly, or an enlarged liver, with infectious mononucleosis, it does not carry the severe ramifications that splenomegaly does in athletes. There are hepatic complications because hepatocellular enzyme levels are elevated two to three times that of normal in 95% of patients, and they can take as long as 1 mo to return to normal levels.[7,30]

Other potential complications of mononucleosis are related to the central nervous system (CNS), including seizures, peripheral neuropathy, aseptic meningitis, meningitis, cranial nerve palsy, and Guillain-Barré syndrome.[7]

Group A α-hemolytic streptococci, cytomegalovirus, HBV, rubella, and primary HIV infection are all options to consider and rule out when diagnosing mononucleosis.

Referral and Diagnostic Tests

A patient presenting with a history of malaise combined with a sore throat and fever should be referred to a physician, especially if the symptoms are present for a number of days.

Patients suspected of having infectious mononucleosis often present with mild **leukocytosis**, which is also common in a number of other illnesses.[7] A strong indicator for EBV includes a blood count indicating **lymphocytosis**; a low or falling hematocrit is suggestive of splenic rupture.[31] A more specific blood test, the heterophile antibody test, will show these antibodies in 40% to 60% of patients with mononucleosis within the first week. Another test, the monospot, is based on agglutination, or clumping, of erythrocytes and is slightly more sensitive in detecting the antibodies of infectious mononucleosis than is the heterophile antibody test.[30] This screening test is reliable in up to 90% of patients and is usually positive within 4 wk of onset. However, the monospot test may not be sensitive to the presence of EBV in the early days after infection.[29] False-positive monospot results can occur in the context of other diseases, such as lymphoma, autoimmune disease, HIV, and hepatitis.[30]

Treatment and Return to Participation

The standard treatment for mononucleosis is rest and hydration, although complete bed rest is not recommended. More than 95% of patients recover with symptomatic treatment alone.

Research has shown that there is no effective pharmacological treatment for infectious mononucleosis.[29] However, if the pharyngitis is such that it warrants medication, corticosteroids have been shown to relieve pain and prevent airway compromise from swelling. To assist in the management of body aches and fever, acetaminophen is preferred over aspirin because of aspirin's association with **Reye's syndrome**.[30] In addition, patients would be wise to avoid prolonged use of nonsteroidal anti-inflammatory drugs (NSAIDs) during the illness because of the hepatic complications already associated with mononucleosis.

Athletes must be sure that they are reconditioned for sport before they return to competition. Those in contact or collision sports may need 1 mo or more to recover enough to allow the spleen to again fit behind the rib cage for adequate protection.[30] Physicians must consider the details of each case before allowing a full return to activity. A swimmer may return to full activity rather quickly, whereas a diver may still be in danger of spleen injury with a premature return.

Return to full participation following mononucleosis recovery depends on the type of sport (noncontact, contact, collision), return to appropriate fitness levels, and control of symptoms. There is no strong evidence that either physical examination or ultrasonography can reliably determine whether the spleen has returned to normal size, so these measurements should be used with caution.[32] Serial ultrasonography, however, has been found to be useful in determining the spleen's gradual return to normal size following mononucleosis.[32,33]

Mumps

Mumps is a contagious viral disease that manifests with enlarged parotid and salivary glands and on occasion also involves the sublingual or submaxillary glands (figure 14.5). It presents as an acute epidemic that peaks in late winter or early spring and chiefly involves children ages 5 to 15 yr. Children younger than 2 yr are typically immune.[7] A national immunization campaign was intended to eradicate the disease by 2010. However, with a 2006 outbreak in the Midwest involving more than 6,500 people and another outbreak from a 2019 wedding, the disease is still present in the United States. In the 2019 outbreak, there were 62 cases spread over a six-state region. The average patients were men age 35 yr, and 66% of patients had received the two-shot series. The two-dose childhood vaccination was not sufficient to prevent the disease for many.[9,12]

Mumps has a 2 to 3 wk incubation period and is spread through the air via infected droplets as well as through direct contact with contaminated saliva. The disease has been found in saliva 1 to 6 d before onset and up to 9 d after glandular swelling. Mumps also has been found in the urine 6 d before **parotitis** (inflammation of the parotid salivary glands) and 15 d afterward. In addition, the virus may be isolated in the blood of symptomatic patients.[7]

Signs and Symptoms

Chief signs and symptoms of mumps include parotitis, headache, low-grade fever, malaise, anorexia, vomiting, and **nuchal rigidity** in the posterior neck. Common

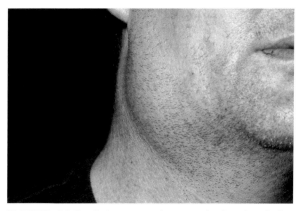

FIGURE 14.5 Salivary and parotid glands of the mouth and neck can become rapidly and painfully inflamed as a result of mumps; note the swelling anterior to the lower earlobe.

Dr P. Marazzi / Science Source

symptoms also include pain with chewing and swallowing, especially swallowing acidic drinks or foods such as orange juice, pickles, or lemons. Within 24 h of sign and symptom onset, the parotid glands swell and become sensitive to palpation. Initially, it is not unusual for only one of the two parotid glands to become swollen, with the second following about 2 d later. A person generally presents with asymmetry in the face and jaw caused by unilateral swelling of the parotid gland. Enlargement of the glands can extend from in front of to below the ear, and the associated skin can become tight and shiny because of the pressure from the swelling.

The complications of mumps include orchitis, oophoritis, **meningoencephalitis**, and pancreatitis. Postpubertal males may experience testicular inflammation, which is typically unilateral. Although this can occur in up to 50% of the adult males with mumps, it is rarely associated with infertility.[34] CNS involvement is relatively uncommon and most often manifests as meningitis or encephalitis, which occur in up to 15% of cases.[34] Encephalitis is thought to be an autoimmune response producing demyelination and has an onset 7 to 10 d after parotitis.

Oophoritis occurs in 7% of postpubertal females with mumps and is more difficult to diagnose; however, it rarely results in fertility issues.[34] Exposure to mumps within the first trimester of pregnancy may induce spontaneous abortion.[7,34]

Because the patient with mumps has a headache, stiff neck, and sometimes low (20-40 mg/dL) cerebrospinal fluid (CSF) glucose levels, it is often mistaken for bacterial meningitis. Fifteen percent of patients with mumps experience CNS involvement but only 1% to 10% manifest symptoms. Although permanent damage, such as deafness or facial paralysis is unusual, it may result from mumps with CNS involvement.

The differential diagnoses for mumps include streptococcal throat infection, encephalitis, meningitis, dental caries, influenza type A, leukemia, **lymphosarcoma**, malignant and benign tumors of the salivary glands, and an obstructed duct in the parotid gland. Epididymitis, orchitis, and ovarian torsion may also be considered.[34]

Referral and Diagnostic Tests

Patients who present with swollen salivary glands, malaise, or low-grade fever are referred to a physician. The diagnosis is largely based on signs and symptoms coupled with a history of recent exposure. Atypical presentations require laboratory confirmation, usually by culturing the mumps virus or discovering the mumps immunoglobulin M (IgM) antibody.[34]

Treatment and Return to Participation

Patients with mumps should be isolated from others until parotid swelling returns to normal. Treatment is based on symptoms. Over-the-counter analgesics or antipyretics are used as necessary to alleviate headache and fever. Patients should avoid acidic foods and beverages and maintain a soft diet to lessen the need for **mastication**. Mumps is typically self-limited, and most patients recover without pharmacological intervention.[31]

Because most symptoms of mumps (e.g., fever, malaise, vomiting, nuchal rigidity, parotitis) seem to resolve within 3 to 10 d, long-term absence from athletic participation is not typical. It is more important to prevent the spread of infection.

Prevention

In 2005, the FDA approved a mumps vaccine (ProQuad) for measles, mumps, rubella, and varicella (MMRV) that causes little systemic reaction. The live virus vaccine, introduced in the United States in 1967, is administered alone or in combination with the MMR or MMRV vaccine. These vaccines are generally administered any time after the first year of life but most typically between age 12 and 15 mo. Current recommendations include a second dose between ages 4 and 6 yr.[9,35]

Rubeola

Also known simply as *measles* or *red measles*, **rubeola** is one of the most highly communicable infectious diseases. Before immunization was available, more than 90% of the population was infected by age 20 yr.[36] Since immunization was introduced, measles cases have decreased 99%, with the residual in the United States attributed to unimmunized or underimmunized children

who have had only one shot. By 2000, measles was said to be eliminated in the United States.[35] There have been measles outbreaks in the United States since 2010, but they are largely attributed to travelers to the country spreading the virus to unvaccinated residents.[36] There are also outbreaks elsewhere in the world, with China and Japan leading Western Europe in outbreaks.[35] The resurgence of measles has been attributed to living in remote communities, misinformation about the vaccine, cultural factors, and insufficient vaccine coverage.

Measles is spread through airborne droplets from nasal or throat secretions of infected people. A lesser means of transmission is through direct contact with soiled articles such as towels, which may contain secretions from those already sick. The incubation period is typically 10 d, but it can range from 7 to 17 d. Measles is most contagious from the 3 to 5 d before the rash erupts through 4 d after eruption.[36]

Signs and Symptoms

Most often, rash is the manifestation of rubeola, and it appears after a **prodromal** fever, most often in days 3 to 7 of the disease. The erythematous rash begins on the face before spreading to the body proper and lasts approximately 4 to 7 d. Other signs and symptoms of measles include conjunctivitis, cough, **leukopenia**, headache, fever, and sore throat. Leukopenia is present beginning with rash onset largely because of a decrease in lymphocytes. Complications can occur because measles suppresses the immune system, allowing opportunistic conditions to take hold. Common infections arising from measles include sinusitis, otitis media, pneumonia, encephalitis, diarrhea, laryngotracheobronchitis, or keratitis, which can lead to blindness.[36]

Differential diagnoses for rubeola are rubella, mononucleosis, influenza, Rocky Mountain spotted fever, and allergic rhinitis. Many childhood diseases have similar presentations and are often the differential diagnoses of each other. Table 14.1 compares several childhood diseases.

Referral and Diagnostic Tests

Patients with a rash indicative of measles are referred for further evaluation. Likewise, those with signs or symptoms of measles before rash onset, such as sore throat, fever, cough, conjunctivitis, or recent exposure, must be referred to a physician. A recent history of measles vaccine does not preclude one from contracting measles. Therefore, a recently immunized person who shows signs or symptoms of measles needs to be referred immediately to a physician.

A diagnosis of measles can be confirmed by the pres-

TABLE 14.1   **Comparison of Childhood Infectious Diseases**

Disease	Incubation (wk)	Mode of transmission	Duration of symptoms
Mononucleosis	2-3	Saliva, air droplets	Up to several months
Mumps	2-3	Saliva, air droplets	Up to 10 d
Rubeola	1-2	Airborne, direct contact	4-7 d
Rubella	2-3	Respiratory secretions, placental blood	3 d
Varicella	2-3	Direct contact, respiratory secretions	1 wk

ence of a measles-specific IgM antibody in the blood, which presents itself 3 to 4 d after onset of the measles rash. A nasopharyngeal swab is also used to identify the antigen but is less commonly used than the blood test.[36]

Treatment and Return to Participation

Because no antiviral remedy for measles is currently available, the best treatment is supportive and symptomatic care. Rubeola is largely self-limiting, but analgesics and antipyretics may help alleviate symptoms.[36] If the patient has accompanying bacterial complications, such as conjunctivitis, otitis, sinusitis, or pneumonia, antibacterial therapy may be warranted.

Mortality rates for measles are low, but pneumonia and encephalitis are complications of the disease in children younger than age 5 yr. For athletes, activity during the contagious stages is discouraged.

Prevention and Public Health Implications

Measles is one of the most easily communicable diseases and one of the deadliest childhood illnesses, yet it is vaccine preventable.[37] People born after 1957 are encouraged to obtain immunization for measles. A single injection of the live measles virus is often administered in conjunction with two other live viruses (mumps and rubella) and reduces susceptibility to measles by 94% to 98%; a second dose may elevate immunity to 99%.[9,35,38] The two-dose vaccine is recommended to offset the possibility of immunization failure. Most often, the MMR initial dose is given at age 12 to 15 mo, with the second dose administered at the onset of school (ages 4-6 yr), although if exposure risk is high, the second dose can be delivered as soon as 4 wk after the first.

Measles is a reportable disease. Reporting to the local agency within 24 h of diagnosis can improve chances of controlling disease spread. Typically, patients are not quarantined, but it is a good idea to isolate school-aged children and athletes while they are contagious.

Rubella

Rubella, once known as *German measles* and also called *three-day measles*, is an acute contagious virus that has mild symptoms in children and adults but can cause death or profound congenital defects in infants born to mothers infected during the first trimester of pregnancy. In the United States in 1969, nearly 58,000 rubella cases were reported. Since 2001, there have been fewer than 20 cases per year, largely owing to vaccination. Internationally, rubella still exists, as there were more than 304,000 cases reported in Europe in 2003. Global rubella vaccination was reported to be at 70% in 2020.[39]

Rubella is acquired through the upper respiratory tract or through placental blood exchange with a mother infected in early pregnancy. Exposure to rubella during pregnancy can cause spontaneous miscarriage, stillbirth, or profound effects on the fetus. A female infected with rubella early in pregnancy has a 90% chance of passing congenital rubella syndrome (CRS) to the fetus, which can cause congenital birth defects. Despite the increased

 RED FLAGS FOR RUBELLA

Rubella is profoundly dangerous to the unborn fetus of expectant mothers because exposure during the first trimester of pregnancy can cause the following to the fetus:

- Spontaneous miscarriage
- Intrauterine death
- Stillbirth
- Deafness
- Intrauterine growth retardation
- Mental retardation
- Behavior disorders
- Bone radiolucencies
- Diabetes mellitus
- Cardiac defects

vaccine presence internationally, there are still about 110,00 cases of CRS globally.[37,39] Obviously, great care must be taken to ensure that pregnant women are safeguarded from exposure.

Signs and Symptoms

Rubella has a 12 to 24 d incubation period, and patients present with a low-grade fever (<38.3 °C [101 °F]) that is often transient, a mild rash, lymphadenopathy, conjunctivitis, cough, headache, and joint pain (arthralgia). The rash usually lasts 2 to 3 d and is a blotchy eruption that has its origin on the face and spreads to the trunk and limbs (figure 14.6).[31,39,40] Mild rose-colored spots may appear on the palate, and although the pharynx may be bright red, the throat is not typically sore. Swelling of specific glands, including the suboccipital, postauricular, and postcervical glands, precedes the rash by 5 to 10 d and may be first noted by the patient when washing their hair or by the athlete when putting on a helmet. On occasion, the patient has splenomegaly and hepatitis in conjunction with the rash. Arthritis can be involved as a complication, especially in women.[7]

Differential diagnoses of rubella include allergic reactions, scarlet fever, secondary syphilis, mononuclear viral infections, and Kawasaki's disease (see chapter 7).

Referral and Diagnostic Tests

Any unimmunized person with a history of exposure who presents with rubella symptoms is referred to a physician for confirmation. Diagnosis of rubella is often made based on the combination of glandular swelling and the onset of facial rash. A history of immunization or recent exposure may expedite disease confirmation or rule it out. Serological testing can confirm the disease by revealing a fourfold increase in specific antibodies.[7]

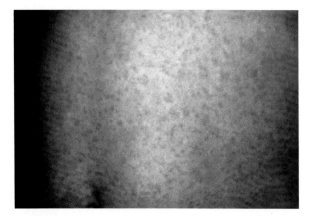

FIGURE 14.6 Rubella lesions.
Centers for Disease Control and Prevention / Science Source

Treatment and Return to Participation

There is no known antiviral treatment for rubella after the disease is present. Most patients do well with supportive care.

Rubella is a mild illness, and symptoms rarely last more than 3 to 4 d. However, the person is contagious from day 7 of exposure through day 21 after the last known exposure and should be isolated from pregnant women.

Prevention and Public Health Implications

The MMR immunization provides protective antibodies to 90% to 95% of those immunized at age 1 yr, with 99% protected by the second vaccination.[37] Also, adult women should practice birth control for at least 3 mo after vaccine receipt. Congenital rubella has been a reportable disease in the United States since 1966.

Chicken Pox and Shingles

Varicella-zoster virus causes varicella (chicken pox) and herpes zoster (shingles). Chicken pox is a viral, readily communicable disease (figure 14.7a). It was one of the most common childhood diseases in the United States, and children tend to contract the disease before beginning school. Ninety percent of cases of varicella occur within 10 to 20 d of exposure.[41]

Shingles, also known as herpes zoster (see figure 14.7b), is a reactivation of varicella disease in the dorsal ganglia. The dorsal ganglia are a group of nerve cell bodies that exit the spinal cord posteriorly and provide sensation to specific regions of the body. Both diseases are problematic to the **immunosuppressed patient**. Ninety percent of unvaccinated contacts become infected, making varicella extremely contagious to the unprotected person.[31]

Although both varicella and herpes zoster have similar methods of transmission, varicella is much more contagious. These infections are spread by direct person-to-person contact, by respiratory secretions seen in varicella only, by direct contact with vesicle fluid, or indirectly by vesicle fluid on soiled articles such as towels or jerseys. Sports in which there are more opportunities for skin-to-skin contact, such as wrestling, carry a greater risk of infection transmission. In a 15 yr study on collegiate wrestlers, 5% of dermatological issues were attributed to varicella-zoster virus.[42] Scabs themselves are not transmittable sources of the infection.

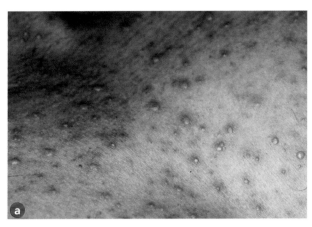 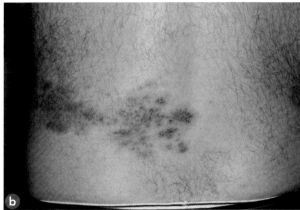

FIGURE 14.7 *(a)* Varicella, or chicken pox, lesions. *(b)* Herpes zoster, or shingles, lesions.
The Division of Dermatology at Brody School of Medicine, East Carolina University

Signs and Symptoms

Chicken pox begins rapidly with a headache and a maculopapular rash that gives rise to vesicles within hours of onset. The lesion is described as a dew drop or a vesicle on an erythematous base. New lesions develop over about 4 d and start as erythematous papules progressing to vesicles. The subsequent vesicles last 3 to 4 d and represent the time of highest contagiousness. These lesions are of varying size, shape, and age and quickly rupture to form crusts. The patient usually has a combination of papules, vesicles, and crusts all at once. Lesions may occur anywhere on the body, but they tend to cluster on covered, rather than exposed, areas. Lesions begin on the trunk and face, eventually spreading to the extremities, but it is also common to find lesions on the scalp, buccal mucous membrane, conjunctiva, and axilla. Other findings include intense itching, headache, fever, chills, malaise, and backache.[31,41]

As with chicken pox, herpes zoster presents with a vesicular rash. However, in herpes zoster, these vesicles follow the track of one or more sensory nerve roots. They give rise to patterns following specific dermatomes and most often are unilateral (see figure 10.6). In patients with herpes zoster, pain severity and paresthesia along the rash increase with the patient's age. Patients are typically contagious from a few days before the rash to until the vesicles have scabbed over.

Differential diagnoses for varicella and herpes zoster include impetigo, scabies, urticaria, smallpox, acute nerve root injury, and an allergic drug rash.[41]

Referral and Diagnostic Tests

People who present with complaints associated with varicella or shingles are referred to a physician. Symptoms tend to be more severe in adults, and they may mimic myocardial infarction, pleurisy, acute abdominal pain, or migraine, depending on the outbreak location.

In general, laboratory tests are not warranted, but a complete blood count (CBC) may reveal leukopenia and **thrombocytopenia**.

Treatment and Return to Participation

Although varicella is self-limiting, acyclovir (Zovirax) is often prescribed. Valacyclovir (Valtrex) and famciclovir (Famvir) are used to treat herpes zoster.[41] If acyclovir is administered within 48 h of initial rash, it alleviates symptoms, shortens their duration, and lessens recurrent outbreaks. Other treatments for varicella combat pruritus and superinfection. Simple calamine lotion is an excellent agent to diminish itching associated with varicella, as is a colloidal starch bath. Antibiotics also may be needed to help prevent secondary bacterial infections.

Collegiate athletes may return to participation when all lesions have a firm, adhered crust and there is no evidence of a secondary bacterial infection (see the NCAA and NFHS Participation Regulations for Wrestlers With Bacterial Infections sidebar in chapter 16).[1] Scholastic athletes follow the same return-to-participation guidelines as those with herpes simplex virus: 10 to 14 d of antiviral medication and no new lesions within 48 h.[4,43] Athletes may return to participation when fully asymptomatic, and they may engage in noncontact (and nonswimming) activities as long as they have no vesicles and feel well. Activities in the water should be avoided until patients are cleared by a physician.

Prevention and Public Health Implications

Since 2005, the FDA-approved MMRV two-dose vaccine has proven effective in preventing varicella. However, individuals born before approval of the MMRV vaccine could have had the two-dose vaccine specific to varicella, the live attenuated Varivax.[44] Immunization within 3 d of exposure will lessen disease symptoms and duration. It should be noted that some studies found an increased risk of febrile seizures in a small percentage of children age 12 to 23 mo with the MMRV vaccine compared with the traditional MMR vaccine. In response, the CDC Advisory Committee on Immunization Practices (ACIP) recommends (1) administration of the MMR vaccine and a separate varicella vaccine for dose 1 and (2) considering using the MMRV vaccine as a second dose under advisement of a pediatrician.[44] Interestingly, varicella vaccination is not a routine childhood prevention strategy in Europe, although studies are underway to determine whether this practice should continue.[45]

The Shingrix vaccine is available for the prevention of herpes zoster but not for treatment. It is a two-dose drug that is approved for people older than age 50 yr.[44]

Varicella is not a reportable disease. Affected children must be isolated from school, public spaces, and medical offices until the lesions have scabbed over. Likewise, adults must not have contact with others until their vesicles dry. Extra caution is maintained with athletes involved in contact or collision sports because vesicles can "unroof" and secrete fluid infected with the virus.

Hepatitis A to D

The liver is the largest organ in the body, and it functions primarily as the central organ of glucose homeostasis. It lies protected chiefly by the lower right ribs in the upper right abdominal cavity (figure 14.8). This four-lobe organ secrets bile to facilitate fat digestion, and it has metabolic functions as well. The liver also assists in amino acid and carbohydrate metabolism, fat-soluble vitamin storage (A, D, E, K), phagocytosis, and detoxification of potentially harmful substances. Damage to the liver has profound repercussions for many body functions.

Hepatitis, translated literally, means inflammation of the liver. Hepatitis is characterized by diffuse necrosis affecting the smallest secretory units of the liver.[7] The many varieties of the disease are differentiated by letters, mechanisms of acquisition, and lasting sequelae. Table 14.2 compares the common hepatitis viruses. The diseases are typically abbreviated to HAV (hepatitis A virus), HBV, HCV, and so on. The emphasis in this chapter is on hepatitis A, B, C, and D; hepatitis E and hepatitis G typically do not affect the healthy population, occurring more often in endemic countries or immunocompromised patients.

In general, hepatitis can be caused by certain bacteria or viruses, in addition to some drugs, toxins, and excessive alcohol abuse. HAV and HEV are infectious and highly contagious forms of the disease associated with poor sanitation and oral–fecal transmission. HBV, HCV,

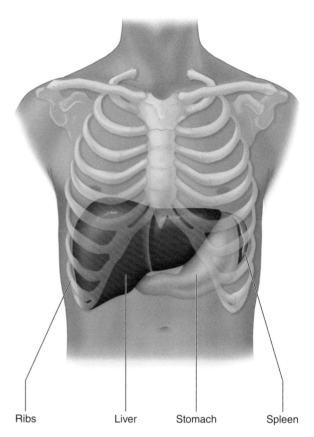

Ribs Liver Stomach Spleen

FIGURE 14.8 The liver in its normal anatomical position is well protected by the lower right ribs.

and HDV are varieties of serum hepatitis and are transmitted via parenteral (blood) or sexual contact; these forms can lead to chronic conditions. In 2020, the CDC reported 9,952 new cases of HAV in the United States (up from 1,781 in 2013) and 11,635 newly reported incidences of HBV, a substantial increase over the 2013 report of 3,050. Whereas HAV and HBV showed small declines over the 2009 to 2013 reporting period, HCV rose to 4,798 in 2020.[46] Injectable drug use has been the culprit for up to 60% of the new cases of HCV, with most acute HBV cases from the same cause. Household contact and sexual contact had equal roles in the transmission of HBV.[31,46]

Signs and Symptoms

Viral hepatitis has an incubation period of 2 wk to 6 mo and has several phases, each marked by specific signs and symptoms, except phase 1, in which patients are asymptomatic. In the prodromal stage (phase 2), the patient could experience malaise, fatigue, upper respiratory infection, anorexia, nausea, vomiting, mild abdominal pain, myalgia, or arthralgia.[47] Some patients have accompanying headache, fever, and rash. When jaundice occurs, it typically manifests 5 to 10 d after

TABLE 14.2 **Comparison of Hepatitis Viruses**

Disease	Incubation	Transmission	Notes
Hepatitis A (HAV)	30 d	Oral–fecal contact, crowding, poor sanitation, contaminated food or water	Clinical illness more severe in adults than children
Hepatitis B (HBV)	6 wk to 6 mo (average is 12-14 wk)	Infected blood and blood products; sexual contact; virus is present in saliva, semen, and vaginal secretions	Chronic HBV creates a high risk of cirrhosis and liver cancer
Hepatitis C (HCV)	6-7 wk	Intravenous drug use, body piercing, multiple sex partners	High coinfection rate among patients with HIV; highest mortality
Hepatitis D (HDV)	30-150 d	In the United States, primarily by intravenous drug use	Best prevented via HBV vaccine

Note: HIV = human immunodeficiency virus.

the prodromal symptoms present and peaks within 1 to 2 wk. Phase 3—the icteric phase—is typically marked by patients presenting with pale stools and dark urine. Icteric means "pertaining to jaundice," and this phase is when jaundice appears. The chief complaints besides jaundice are gastrointestinal symptoms, malaise, and hepatomegaly.[47] The final phase (phase 4) is a 2 to 4 wk recovery and convalescent phase marked by a state of well-being, return of appetite, and disappearance of fatigue and pain. General recovery is based on the specific virus, but the acute illness typically subsides within 2 to 3 wk. Some patients have few of these signs but instead experience a lingering, unexplainable fatigue. Taking a good and thorough history is critical because each type is distinguished by its method of transmission.

Differential diagnoses may include EBV, herpes simplex, URI, cholecystitis (gallstones), pancreatitis, influenza, and infectious mononucleosis.[31]

Referral and Diagnostic Tests

Patients with unexplainable fatigue are referred to a physician for further evaluation. Physical findings include an enlarged liver and jaundice, but if these occur, it is later in the disease progression. Blood and urine tests reveal a normal to low white blood cell (WBC) count, mild proteinuria, and bilirubinuria in patients with jaundice.[7] Each type of hepatitis has its own antigen that will be assessed to ascertain the specific virus type and the treatment plan.

Treatment and Return to Participation

Hepatitis typically resolves spontaneously within 4 to 8 wk but can have lasting sequelae. Until the patient has completely recovered, alcohol is avoided and sex partners are limited. To prevent possible spread, household members receive immune globulin and initiation of vaccine as appropriate. Physician follow-up for hepatitis requires thorough management to ensure complete resolution of the disease; specialists in gastroenterology or hepatology are often involved.

Athletes who participate in collision sports may need additional laboratory tests to determine any residual effects of the disease before resuming full activity.

Prevention and Public Health Implications

HAV and HBV can be prevented by vaccination and good personal sanitation measures, such as handwashing after bowel movements and after contact with contaminated linens, clothing, patients, or utensils. The athletic trainer must routinely adhere to universal precautions when working with athletes with open wounds or when cleaning up body fluid spills.[90] HBV and HCV can be transmitted via contact during competition, so return-to-play decisions must be made individually by athlete and type of sport.[48,49] Sexually transmitted hepatitis can be prevented by using prophylactic barriers.

All cases of acute hepatitis need to be reported to local or state health agencies after diagnosis.

Hepatitis A

HAV is caused almost exclusively by poor sanitation because it is transmitted via oral–fecal contact. Outbreaks occur most often in crowded areas and through contaminated food or water. Transmission of HAV through food is typically via milk, sliced meat, shellfish, and salads.[50] In HAV, patients present with mild flu-like symptoms. In the icteric phase, they have dark urine, pale stools, and jaundice. Jaundice is present in 70% to 85% of adults with acute-onset HAV.[50] Forty percent of patients also have abdominal pain and pruritus (itching). Although the acute phase of HAV lasts up to 3 wk, convalescence is prolonged, and relapsing HAV is common. Treatment consists of supportive care for the side effects. HAV is self-limiting and rarely causes death. A vaccine for HAV has been available since 1995, and it is nearly 100% effective after two doses.[50]

Hepatitis B

HBV is a worldwide health care problem. Nearly one-third of the global population has been infected with HBV, and about 880,000 to 1.89 million individuals will have lifelong HBV.[51]

Transmission of HBV is primarily by sexual activity, and high-risk groups include those with multiple sex partners, intravenous drug users, men who have sex with men, and individuals engaging in piercing or tattooing. HBV is also spread by contamination with blood and body fluids (which are occupational hazards for health care workers) or from an infected mother to her unborn child. It is commonly contracted through exposure to blood, saliva, semen, vaginal secretions, urine, and feces.[51] This hardy virus can live for an extended period outside the human host, including on inanimate objects such as toothbrushes, utensils, and medical supplies.[31] HBV is approximately 100 times easier to contract than HIV.[49] HBV has been shown to be transmitted among football players and sumo wrestlers.[52,53] The 1982 licensure of the HBV vaccine has made a considerable difference in spread; in 1996, the United States recommended vaccination for adolescents who missed the immunization as a child.[8,9]

Signs and symptoms of HBV follow the other versions of hepatitis, and treatment is centered on preventing further sequelae from the disease. Although people can recover from HBV, recovery is protracted. The acute phase lasts approximately 6 mo, with potential for the chronic state to last years. Patients with either HBV or HCV are more susceptible to chronic infection, cirrhosis, and liver cancer than those with other types of hepatitis.[31]

Most athletes in noncontact sports who contract acute HBV are allowed to participate in athletics depending on clinical signs and symptoms. In the absence of fever or fatigue, there is no evidence that intense training is contraindicated. In close-contact sports, such as wrestling or boxing, however, athletes with acute HBV need to refrain from participation until they are not infectious.[19] The risk of transmission to others is limited but is higher compared with HIV.[7,31] As a precaution against infecting others, athletes who develop chronic HBV should not participate in close-contact, combative sports. Chronic HBV is a nationally reportable disease.

Hepatitis C

Although HCV is less prevalent than HBV, approximately 50% to 84% of patients remain chronic carriers of HCV.[47] This is a dangerous variety of the virus and is the cause of liver disorders. Close to 20% of chronic HCV carriers will develop cirrhosis over 20 to 30 yr; of these cases, up to 2.5% will also develop hepatocellular carcinoma.[54]

Common transmission routes for HCV involve intravenous or intranasal drug use (60%) or multiple sex partners (20%); the remaining transmission comes from needlesticks, maternal–fetal transmission, and unknown etiology.[31,54] At present, there is no known prevention method for HCV other than avoiding risky behaviors. HCV is a nationally reportable disease.

HCV is the most likely hepatitis virus to fluctuate for several months or years, and HBV is likely to have a higher mortality rate than HAV or HCV. Chronic hepatitis occurs most often with HBV; 5% to 10% of patients have persistent inflammation and cirrhosis and are subclinical chronic carriers.[7]

Hepatitis D

HDV, or delta virus, is linked to HBV but is structurally dissimilar to HAV, HBV, and HCV. It is far less common than other hepatitis viruses.[55] Transmission is via sexual contact and injection drug use. Recipients of multiple blood products are particularly at risk of HDV, but transmission is less efficient for HDV than for HBV.[47] As a separate disease, HDV presents with symptoms similar to those of other hepatitis viruses, but it has a shorter incubation period (21-45 d).[55] There is no vaccine for HDV, but HBV immunization also prevents HDV.

Streptococcal Infections

Streptococci (strep) are small, spherical, gram-positive chains of bacteria commonly found in human tissue. Various types of streptococci are typically found in the gastrointestinal tract, throat, respiratory system, vagina, and skin. The presence of streptococcal bacteria does not in itself indicate infection, and it only poses a problem when these bacteria occupy areas outside of their usual habitat. Streptococcal infections are, however, among the most common, yet dangerous, infections known to humans.[7] Table 14.3 compares the various streptococcal bacteria, their normal habitats, and related illnesses.

Clinical Tips

Hepatitis B Immunization

Hepatitis B vaccine is given as a series of three shots over 9 mo and is highly recommended for all health care workers.

Streptococcal infections are a group of microbially similar pathogens that have unique characteristics. They are categorized into groups A, B, C, D, and G, with groups A, B, and D being most common (table 14.4). Certain streptococci in groups C and G are resistant to bacitracin therapy and are naturally found in the human intestinal tract, skin, pharynx, and vagina. These can attack their host and cause a variety of problems, including pneumonia, cellulitis, impetigo, sepsis, and pharyngitis. This chapter provides an overview of groups A, B, and D; most of the common streptococcal infections are discussed in chapters covering the system related to infection.

Streptococcal infections can have a carrier or non-active state.[56] The term *carrier state* is used to refer to the presence of streptococci in tissues that have no sign of infection. Those with acute infections show physical signs of streptococcal bacteria invading tissues, and the delayed state becomes apparent approximately 2 wk after an overt streptococcal infection. Streptococcal infections are communicable diseases and are primarily spread by person-to-person contact, but they also have been contracted from infected food or water.[56]

Group A Streptococcal Infections

Group A streptococcus (GAS) infections are caused by group A β-hemolytic streptococci (*Streptococcus pyogenes*) and fall into two categories: **suppurative** and **nonsuppurative**. Suppurative infections are derived from invading bacteria that produce necrosis and cause acute inflammation, whereas nonsuppurative diseases occur in tissues remote from the original bacterial attack. Examples of the former are tonsillitis, streptococcal pharyngitis (strep throat), impetigo, myositis, pneumonia, toxic shock syndrome (TSS), and cellulitis. TSS became known in 1978 for its occurrence among women using highly absorbent tampons and keeping them in too long during their menstrual cycles. Fewer than 50% of TSS cases are attributable to tampon use, and this syndrome has been uncommon in recent years but still occurs. TSS is caused by either GAS or *Staphylococcus aureus* (see next section), and it is preventable by good hygiene in wound care and tampon replacement.[57] Nonsuppurative infections include rheumatic fever and acute poststreptococcal glomerulonephritis.[56] *S. pyogenes* skin infections tend to occur more often in the summer or in climates

TABLE 14.3   **Comparison of Streptococcal Infections**

Bacterium	Normal location	Diseases or illnesses caused
Streptococcus agalactiae	Raw milk	Meningitis in newborns; endometritis and fever in postpartum women
Streptococcus bovis	Alimentary tract of cattle	Endocarditis
Streptococcus equisimilis	Upper respiratory tract	Pneumonia, osteomyelitis, endocarditis, bacteremia
Streptococcus mutans	In dental cavities	Dental caries, endocarditis
Streptococcus pneumoniae	Upper respiratory tract	Pneumonia, meningitis, conjunctivitis, endocarditis, periodontitis, otitis media, septic arthritis, osteomyelitis
Streptococcus pyogenes	Upper respiratory tract	Scarlet fever, septic sore throat, impetigo, toxic shock syndrome, necrotizing fasciitis
Streptococcus viridans	Upper respiratory tract	Endocarditis

TABLE 14.4   **Categories of Common Streptococcal Infections**

Group	Common streptococcal infections
A	Pharyngitis, impetigo, pneumonia, cellulitis, otitis media, sinusitis, meningitis, rheumatic heart disease, necrotizing fasciitis
B	Neonatal, maternal, and cutaneous infections in persons with diabetes
C and G	Respiratory infections, pneumonia, cutaneous infections
D	Bacteremia associated with gastrointestinal cancer, urinary tract infection, endocarditis, meningitis, otitis media, pneumococcal pneumonia

🚩 RED FLAGS FOR NECROTIZING FASCIITIS

Necrotizing fasciitis has a mortality rate as high as 80%. Signs and symptoms include the following:

- Pain disproportionate to the severity of the injury or wound
- Rapid deterioration of the wound over the first 24 to 48 h
- Rapidly changing skin surface over the injury or wound (e.g., color, integrity)
- Fever
- Respiratory difficulty or failure
- Possible mental confusion

where it is warm year-round, when more skin is exposed and the likelihood of abrasions, cuts, or bites is higher.[56]

One form of GAS, group A β-hemolytic streptococcus (GABS), popularly referred to as *flesh-eating bacteria*, causes a form of gangrene called **necrotizing fasciitis**. This has created interest because infection in previously healthy people can rapidly become critical, requiring hospitalization and surgical debridement of the infected skin. Other forms of streptococcal and staphylococcal infections also have been known to cause necrotizing fasciitis.[58] Other names for this affliction are *hemolytic streptococcal gangrene*, *acute dermal gangrene*, *suppurative fasciitis*, and *synergistic necrotizing cellulitis*.

Necrotizing fasciitis is a rare and severe condition in which an infection progressively invades the skin, fascia, and blood supply. The frequency of cases has risen, most likely owing to an increase in immunocompromised patients.[58] The mortality rate of necrotizing fasciitis is 20% to 80% and is related to age and overall health at the time of infection.[56] Transmission occurs through a break in the skin and subsequent contact with a carrier of GAS. Inanimate objects are not likely to transmit GAS, and necrotizing fasciitis is not necessarily contagious between people as is methicillin-resistant *S. aureus* (MRSA). The condition is progressive, and it rapidly spreads via the fascial tissues to contiguous areas of the body. It may begin in a region distant from the original insult, and it may be caused by a minor invasion of the skin, such as an insect bite, an injection site, or a boil or minor scrape, or by surgical procedures or cauterizations. It has also been discovered when a seemingly minor wound is contaminated with salt water.[58]

The main symptom associated with necrotizing fasciitis is disproportionate pain for the size and apparent severity of the wound or incision combined with a rapid degeneration within the first 24 to 48 h. Open wounds can be further inspected to reveal yellow-greenish necrotic fascia, and closed tissue will reveal the same result through an incision.[58] Other key signs are putrid discharge, gas production from the wound, and the lack of normal tissue inflammatory healing. Accompanying signs include fever and respiratory difficulty and, on occasion, the patient presents in a delirious or confused state. If necrotizing fasciitis is left untreated, septic shock, renal failure, limb loss, or death could occur. Early treatment is surgical debridement, and it is a surgical emergency because it is often a limb- or lifesaving procedure. Antibiotic therapy is considered, as is hyperbaric oxygen therapy.[58] The incidence of necrotizing fasciitis is on the rise, owing largely to the rising number of patients with chronic issues that affect their immune systems, such as those with diabetes, cancer, HIV, alcoholism, and vascular insufficiency. The average age of patients with this condition is ages 38 to 44 yr.[58]

Group B Streptococcal Infections

Group B β-hemolytic streptococci (GBS) cause infections, endocarditis, septic arthritis, postpartum sepsis, pneumonia, meningitis, osteomyelitis, and soft-tissue infections. These infections are uncommon in adults; however, they are also opportunistic and occur in patients with lowered resistance.[59] GBS is indigenous to the upper respiratory, gastrointestinal, and female genitourinary tracts. In older adults, GBS is strongly linked to congestive heart failure.

Group D Streptococcal Infections

Group D streptococcal infections includes two distinct bacteria: enterococcal and nonenterococcal species. These streptococci are commonly found in the gastrointestinal system (e.g., *Streptococcus bovis*), but they can also cause bacterial endocarditis, urinary tract infection, abdominal sepsis, cellulitis, and wound infections.[60]

Signs and Symptoms

Because streptococci can attack almost any system, the signs and symptoms are not unique to this group of infections but to the body system affected. For example, pneumonia will have signs and symptoms unique to that infection, as will cellulitis; both are vastly different in presentation, yet both are caused by a streptococcal infection. The most common streptococcal presentation is pharyngeal infection from group A; strep throat presents with a bright-red pharynx, fever, sore throat, lymphadenopathy, and tonsillar exudates (see chapter 12).

Referral and Diagnostic Tests

Patients exhibiting any signs of infection must be referred to a physician. Patients may present with symptoms or signs remote from the origin of the infection, as is the case in nonsuppurative infections. Laboratory blood

Clinical Tips

Signs of Infection

Signs of infection include localized redness, heat, and swelling. Presence of a fever is also an indicator of infection, as is pain and general malaise.

tests showing a WBC count of 12,000 to 20,000/μL with 75% to 90% neutrophils indicate a streptococcal infection. See table 2.4 for normal CBC values. Tissue or blood culture can determine the specific cause of the infection (e.g., GAS, GBS), which in turn can dictate treatment.[56,60] Depending on the infection, urine or CSF may be tested.[59] A CBC sample cultured overnight and evaluated by microscopic examination provides confirmation, whereas the absence of streptococcal bacteria indicates other pathology.

Treatment and Return to Participation

The best medicinal treatment for streptococcal infections depends on the exact group and target tissue of the infectious agent. Patients must complete the course of their medication for complete effectiveness. Depending on the disease, isolation may be required (e.g., scarlet fever), and any materials soiled with residue from the infection or infected person are handled as infectious waste to prevent all types of streptococci from spreading.

The prognosis for return to activity after a confirmed streptococcal infection depends on the symptom severity and duration, tissues involved, speed of diagnosis and treatment, and disease progression. Certain streptococcal infections, such as impetigo, require absence from participation until the skin has completely healed (see chapter 16).[1,4,43]

Prevention of streptococcal infections includes proper sanitation, personal hygiene, and isolation of contagious persons until the period of communicability has passed.

Staphylococcal Infections

S. aureus, the main culprit of staphylococcal infections, is found in up to 80% of healthy adults intermittently and up to 30% are permanent carriers or colonized. Most commonly, the bacteria are found in the nares, but they can also be found in the throat, axilla, and rectum.[61] Staphylococcal organisms are grape-like clusters of gram-positive bacteria that cause a tremendous number of infections in nearly every human body system. Table 14.5 compares staphylococcal infections, their normal environments, and the ailments most often caused. Immunocompromised patients, especially those with influenza, chronic pulmonary disorders, chronic skin conditions, diabetes mellitus, and surgical incisions, are prone to staphylococcal infections. Transmission is commonly through hand-to-hand contact during patient care and also by airborne transmission. In athletics, the biggest culprits are those associated with seemingly benign skin wounds and postsurgical infections.

Certain types of staphylococcal infections are caused by ingestion of infected or undercooked food. TSS, previously described, is another preventable condition that results from a staphylococcal or GAS infection.[57]

An emerging problem with staphylococcal infections is the impediment to treatment with antibiotics, specifically MRSA. The two most discussed are health care–associated MRSA (HA-MRSA) and community-acquired MRSA (CA-MRSA). In the active population, CA-MRSA is typically the culprit in staphylococcal infections. The first report of a CA-MRSA infection in athletes was in 1993, and such reports have risen steadily since then.[62] At present, the low estimate is that

TABLE 14.5 **Comparison of Staphylococcal Infections**

Bacterium	Normal location	Diseases or illnesses caused
Staphylococcus aureus	Skin, mucous membranes (nose, mouth); produces golden-yellow pigment	Boils, carbuncles, internal abscesses; toxins cause food poisoning, toxic shock syndrome
Methicillin-resistant *S. aureus* (MRSA)	Same as for *S. aureus*	Same as for *S. aureus*
Vancomycin-resistant *S. aureus*	Becomes serious in nosocomial infections	Same as for *S. aureus*
Staphylococcus epidermidis	Skin	None
Staphylococcus hominis	Frequently recovered in skin	Causes no known diseases
Staphylococcus saprophyticus	Anal area, genitals, nose, mouth	Urinary tract infection

annually, there are 120,000 people treated for MRSA and 20,000 MRSA-associated deaths.[63] CA-MRSA is treatable if recognized and diagnosed in its early stages; with prophylactic treatment, its postsurgical infection rate is decreasing.[64]

Signs and Symptoms

Most CA-MRSA infections begin in a manner similar to other streptococcal infections, as a small lesion similar to a pimple, a mosquito bite, a recent injury or abrasion, or a wound from surgery. The wound quickly enlarges and becomes inflamed and quite painful. Patients may have a low-grade fever that increases as the body fights the infection. The seemingly small infection is painful beyond expectation for the type of pain a similar wound would cause. As the infection increases, so does the size of the infected area. In athletics, it is not unusual for outbreaks to occur among teammates.[62,65]

Referral and Diagnostic Tests

A patient who presents with a wound that shows signs of infection, such as heat, swelling, and redness, and is accompanied by pain is referred to a physician. Wounds that rapidly deteriorate or become enlarged are suspect. Unaware that they are fighting a serious condition, patients often try to drain the infection themselves and delay seeking treatment. Any patient with a postoperative wound needs to be especially diligent in cleaning and inspecting the wound and must immediately report any increase in pain, swelling, or fever.[64]

 RED FLAGS FOR CA-MRSA

Systemic treatment and hospitalization for CA-MRSA may be required if two of the following signs are present:[62,66]

- Temperature above 38 °C (100.4 °F) or below 36 °C (96.8 °F)
- Tachypnea above 24 breaths/min
- Tachycardia above 90 beats/min
- WBC count either above 12,000 cells/μL or below 400 cells/μL

Treatment and Return to Participation

If an infection is detected and the patient is referred early enough in infection development, a physician may be able to incise and drain it to prevent further problems. The release of infectious materials, coupled with an antibiotic and proper hygiene, may be enough to prevent MRSA.

If the patient is a staphylococcal carrier or has a history of resistance to penicillin treatment, other medications may be needed to eradicate the infection. The current antibiotic therapy for outpatient treatment is dependent on the *Staphylococcus* strain and infection severity. Effective medications are clindamycin, doxycycline, or linezolid.[62,64] Hospitalization may be required for the patient with high fever and pain unmanageable with outpatient medications.

Vehicles for Transmission of CA-MRSA in the Athletic Setting

- Towels
- Water bottles
- Hydrocollator pad covers
- Elastic wraps
- Weights (handheld and bars)
- Tubs of balms
- Tape-cutting devices
- Bell and diaphragm of a stethoscope
- Ultrasound applicator head
- Rehabilitation equipment
- Freezable gel packs
- Paraffin baths
- Ice scoop (if left in the ice machine)
- Applicator pads for electrical stimulation modalities
- Cryotherapy devices (e.g., Game Ready)

Note: CA-MSRA = community-acquired methicillin-resistant *Staphylococcus aureus.*

An athlete confirmed to have MRSA cannot engage in contact athletic activity until proven infection free. Communal areas, including weight rooms and athletic training clinics, need to be sanitized after every patient use.[1,43,65]

Prevention

Soap and water go a long way in the initial cleaning and disinfecting of wounds. The soap Hibiclens (Mlnlycke Health Care) is often prescribed for daily use for patients with infection. Athletes must thoroughly clean abrasions and turf burns as soon as possible after they occur and follow-up with hot water and soap in the shower; finally, the wounds must be covered with a sterile dressing. Daily cleaning and inspection of wounds will indicate if an athlete may be slower to heal or prone to infection. To prevent further colonization in an individual who is a carrier, an antibiotic is prescribed for 5 to 7 d. A study involving more than 38,000 surgical patients demonstrated that rates of postoperative infection can be lessened dramatically by a presurgical preventive approach. Patients were screened for *S. aureus* via a nasal or buccal (mouth) swab at least a week before surgery. Those who had a positive result as a carrier for *S. aureus* were given intranasal mupirocin and asked to bathe with chlorhexidine for each of the 5 d before surgery. Those who were not identified as a carrier bathed in chlorhexidine the night before surgery and were given a dose of cefazolin.[61]

Sexually Transmitted Diseases and Infections

Sexually transmitted diseases and STIs are a group of infectious diseases that are transmitted through body secretions from an infected partner. There are documented rare occasions in which a STI may be contracted in a nonsexual fashion, such as through occupational hazard (e.g., needlesticks) or dental care (e.g., an infected health care provider); and a fetus can acquire a STI through the maternal placenta before or during birth.

The presentation and detection of STIs differ for each sex and are covered in detail in chapter 9.

Clinical Tips

Vector Transmission of Disease

Organisms that transmit disease from one animal host to another are called *vectors*. For example, mosquitoes are vectors for the transmission of encephalitis from small creatures, usually birds and rodents, to humans.

Encephalitis

Encephalitis, translated literally, means "inflammation of the brain." In general, encephalitis is caused by a viral infection, but it can also be a sequela of immunizations or vaccines. The same organisms responsible for aseptic meningitis are also responsible for encephalitis, although their relative frequencies differ.

Encephalitis takes two forms: primary and secondary with complications from a viral infection. Primary encephalitis is caused by a direct viral invasion of the brain and spinal cord. The virus can be sporadic or epidemic. Sporadic infection arises from herpes simplex, varicella-zoster virus, measles, mumps, and other viruses.[7,67] Epidemic encephalitis is typically caused by mosquito-borne arboviruses, except for the Zika virus. **Arboviruses** are a large group of viruses recovered largely from bats, rodents, and arthropods (e.g., insects and crustaceans). Disease is typically transmitted by blood-feeding insects such as mosquitoes and ticks. These arboviruses are also known as distinct disorders: eastern and western equine encephalitis, both named after the horses that are also attacked by the virus; St. Louis and La Crosse viruses, which are named for the areas of the United States where they were first discovered; and West Nile virus. Zika virus, also an arbovirus caused by a mosquito, does not cause encephalitis, and it is covered after this section.

Secondary encephalitis is typically a complication of a viral infection in another part of the body that then enters the brain. All forms of encephalitis have a similar presentation that may begin as a minor illness with headache and fever but then develop more serious symptoms. Whereas primary encephalitis is more serious, the secondary form is more common. People often do not seek medical care because of the milder nature of secondary encephalitis; therefore, physicians see more cases of primary encephalitis.[67]

Although encephalitis is rare, it is the most common mosquito-borne disease in the United States. The mortality rate varies with the source of the virus. Insect-borne sources might cause low morbidity one year but severe mortality the next. Domestic arboviral disease infections are rising, with 2020 having had the highest incidence. The number of infections in 2020 was greater than the average annual occurrence in the past decade, with July through September having the highest rate.[68]

Birds are the conduit that spread the virus to mosquitoes through their food chain. A newly infected bird carries high levels of the virus in its bloodstream before developing immunity. Mosquitoes that feed on these birds become lifelong carriers of the disease. Carrier mosquitoes then easily pass the infection on to more birds, which in turn spread it to more mosquitoes.

Although most mosquitoes would choose birds over mammals for their primary food source, they do attack humans and other warm-blooded creatures. The risk is highest during the warm months when birds and mosquitoes reproduce. The ease of modern travel has also contributed to a slight rise in some vector-borne diseases. Travelers can bring back infected mosquitoes from their trips to their home. Because many athletes practice in the late afternoon and early evening during the warmer months, their activity coincides with the highest mosquito activity, so their risk is highest.[68,69] In addition, mosquitoes congregate in bodies of water, however small. This makes puddles of water from a hydration station or a discarded water bottle a haven for these pests.

Eastern equine encephalitis is the most serious viral encephalitis found in North America, primarily in the eastern United States. It affects horses, as its name suggests, and humans. Western equine encephalitis also affects horses and humans and is prevalent in the central and western plains. It is a serious variety of encephalitis but is not fatal as often as the eastern variety. Both are rare in the United States.[67] In 2020, 31% of people in the United States infected with eastern equine encephalitis died.[68]

The St. Louis variety, first discovered in the Midwest, is third in infections, behind La Crosse and West Niles.[68] La Crosse encephalitis is one of the few mosquito-borne viruses common in hardwood forests and is primarily found in the upper Midwest. It is transmitted to mosquitoes via chipmunks and squirrels rather than birds. However, the West Nile virus, with activity in all 50 states, attracts the most media attention. *Culex*, *Aedes*, and *Anopheles* mosquitoes are the primary culprits for West Nile virus, which was first reported in Africa, Europe, and Asia and reached the United States in 1999.[70]

West Nile virus has been transmitted through blood transfusions, through donated organs, and through breastfeeding and during pregnancy from mother to fetus. First reported in New York, West Nile virus is now found coast to coast. It has been found in humans and in birds, horses, dogs, squirrels, and bats.[70] Prevention strategies have proven effective.

Although symptoms of West Nile encephalitis are generally mild, the disease can become severe, especially in older people and those with a weakened immune system.[70]

Signs and Symptoms

Signs and symptoms of mosquito-borne encephalitis generally appear within 5 to 15 d of being bitten by an infected mosquito. Presentation is unique to the virus type. For example, patients with St. Louis encephalitis have dysuria and pyuria, whereas individuals with West Nile encephalitis suffer from extreme lethargy.[70] In general, signs and symptoms of encephalitis include sudden fever, headache, vomiting, photophobia, stiff neck

and back, confusion, drowsiness, clumsiness, unsteady gait, and irritability. Infection resulting from a virus (e.g., varicella-zoster virus, EBV, measles, and mumps) includes rash, lymphadenopathy, parotid enlargement, and hepatosplenomegaly.[67] Symptoms that require emergency treatment include loss of consciousness, seizure, poor responsiveness, muscle weakness, memory loss, sudden and severe dementia, impaired judgment, coma, and paralysis.[31]

Differential diagnoses for encephalitis include bacterial meningitis, brain abscess, parasitic diseases, metastatic tumors, and collagen diseases.

Referral and Diagnostic Tests

Encephalitis is potentially serious and life-threatening. Early referral to a physician or hospital emergency department may be necessary. The cardinal symptoms for immediate referral include severe headache, stiff neck, photophobia, and mental disturbances.[70] Because the origin of encephalitis can be autoimmune, bacterial, fungal, or vector-borne, a thorough history is paramount. History of travel, immunizations, proximity to infectious people, and outdoor activity can all provide critical information to distinguish the variety of encephalitis.

The keystone diagnostic test is CSF examination and analysis. Neuroimaging studies, magnetic resonance imaging (MRI), computed tomography (CT) scan, both with and without contrast, and often an electroencephalogram (EEG) may be performed as well. Both MRI and CT imaging may show edema or increased signal, indicating vector-borne virus.[67] An EEG is a graphic record of the electrical activity of the brain. Electrodes are placed on the patient's scalp to measure electrical waves, frequencies, and amplitudes. These tests help identify or exclude alternative diagnoses. They also determine whether the disease process is focal or diffuse.

Treatment and Return to Participation

Viruses are not responsive to antibiotics. Antiviral agents, such as acyclovir, which is used only in the early stages for the herpes simplex virus, are geared toward symptom management and maintenance of body systems. Management includes adequate nutrition, ventilation, and hydration. Control of seizures and cerebral edema, along with prevention of secondary infection, may be necessary.[67,70]

The overall prognosis for recovery is good, depending on the infecting source and the speed with which treatment is begun. Some cases are mild and the patient experiences a full recovery. In severe cases, however, permanent impairment or death is possible within 48 h despite early treatment. The acute phase of the infection may last 1 to 2 wk. Resolution of fever and neurological symptoms may be sudden or gradual. Neurological symptoms may require many months of treatment before full recovery, and rehabilitation with speech therapy is often required.

Prevention and Public Health Implications

All cases of encephalitis caused by an arbovirus should be reported to the local public health authority. Each state authority is allowed to determine whether to report these diseases immediately, within 1 working day, or within 1 wk.[71]

Prevention of many forms of secondary encephalitis caused by a viral infection in another part of the body, such as mumps, chicken pox, rubeola, or rubella, is best achieved through immunization.

Public health measures that control mosquitoes can reduce the incidence of many types of viral encephalitis. Effective local mosquito control includes the use of appropriate pesticides and cleanup of containers with standing water that may offer breeding sites.[69] Common containers that may hold enough water to breed mosquitoes include discarded cups and water bottles, football sleds, flowerpots, tire swings, and birdbaths. Individual prevention measures include wearing a hat, wearing long pants with the pant legs stuffed into socks, and avoiding scented lotions and perfumes, habitats, and times of day mosquitoes are most active.[72] In addition, liberal use of an EPA-registered insect repellent, including ones that contain DEET (*N,N*-diethyl-*m*-toluamide), or picaridin or citronella oil on the face, neck, ears, and arms is useful.[72]

Zika Virus

The Zika virus is another arbovirus but not one that causes encephalitis. It is related to yellow fever, dengue, West Nile, and St. Louis encephalitis viruses.[73] The consequences of Zika virus include loss of pregnancy, the birth defect microcephaly, and ocular defects.[74] Microcephaly is caused by defective brain development, resulting in an unusually small head. Other environmental and genetic causes for microcephaly include exposure to drugs or radiation, fetal alcohol syndrome, and some infections. Approximately 14% of babies exposed to Zika in the womb reportedly have health challenges associated with the virus, and mothers infected in the first trimester of pregnancy seem to be at highest risk of delivering babies with microcephaly.[74]

The *Aedes* mosquito has been identified as the carrier of the Zika virus, and it has two varieties: *Aedes aegypti* and *Aedes albopictus*.[73] The former is an African native, but it is found globally in tropical and subtropical areas. The latter is originally from Asia, and it is most known for being transported internationally in used tires. Both are found in the United States, although *A. albopictus* has a broader inhabitance. Zika virus disease peaked in 2016 for both the U.S. and its territories, with over 41,000 cases, but dipped to 60 total cases in those regions in 2020.[75]

Zika is named after an area in the Ugandan forest in Africa where it was first discovered in 1947. The first human transmission was in 1952, but it was not until February 2016 that it was truly recognized as a public health emergency by the WHO.[73] Once infected, humans can spread the virus. Zika has been found in blood, breast milk, and semen of infected people, and it can spread by maternal–fetal transmission and laboratory exposure.[73,76] A high correlation between Zika virus and Guillain-Barré syndrome has been observed. In 2021, a proposed vaccine prompted antibody responses in 80% of those who received two doses in phase 1 of that study.[77]

Signs and Symptoms

Unfortunately, many patients are unaware they have the Zika virus. It is believed that signs include a fine maculopapular diffuse rash, fever, and conjunctivitis. Symptoms can include joint or muscle pain and a headache.[73] Symptoms emerge within 2 wk of infection. The virus remains in the blood of infected people for about a week and longer in the semen.[75] One case demonstrated Zika virus was present in semen over 2 mo after symptom onset. Symptoms are mild and last less than a week. Differential diagnoses for Zika virus include GAS infections, malaria, rubella, measles, and dengue.[73,75]

Referral and Diagnostic Tests

Patients should be referred to a physician for evaluation if they have symptoms of Zika virus and a history of travel to countries with high Zika infection or a history of outdoor activity in areas known to have *Aedes* mosquitoes and reported infections. Although there is no commercially available test for Zika virus, assessment is done to rule out other conditions. Laboratory examination includes serological testing. Specifically, testing using reverse transcription polymerase chain reaction or enzyme-linked immunosorbent assay, depending on the time of symptom onset, is most reliable.[73] Zika virus has been found in urine more than 10 d following symptom onset.[73] Fetal ultrasonography and amniocentesis may be used in pregnant women with symptoms, although there is no reliable research supporting amniocentesis.

Treatment and Return to Participation

Because up to 80% of patients with Zika virus infection are unaware that they have it, return to participation may be unaffected.[75] For those with symptoms, appropriate fluid replacement is recommended, as is acetaminophen for pain and fever control. NSAIDs are not recommended because of the association of hemorrhagic consequences with similar conditions, such as dengue fever.[73]

Prevention and Public Health Implications

Prevention of the Zika virus begins with eliminating anything that may attract mosquitoes in general. Insect repellent should be the top layer, over hats, over clothing, and over sunscreen. In addition to the measures previously discussed for encephalitis prevention, public education is paramount. Use air conditioning or screened windows when indoors. Keep vegetation trimmed and grasses cut; cover, dump, or treat any vessel that can hold water to eliminate larva infestation.[69,71]

Men with a pregnant partner should use barrier protection to ensure that Zika virus is not transmitted. Women who are pregnant or anticipating a pregnancy should use extra caution, especially when determining travel to areas that host the *Aedes* mosquitoes.[74,75] Zika virus is a notifiable disease in the United States.

Viral Meningitis

Viral or aseptic **meningitis** is the most common form of meningitis, an inflammation of the meninges and CSF surrounding the brain and spinal cord (see figure 10.2 for an illustration of these structures).

Even though viral meningitis is a benign, self-limiting illness, it is associated with 26,000 to 42,000 hospitalizations each year in the United States.[31] It is generally less severe than bacterial meningitis and is rarely fatal in adults with normal immune systems. Care focuses on management of symptoms, which typically last 7 to 10 d before complete recovery.

Several viruses cause meningitis, including **enterovirus**, arboviruses, mumps, varicella-zoster virus, influenza viruses, and herpes simplex virus. Arboviruses such as West Nile can also cause viral meningitis.[68,70] The most common causative agent is enterovirus. Enteroviruses are a group of RNA viruses that can cause diseases in humans; they are typically found in respiratory secretions and stools of infected people. Other causes of infection can be bacteria, parasites, and drug use.

The organisms that cause viral meningitis are contagious. An enterovirus is most commonly spread through direct contact with respiratory secretions, such as the saliva, sputum, or nasal mucus, of an infected person. The typical pathway for infection occurs by shaking hands with an afflicted person or by touching something that the person has handled before rubbing the nose, mouth, or eyes. Kissing an infected person on the mouth can also spread the disease.[74]

In temperate climates, most cases are seen in the summer and early fall. The incubation period for an enterovirus is generally between 3 and 7 d from the time of infection until symptoms develop. An infected person can spread the virus to someone else during a period of about 3 d after infection until approximately 10 d after symptoms develop.

Viral meningitis has been transmitted among athletes. In 2014, eight football players and two siblings of the athletes sought treatment at an emergency department. All were diagnosed with viral meningitis, and all survived.[78] In 1989, 25% of students and staff at a high school suffered an outbreak of an enterovirus-like illness. Twenty-one percent were diagnosed with viral meningitis; of them, the highest rates of infection were among members of the football team.[79] Another high school group traveling to Mexico became ill after swimming in the ocean. Of the 25 group members, 21 contracted meningitis, most likely because of improper sewage dumping into the sea.[80] These three examples are a few among many reports of groups of active people contracting meningitis. They highlight the importance of proper hygiene and early recognition of an infectious condition.

Signs and Symptoms

Signs and symptoms of acute viral meningitis are common to all pathogens. Often the disease is accompanied or preceded by a nonspecific malaise or upper respiratory infection. Viral meningitis is similar in presentation to meningococcal infections because it appears with a sudden high fever, headache, and cervical rigidity. Nausea, vomiting, and diarrhea are found in more than 50% of patients.[81]

Other conditions to rule out include bacterial meningitis, migraine, Lyme disease, varicella-zoster, and systemic lupus erythematosus.[31]

Referral and Diagnostic Tests

The three indicators of viral meningitis that occur abruptly and develop rapidly are severe headache, high fever, and stiff neck. These indicators should alert the

 RED FLAGS FOR MENINGITIS

Warning signs of meningitis that warrant immediate referral include the following:

- Severe headache
- High fever
- Stiff neck

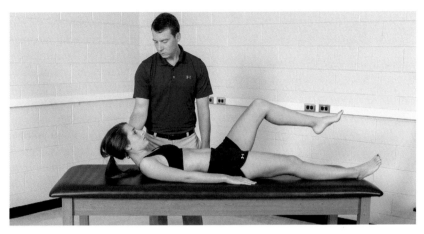

FIGURE 14.9   Brudzinski's sign involves passive neck flexion, thereby elongating the spinal cord. A positive sign is increasing localized pain, radiating in the lower extremity, or voluntarily flexing the hip or knee to alleviate spinal cord pressure; either action can indicate meningeal or nerve root irritation.

health care provider to the need for immediate referral to a physician or hospital emergency department. Applying stress on the spinal cord through Brudzinski's sign (figure 14.9) or Kernig's sign can exacerbate pain in the meninges, but it is not as definitive an indicator of the disease as is a stiff neck.[7] These two signs are often described with many varieties in positioning, but the chief result is an elongated neural tube along the spine, resulting in pain.

In the early stages, it is impossible to separate viral meningitis from acute bacterial or meningococcal meningitis without laboratory studies. It is necessary to examine the CSF to distinguish between the two infections as well as to rule out differential diagnoses. CSF is obtained through a spinal tap, which is also known as a lumbar puncture (see chapter 2). With viral meningitis, the spinal fluid on gross inspection is usually clear to the naked eye; no organisms are seen on microscopic examination, and they cannot be cultured. The glucose content also is normal.[81,82]

Treatment and Return to Participation

Once a diagnosis of viral meningitis is made, treatment is supportive. It consists of symptom management with bed rest, increased fluids, analgesics, and medications to prevent or relieve nausea and vomiting. Antibiotics are not helpful with a viral disease.

Prevention and Public Health Implications

Although aseptic or viral meningitis is the most common type of meningitis, in 1999 the CDC dropped it from the list of illnesses that need to be reported to the agency. It is

---

CONDITION HIGHLIGHT

Bacterial Meningitis

Acute bacterial meningitis is a potentially life-threatening illness that develops quickly. Because it is prevalent in areas of close living, such as military barracks and college dorms, many colleges require vaccination before admission. The bacterium is carried in respiratory and pharyngeal tissues and spread by air and mouth contact either with an infected person or with something the infected person ate or drank from (e.g., shared utensils, cups, beverages).[82] The condition begins as a harmless headache, accompanied by a stiff neck, rash, and, eventually, a high fever. Because the meninges are involved, the patient can experience concussion-like symptoms, including confusion, drowsiness, personality changes, and irritability. People with these signs and symptoms should be referred to a health care provider for immediate follow-up because bacterial meningitis can progress quickly, leading to limb amputation, coma, or death. Diagnosis is made via CSF examination through a lumbar spinal tap, and most health care providers will treat these symptoms as bacterial meningitis until a different diagnosis is confirmed. Treatment involves hospitalization and antibiotics. Bacterial meningitis is a health risk to the public and is a reportable disease.

RED FLAGS FOR BACTERIAL MENINGITIS

- Headache increasing in severity is the first symptom, typically frontal or retroorbital
- Rapid onset of symptoms
- Fever up to 40 °C (104 °F)
- Nausea and vomiting, especially in the early stages
- Confusion
- Drowsiness, progressive lethargy
- Convulsions or seizures more common in children, especially with influenzal meningitis; rare in adults
- Cervical rigidity
- Positive Brudzinski's sign
- Positive Kernig's sign
- Skin rash, especially near the armpits or on the hands or feet
- Rapid progression of small petechiae under the skin
- Malaise
- Irritability
- Photophobia
- Muscle aches

still reportable to some state public health agencies. The time period within which to report a case or suspected case of aseptic meningitis varies from state to state but is usually within 1 wk. The National Enterovirus Surveillance System is in place to gather information about enterovirus detection and outbreaks from state public health agencies, private laboratories, and treating physicians.

The most effective way to prevent enteroviral disease is adherence to good hygiene practices that include frequent and thorough handwashing and avoidance of shared utensils and drinking containers. In institutional settings, washing objects and surfaces with a dilute bleach solution (as described in the beginning of this chapter) can be effective in destroying the virus. Other preventive methods encompass the mosquito prevention techniques mentioned earlier.

Acute Bacterial Meningitis

Unlike viral meningitis, acute bacterial meningitis is a potentially life-threatening infection of the meninges and the CSF. Four types of bacteria account for more than 80% of all cases: *Streptococcus pneumoniae* (the most common cause of bacterial meningitis in adults), GBS, staphylococci, and *Neisseria meningitidis* (a meningococcus).[7] Incidences of pneumonia and meningococcal meningitis are decreasing as a result of increased vaccinations targeted to prevent them.

The health care provider needs to fully appreciate the severity of meningitis: If left untreated, it is fatal in 50% of the cases.[82] The disease is expressed most commonly either as *meningococcal meningitis*, an inflammation of the membranes surrounding the brain and spinal cord, or as *meningococcemia*, a serious infection of the blood. Meningococcemia blood infections are caused by gram-negative *N. meningitidis* but do not present with associated meningitis.[7]

Meningococcal meningitis can result in permanent brain damage, hearing loss, learning disability, limb amputation, kidney failure, or death. Meningococcal disease is spread by the exchange of respiratory and throat secretions through such activities as coughing or kissing. Sometimes, however, bacteria have spread to other people who have had close or prolonged contact with a patient with meningitis caused by *N. meningitidis*.[83] People in the same household (e.g., college students living in dormitories) or anyone in direct contact with a patient's oral secretions from coughing, sneezing, kissing, or oral contact with shared items (e.g., cigarettes, hookah mouthpieces, or drinking glasses) would be considered at increased risk of acquiring the infection. People who qualify as close contacts of a person with meningitis caused by *N. meningitidis* should receive prophylactic antibiotics to prevent them from getting the disease. *N. meningitidis* has been found in the nasopharyngeal passages of about 10% of uninfected adults.[84] Although these people carry the bacteria in their nose and throat without signs of illness, they can spread the disease to others.

Signs and Symptoms

As stated earlier, meningitis strikes suddenly; therefore, early diagnosis and treatment are especially important. All forms of acute meningitis, bacterial or viral, have common symptoms that may also be mistaken for influenza. This disease has also been erroneously dismissed as torticollis because of its proclivity for stiff neck.[84] Patients complain of a respiratory illness or sore throat, followed by fever, headache, and a stiff neck.[31] Other symptoms can include confusion, irritability, delirium, and coma.[82] In children, projective vomiting and seizures may be present. Symptoms can develop over several hours or a few days, but only 44% of adults with bacterial meningitis presented with the classic diagnostic trio of headache, fever, and neck stiffness.[82] Another anecdotal observation

TABLE 14.6 Cerebrospinal Fluid Values and Indicators

Parameter	Normal value	Notes
Pressure	50-80 mm (H_2O)	High: Acute bacterial meningitis, cerebral hemorrhage, perhaps Lyme disease
Appearance	Clear	Cloudy: Infection, meningococcal meningitis Red: Cerebral hemorrhage, obstruction Orange: High protein, old bleeding
Protein	20-45 mg/dL	High: Tumors, trauma, infection, inflammation, acute bacterial meningitis, Guillain-Barré syndrome
Glucose	40-70 mg/dL	Low: Acute bacterial meningitis, hypoglycemia, infection, cancer High: Hyperglycemia
Leukocytes	Up to 5 cells/µL	500-10,000: Acute bacterial meningitis 0-500: Lyme disease 0-100: Guillain-Barré syndrome Presence of red blood cells: Cerebral hemorrhage

Based on Porter Kaplan (2018); Ferri (2023); R. Hasbun, "Meningitis," Medscape, last modified February 16, 2016, http://emedicine.medscape.com/article/232915-overview.

is not to dismiss headache and stiff neck complaints from athletes the first few days in a sport requiring a helmet, as the helmet adjustment period can often lead to headaches. Be certain to ask history questions germane to other signs or symptoms of meningitis.

With a careful review of the patient's clinical history and a physical examination that notes the sudden onset of severe headache accompanied by high fever and lethargy or confusion, a diagnosis of bacterial meningitis is not difficult.

Referral and Diagnostic Tests

Bacterial meningitis is a medical emergency. A satisfactory outcome depends on the speed with which treatment is begun. As with viral meningitis, the three indicators that occur abruptly and rapidly are severe headache, high fever, and stiff neck, but they are not always present. Because Kernig's and Brudzinski's signs are positive in approximately 50% of patients with meningococcal disease, the practitioner should consider using them as clinical noninvasive tests.[7,84]

Diagnosis is based on clinical history, physical examination, and specific diagnostic tests. The definitive diagnosis of bacterial spinal meningitis is made by examination of CSF (table 14.6) obtained through a lumbar puncture (see chapter 2); opening pressure of the CSF will be elevated (>180 mm H_2O). On visual inspection, the CSF appears cloudy or purulent. Further evaluation of the CSF includes culture, protein, glucose, and WBC count.[82] Other key laboratory tests include blood cultures, chest radiograph, and electrolyte and glucose measure-

ment. CT or MRI brain scanning may also be desirable.

Treatment and Return to Participation

Bacterial meningitis can be treated effectively with a number of antibiotics. Treatment is two pronged. First, because of the severity and emergent nature of the disease, antimicrobial treatment is started before the results of CSF cultures are known. Once the specific pathogen is identified, specific intravenous drug therapy is begun. Second, other associated complications, such as hearing loss, brain swelling, shock, convulsions, and dehydration, must be addressed with appropriate supportive treatment and drug therapy.[84,85]

The prognosis for bacterial meningitis depends on several factors, including the type of infecting organism and the speed with which medical treatment is initiated. Untreated bacterial meningitis can be fatal. The mortality rate for uncomplicated meningococcal meningitis and *H. influenzae* meningitis is about 5%. Meningococcal infections in the United States still cause about 500 deaths a year.[82] In general, early and effective treatment leads to recovery with no residual symptoms. Late or inadequate treatment may result in permanent damage. Common sequelae include memory impairment, decreased intellectual function, hearing loss, dizziness, seizures, and gait disturbances.[84]

Return to participation will depend on the complete resolution of symptoms and medical clearance from the treating physician or medical team.

Prevention and Public Health Implications

Anyone exposed to meningococcal meningitis who has face-to-face contact (family member, housemate, teammate) should begin **prophylaxis**. Appropriate medications range from rifampin to ciprofloxacin. Rifampin is targeted to children and tends to turn body fluids orange. A better choice for athletes is ciprofloxacin, a one-dose pill that assures compliance.[7] At the national level, meningococcal meningitis is a reportable disease. State and local public health agencies also have their own guidelines for reportable diseases. Universities typically have guidelines for proper reporting procedures. Notification to local, state, and national agencies is usually done through the hospital or treating physician. Meningococcal infections require immediate reporting to the public health department.[22]

There are currently six vaccines available to prevent meningococcal conditions, and each covers specific subgroups of the infection.[82,85] The patient's age, health status, and risk evaluation all matter in determining which vaccine is most appropriate. The vaccine is 85% to 100% effective in preventing disease in older children and adults. The CDC, the American College Health Association, and the American Academy of Pediatrics recommend that parents and college students, particularly freshmen who plan to live in dormitories, learn about meningococcal disease and the potential benefits of vaccination. Other college undergraduates wishing to reduce their risk may also choose to be vaccinated. The CDC has issued updated vaccination criteria for meningococcal meningitis. The ACIP recommends the quadrivalent meningococcal conjugate vaccine for all people ages 11 to 18 yr and for people ages 2 to 55 yr if they are at increased risk of meningococcal disease.[85]

Summary

Infectious diseases commonly attack every system in the human body, but most are largely preventable. People who take advantage of immunizations and follow universal precautions will protect themselves from most common infectious diseases. The athletic trainer must consider infectious diseases when working with patients who have fever, unexplained fatigue, or a skin abrasion that does not heal in order to ensure that they get the best care possible and to protect other individuals who may have been exposed to an infectious agent.

Apply It!

Go to HK*Propel* to complete the case studies for this chapter.

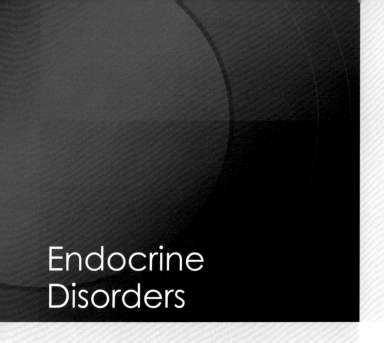

Endocrine Disorders

15

OBJECTIVES

At the completion of this chapter the reader should be able to do the following:

1. Summarize the effects of the endocrine system on the body.

2. Describe prevention strategies for type 2 diabetes mellitus.

3. Determine and understand diabetic emergencies.

4. Recognize and refer patients with signs and symptoms of a malfunctioning thyroid.

An endocrine organ or gland creates and secretes hormones directly into the bloodstream to influence tissues throughout the body. In turn, hormones regulate metabolism, growth, and reproductive functions. When the endocrine organ or gland dysfunctions, the effects on other areas of the body can be catastrophic. There are hundreds of conditions related to the effects of hormones on tissues that can profoundly affect physically active people. This chapter focuses on the more common endocrine disorders of pancreatitis, diabetes, and thyroid gland disorders.

Endocrine Disorders

Endocrine glands secrete hormones directly into the bloodstream, allowing specific body functions to occur. The disorders discussed here are related to the pancreas, a gland with both exocrine and endocrine functions, and the thyroid. The pancreas lies with its ends laterally touching the spleen and the duodenum of the small intestine medially (figure 15.1). The chief functions of the pancreas are to secrete bicarbonate to protect the duodenum from gastric acid and to produce insulin, glucagon, and somatostatin from the endocrine glands, called **islets of Langerhans**. The normal pancreas has between 500,000 and several million islets. The islets comprise four cell types, but only the two primary cell types, alpha and beta, are discussed here. Alpha cells produce glucagon, whereas beta cells secrete insulin.

When serum glucose (blood sugar) is high, the beta cells are stimulated to produce insulin. The secreted insulin then allows muscle, blood, and fat cells to absorb glucose out of the blood and store it in muscle and the liver as glycogen, effectively lowering blood sugar to normal ranges. The alpha cells of the islets of Langerhans

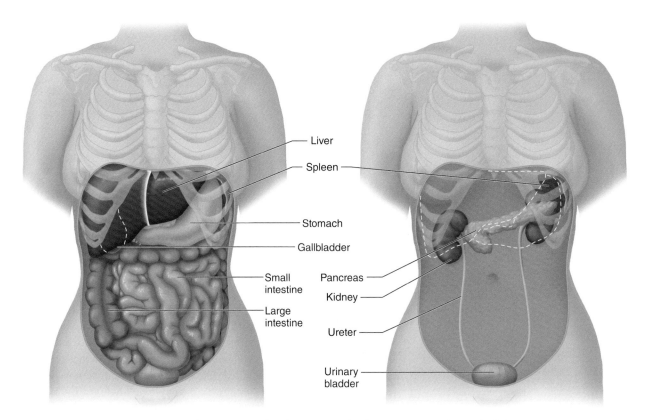

FIGURE 15.1 The pancreas is the primary gland secreting the hormones insulin and glucagon.

secrete glucagon, which has the opposite effect of insulin. If blood sugar is low, glucagon is secreted where it has the most effect—the liver. Glucagon stimulates liver cells to break down stored glycogen into glucose and release it into the bloodstream, increasing serum levels of glucose. Glucagon also stimulates muscle to manufacture glucose from stored protein by means of gluconeogenesis. The human body functions best when glucose levels are relatively constant within the bloodstream. Because most body functions rely on glucose in some form, severely fluctuating levels can have profound sequelae.

Pancreatitis

Acute pancreatitis is an inflammatory process of the pancreas with intrapancreatic activation of enzymes. It is one of the most common gastrointestinal causes of hospitalization in the United States.[1] In 40% of cases, pancreatitis is caused by blockage of the biliary tract by gallstone formation (**cholelithiasis**), but an additional 35% of acute cases can be attributed to alcohol abuse.[1] Untreated gallstones can lead to a 32% to 61% risk of reoccurrence, which could trigger acute pancreatitis.[2] In general, more males than females present with acute pancreatitis, but males tend to have the condition as a result of alcohol, whereas females tend to experience biliary-tract obstruction. Several medications (gluco-

corticoids, diuretics, hormones) have been implicated in pancreatitis as well.[3] African Americans have 3 to 10 times higher risk of pancreatitis than any other racial group.[4]

In athletes, acute pancreatitis has been attributed to anabolic-androgenetic steroid use or abuse[5-8] and growth hormone (injected subcutaneously).[5]

Signs and Symptoms

Patients with pancreatitis typically present with sudden-onset abdominal pain in the epigastric area and occasionally radiating to the back. The pain has been characterized as beginning dull and steady and increasing with time, and patients may have severe nausea and vomiting.[4] The majority of patients with acute pancreatitis present with fever and abdominal distention. Tachycardia, hypotension, and dyspnea are not uncommon.[4] On examination, patients typically guard their abdomen because of the extreme pain, possible fluid or blood within the abdominal cavity, and discomfort with palpation of this area. Bowel sounds are hypoactive in patients with pancreatitis. Chapter 8 presents a basic assessment of the abdomen.

Several diseases can present with abdominal pain, and they should be considered when assessing for pancreatitis. These include peptic ulcer disease, intestinal obstruction, early acute appendicitis, bowel obstruction, cholecystitis, pneumonia, and heart attack. The history, physical examination, and laboratory results will help differentiate these problems.[9]

Referral and Diagnostic Tests

People with acute nontraumatic abdominal swelling or pain accompanied by fever should be referred to a physician or the emergency department for further evaluation. Patients often require hospitalization for pain control and treatment of pancreatitis.

History and physical examination are paramount in the assessment of these patients. Alcohol intake history is important to help elucidate a cause for the inflamed pancreas. Pancreatitis presents with elevated enzymes produced by the pancreas, including lipase and amylase. Of the two enzymes, lipase is more sensitive. Further testing, including blood count, liver enzymes, and glucose and serum calcium levels, is important in the initial workup. Abdominal radiographs, ultrasound, or computed tomography scans are appropriate for diagnosis.[3] They help to evaluate not only for inflammation of the pancreas, intestines, gall bladder, and liver but also for any potentially obstructing stones or cancers.

Treatment and Return to Participation

Pancreatitis requires hospitalization. Food is avoided because it may irritate the pancreas and therefore slow healing. Maintenance of intravascular volume with intravenous fluids is critical because patients with pancreatitis tend to have a total body water deficit. Pain control is provided with medications, such as meperidine (Demerol). Surgical consultation may be warranted if there is evidence of gallstone pancreatitis. Patients with severe acute pancreatitis typically require intensive care and may be intubated and sedated to manage pain.

Prognosis varies with the severity of the illness. Overall mortality for acute pancreatitis approaches 5% to 10% of patients.[3] Individuals with a history of alcohol abuse commonly have recurrent bouts of pancreatitis, leading to chronic pancreatitis. People with chronic gallstone attacks are especially susceptible to pancreatitis and should be counseled to have the stones removed preemptively. There is also a documented higher risk of acute pancreatitis for patients with type 2 diabetes mellitus (DM), and successful management of DM may alleviate the chances of contracting pancreatitis.[10]

Diabetes and pancreatic insufficiency are common complications following acute pancreatitis, occurring in 20% of patients.[1] Individuals need to be counseled on triggers for an acute attack and assessed for common sequela of the condition. Patients recovering from pancreatitis will need to refrain from competition until the acute phase has resolved. Because the pain associated with pancreatitis is so great, it will not allow the patient to make any sudden movements. Once the cause of pancreatitis is identified, it should be treated appropriately.

Diabetes Mellitus

DM is a disease in which the body cannot produce or use insulin effectively. This disease affects 11.3% of the U.S. population, or roughly 37 million people. An additional 96 million Americans have prediabetes, with 38% of adults unaware they have the condition. The risk of death among patients with diabetes is nearly twice that of individuals without the disease in the same age range.[11] There are more than 88 specific classifications for DM, but here we focus on types 1 and 2.[3]

- Type 1 DM, formerly called *insulin-dependent diabetes mellitus*, is an autoimmune condition characterized by the body's inability to produce insulin, which is needed for the proper use and storage of carbohydrates. Insulin is released by the pancreas to regulate blood sugar. Type 1 DM accounts for roughly 10% of the total number of cases, and its onset usually occurs in people younger than age 20 yr.

- Type 2 DM, formerly called *non–insulin-dependent diabetes mellitus*, comprises the remaining 90% of cases.[9] This form of DM is related to the body's inability to use insulin effectively because of a combination of insulin resistance and an overall decrease in insulin production. In addition, 89.9% of people diagnosed with type 2 DM are obese (body mass index >25 kg/m^2).[11]

Diabetes incidence is known to increase with age. Diabetes is the leading cause of end-stage renal disease in the United States and is a primary cause of blindness and foot and leg amputations in adults. More than 102,000 people with diabetes die annually because of complications of the disease.[12] Diabetes is also known to cause **neuropathy** (nerve damage) in up to 70% of patients. People with diabetes are twice as likely to develop cardiovascular disease as those without diabetes.[13]

Type 1 DM is caused by autoimmune-mediated destruction of pancreatic beta cells, which are responsible for producing insulin. There appears to be a hereditary link in people with type 1 DM. Other factors have been postulated to induce type 1 DM, including viral infections, toxins, and other environmental factors. Although there is a genetic predisposition for developing type 2 DM, several physical factors also put a person at increased risk of the disease. Type 2 DM results more from an insulin resistance syndrome. In addition to environmental and physiological reasons for insulin resistance, the main cause is excess body fat (body mass index >25 kg/m^2) linked primarily to a sedentary lifestyle and consumption of excess calories.[14] Females can also be affected by gestational diabetes, which usually occurs in the third trimester of pregnancy and typically resolves in the postpartum period. These females are more likely to develop type 2 DM later in life. Uncontrolled high blood pressure and high cholesterol are also risk factors for type 2 DM, as is being older than age 45 yr. Certain racial and ethnic populations are at increased risk of diabetes, including Native Americans, African Americans, Asian Americans, and Hispanic Americans. Other causes of type 2 DM are Cushing's syndrome, pancreatic disorders (e.g., pancreatitis), or prolonged use of medications, including glucocorticoids.[13]

 RED FLAGS FOR SIGNS AND SYMPTOMS OF DIABETES

Undiagnosed diabetes is dangerous because it can result in coma, convulsions, permanent brain injury, and possible death. Recognizing the following signs and symptoms, particularly when they present together, can lead to early diagnosis:

- Polyuria (increased urination)
- Polydipsia (excessive thirst)
- Polyphagia (persistent hunger)
- Tingling, pain, or numbness in hands or feet (type 2 diabetes)
- Blurry vision
- Cuts or bruises slow to heal
- Fatigue
- Weight loss, even when eating more (type 1 diabetes)
- Incoordination

Signs and Symptoms

There is usually a prolonged, albeit unknown, period when people with type 2 diabetes have hyperglycemia but do not have any clinical symptoms. Later in the disease process, as the body can no longer compensate for the elevated sugar load, symptoms begin. The most common initial symptoms are listed in the Red Flags for Signs and Symptoms of Diabetes sidebar. All of these symptoms are attributable to elevated glucose levels in the bloodstream. Overtreatment of diabetes or inadequate food intake can cause **hypoglycemia**, which is also dangerous. Hypoglycemia is defined as low levels of glucose in the blood, clinically below 60 mg/dL, and further clarified as less than 50 mg/dL in men, less than 45 mg/dL in women, and less than 40 mg/dL in infants and children.[15]

Differential diagnoses of diabetes include diabetes insipidus, stress hyperglycemia, and diabetes secondary to medications, pancreatic disease, and possible hormonal excess.

Referral and Diagnostic Tests

Individuals with signs or symptoms consistent with diabetes or those who have risk factors are referred to a physician. Three tests of blood glucose levels can be performed to confirm the diagnosis of diabetes: fasting plasma glucose (table 15.1), hemoglobin A_{1c} (HbA_{1c}), and oral glucose tolerance testing. In addition, a random blood draw, performed without regard to food intake, that yields a blood glucose level equal to or greater than 200 mg/dL, associated with weight loss, polyuria, and polydipsia, indicates DM. All three criteria can diagnose diabetes, but one positive test must be confirmed on the following day by another one of the tests.[17] A fasting blood glucose level between 100 and 125 mg/dL is consistent with the diagnosis of prediabetes.

CONDITION HIGHLIGHT

Hyperglycemia and Hypoglycemia

Hypoglycemia can also affect athletes without diabetes, as many athletes show up to practice or events without having consumed the proper nutrition for the session they are about to endure. The symptoms of hypoglycemia are numerous and include sweating, palpitations, hunger, tremors, confusion, nausea, headache, fatigue, slurred speech, inappropriate behavior, and incoordination.[15] Health care providers must recognize these symptoms in patients because if left uncorrected, hypoglycemia can result in coma, convulsions, permanent brain injury, and possibly death. *Hyperglycemia* is another risk factor for people with diabetes; it has a variety of symptoms such as polyuria, polydipsia, fatigue, nausea, and elevated blood sugar. It has been reported that athletes with type 1 diabetes sometimes run chronically hyperglycemic to decrease the risk of exercise-induced hypoglycemia, which will increase their risk of infection. On-site health care providers should be aware of which athletes have diabetes and their increased risk of infection from cuts and abrasions. For conscious patients with diabetes, treatment for hypoglycemia includes providing sugar-laden (not diet) drinks, such as orange or apple juice, or hard candy. Glucagon is a drug administered via nasal inhalation for severe hypoglycemic reactions and should be available on-site for patients with diabetes.[14]

CONDITION HIGHLIGHT

Diabetic Ketoacidosis

Diabetic ketoacidosis (DKA) can be the first overt sign of undiagnosed diabetes (25% of cases), but it can also occur with mismanaged diabetes (25%) or a concomitant infection (40%).[16] This is a life-threatening, acute response to hyperglycemia or uncontrolled DM. In DKA, there is systemic hypovolemia, extremely high serum glucose, and breakdown of fatty acids, creating acidosis. If left unattended, coma and death follow.[16] Early signs of DKA include polyuria, polydipsia, weakness, nausea, vomiting, altered consciousness, and a history of noncompliance with insulin therapy. As DKA progresses, tachypnea, tachycardia, decreased reflexes, and dry skin and mucous membranes signal a dangerous spiral for the patient. Recognition is critical at this point. The patient requires intravenous fluids, insulin, and electrolyte rebalancing.[16] If discovered in time, DKA is largely reversible, but the patient must be educated about better self-regulation of their glucose or insulin levels. DKA primarily occurs in type 1 diabetes but is not uncommon in type 2 diabetes.

Another common blood test is for glycated hemoglobin, or HbA_{1c} (table 15.2). This test identifies the concentration of glucose in plasma over time, typically 3 mo. The 2022 American Diabetes Association Standards of Medical Care for Diabetes recommends a level at or below 6.5% as a criterion for the diagnosis of diabetes.[19] Once diabetes is diagnosed, HbA_{1c} can be used periodically in conjunction with other tests to monitor plasma glucose levels. For every percentage decrease in HbA_{1c}, individuals with diabetes have a 40% reduction in the occurrence of microvascular complications (including damage to nerves, kidneys, and eyes).[14,18]

Once the diagnosis is confirmed, those caring for people with diabetes, especially athletes, need to be well versed in the signs and symptoms of hyperglycemia and hypoglycemia. See the Comparison of Signs and Symptoms for Hypoglycemia and Hyperglycemia sidebar.

Although exercise is important to treating and controlling diabetes, there are also inherent risks for people with diabetes who do exercise.[20] Hypoglycemia usually presents several hours after exercise, but it can happen during competition or as a result of an overuse of insulin. People can have reactionary hypoglycemia, brought about by improper nutrition and exercise or fasting and exercise.[21] These individuals need to be counseled about making better nutritional choices. The treatment for hypoglycemia is to ingest glucagon or carbohydrates; the treatment for hyperglycemia is to receive a measured dose of insulin prescribed for that patient.

TABLE 15.1   Fasting Plasma Glucose Levels

Result	Blood glucose serum level (mg/dL)
Normal	<100
Prediabetes	100-125
Diabetes	≥126

*mg/dL = Milligrams of glucose in 100 milliliters (1 deciliter) of blood. *Hypoglycemia* is defined as less than 60 mg/dL, and *hyperglycemia* is defined as greater than 180 mg/dL.

Data from ADA (2022).

TABLE 15.2   Glycated Hemoglobin/Hemoglobin A$_{1c}$

Result	HbA$_{1c}$/A$_{1c}$ (%)
Normal	<5.7
Prediabetes	5.7-6.4
Diabetes	≥6.5

*mg/dL = Milligrams of glucose in 100 milliliters (1 deciliter) of blood. *Diabetes* is defined with an A$_{1c}$ of 6.5% or higher

Data from ADA (2022).

Comparison of Signs and Symptoms for Hypoglycemia and Hyperglycemia

Hypoglycemia (<60 mg/dL)
- Palpitations
- Tachycardia
- Anxiety
- Hyperventilation
- Blurred vision
- Shakiness
- Weakness
- Diaphoresis
- Nausea
- Confusion
- Behavior changes
- Hallucinations
- Hypothermia
- Seizure
- Coma

Hyperglycemia (>180 mg/dL)
- Weakness
- Polyuria
- Altered vision
- Weight loss
- Dehydration
- Polydipsia
- Hyperventilation
- Hypotension
- Cardiac arrhythmia
- Stupor
- Coma

Treatment and Return to Participation

Patients with diabetes, whether type 1 or 2, need to be under the care of a physician because of the many complications that can arise if diabetes is not controlled. Athletes with diabetes are more prone to tendinopathies, shoulder adhesive capsulitis, and articular cartilage diseases, and they have more surgical complications. Athletic trainers and others caring for athletes with diabetes must be aware of possible difficulties with routine healing and tendencies toward chronic musculoskeletal pathologies.[22] Because there are so many people with diabetes in the United States, most primary care physicians can manage the disease without the assistance of specialists. If referral is needed, as may be true for most people with type 1 diabetes, an endocrinologist or diabetologist would be appropriate. The care of the person with diabetes requires a multidisciplinary approach. Patients may be referred for nutritional counseling, exercise prescriptions, yearly eye examinations, and routine podiatric care.

The overall goal in the treatment of diabetes is to decrease the end-stage effects, such as renal disease and failure, coronary artery disease, blindness, and stroke. In addition to medications, diet, and exercise to improve glucose control, other conditions common to people with diabetes need to be treated, including hypertension, elevated cholesterol and triglycerides, and tobacco abuse. If further complications arise, nephrologists, cardiologists, podiatrists, or other appropriate specialists are consulted.

The treatment for diabetes is multifactorial. At the cornerstone of therapy is education about the disease, sound nutrition, and increased physical activity. Lifestyle modification has been shown to delay or prevent diabetes onset.[20,23,24]

Development and progression of complications decrease immensely with intensive treatment of diabetes and its associated conditions. If diabetes is not treated intensively, patients can expect many complications as the disease progresses. Neuropathy, or decreased and sometimes painful sensation in the extremities, is very common and can lead to eventual amputation. Infections are more common in patients with diabetes and are much more difficult to control if blood sugars are not optimized. Surgical complications, such as delayed healing or grafting failure, can occur in patients with uncontrolled diabetes.[20,22,23]

For the active patient, sound knowledge of the disease, medications, and dietary habits is critical to control blood sugar while training and competing. Wounds in people with diabetes tend to heal more slowly than in those without diabetes; however, excellent control of blood sugars can almost negate this disadvantage. Common athletic wounds, such as blisters and calluses, need more diligent care in athletes with diabetes. These seemingly harmless lesions can lead to infections or chronic ulcers if not properly cared for. In the worst case, a patient may have to undergo amputation because of an inability to control

Clinical Tips

Diabetes Insipidus

Although it has the word *diabetes* in its title, diabetes insipidus is a rare metabolic condition that affects the fluid balance in the body and results in excessive urination (polyuria) and thirst (polydipsia). Although both type 1 and type 2 DM can present with polyuria and polydipsia, these two conditions affect glucose metabolism. Patients with diabetes insipidus display typical glucose ranges but pass copious amounts of urine daily and can easily become dehydrated.

There has been recent discussion about changing the term *diabetes insipidus* to two different acronyms. In a 2022 position paper, a group of leading international endocrine associations proposed the terms *arginine vasopressin deficiency (AVP-D)* and *arginine vasopressin resistant (AVP-R)* to denote central (cranial) and kidney-related etiologies, respectively.[26] This is because diabetes insipidus is related to the hormone AVP either having inadequate production by the hypothalamus (and stored in the pituitary gland) in the brain or resistance in the kidney. The group suggested that the term *diabetes insipidus* is antiquated and it is time to label the condition by the origin of the cause (brain [AVP-D] or kidney [AVP-R]).

ulcers caused by simple friction. Active patients with diabetes should inspect their feet daily and, if necessary, the athletic trainer should participate.[23] Identifying and eliminating the underlying cause of lesions is important to preventing further damage; causes can include socks, shoe wear, and gait variations. Education and a collaborative approach between the athlete and the medical care team is essential to the patient's longevity and safety, especially in the adolescent athlete with diabetes.[24,25]

Type 1 diabetes is not preventable. However, type 2 diabetes onset and severity can be greatly decreased, if not eliminated, with adequate exercise and a proper diet.

Type 1 Diabetes Mellitus

The goal of treatment for type 1 DM is to maintain a normal blood sugar level and to prevent complications that occur when blood sugar remains elevated. In people with type 1 diabetes, this is achieved with insulin because their insulin production is decreased. Patients must monitor their blood sugar and adjust insulin levels to meet their specific needs. Traditionally, this entails two or more self-injections of insulin daily. Many types of insulin are available. Rapid-acting insulin (lispro, glulisine, or aspart insulin) begins to work in as little as 5 to 10 min and lasts

up to 4 h. Regular, or short-acting, insulin begins to work in 30 min and lasts up to 6 h. Intermediate-acting insulin begins to work 2 h after injection and lasts up to 18 h. An inhaled rapid-acting insulin powder (Afrezza) was approved by the U.S. Food and Drug Administration in 2014, and is classified as rapid acting because it peaks at 15 min and returns to baseline within 2.5 h. By comparison, regular subcutaneously injected insulin has onset within 30 min and peaks at 2.5 to 5 h.[14] There is also long-acting insulin (glargine or detemir) that has no peak of activity and will last up to 24 h, which allows the patient to have a basal level of insulin much like an individual without diabetes. With new types of insulin appearing nearly annually, patients with diabetes must discuss their individual needs and challenges with their physician.[14] The type of insulin used must be tailored to each person and is commonly based on eating habits, exercise schedule, and convenience. With many collegiate athletic departments hiring full-time registered dietitians, some college athletes have on-site counseling about the types of food necessary for sustained competition for their diabetes concerns and sport demands. Other physically active people can use the resources available through their physician or publicly accessible websites, such as the American Diabetes Association.

Patients with type 1 diabetes need to carry testing strips and a glucometer to measure their blood sugar levels (figure 15.2). They must also always carry their own insulin. The on-site health care provider must be thoroughly familiar with the type of insulin the patient uses, the regular schedule of injections and dosage used, and proper storage and disposal of insulin and needles. Insulin should never be stored in extreme heat, in direct sunlight, or in an area with high or low temperatures, such as a freezer or the glove compartment of a car. It is common for some sporting events to last an entire day and for athletes not to have access to proper nutrition. Athletic trainers must encourage their patients with diabetes to relay blood sugar levels to them daily and more often if the situation warrants it. It is also crucial to carry an emergency supply of appropriate food and glucagon for patients with diabetes in the event of an emergency.

Patients with type 1 diabetes must be aware of their blood sugar level before competition. Ideally, preparticipation blood sugar levels should range from 120 to 180 mg/dL. Participation is postponed for athletes with blood sugar above 200 mg/dL and ketones in their urine or if their blood sugar is over 300 mg/dL and supplemental insulin is administered. If the athlete's blood sugar level is less than 100 mg/dL, a preparticipation snack is administered.[23,25] Without insulin, skeletal muscle does not take up glucose and it will burn fat for energy, leading to ketoacidosis. Also, patients with diabetes cannot control the amount of circulating insulin in the blood, and the exercising muscle uses the insulin to take up the glucose, leading to hypoglycemia. To prevent hyperglycemia or

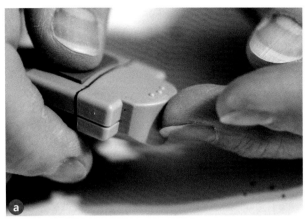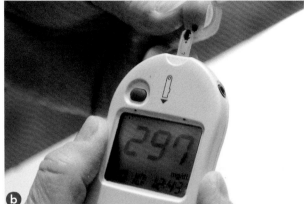

FIGURE 15.2 Using a glucometer, *(a)* the patient with diabetes pricks the distal side of their finger with a single-use needle and *(b)* places the resulting blood drop on a strip that inserts into the glucometer and registers the amount of glucose in the blood.

hypoglycemia, people who exercise should be familiar with their blood glucose concentrations and how they vary with different types of activity.[20,24,25]

There are many types of insulin on the market. Rapid, intermediate, and long-acting human insulin are all used to treat diabetes. Although all could be beneficial in the active population, the choice depends on the type, intensity, and duration of activity. Many people using insulin on a regular basis prefer to use continuous subcutaneous insulin infusion (CSII), also referred to as an *insulin pump*. CSII was introduced in the 1970s, and an estimated 450,000 adults use these devices today.[27] The pump is a pager-sized device that can be worn on a belt and is attached by a soft plastic catheter in the skin (see figure 3.6). CSIIs use subcutaneous sensors that measure interstitial glucose levels every 1 to 5 min, they send alarms to notify the wearer when glucose levels are at either end of the spectrum, and they can be monitored via a cell phone.[27] The pump can administer regular basal doses of insulin as well as insulin needed around mealtimes. There are also continuous glucose monitors (CGMs), which use similar technology, a catheter and pump. CGMs allow insulin to be given with the push of a button, and they omit the need for individual injections. They are no longer cumbersome, and advances in pump technology have provided pumps that can be worn even while swimming if placed in a waterproof pack. Although they are convenient, CGMs have some drawbacks. There is a lag time between measuring blood glucose levels with the pump and measuring with a fingertip stick, which can lead to overtreatment of hypoglycemia. CSIIs and CGMs should not be worn in contact sports because they can be damaged and they can also injure the athletes or their competitors.[28] A pump can be reconnected after the competition is over.[24] Should blood glucose fall below a specified level and the patient fails to deliver insulin, the pump will stop insulin delivery, which will prevent blood glucose falling even further. Although the pump is 69% smaller than other units, it is also more accurate than earlier sensors.[27]

Type 2 Diabetes Mellitus

The treatment for type 2 diabetes is based on increased physical activity and proper nutrition. These two factors help all patients with diabetes and, in the early stages, they may be the only treatment needed. If diet and exercise are not enough to control the patient's blood sugar levels, then medication is needed. Patients with type 2 diabetes have access to an array of oral medications that can help control blood sugar levels. Medications called **sulfonylureas** are a first-line treatment for type 2 diabetes, but they may cause hypoglycemia, especially in individuals who are more active. Sulfonylureas work by stimulating the beta cells of the pancreas to release insulin. Another class of agents is the **biguanides**, such as metformin, which decrease glucose production by the liver and reduce insulin resistance so glucose is absorbed by the muscles.[29] Patients with impaired renal function are at risk of lactic acidosis, a potentially deadly side effect, when they take metformin, and it is therefore not recommended for them. The thiazolidinediones increase insulin sensitivity in the muscle, liver, and adipose tissue, allowing for better deposition of glucose. If these measures fail, insulin therapy may be needed.[29]

Although type 2 DM is rare in competitive athletes, it occurs in obese adolescents in shocking numbers. Athletic trainers caring for middle school and high school athletes should be aware of the treatment options for diabetes. Athletic trainers should also be aware of risky behavior that may occur in athletes engaging in certain sports. Some sports emphasize being a certain body weight, and athletes may withhold insulin to decrease body weight rapidly to make their weight requirement; this can have deadly consequences.[28]

Thyroid Gland Disorders

The **thyroid gland** is an endocrine gland that lies anterior to the trachea in the neck and has an isthmus that joins two lateral lobes (figure 15.3). It is chiefly responsible for the synthesis of thyroxine (T_4) and triiodothyronine (T_3), reactions, which are stimulated by thyroid-stimulating hormone (TSH) from the anterior pituitary gland. The effects of thyroid hormones include protein synthesis in virtually every body tissue and increased oxygen consumption.

Assessment of the thyroid gland involves palpation of the gland along the anterior aspect of the neck (figure 15.4). Correct finger placement is on the gland from an anterior approach while palpating for symmetry, swelling, edema, or pain. The trachea may be displaced laterally by one thumb while the other thumb assesses the gland. Typically, adults will not have a palpable thyroid gland. Abnormalities include enlarged lobes, tenderness, or lumps.

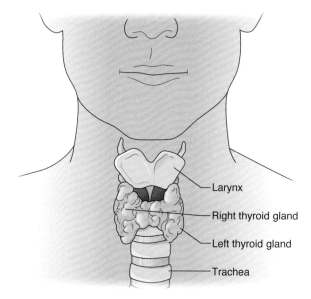

FIGURE 15.3   The thyroid gland.

Hyperthyroidism

Hyperthyroidism is characterized by a hypermetabolic state that is caused by excess production of thyroid hormones from the thyroid gland. It affects roughly 1 in 50 women and 1 in 500 men throughout their lifetimes, with a peak between ages 30 and 50 yr.[3]

Hyperthyroidism is often called **Graves' disease** because Graves' disease is the cause of nearly 90% of all hyperthyroid cases.[9] It is an autoimmune disorder characterized by a diffuse toxic **goiter**, or enlargement of the thyroid gland (figure 15.5). There is a familial predisposition to Graves' disease, but the exact etiology is unknown. It appears that an autoantibody forms and causes an imbalance in TSH production. Other causes of hyperthyroidism include toxic multinodular goiter, toxic thyroid **adenoma**, subacute thyroiditis with transient hyperthyroidism, and factitious hyperthyroidism.[30]

Signs and Symptoms

The signs and symptoms of hyperthyroidism are vast. Common symptoms include increased heart rate, heart palpitations, difficulty concentrating, shakiness, nervousness, gastrointestinal disturbances (excess gas, frequent normal bowel movements, or diarrhea), eyelid retraction, depression, menstrual irregularities, panic or anxiety attacks, weight loss despite a good appetite, and increased sweating.[9] Athletes can also present with fatigue and muscle weakness leading to impaired performance.

The physical findings of hyperthyroidism include brisk reflexes, tremor, anxiety, reddening of the palms, elevated heart rate, and occasionally an irregular heart rhythm, such as atrial fibrillation. Patients also usually have an enlarged or swollen thyroid gland. Because of swelling that accumulates behind the globe of the eye, patients may present with exophthalmos or a bulging out of the eyes (figure 15.6). Other eye symptoms include diplopia and blurred vision.[13]

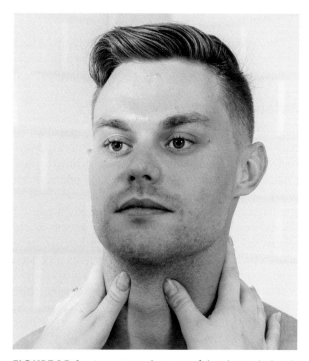

FIGURE 15.4   Anterior palpation of the thyroid gland. Note that the right thumb displaces the trachea while the left is palpating for tenderness, swelling, or asymmetry.

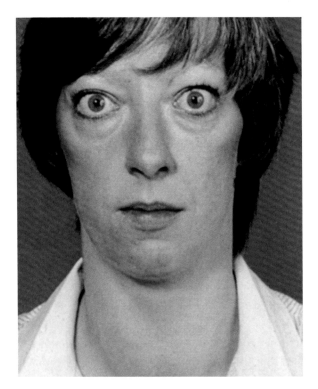

FIGURE 15.5 Hyperthyroidism is also called Graves' disease. Note the swelling in the thyroid region as well as the exophthalmos of the eyes.

Biophoto Associates / Science Source

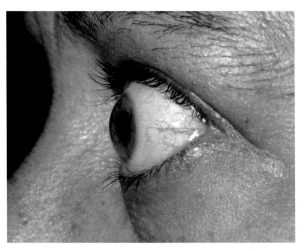

FIGURE 15.6 Exophthalmos associated with hyperthyroidism.

Dr P. Marazzi / Science Source

The differential diagnoses of hyperthyroidism include anxiety, DM, myasthenia gravis, premenopausal state, metastatic neoplasms, and pheochromocytoma.

Referral and Diagnostic Tests

Individuals who appear to have an enlarged thyroid gland, bulging eyes, and symptoms associated with hyperthyroidism are referred to a physician. Those with hyperthyroidism can be initially evaluated by their primary care physician and then referred to an endocrinologist who specializes in diseases of the thyroid if needed. A surgical referral may be needed if part of the treatment would require removal of the thyroid gland. A patient who presents with an acute exacerbation of thyroiditis may need to be admitted to the hospital for further management.

The diagnosis of hyperthyroidism is usually made based on a complete history, a physical examination, and a simple blood test to check the TSH level. If TSH is elevated, additional testing can be done, including a free T_3 index and a free T_4 index. These tests measure the thyroid hormone that is not bound to protein and is typically elevated in patients with hyperthyroidism. Because hyperthyroidism can be an autoimmune disorder,

the autoimmune status of the patient is assessed via the enzyme-linked immunosorbent assay test.[30]

Imaging studies also can be performed to help differentiate types of hyperthyroidism. The test used most often is a 24 h radioactive iodine uptake scan.[3,30] The radioactive iodine is taken up by the thyroid gland and has dissimilar appearances on the scan as a result of differences in uptake by healthy and diseased tissues, which helps determine the underlying cause of hyperthyroidism.

Treatment and Return to Participation

Treatment for hyperthyroidism centers on controlling the patient's symptoms and slowing the overactive thyroid gland. The three ways to manage the thyroid gland are medications, radioactive iodine, and thyroid surgery. To control symptoms, especially increased heart rate and tremors associated with hyperthyroidism, patients are typically given β-blockers, also commonly used to treat hypertension. These medications are used in the acute presentation and are usually withdrawn after definitive treatment of the overactive thyroid.[9] Those taking care of athletes must know that β-blockers are banned substances in several governing bodies for sports such as archery and shooting.

Other medications typically used to treat hyperthyroidism include propylthiouracil and methimazole. These medications inhibit the production of thyroid hormone. They are usually given for 6 to 24 mo and are typically used as adjunctive therapy before thyroid surgery or radioactive iodine treatment. While the patient is taking these medications, free T_3 and T_4 indexes are checked to determine how well these agents are working. Radioactive iodine ablation of the thyroid is common in the United

Thyroid Cancer

Although rare, thyroid cancer is rising in the United States. It is three times more prevalent in women than men and occurs most often in people in their 30s to 40s.[31,32] There are six different types of thyroid cancers, with papillary carcinomas representing 80% of all varietals, and exposure to radiation is the primary risk for this type. Thyroid cancer presents as a painless, palpable nodule and often found on an annual physical examination. It is diagnosed via ultrasound and fine-needle aspiration biopsy. As with other cancers, thyroid cancer is staged, and treatment options are based on the cancer stage (well-defined tumor versus metastasis). Long-term survival is 90% if caught and treated appropriately, but the patient will likely take lifelong medication if the cancer abrupted the hormone function of the thyroid.[32]

States, and it is an effective and safe treatment for patients who are not pregnant. A single dose of radioactive iodine returns roughly 80% of patients to a normal state.[30] Thyroid surgery is usually limited to those with very large goiters that may be causing obstruction, abnormal-appearing thyroid nodules, or pregnant females. It is rarely used in the United States because the other treatments are effective and, in general, have fewer adverse effects.

After successful treatment of hyperthyroidism, many people will need to take lifelong thyroid replacement therapy because the gland itself may be incapable of producing thyroid hormone. Patients with a history of treated hyperthyroidism must be checked annually with blood tests to determine the functional status of their thyroid. Return to full participation is generally not problematic.

Hypothyroidism

Hypothyroidism is a metabolic condition caused by thyroid hormone deficiency. It is more prevalent in women, has increased frequency with age, and has a genetic predisposition.[9,33]

Of the many causes of hypothyroidism, 95% are classified as primary hypothyroidism—that is, the origin of the problem involves the thyroid itself. The most common cause of primary hypothyroidism is an inflammatory disorder of the thyroid gland called Hashimoto's disease. Hashimoto's is the most frequent cause of goiter in the United States and is characterized by a lymphocytic infiltration of the thyroid gland.[33]

Another common cause of primary hypothyroidism is previous treatment for hyperthyroidism, such as radioactive iodine ablation or surgery to remove the thyroid. These treatments lead to intentional destruction of the thyroid gland; the patient then requires supplemental thyroid hormone replacement. In addition, medications such as lithium and interferon can cause hypothyroidism. The thyroid gland can be infiltrated by abnormal tissue caused by diseases, such as sarcoidosis and **amyloidosis**, which can then result in hypothyroidism.

Causes of secondary hypothyroidism include cancers of the pituitary or hypothalamus.

Signs and Symptoms

Hypothyroidism usually presents with signs and symptoms that develop over a prolonged period and represent a slowed metabolic state. The most common symptoms include weakness, fatigue, dry or coarse skin, cold intolerance, weight gain, and swelling of the tongue leading to thickened or slurred speech. Other symptoms include dry and coarse hair, hair loss, constipation, depression, vocal hoarseness, carpal tunnel syndrome, and memory impairment.[13,33]

Active patients, especially those involved in athletics, may prove difficult to diagnose in the early stages of hypothyroidism because of common muscle fatigue and overuse injuries that may be attributed to delayed-onset muscle soreness.

Physical findings in hypothyroidism are nonspecific and include bradycardia (slow heart rate), low blood pressure, hair loss (especially the outer third of the eyebrows), dry skin, and decreased reflexes.[33] The thyroid gland may feel enlarged on palpation.

The differential diagnoses for hypothyroidism are based primarily on the symptoms and include Addison's disease, depression, fibromyalgia, chronic fatigue syndrome, anemia, goiter, menopause, and viral infections such as infectious mononucleosis.[9]

Referral and Diagnostic Tests

A patient who has many musculoskeletal complaints, does not respond to typical treatments in the expected time frame, and experiences persistent, unexplained fatigue should be referred to a physician to rule out hypothyroidism.

Because of the vague symptoms of the initial stages of hypothyroidism, athletic trainers need to be suspicious of the possibility for this disease if no other plausible explanations exist. Evaluation for elevated TSH level is the first laboratory test for hypothyroidism. Determination of the free T_4 level can also help in the diagnosis and in differentiating between primary and secondary hypothyroidism.[33] There are no imaging studies to aid in the diagnosis of primary hypothyroidism, but evaluation of the pituitary gland by MRI or ultrasound is appropriate when a secondary cause is suspected.

Treatment and Return to Participation

When the diagnosis is made, treatment can start by replacing thyroid hormone with levothyroxine. The starting dose is based on the patient's weight, age, and other medical problems. The dose can then be titrated, as needed, with the goal of returning TSH levels to normal ranges. Blood samples to check TSH levels should be drawn every 4 to 6 wk to help with the titration. The medication is generally safe but needs to be monitored, especially in older adults and in those with heart conditions, because too much medication can elevate the heart rate and have deleterious effects on certain heart conditions.[33]

The prognosis for patients with primary hypothyroidism and their prospects for return to activity are excellent because symptoms of the disorder improve immensely, if not completely, with medication. Follow-up to ensure the proper dosage of levothyroxine is imperative. The prognosis for patients with secondary hypothyroidism depends on the underlying cause.

Summary

Conditions affecting the endocrine system can often present across body systems, but most can be treated if diagnosed early enough. Ensuring that the preparticipation physical examination contains questions related to changes in this system is one way to achieve early detection. Diagnosing diabetes is just the beginning of treatment, as patients must be carefully counseled and educated about the gravity of attending to their condition, especially in preseason and tournament activity. Being attentive to signs and symptoms affecting the endocrine system is key to early detection of any disorder.

Apply It! Go to HK*Propel* to complete the case studies for this chapter.

Dermatological Conditions

Dermatological conditions in active people are common and are a major reason that many athletes miss practice or competition. In a national survey of U.S. high school athletes from 2009 to 2014, nearly 500 dermatological conditions were reported. Wrestling accounted for 73.6% of infections, followed by football at 18%. Nearly 70% of the infections were bacterial (including impetigo and staphylococcal and streptococcal infections), and 28.4% were fungal (tinea).[1] Although most dermatological conditions originate from skin-to-skin contact and resultant transmission, some may involve respiratory or airborne transmission. Others may result from allergic reactions, cancer, or insect bites. The five main types of dermatological conditions are general, bacterial, viral, fungal, and parasitic. This chapter reviews pertinent anatomy and discusses signs and symptoms, referral and diagnostic tests, and treatment and criteria for return to participation for simple dermatological conditions.

Overview of Anatomy and Physiology

The skin, or integument, is the largest organ of the body and can be divided into three layers: the **epidermis**, the dermis, and the subcutaneous tissue or hypodermis (figure 16.1). The epidermis is composed of up to five layers from deep to superficial: stratum basale, stratum spinosum, stratum granulosum, stratum lucidum (found only in the soles of the feet and palms of the hands), and stratum corneum.

Each layer of the epidermis, except for the stratum basale, is composed of dead cells. The epidermis is the body's primary protective shield; it constantly forms new cells and sloughs off old ones, and it produces a protective pigment known as melanin. The dermis, which is composed of a papillary layer and a reticular layer, contains a variety of vascular and sensory structures,

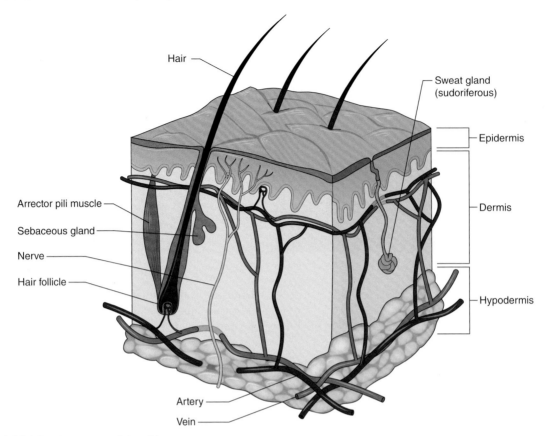

FIGURE 16.1   Anatomy of the skin.

hair follicles, nails, and sebaceous, sudoriferous, or sweat glands. Finally, the hypodermis is made up of connective tissue, which binds the dermis to the deeper structures, and adipose tissue, which provides insulation and cushioning. Together the epidermis, dermis, and hypodermis make up the integumentary system.

The integumentary system serves as the interface between the body and the external environment. This dynamic system serves as a barrier against invading organisms and outside influences such as ultraviolet (UV) radiation, toxic chemicals, thermal changes, and penetrating forces. At the same time, it allows people to sense and to adapt to the environment in terms of thermoregulation, fluid loss, proprioception and kinesthesis, force dissipation, synthesis of vitamin D, and cutaneous absorption of gases, UV light, and toxins. Finally, the skin plays an important role in human communication by helping people convey emotions through changes in skin color and texture and through facial expression.

Nails are made up largely of keratin and are found on the dorsal surfaces of all fingers and toes. The nail is a hard, clear surface that presents a pink color from the underlying highly vascular epithelial cell layer (figure 16.2). The lunula lies at the proximal end of all nails. It is a moon-shaped, white opaque layer that protects the nail matrix, which in turn produces new keratinized cells. The nail fold surrounds the lateral and proximal nail and hooks onto the nail bed. It is in this area that certain bacterial conditions arise.

Clinical Tips

Informed Consent

The health care provider should ask the patient for permission to touch them if contact is necessary to fully view the area.

Evaluation of the Skin

The goal of a skin examination by the health care provider is to identify, or attempt to identify, unknown skin lesions to determine the need for referral, need for treatment, or activity status (i.e., to allow participation or to withhold from participation), and to prevent transmission among athletes. New or previously undiagnosed lesions must be diagnosed and treated or, at minimum, carefully watched for changes. A history and a visual inspection can be very revealing; exactly how revealing depends on the patient's history, the quality of the visual inspection, and the patient's willingness to be truthful in either reporting or trying to hide a skin lesion. The athletic trainer should be suspicious of an athlete-patient wearing a wrap or a bandage that the athletic trainer did not apply. When asking the patient to disrobe for a skin inspection, all tape, wraps, and bandages should be removed. Wrestlers have been known to self-abrade (e.g., using sandpaper) or to apply caustic chemicals (e.g., bleach) to skin lesions to hide or remove the infection.

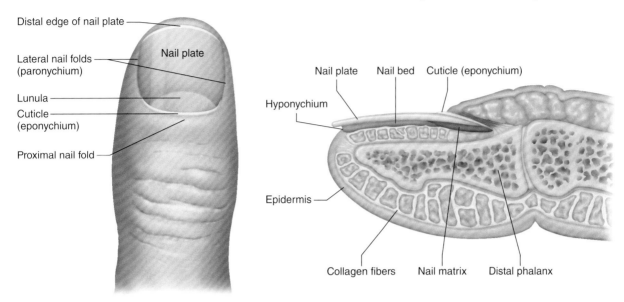

FIGURE 16.2 Anatomy of the nail.

When working with athletes whose sports put them in close skin-to-skin contact, such as wrestlers, a skin examination should be performed often enough to detect newly forming and potentially contagious lesions early enough to initiate treatment and to prevent transmission to others. Weekly skin examinations are considered the norm; however, when the possibility of an active outbreak exists, they should be performed often enough to detect new lesions immediately, thereby shortening the course of the outbreak among team or family members. For athletes, specific league rules may require that full-body skin examinations be performed at specified intervals; however, compliance with league rules should be viewed by the athletic trainer only as the minimal standard, especially when more frequent inspections are warranted.

A skin inspection should be conducted in a well-lit room that provides a private, respectful environment. For full-body examination, males should be wearing only shorts, while females should be wearing shorts and a sports bra or swimsuit top. Whenever possible, a health care provider of the same sex should conduct the examination. Begin the examination by obtaining a patient history. Ask if the patient has any skin problems to report and if they have felt ill or have nausea, fever, body aches, or fatigue. These symptoms may be especially indicative of viral or bacterial infections. The visual inspection is conducted with the patient standing erect, feet shoulder-width apart, arms abducted to 90°, and palms forward with hands open. Avoid touching the patient whenever possible; however, this may be unavoidable when examining specific body parts, especially the scalp. If contact is necessary, athletic trainers should wear gloves and should change them and disinfect their hands between patients to avoid cross-contamination. Begin a systematic inspection of the patient, including all aspects of the upper and lower extremities and the torso, including the axilla, neck, face, and scalp. The scalp is especially important because hair may conceal active infections. Patients should be able to adjust their neck and move their hair to facilitate the inspection, but the on-site health care provider may have to physically part the hair to visualize the scalp.

The athletic trainer should look for any abnormalities and should note specifically the pattern, color, and location of all lesions:

- *Pattern:* Does the lesion appear scratched, raised, depressed, or in groups or clusters, and is it bullous, moist, dry or crusted, or draining fluid?
- *Color:* What is the color of the lesion, the surrounding tissue, and the fluid or crust, and is the color uniform with well-defined borders and symmetry?
- *Location:* Is the lesion above or below the hairline on the scalp, on or near the genitals, or on or near the mouth?

The athletic trainer is usually the first clinician to evaluate a dermatological lesion on a patient. A **lesion** is synonymous with abnormal tissue. The key is to look for tissue abnormal to the surrounding area. A freckle is also one form of a lesion. Lesions are typically in the very early stages of development and can be difficult to differentiate without microscopic or laboratory testing. Because these types of diagnostic procedures are beyond the scope of many health care providers, the athletic trainer must use sound clinical judgment when determining the appropriate course of action for patients with dermatological conditions.

When referral to a medical doctor for evaluation and treatment is necessary, the health care provider must understand the patient's signs and symptoms and be able to effectively describe findings to the physician using dermatographical nomenclature. The terminology used to describe the appearance of a skin lesion or condition is very specific (figure 16.3). The athletic trainer must have the

Primary lesions: Caused by a condition or a disease

---Nonpalpable---

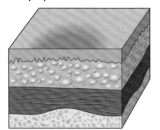

Type: Macule
Description: A flat area on the skin that is usually lighter or darker in color than the surrounding skin
Examples: Freckles, petechiae, vitiligo, café au lait spots

---Palpable and solid---

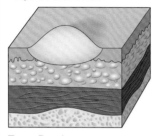

Type: Papule
Description: A small bump, palpable and circumscribed, and less than 5 mm in diameter; may be pigmented, erythematous, or flesh-toned
Examples: Elevated nevus (mole), prickly heat, psoriasis, melanoma

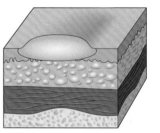

Type: Wheal
Description: A temporary elevation of the skin that itches, with a smooth surface, and is light pink to pale red in color; caused by acute inflammatory reaction in the skin; may appear, disappear, or change form abruptly within minutes or hours
Examples: Urticaria, anaphylaxis

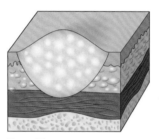

Type: Tumor
Description: A swelling or enlargement, any mass lesion; may be either malignant or benign
Examples: Lipoma, inflammatory reaction

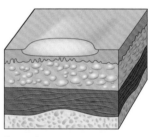

Type: Plaque
Description: A flat, raised patch on the skin or other tissue
Examples: Psoriasis, dental plaque

---Palpable and fluid-filled---

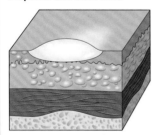

Type: Vesicle
Description: A small blister (up to 5 mm in diameter); filled with clear fluid
Examples: Herpes simplex (early stages), common blister

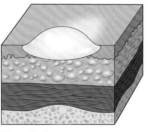

Type: Bulla
Description: A thin-walled, fluid-filled blister larger than 5 mm
Example: Impetigo

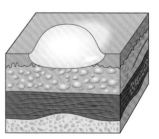

Type: Pustule
Description: An elevated, well-circumscribed lesion filled with white blood cells (WBCs) or bacteria
Examples: Acne vulgaris, herpes simplex, herpes zoster

> continued

FIGURE 16.3   Common skin lesions.

Secondary lesions: Caused by external forces

Damaged or diminished skin surface

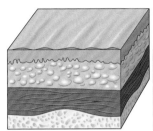 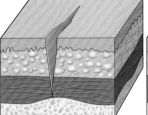 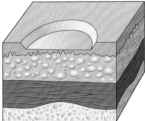 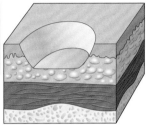

Type: Excoriation
Description: An abrasion of the outer layers of the skin due to scratching, rubbing, chemical irritant, burns, or trauma
Examples: Abrasion, scratched skin

Type: Fissure
Description: A cleft, groove, or split through all epidermal layers of skin
Example: Athlete's foot

Type: Erosion
Description: Loss of epidermis that does not extend into dermis
Example: Ruptured chicken pox vesicle

Type: Ulcer
Description: Loss of skin through the epidermis or mucous membranes; begins with inflammation and leads to necrosis and sloughing of damaged and dead tissue; healing results in scar formation; not unique to skin
Examples: Stasis ulcer, herpes simplex

Augmented or increased skin surface

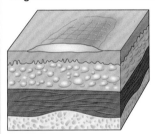 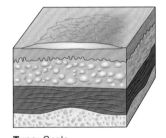 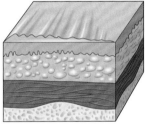

Type: Crust
Description: Dried plasma, serous exudates, blood, or debris on the surface of damaged or absent outer skin layers; fluid is often honey colored
Examples: Impetigo, eczema, seborrhea

Type: Scale
Description: Flakes or plates on the skin; may vary in size, thickness, and consistency
Examples: Psoriasis scale (compact and thick), pityriasis rosea scale (thin and small)

Type: Lichenification
Description: Epidermal thickening and roughening of the skin with increased visibility of skin surface furrows
Example: Chronic atopic dermatitis

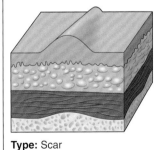 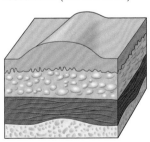

Type: Scar
Description: A permanent fibrotic change of tissue that forms to replace lost epidermal and dermal tissue
Examples: Surgical scar, acne scar

Type: Keloid
Description: An exaggerated response to tissue insult resulting in obvious, permanent, and raised scar tissue
Examples: Postsurgical scar, postacne scar

FIGURE 16.3   *> continued*

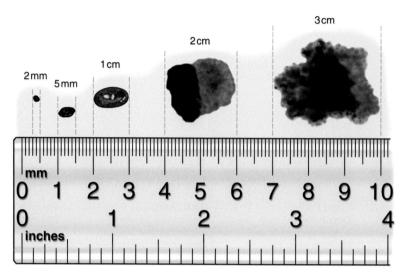

FIGURE 16.4 Comparison of lesion size.
© Katie Walsh Flanagan

knowledge and resources necessary to make these distinctions. It is much easier and more efficient to describe the lesion as a *fissure* rather than as a "linear loss of epidermis and dermis with sharp, defined borders." The clinician must also understand that these terms are important to the description and are not a specific diagnosis.

Dermatitis, for example, is an inflammation of the skin or dermal layers and can result from a variety of dermatological conditions with various causes. The term *dermatitis* merely indicates a general inflammation of the skin, whereas **contact dermatitis** indicates an inflammation of the skin caused by direct contact with a specific allergen, and **actinic dermatitis** indicates inflammation of the skin from exposure to sunlight or another irritating light source.

Another way to describe dermatological conditions is by referencing the area of skin affected. Most physicians use millimeters to describe the width or breadth of a condition, but centimeters are used for larger surface areas. As a point of reference, 1 in. is equal to 25.40 mm or 2.54 cm (figure 16.4).

Urticaria

Urticaria is a group of distinct skin conditions characterized by itchy, wheal-and-flare skin reactions, commonly known as *hives*. Urticaria is a common skin pathology. When histamine is released from mast cells, it produces a characteristic triple response: vasodilation causing local erythema, erythematous flare beyond the local erythema, and leakage of fluid causing local tissue edema (figure 16.5). Urticaria can occur with or without **angioedema** (subcutaneous or submucosal acute swelling), but up to 50% of patients present with both conditions.[2] Most cases are acute and can last up to a few weeks. The causes of urticaria are wide ranging and include the following:

allergies to foods (e.g., shellfish, nuts, and eggs), food additives (e.g., salicylates, dyes, and sulfites), or drugs (e.g., penicillin, aspirin, and sulfonamides); bacterial, viral, and fungal infections; and allergens, such as pollens, mold, and animal dander. Internal disease, physical stimuli (e.g., dermatographism, exercise, cholinergic agents, cold, and sun), skin diseases, hormones that occur during pregnancy, and genetic predisposition can also trigger urticaria. The underlying cause of acute urticaria cannot be determined in about 50% of cases.[2] A rarer variety of the condition is chronic urticaria, which arises from chronic infection, intolerance to food additives, or autoreactivity. A typical hive is an intensely itchy erythematous or white edematous area. A discussion of general urticaria and specific conditions follows.

RED FLAGS FOR ANAPHYLACTIC SHOCK

General urticaria may also indicate anaphylactic shock. Any patient with the following signs or symptoms should be referred to a medical facility immediately:

- Facial edema
- Swollen tongue
- Respiratory distress
- Stridor
- Difficulty talking
- Difficulty swallowing
- Hoarseness
- Hypotension
- Syncope or near syncope

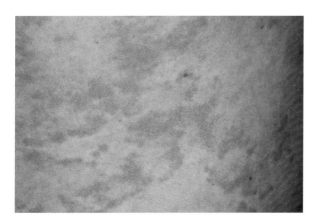

FIGURE 16.5   Urticaria, seen here in various stages of formation, is a local erythemic reaction to exercise, temperature changes, drugs, or allergies.

The Division of Dermatology at Brody School of Medicine, East Carolina University

Signs and Symptoms

General urticaria may develop at any age and is extremely common. The characteristic appearance described previously is easy to diagnose, and most cases are self-limiting, lasting from a few hours to a few weeks. The lesions are usually very itchy, or **pruritic**, but the intensity may vary. Also, the size may range from small, 2 mm lesions, to very large areas. They last 20 min to 3 h and can disappear and reappear in other areas.[2] This pattern repeats itself for up to 48 h.

Referral and Diagnostic Tests

Referral to a physician is appropriate if symptoms persist for an extended period and if they interfere with daily activities. Immediate referral to a medical facility is necessary if a patient shows signs or symptoms of **anaphylactic shock**. Diagnostic testing to determine the exact cause of urticaria can be highly expensive and ongoing, commonly with no resolution.

Treatment and Return to Participation

The most effective treatment for urticaria is to determine and eliminate the cause or allergen, but this is often extremely difficult. Most patients will need an oral nonsedating antihistamine, such as loratadine (Claritin) or fexofenadine (Allegra), because the sedating antihistamines may impair performance. Another popular antihistamine commonly used for urticaria is cetirizine (Zyrtec). Although cetirizine has mild sedative properties, they are not as severe as the sedating antihistamines. If the aforementioned antihistamines are unsuccessful, short-term use of glucocorticoids (steroids) has been

effective.[3] In emergencies in which the patient's airway is compromised, epinephrine (EpiPen) injection prescribed for that patient may be warranted (see chapter 3). Most cases resolve spontaneously and have a good prognosis. The patient may return to participation once stable and comfortable. The best prevention for most urticarial conditions is to determine and eliminate the cause or allergen if possible.

Dermatographism

Dermatographism is one form of urticaria induced by rubbing or stroking the skin or by rubbing of the skin with clothing. The exact cause is unknown, but recent infections or medications appear to be the most common cause. The hives develop within 1 to 3 min of stroking the skin and resolve in 30 to 60 min. Patients with dermatographism will experience periods of reactivity during their lifetime, but this condition is more common in younger adults.[4]

Signs and Symptoms

Dermatographism presents with blanching and associated linear edema and erythema (figure 16.6). The condition can occur on any part of the body because it does not matter if the skin is covered by clothing or equipment. However, friction caused by clothing or equipment may induce a dermatographical reaction.

Referral and Diagnostic Tests

If a patient presents with signs of dermatographism, referral may be warranted when the reaction is either severe or prolonged. The common test for this condition is to use a tongue blade to draw a line on the area to see the response. Any raised or discolored reaction is considered

Clinical Tips

Sedating Antihistamines

The following antihistamines have a sedating effect that may be counterproductive to athletic participation:

- Diphenhydramine (Benadryl)
- Hydroxyzine (Atarax)
- Dimenhydrinate (Dramamine)
- Promethazine (Phenergan)
- Brompheniramine (Dimetapp Allergy)
- Chlorpheniramine (Chlor-Trimeton)
- Clemastine (Tavist)
- Cyproheptadine (Periactin)

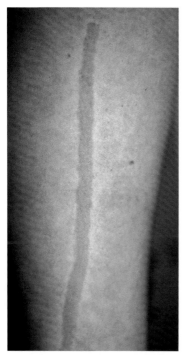

FIGURE 16.6   Drawing on the skin provided this reaction in a patient with dermatographism.

The Division of Dermatology at Brody School of Medicine, East Carolina University

positive for dermatographism. No other diagnostic tests are needed.

Treatment and Return to Participation

Treatment ranges from conservative use of topical agents to use of oral antihistamines as described for general urticaria. As with urticaria, dermatographism is not infectious or contagious. The prognosis is excellent, and participation in activities and sports is not restricted. If the allergen is associated with the uniform or equipment needed to participate, it would be wise to alter the allergen within safety rules to prevent recurrence. Another means of preventing dermatographism is to wear a barrier between the allergen and the skin.

Cholinergic Urticaria

Cholinergic urticaria is caused by a physical stimulus. It was once thought to be triggered by heat, but the irritant is actually sweat.[5] Cholinergic urticaria usually develops in younger patients between ages 10 and 30 yr and typically resolves within 30 to 90 min. Ninety-six percent of patients diagnosed with cholinergic urticaria are male.[5] This reaction consists of hives 1 to 4 mm in size with surrounding erythema, occurring during or

shortly after the patient experiences exposure to heat or overheating of the body during exercise or stress. In addition to exercise, other inducers are hot food, emotional distress, and exposure to hot water or a hot tub or sauna.[6] This reaction typically occurs within 2 to 20 min of exposure but may be delayed for up to 1 h. Signs and symptoms are induced by the parasympathetic nervous system release of acetylcholine and may last up to 3 h.[3]

Signs and Symptoms

Symptoms of cholinergic urticaria include itching, burning, tingling, warmth, or irritation of the skin that appears following any event that raises the core temperature or elicits sweating. Cholinergic urticaria can occur anywhere on the body. Systemic symptoms of wheezing, angioedema, or hypotension may also occur. Patients with this disorder have a higher core temperature than normal.

Referral and Diagnostic Tests

The athletic trainer refers the patient with symptoms of cholinergic urticaria to a physician for definitive diagnosis, which is typically made by history and clinical examination. The patient may also exercise in place or on a stationary bicycle for about 10 to 15 min while being observed for 1 h for the development of hives. This exercise will help establish the diagnosis and is done only under the supervision of a physician at a medical facility.

Treatment and Return to Participation

Treatment consists of limiting strenuous exercise, stressful environments, and hot showers. Antihistamines may help before exercise, but most often a strong sedating antihistamine is needed. Rapid cooling upon the first signs or symptoms of cholinergic urticaria has also been effective in slowing hive progression.[5] The athlete may also shower with hot water to induce a reaction, deplete the histamine stores, and begin a refractory period of about 24 h. Athletes known to be reactive should always exercise with someone else in case exercise anaphylaxis occurs.

Only a few cases of cholinergic urticaria spontaneously resolve because most of these patients will have persistent symptoms. Return to participation depends on the development of any additional symptoms, especially exercise-induced anaphylaxis.

Cold Urticaria

Cold urticaria is a reactive disorder that manifests as hives after exposure to cold. It is the most common form of physical urticaria.[3] Cold urticaria can occur often in athletes because ice baths and ice therapy are a common treatment modality. There are two forms of cold urticaria: acquired and hereditary. The former occurs after exposure to cold, with hives appearing rapidly. Hereditary cold urticaria has a slower onset, with reactions appearing up to 24 to 48 h after exposure.[5] Likewise, symptoms last longer, up to 48 h, with hereditary cold urticaria.

Signs and Symptoms

A patient with cold urticaria usually develops hives within 5 min of exposure to ice, cold water, or a sudden drop in air temperature. These lesions may last 1 to 2 h after removal of the stimulus. Systemic symptoms of generalized urticaria, angioedema, or anaphylaxis may also develop. Urticarial vasculitis, cholinergic urticaria, Raynaud's phenomenon, and dermatographism are all differential diagnoses for cold urticaria.

Referral and Diagnostic Tests

The athletic trainer refers any patients with extreme reactions to cold to a physician for definitive diagnosis and evaluation for other systemic symptoms. Diagnosis is made in the physician's office by applying ice to the skin for 1 to 5 min or by exposing the forearm to cold water (0-8 °C [32-46 °F]) for 5 to 15 min and monitoring for hives (figure 16.7). This is recommended only under the supervision of a physician in a medical facility because systemic symptoms and anaphylaxis may develop.[7]

Treatment and Return to Participation

Treatment and prevention of cold urticaria consist of avoiding sudden decreases in temperature and reducing or avoiding exposure to cold water or ice. The antihistamine cyproheptadine and the tricyclic antidepressant

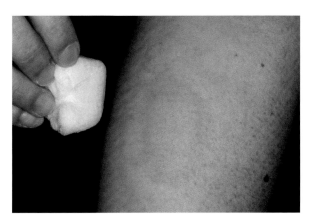

FIGURE 16.7 Cold urticaria hive reaction.

The Division of Dermatology at Brody School of Medicine, East Carolina University

doxepin have been shown to help suppress this reaction. Symptoms in most patients will resolve spontaneously. For those using cryotherapy to reduce the pain and inflammation of an injury, placing a barrier between the ice and the skin can help ameliorate symptoms of cold urticaria. Return to participation depends on the development of any other symptoms, such as angioedema, general urticaria, or anaphylaxis. If the reaction is local, the patient may return to participation if no other symptoms have developed within the next 1 to 2 h. If generalized symptoms develop, return to participation should be determined by a physician.[7]

Solar Urticaria

Solar urticaria is manifested by hives that occur within minutes of exposure to UV light and resolve within 1 to 3 h.[8]

Signs and Symptoms

The obvious sign of solar urticaria is the sudden onset of hives precipitated by exposure to UV light. Systemic reactions such as syncope have occurred but are rare. Syncope typically occurs in adults ages 20 to 40 yr and slightly more commonly in females shortly after sun exposure.[8]

Referral and Diagnostic Tests

The diagnosis of solar urticaria is based on the obvious hive or wheal formation and quick resolution. Further diagnostic testing includes phototesting and UV sleeve testing. UV sleeve testing exposes a section of skin to a given amount of UV light. The reaction determines whether the patient is reactive to that range of UV light. Polymorphous light eruption, sunburn, and photoallergic drug reaction are the differential diagnoses for solar urticaria.

Treatment and Return to Participation

Treatment consists of antihistamines, liberal use of sunscreen, hats and long-sleeved clothing, and graded exposure to UV light. Prognosis is unknown, but immediate return to play is reasonable if no systemic symptoms, such as angioedema, syncope, or anaphylaxis, have occurred.[8] A return to outdoor activity should include the use of appropriate sunscreens.

Prevention

Prevention of solar urticaria consists of decreasing the amount of sun-exposed skin, using sunscreen, and wearing long sleeves, pants, and hats when possible. Most sunscreen agents absorb the ultraviolet B (UVB) radiation (290-320 nm) responsible for the development of hives; however, sunscreens that contain avobenzone (also known as Parsol 1789) will absorb UVA I and UVA II wavelengths (340-400 nm and 320-340 nm, respectively), and sunscreens containing menthyl anthranilate and oxybenzone will absorb UVA II wavelengths.[9] All of these wavelengths are linked to hives and other skin injuries related to sun exposure.[3]

Epidermoid Cysts

Epidermoid cysts, also known as sebaceous, epidermal, or **keratinous cysts**, are very common from youth to middle age. These cysts may occur anywhere on the body, but the most common sites are the face, scalp, neck, and trunk.[10] Because they are all epidermoid tissue, the term *epidermoid cyst* is favored over *sebaceous cyst*, which indicates the cyst is only sebaceous in nature. Recall that the term *sebaceous* is related to sebum (oil in the skin), which is secreted near sweat (sudoriferous) glands. Epidermoid cysts have a thin wall filled with a white keratin material produced by the epithelium. One of the more common epidermal cysts is the **pilonidal cyst** that can form in the sacrococcygeal area of the lower back. Epidermoid cysts are slow growing, movable, and nontender (figure 16.8).

Signs and Symptoms

Cysts range in size from a few millimeters to several centimeters. They are usually soft, round, flesh-colored, mobile, and smooth and have some communication with the surface. Some originate from **comedones**, and these are usually found on the back. The cyst wall may rupture, and the keratin creates an inflammatory reaction within the dermis. They can become inflamed or infected; if they do, they become painful. Epidermoid cysts may reabsorb or recur. They do not itch or cause a localized increase in temperature. The differential diagnoses for **sebaceous cysts** include abscess, acne, boil, ganglion, and skin tumor.

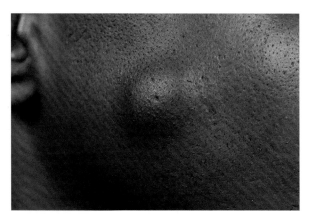

FIGURE 16.8   Sebaceous cyst.
Girand / Science Source

Referral and Diagnostic Tests

The athletic trainer refers to a physician any athlete with skin swelling contained within a specific area or a cyst that does not diminish in size or is problematic because of its location. No specific diagnostic tests are needed, but referral is necessary so that the physician can incise and drain the cyst.

Treatment and Return to Participation

Asymptomatic cysts require no treatment. Symptomatic cysts may be treated by injecting them with triamcinolone or using oral antibiotics.[10] Should surgical intervention be required, a physician may incise and drain the cyst, although some require excision. The physician opens the cyst with a No. 11 blade, and the keratin material is expressed through the opening. A No. 1 curette is then used to remove the remaining excess material, and the wall is removed by either expressing the cyst edges or grasping the wall with small forceps. Infected cysts may require placement of a gauze drain after excision; the drain remains in place for 7 to 10 d. An oral antibiotic regimen may also be prescribed.[11-13]

CONDITION HIGHLIGHT

Pilonidal Cysts

Pilonidal cysts are located distal to the coccyx, are more common in men than women, and tend to occur during the late teen years to early 20s.[11] The theory is that hair follicles can break off during normal sitting and bending and create a pit that becomes inflamed. Unless it drains naturally, the cavity forms an abscess and becomes infected. The patient presents with a swollen, painful lesion 4 to 5 cm posterior to the anal opening. There may be drainage.[11] As with other epidermoid cysts, a furuncle or carbuncle is a differential diagnosis. It is not uncommon for a pilonidal cyst to reoccur. Both referral and treatment are in line with other epidermoid cysts, as discussed.

Epidermoid cysts often recur. Sport participation is not restricted other than to prevent secondary infection.

Dermatitis

The term *dermatitis* is used loosely. Dermatitis means inflammation of the skin, and the large variety of causes is beyond the scope of this chapter. This chapter discusses two conditions: eczema and psoriasis.

Eczema and Atopic Dermatitis

The term *eczema* is often used synonymously with *dermatitis* and is the most common inflammatory skin disease. Whereas eczema itself often indicates vesicular dermatitis, some refer to it as *atopic dermatitis*.[14] Atopic dermatitis is a dermatological reaction caused by environmental and genetic factors.[6] It is the most common inflammatory skin condition in children. There are both intrinsic and extrinsic causes of atopic dermatitis. Whereas the intrinsic form is not well understood, the extrinsic causes include allergic reactions to food and airborne allergens (e.g., mold, dander). Atopic dermatitis has been thought to be an immunological disturbance resulting in immunoglobulin E (IgE) sensitization.[14] IgE is responsible for the release and production of many inflammatory substances, and it can cause over- or underproduction of reactionary enzymes that manifest in atopic dermatitis and other inflammatory responses. Atopic dermatitis has shown genetic tendencies.[3,6] It affects an estimated 17% of the pediatric population in the United States.[14] If left alone, most eczematous lesions will resolve, but patients are rarely able to avoid scratching.

Signs and Symptoms

Eczema consists of three stages: acute, subacute, and chronic. More often, the acute and subacute stages are seen in infants and young children, and the chronic presentation is found in adults. The acute stage consists of a red swollen plaque with small vesicles. These lesions are very itchy, appear within days after exposure, and last for days to weeks. The subacute stage consists of erythema and scales of various degrees, which may also itch. The chronic stage consists of thickened skin with increased skin markings and moderate to intense itching.[14]

Differential diagnoses include contact irritants (e.g., poison ivy), topical medicines (including neomycin), fungal infections, nutritional deficiencies, **dyshidrosis**, scabies, and habitual scratching. Other conditions to consider are herpes simplex virus (HSV), psoriasis, systemic lupus erythematosus (SLE), or discoid lupus erythematosus.[3]

Referral and Diagnostic Tests

Referral to a physician is warranted for a patient exhibiting increasing or persistent symptoms consistent with eczema. Patch testing may be useful to determine specific allergens. This testing involves covering the skin with various patches of allergens for 1 to 2 d to determine which ones cause an allergic response.[15]

Treatment and Return to Participation

The most important treatment for eczema is removal from the allergen if possible. Because one of the consequences of atopic dermatitis is extremely dry skin, proper skin care is paramount. Patients must be counseled to bathe properly with mild soap (e.g., Dove) and to dry their skin and immediately apply emollient skin lotion.[14] Topical steroids are appropriate for up to 2 wk following an acute onset. Antihistamines may be used to reduce itching, and antibiotics should be started if there are signs of infection. Systemic steroids may be needed to control the inflammation, but their use is controversial.[14]

The prognosis of eczema depends on the severity of the reaction. Unless the reaction is severe or a significant infection has developed, the patient may return to participation without restriction.

Psoriasis

Psoriasis is a genetic, chronic, and recurring disorder that often begins during childhood. It is a benign but lifelong condition with remissions and execrations, and it can be resistant to treatment.[16] Psoriasis is a scaling, papular infection similar to eczema but without the epithelial eruptions, wet areas, and crusts. It is a hyperproliferation of *keratinocytes*, which form the tough outer protective layer of the skin, and affects an estimated 2.2% of the U.S. population.[16] Psoriasis is more common in Caucasians, and the average age of onset is 28 yr. It is believed to be associated with the immune system, and it can be triggered by trauma, infections, or certain medications.[6] Psoriasis has a gradual onset and usually has chronic remission and recurrence rates that vary in frequency and duration, but permanent remissions are rare. There are over a dozen types of psoriasis that affect the nails, joints (psoriatic arthritis), scalp, and eyes. The most common form is plaque psoriasis, simply called *psoriasis*.

Approximately 10% to 30% of patients with psoriasis also experience psoriatic arthritis.[16,17] The exacerbation–remission cycle common to this skin disorder may coincide with the arthritic component. Most often, the distal interphalangeal joints of the fingers and toes are affected. Compared to rheumatoid arthritis (RA), psoriatic arthritis tends to enter remission more often and more rapidly than RA, and it lacks the typical joint nodules associated with RA. Psoriatic arthritis may progress to chronic, disabling arthritis, so complaints of joint pain in patients with psoriasis must not be overlooked.[17]

Signs and Symptoms

The distinctive lesion of psoriasis is a silvery white plaque with surrounding erythema with distinct borders (figure 16.9). The lesions usually begin as small, red, scaly papules that coalesce into round or oval plaques except in the skin folds, where they appear as deep red, macerated plaques. These lesions are most common on the extensor surfaces, such as the elbows and knees, but they are also very common on the scalp, fingernails, toenails, gluteal clefts, and previous sites of trauma. Psoriasis can also present with pain and itching at the site.

Forms of psoriasis may develop other than the general chronic plaque type just described. Another common form is scalp psoriasis. The scalp, which may be the only site affected, has a thick, erythematous, silvery scale in multiple areas. This lesion may extend onto the forehead. Psoriasis of the nails is another type and is demonstrated by pitting of the nails.

Other differential diagnoses for psoriasis are as follows: streptococcal infections, pityriasis rosea, SLE, seborrheic dermatitis, RA, squamous cell carcinoma (SCC), secondary syphilis, candidiasis, pancreatic tumors, or drug eruptions generally caused by β-blockers, gold, or methyldopa.[16]

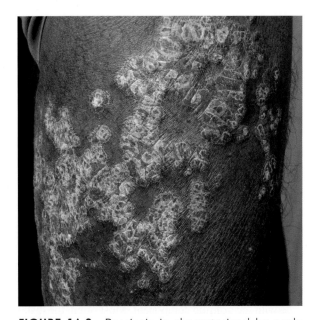

FIGURE 16.9 Psoriasis is characterized by scaly erythematous patches with silvery scales on the top.

Science Photo Library / Science Source

Referral and Diagnostic Tests

Any person suspected of having psoriasis is referred to a physician for medical evaluation and initiation of treatment. The clearly defined, dry, silvery scales are quite distinguishable and unique to psoriasis. Although diagnosis is rarely difficult, testing includes a complete blood count, including erythrocyte sedimentation rate, and a *Streptococcus* screening. Testing for rheumatoid factor is indicated if psoriatic arthritis is suspected. On occasion, biopsy of the lesion may be necessary to confirm the diagnosis and rule out other disorders.[16]

Treatment and Return to Participation

Treatment for psoriasis is complicated and involves many options, from systemic to topical medications, stress reduction, phototherapy, and changing climate.[16] The American Academy of Dermatology put forth treatment recommendations that therapy be tailored for each patient. Multiple medications are approved by the U.S. Food and Drug Administration (FDA) for psoriasis treatment. The physician must clearly inform the patient of possible contraindications to and side effects of the treatment. Therapy should be tailored to the patient's level of discomfort and inability to perform activities of daily living. Pharmaceutical treatment includes methotrexate for as long as tolerated and cyclosporine intermittently.[18] First-line treatment options are topical steroids, such as calcipotriol (Dovonex), anthralin ointment, and targeted UV light. Exposure to sun, sea bathing, and combination therapy with vitamin D have been successfully prescribed. Lubricating creams, including hydrogenated vegetable oil, white petrolatum, and crude coal tar, combined with exposure to UV light (280-320 nm) have been effective.[6] Oral steroids are contraindicated because of their side effects, which include severe exacerbations of psoriasis.

The prognosis for psoriasis is determined by the extent of the disease and whether the arthritic component is present. Traditionally, more severe attacks coincide with an earlier disease onset. Return to activity depends on whether arthritis is involved and on the degree of debilitation. Most likely the patient will have no restrictions, but close follow-up is recommended to prevent flare-ups.

Environmentally Induced Dermatological Conditions

Skin Cancer

The inclusion of skin cancer in this chapter is not intended to provide definitive diagnosis but to encourage athletic trainers to recognize suspicious lesions and make timely referrals for treatment. Two types of skin cancer are discussed: nonmelanoma and melanoma. Each has subcategories based on the tissue invaded.

Nonmelanoma Skin Cancers

Nonmelanoma skin cancer (NMSC) is the most common skin cancer in humans worldwide. NMSC can be classified into two categories depending on which type of cell is affected: basal cell carcinoma (BCC) or SCC. Both arise from keratinocytes. BCCs comprise 80% of NMSCs, whereas SCCs comprise 20%.[19,20] Together, approximately 5.4 million new cases of BCCs and SCCs are diagnosed each year in the United States. Because of the rising incidence of this largely preventable form of cancer, the National Collegiate Athletics Association (NCAA) issued a sports medicine guideline in 2012 that addresses safety from sun exposure.[21,22]

Whereas BCCs rarely metastasize and are infrequently fatal, SCCs may lead to significant mortality if left untreated. **Actinic keratoses** are precursors to SCC and are the most frequently treated lesions in humans. Actinic keratoses are typically characterized as being "precan-cers" or premalignant because of the presence of atypical keratinocytes confined to the epidermis. They are rough patches of skin that appear on sun-exposed surfaces. Treatments of actinic keratoses include topical creams, photodynamic therapy, chemical peel, and laser surgery.

An estimated 3 million new cases of NMSC are diagnosed each year in the United States.[19] The number of skin cancer cases in the United States has surpassed the number of cases of all other cancers combined. Since 1987, the incidence of BCC has increased by 145%, and diagnosed SCC rose 263% in the same period. Approximately one in five Americans will develop skin cancer during their lifetime; more than 95% of these cases will be NMSC.[19,20]

The most significant risk factor for developing NMSC appears to be a fair complexion, blonde or red hair, and light eyes.[19] Other risk factors include environmental exposures, such as chronic or intermittent sun exposure, tanning bed use, radiation therapy, and smoking. The effects of sun exposure cannot be overstated. In a consensus report, the European Academy of Dermatology and Venereology found that the occupational risk of

CONDITION HIGHLIGHT

Predisposition for Melanoma

- *Moles:* A mole is a benign skin tumor. Certain types of moles increase a person's chance of getting melanoma. People with many moles and those who have some large moles have an increased risk of melanoma.

- *Fair skin:* People with fair skin, freckling, light hair, or blue eyes have a higher risk of melanoma, but anyone can get melanoma.

- *Congenital melanocytic nevi:* People with moles present at birth have a higher risk of melanoma.

- *Personal or family history:* Approximately 10% of people with melanoma have a close relative (e.g., mother, father, brother, sister, child) with the disease. A strong family history of breast and ovarian cancer could mean that certain gene changes or mutations are present. Men with this gene change have a higher risk of melanoma.

- *Immune suppression:* People who have been treated with medicines that suppress the immune system, such as transplant recipients, have an increased risk of developing melanoma.

- *Ultraviolet radiation:* Too much exposure to UV radiation is a risk factor for melanoma. The main source of such radiation is sunlight. Tanning lamps and booths are other sources.

- *Age:* About one-half of melanomas occur in people older than age 50 yr, but younger people are also susceptible.

- *Sex:* Men have a higher rate of melanoma than women.

- *Xeroderma pigmentosum:* People with this rare, inherited condition are less able to repair damage caused by sunlight and are at greater risk of melanoma.

- *Past history of melanoma:* A person who has already had melanoma has a higher risk of getting another melanoma.

Adapted from American Cancer Society (2022); "Melanoma Skin Cancer Causes, Risk Factors, and Prevention," American Cancer Society, last modified August 14, 2019, https://www.cancer.org/content/dam/CRC/PDF/Public/8824.00.pdf.

Skin Terms

Recall that the squamous cells comprise the middle layers of the epidermis; they continuously shed to give way to new cells. Deeper than that is the basal cell layer of epidermis that lies closest to the dermis (then the adipose layer). Basal cells also move up and change over time, becoming squamous cells. The basal layer produces melanocytes that give skin its pigment. Melanoma occurs when the melanocytes become cancerous.

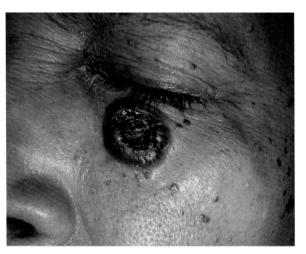

FIGURE 16.10 Nodular basal cell carcinoma.
Rasika Pereira/Medical Images

developing BCC was 43% higher for outdoor workers than for their counterparts working indoors. SCC carried double the risk to the outdoor workers.[23] In addition, a history of immunosuppression, scars, ulcers, or burns will also increase the chances of developing NMSC. Unlike melanoma, there is no genetic predisposition to NMSC.[24]

Basal Cell Carcinoma

BCC is the most common skin malignancy and occurs twice as often in males as in females. The incidence of BCC increases with age, and it is nearly 100-fold higher in those age 55 to 79 yr than those age 35 yr or younger.[24] It is the least likely cancer to metastasize to other areas.

There are many types of BCC. The most commonly occurring types are as follows:

- Nodular BCC
- Superficial BCC
- Pigmented BCC
- Morpheaform BCC

The first two are discussed next.

Nodular BCC is the classic and most common type, comprising 50% to 54% of all BCCs. It typically presents as a pearly, translucent pink papule with central telangiectasias on the head and neck regions, with a predilection for the nose (25%-30%).[24] A central ulceration with bleeding, crusting, and rolled borders may develop in this tumor (figure 16.10), and it usually remains asymptomatic and rarely metastasizes. The nodular BCC may be mistaken for a benign nevus (plural, nevi) or an acneiform lesion.

Superficial BCC comprises 9% to 11% of all BCCs and usually is found in patients younger than those who have nodular BCC. This type presents as an asymptomatic, erythematous, scaly plaque that enlarges very slowly and typically occurs on the trunk or extremities. Superficial BCC may grow to be as large as 15 cm in diameter without ulceration or bleeding. It may be mistaken for psoriasis or a SCC in situ.

Squamous Cell Carcinoma

The incidence of SCC has risen over the last several decades at a rate of 3% to 10% per year, with more than 500,000 cases diagnosed yearly in the United States. SCC is associated with higher mortality in Caucasians, older adults, and males.[25] Classic invasive SCC is discussed next.

Classic Invasive Squamous Cell Carcinoma

SCC occurs on the mucous membranes as well as on sun-exposed skin. SCCs generally arise from actinic keratoses, which are considered premalignant precursors. Actinic keratosis presents as an erythematous crusted papule on sun-damaged skin. It is often recognized more easily by touch as a rough or sharp area felt on the skin rather than by sight (figure 16.11). The presence of an actinic keratosis indicates that skin has been sun-damaged and skin cancer may develop. The most common sites of occurrence include the head and neck, dorsal hands, lower lip, and genitalia. SCC commonly develops as a hyperkeratotic erythematous nodule or plaque on sun-damaged skin. Sites with a higher associated risk of metastases include the lip and ear as well as sites with scarring or inflammation.

Signs and Symptoms

Patients presenting with possible basal cell cancer must have a lesion with a pearly appearance. Often there is a central depression or ulceration and perhaps crusting or bleeding from the lesion.[24] The skin texture feels rough over the lesion. There may be scaling or crusting.[26] Lesions are different from surrounding skin, are slow growing, and occur on areas most often exposed to the sun (e.g., nose, lips, ears, hands, forearms).

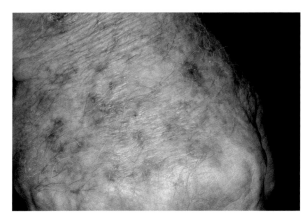

FIGURE 16.11 Actinic keratoses are often precursors of cancer. Because they are recurring rough patches of skin, they are discovered more often by feel than by sight.

The Division of Dermatology at Brody School of Medicine, East Carolina University

Referral and Diagnostic Tests

Patients with lesions that are unusual are referred to a dermatologist. Suspicious lesions are biopsied and staged.

Treatment and Return to Participation

Although the standard treatment of NMSC is surgical excision, cryosurgery or electrodesiccation and curettage are acceptable treatment options for appropriately selected tumors. Mohs micrographic surgery offers the highest cure rate for those at high risk.[27] Mohs surgery is best for NMSCs that are recurrent, exhibit an aggressive histology, are larger than usual (>2 cm), or are located at sites that require tissue conservation. Mohs surgery is an office procedure in which the physician cuts around the tumor with a small scalpel, using local anesthesia, and evaluates the margins of the tumor to be certain there are no remaining cancer cells. Other treatment modalities include radiation therapy, photodynamic therapy, laser ablation, topical chemotherapy (typically 5-fluorouracil or imiquimod), and systemic retinoid therapy.

Suspect but not confirmed lesions are often treated by a regimen of topical chemotherapy, followed by photodynamic therapy. The purpose of this treatment is to remove the most superficial layers of the skin, most likely taking with it the damaged, possibly precancerous aspects of it. The topical cream is applied to lesions and reacts to nontypical cells. During the treatment period (typically 1-2 wk), patients are cautioned to remain out of the sun because the chemotherapy reacts to sunlight. Patients will report a gradual reddening of the skin, followed by possible open sores resembling fever blisters. The subsequent photodynamic therapy reacts to the topical cream;

although this treatment lasts only up to 30 min, the burn effect of the light continues for 24 to 48 h. During this time, the patient will report deepening reddening of the skin, tightness, and eventually peeling. It is imperative to avoid sunlight, even from windows, for the first several days after photodynamic therapy.[24,26] A biopsy may be performed after the chemotherapy or photodynamic care if lesions are still present or suspected.

Melanoma

Melanoma is a skin cancer arising from melanocytes. **Melanocytes** are found in the stratum basale (deepest layer of the epidermis), eye, inner ear, meninges, heart, and bone. They produce the pigmentation in skin, also known as **melanin**. Melanoma is not limited to the skin; it is also found in the nails, mucosa of the oral and genital cavities, and conjunctiva of the eye.[6] The risk of melanoma increases with people exposed to UV light from either the sun or tanning beds. Other risk factors are age, sex (male), immunocompromised status, presence of many moles, and family history of melanoma.[28] The American Cancer Society listed nearly 100,000 newly diagnosed cases of melanoma in the United States in 2022 and attributed it to more than 7,600 deaths.[28] Melanoma is 20 times more prevalent in Caucasians than in African Americans and also in women ages 15 to 29 yr, and the trunk is the most common site. The most susceptible individuals have fair skin and blue eyes, sunburn easily, had multiple sunburns at an early age, and have a personal or family history of skin cancer.[28] Because 40% to 50% of malignant melanomas arise from pigmented moles, people with moles or freckles should be especially cautious.[3]

Melanoma is recognized as a public health issue because of its rising incidence and overall mortality rate. Notably, melanoma is one of the most common cancers in young adults.[28,29] Significant attempts have been made to increase public awareness through public sun protection campaigns for the past 25 yr.[29,30]

There are four recognized major types of primary cutaneous melanoma:

- Superficial spreading melanoma (SSM)
- Nodular melanoma (NM)
- Lentigo maligna melanoma
- Acral lentiginous melanoma

The two most common, SSM and NM, are discussed here.

- SSM is the most common type, constituting 70% of all melanomas.[3] The median age of occurrence is in the fifth decade, and it appears most frequently on the trunk in males and on the legs in females. Most notably, SSM has no preference for sun-damaged skin. SSM can arise anew or from an existing mole. It originates as an asymptomatic brown to black macule (see figure 16.3) with irregular or notched borders and color variegation such as red, blue, and white. Bleeding, itching, and ulceration may also be noted.

- NM is the second most common type of melanoma in fair-skinned people and develops most often during the sixth decade of life. It comprises 15% to 20% of all melanomas and occurs twice as often in males as in females.[6] NM may develop at any sun-exposed body site, but it has a predilection for the head, neck, and trunk. It appears as a bluish-black or reddish-pink nodule that has been rapidly enlarging for months. Ulceration and bleeding may ensue. NMs are often misdiagnosed as blood blisters. NM exhibits vertical growth de novo and lacks the typical initial horizontal growth phase demonstrated by the other types of melanoma. Therefore, NM tends to grow thicker, invade deeper, and associate with a poorer prognosis at the time of diagnosis.

It is important to recognize the risk factors for the development of melanoma. Unlike NMSC, risk factors for melanoma are both genetic and environmental. Genetic factors include fair skin, red hair color, a tendency to burn, and a family history of melanoma or atypical (dysplastic) moles or nevi. Environmental factors include intense intermittent sun exposure, sunburn, and geographic residence proximal to the equator. Other risk factors include having more than 50 atypical or large moles, being immunosuppressed, having a history of sunburns or skin cancer, and using tanning beds.[9,23]

Although ocular (eye) melanoma is rare, comprising only 5% of all melanomas, patients with **dysplastic nevi** have a higher risk of ocular nevi. Dysplastic nevi are atypical moles that look different from other, more common forms of mole.

It is known that people who burn easily typically have fair skin, blonde or red hair, and blue eyes, and therefore have a higher risk of developing cutaneous (skin) melanoma. There is also a slight trend of increased ocular melanoma among non-Hispanic Caucasian women in the United States.[31]

Signs and Symptoms

Patients presenting with atypical lesions must have a thorough medical history, focusing on the genetic and environmental risk factors such as a personal or family history of melanoma or atypical moles, fair skin type, a large number of moles, childhood history of sunburns, immunosuppression, and genetic syndromes with skin cancer predisposition. A detailed history about a suspicious lesion should be obtained regarding the following: whether it was present at birth; any changes in appearance; symptoms such as itching, bleeding, burning, or pain; and any other systemic symptoms such as weight loss, fatigue, cough, or headache.

A complete total body skin examination should be performed to rule out any suspicious lesions. Both the American Academy of Dermatology and the American Cancer Society use the ABCDE mnemonic as a guide to better recognize suspicious pigmented lesions.[32] The ABCDE mnemonic is outlined in table 16.1.

Differential diagnoses for melanoma include BCC, SCC, sebaceous carcinoma, dysplastic nevi, vascular lesions, and blue nevus.[33]

Referral and Diagnostic Tests

A mole or lesion should have clear, definitive borders. If it does not or if it falls into any of the ABCDE categories, then the lesion is suspect and the patient needs to be evaluated by a physician. The athletic trainer should refer to a

TABLE 16.1 **The ABCDEs of Melanoma**

Abbreviation	Descriptor	Parameters
A	Asymmetry	A melanoma lesion cannot be "folded in half"; in other words, the lesion does not have equal right and left sections or top and bottom sections.
B	Border	Benign lesions have a distinct border that can easily be traced, whereas malignant lesions may have borders that can fade off and be difficult to trace.
C	Color	Benign lesions have a uniform tan, brown, or black color, whereas malignant lesions may have variegated or multiple (i.e., red, white, and blue) color patterns. In addition, a sudden darkening in color or spreading into normal skin suggests a malignant lesion.
D	Diameter	Benign lesions usually have a diameter of <6 mm, whereas malignant lesions usually have a diameter >6 mm (the size of a pencil eraser when diagnosed), but they can be smaller.
E	Evolving	A mole or lesion looks different from the surrounding area or is changing in shape, color, or size.

physician any athletes with changes in shape, border, or size of a mole or lesion or the development of ulceration or bleeding, all of which are suggestive of melanoma. It is paramount to convey to patients with risk factors and an unusual lesion the urgent need to seek dermatological care, because the prognosis for a patient with melanoma depends on the disease stage at diagnosis.

Diagnosis is typically based on a biopsy performed on a suspicious pigmented lesion. The preferred procedure is an excisional biopsy, where the lesion and the 1 to 3 mm margins are completely excised.[33] The lesion and its border are then evaluated under a microscope via histopathological examination. The pathologist can then clearly identify the types of cells in the lesion. Because the degree of atypia and the depth of invasion may not be uniform in a pigmented lesion, an excisional biopsy decreases the risk of sampling error by allowing the pathologist to examine the entire lesion.[34] Another type of biopsy is an incisional biopsy, also termed a *punch biopsy*, in which only one part of the lesion is inspected microscopically.

Malignant melanomas are staged at the time of biopsy. An accurate staging system that groups patients at similar risk of disease progression and natural history is a necessary tool for the selection of optimal treatments. The staging of melanoma involves determining the tumor thickness and any involvement of the lymph nodes or organs. The system most commonly used to stage cancers is the TNM staging system.[34] TNM stands for primary Tumor, regional lymph Nodes, and distant Metastasis. Each of the three TNM categories has levels designated by the letter, followed by an alpha-numeric digit that are used to denote the invasiveness of the cancer. The combination of the three categories gives rise to a stage.[34] This system was created by both the American Joint Committee on Cancer and the Union for International Cancer Control.

The local, regional, or distant extent of the melanoma strongly correlates with survival. In general, the prognosis for a patient with localized melanoma and no nodal or systemic metastases is favorable. There is a delineation between patients with stage I low-risk melanoma with a depth less than 1 mm and patients with stage II higher risk melanoma with a depth greater than 2 mm. Depth is an indicator of how deep melanoma cells have penetrated into the skin, and the TNM system and clinical (anatomical) and pathological staging are used to determine the patient's prognosis.[9] Stages I and II include localized melanoma with estimated five-year survival rates of 90% to 95% and 45% to 78%, respectively.[34] Involvement of regional lymph nodes (stage III) decreases the survival rate to 24% to 63%, and the presence of distant metastases (stage IV) correlates with only a 7% to 19% survival rate. Other prognostic indicators include sex, age, and anatomic site.[33,34]

Patients diagnosed with malignant melanoma will undergo further testing to include chest radiography, magnetic resonance imaging (MRI), computed tomography scans, and positron emission tomography scans to determine the extent of the cancer.

Treatment and Return to Participation

Although benign moles, freckles, and age spots may provoke suspicion, it is wise to refer any questionable lesion to a medical doctor for inspection and likely a biopsy. If caught early, surgically removed melanoma has a high cure rate, but once it metastasizes to the lymph nodes, the five-year survival rate drops considerably. If organ involvement has occurred through this spread, the survival rate decreases again.[33] Excision includes removing at least 1 cm lateral to the tumor. Large surgical areas may require skin grafts or loss of underlying tissue that could result in deformity of the area involved.

The "gold standard" for treatment of stage I and II primary melanoma is wide local excision with the appropriate margins determined by the depth of the tumor. The purpose of the wide excisional margins is to ensure complete removal of any migratory melanoma cells and to prevent local recurrence. Management options for stage III regional metastatic melanoma include sentinel lymph node biopsy, elective lymph node dissection, and adjuvant therapy by chemotherapy. Current treatment options for stage IV include chemotherapy, radiation therapy, immunotherapy, biochemotherapy, and molecularly targeted therapy.[35]

Prognosis for the patient with melanoma depends on the thickness of the tumor involved. Patients with tumors less than 1 mm have a five-year survival rate of up to 95%, whereas patients with tumors greater than 4 mm thick have an approximately 45% survival rate for the same period.[3,20] The more tissue involved, the longer a patient will need to recover.

Prognosis and return to participation also relate to growth of the tumor in other areas or tissues. A patient with a melanoma contained within one mole will have a return-to-participation rate based on the sutures, the location of surgery, and any additional treatment such as chemotherapy. Melanoma involving organs or the lymphatic system most likely will require cessation or at least a great reduction of activity until the cancer is fully under control.

Prevention

Because of the numerous data linking sun exposure to melanoma and other skin cancers, sun protection is imperative. Sunbathing and the use of tanning beds are discouraged. Sun damage is cumulative, and 80% of

Clinical Tips

Proper Sunscreen Application

- Apply sunscreen at least 20 to 30 min before exposure.

- Use a sunscreen with a high sun protection factor (SPF), as well as one that has water-proof capabilities.

- Apply liberally to all exposed areas, including ears, back of the neck, and the posterior aspect of the legs.

- Reapply often (at least every hour) and after drying off from water activities.

- Realize that the sun does not need to be shining for one to be dangerously exposed to UVA or UVB light, so make using sunscreen a daily habit.

- Use sunscreen even when in the shade; sunlight reflected off water can also damage the skin.

Note: UVA = ultraviolet A; UVB = ultraviolet B.

the damage occurs before age 18 yr.[34] In 2015, the FDA proposed new safety rules for indoor tanning bed use. These restrictions included banning tanning bed usage for individuals younger than age 18 yr and requiring all users to sign a safety statement acknowledging the health risks of using tanning beds.[29] It should be noted that both Australia and Brazil have banned indoor tanning, and 20 European countries forbid tanning bed use among individuals younger than 18 yr.[83]

Sun avoidance during peak midday hours may be impractical for certain people, especially those whose occupations keep them outdoors and patients who practice and participate outside. The public has been slow to embrace the use of sun-protective clothing. Clothing itself is not a prohibitive barrier, as it has been found that clothing typically yields a sun protection factor (SPF) of 5. Clothing with higher SPF values is available. Other protection from the sun includes hats with wide brims that can increase coverage to the face, neck, and portions of the shoulders. Long-sleeved shirts and pants aid in protection, as does wearing gloves when possible during gardening, golf, cycling, and other outdoor activities.

People can be genetically predisposed to melanoma. Overexposure to UV light, even for brief periods, can cause a twofold increase in melanoma incidence, so sun protection is paramount.[19,20] The liberal use of sunscreens with an SPF rating of at least 30 and those effective against UVA and UVB can greatly reduce exposure. Darker skinned people are not immune to melanoma and should be encouraged to follow these precautions as well.

Ideal sunscreens for sport activities are those that are also waterproof and sweatproof. Furthermore, sunscreens need to be applied liberally to the sun-exposed skin to provide even coverage. They need to be applied at least 20 to 30 min before sun exposure and should be reapplied every 1 h or after water exposure.[9] In 2012, the NCAA added a new sports medicine guideline (2S) that addressed sun protection. It states that environmental factors such as latitude, altitude, minimal clouds, and reflective surfaces (water, snow, ice) can increase UV radiation exposure.[22] It also states that more than 250,000 student-athletes practice outdoors, and UV rays can damage unprotected skin in as little as 15 min. The guideline offers protective measures that include avoiding the sun between 10 a.m. and 4 p.m., wearing sun-protective clothing, and using a broad-spectrum sunscreen with an SPF of 30 or higher when outdoors.[22] The National Federation of State High School Associations (NFHS) has yet to publish a position on sun exposure, but prudent athletic trainers would align with the NCAA statement for the safety of athletes.

Sunglasses with UVA or UVB protection help protect the eyes not only from direct sun but also from reflected sunlight. To further protect the eyes from sun-induced damage, choose sunglasses that also wrap around the eyes to prevent light from entering the sides that can be reflected into the eyes. Polycarbonate lenses are recommended for children and athletes because they are the most shatter resistant. Refer to chapter 11 for more information about sun protection for the eyes.

Ultimately, public health campaigns educate people about the importance of being proactive in performing regular skin self-examinations. Through monthly screenings using the ABCDE criteria, one may be able to detect subtle changes in a skin lesion much earlier than at the time of the annual skin examination. Early detection of melanoma yields the greatest chance of a cure. Benign lesions usually appear early in life, and malignant lesions typically arise from preexisting moles or appear spontaneously later in life. If suspicious lesions are recognized during evaluation or during normal daily interactions with athletes, referral to a physician is in order. Annual screening examinations by a board-certified dermatologist are critical for those who have genetic risk factors. It is recommended that everyone have an annual screening beginning at age 40 yr, regardless of risk factors.

Frostbite

Prolonged outdoor cold exposure during sport or recreational activities may lead to frostbite or hypothermia. Hypothermia is a systemic presentation with minimal dermatologic features and is not discussed here. Frostbite is caused by vasoconstriction in response to cold, resulting in freezing tissues of the affected body part. Frostbite occurs most commonly on exposed skin, especially on the ears, nose, cheeks, and wrists.[36] Cold injuries are most prevalent at –25 to –35 °C (–13 to –31 °F). Although the temperature and wind chill factors do not affect the severity of a cold injury, a significant risk factor is a prior cold injury. Intrinsic risk factors for frostbite include fatigue, circulatory impairment, malnutrition, and prior history of cold injury. Extrinsic and environmental risk factors include inadequate or constrictive clothing, wind chill, high altitude, and prolonged exposure to cold or moisture.[37-39] Exposure to environmental cold affects younger athletes more severely than college- and middle-aged people. Athletes with lean body mass and those older than age 50 yr are also at increased risk of hypothermia-related issues.[37-39]

Signs and Symptoms

Because of the body's protective vasoconstrictive mechanism in the cold environment, the core temperature of the trunk is maintained at the expense of the extremities, nose, and ears. Frostbite can occur while in contact with cold surfaces and fluids as well as cold equipment. Because the condition begins at superficial skin levels and progresses to deeper tissues, damage worsens as the exposure continues. This condition is a localized response to a cold environment and is different from hypothermia, which is a systemic reaction to cold whereby the core temperature drops.[38,39] Frostbite is divided into four stages, which are detected only on rewarming.

- *First-degree frostbite (frost nip):* First-degree frostbite exhibits erythema, swelling, cutaneous numbness, and fleeting pain. Localized mild edema is not uncommon. The patient is expected to make a full recovery with only mild residual superficial skin peeling.[38]

- *Second-degree frostbite:* Second-degree frostbite causes marked redness, swelling, and blister formation. It is a full-thickness skin freezing; the outer skin is hard but resilient with pressure to the underlying areas.[38] Although it may heal, the patient may be left with long-term sensory neuropathy and cold sensitivity.

- *Third-degree frostbite:* Third-degree frostbite causes subdermal freezing with destruction of the skin, with the formation of hemorrhagic blisters and hard, waxy skin. This patient will have deep burning pain on rewarming, which can last up to 5 wk.[38]

- *Fourth-degree frostbite:* Fourth-degree frostbite results in loss of the entire body part with full-thickness destruction of the skin, muscle, tendon, and bone. Severe injury to this degree usually requires amputation. Visual signs and symptoms include edema, redness, or mottled gray or white skin and accompanying numbness, tingling, or burning. Limited range of motion and cold, hard skin are also signs of fourth-degree frostbite.[37,39]

Referral and Diagnostic Tests

Frostbite injuries are usually easily recognizable because of the clinical history and presentation. Determining the degree of a cold injury may be more challenging; however, radiological evaluation such as MRI, radiography, and bone scan may help determine the extent of a cold injury.

Treatment and Return to Participation

The key goals in treating frostbite are removing the patient from cold exposure, rewarming the tissues, and restoring circulation. Rewarming should be achieved slowly at room temperature or by placement next to another person's skin. In an emergency, when transportation to a medical facility is imminent, wrap the tissue in dry towels or blankets to ward off further exposure to cold.[38] If using water to rewarm, use circulating water temperatures not exceeding 37 to 39 °C (98.6-102.2 °F).[37,39] Warming is continued for 15 to 30 min or until tissue is thawed. It is not advisable to apply dry heat to the frozen extremity or to rub it. It is important to complete core body rewarming and to completely rehydrate the patient before attempting limb rewarming in order to avoid sudden shock and hypotension. The affected tissue should not be allowed to refreeze once the rewarming has begun, as necrosis could result.[36,38,39]

Standard therapy consists of local wound care of the frostbitten area. Superficial blisters may be gently debrided to avoid further contact with the inflammatory mediators in the blister fluid. A tetanus prophylaxis should be administered, if outdated. Other therapies include administration of topical aloe vera, which inhibits the inflammation in superficial frostbite. Thrombolytic therapies including heparin are useful, as are anti-inflammatory agents such as aspirin and pentoxifylline.

Prevention

Active people who participate at high elevations or in winter-like conditions need to prepare for the weather by wearing equipment designed for the conditions. High-quality hiking boots and appropriate gloves are two of the critical items needed for adverse conditions. Individuals who participate in colder weather should wear layers of clothing with wicking layers against the body, a middle layer that offers insulation, and a wind and water barrier as the outermost layer. Because wind can greatly affect colder temperatures, a windbreaker is one of the most critical pieces of protective gear. Other ways to prevent frostbite include maintaining proper nutrition and hydration status and avoiding standing still for long periods of time.[22,36,39] Alcohol, nicotine, and certain drugs affect a person's ability to adapt to colder environments and should be avoided.

Bacterial Conditions

Bacterial skin disorders include impetigo, abscesses, folliculitis, furuncles or boils, carbuncles, and paronychia or onychia. Healthy skin has many different bacterial and fungal organisms that are usually held in check and do not cause infection. However, if bacteria, often *Staphylococcus aureus* or *Streptococcus pyogenes*, are introduced into a break in the skin, they may begin to secrete toxins or interfere with cellular function, thereby producing symptoms.

S. aureus and *S. pyogenes* are responsible for most bacterial dermatological conditions. Bacterial and viral conditions may coexist within the same infection and complicate diagnosis and treatment. It is important to note that individuals are not immune to a particular bacterial infection after recovery. Given the right conditions, infection is possible again.

The NCAA and the NFHS provide oversight of collegiate and scholastic sports, respectively. Both organizations have singled out the bacterial infections of impetigo, folliculitis, furuncles, carbuncles (including methicillin-resistant *S. aureus* [MRSA]), and staphylococcal diseases for particular restrictions.[22,40-42] In wrestling, time lost because of skin conditions accounted for 12% of time lost in the sport for collegiate wrestlers.[43] Although the rules regarding infectious skin conditions

are meant especially for wrestlers, they apply to all athletes. Protecting others from infection is paramount, as is protecting the health and welfare of the infected athlete. These guidelines will be reiterated for each transmittable skin infection discussed in this chapter.

Impetigo

Impetigo is a highly contagious skin disorder caused by either *S. aureus* or *S. pyogenes*, with *S. aureus* accounting for the majority of the infections. Impetigo is one of the most common bacterial infections in children and occurs most often in warm temperatures and humid areas.[44] Infection usually occurs in areas of previous skin disease or injury, such as sites of eczema, insect bites, varicella, or abrasion. Earlier damage to the skin by abrasion opens a pathway for invading bacteria, leading to impetigo. It is transmitted by skin-to-skin contact, with combative sports having a higher incidence of transmission than other activities.[1] Each year, it prevents many athletes from participating. Impetigo is self-limiting and typically heals within 2 to 3 wk without scarring.[44] It is readily transmitted with skin-to-skin contact, as evidenced by a 2014 high school outbreak from a wrestling meet that hosted 24 schools. Of the 47 athletes who were subsequently infected, 47% contracted impetigo. The original contagion was an athlete who was allowed to illegally participate with uncovered lesions.[45]

Signs and Symptoms

Athletes with impetigo generally are afebrile, but they may have localized lymphadenopathy. The two types of impetigo are nonbullous and bullous. The nonbullous form (about 70% of cases) typically appears as a yellow or honey-colored, crusted lesion on an erythematous base (figure 16.12). Bullous impetigo first presents with moist, red skin that resembles a burn and progresses to

NCAA and NFHS Participation Regulations for Wrestlers With Bacterial Infections

The following regulations apply to participation with the bacterial conditions of impetigo, folliculitis, furuncles, carbuncles, and staphylococcal diseases, including community-acquired MRSA:

- Completion of at least 72 h of antibiotic therapy.
- No new lesions for 48 h before participation.
- No moist, draining, or exudative lesions at time of participation.
- Active purulent lesions *shall not* be covered to participate.
- A Gram stain of exudate from questionable lesion is required if available.*

*NCAA regulation only (not NFHS).

Adapted from NCAA (2019); National Federation of State High School Associations (2022).

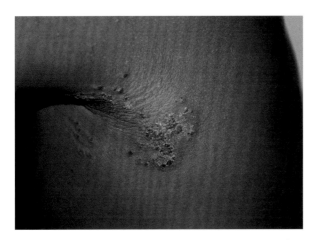

FIGURE 16.12 Nonbullous impetigo presents with a honey-yellow crust covering the lesion.

DermPics / Science Source

flaccid small to large vesicles that appear filled with clear or yellow fluid.[44] Both bullous and nonbullous forms present lesions that may be small and pea-shaped or large and blister-like in appearance, or they may appear as ribbon-like strands.

Lesions of impetigo eventually erupt, leaving purulent discharge to dry on the skin. They are painless yet pruritic, which exacerbates and spreads the infection to other areas. The face, arms, legs, and trunk are the most common sites for impetigo. Differential diagnoses for impetigo include HSV, varicella-zoster virus, insect bites, and tinea infections.[44]

Referral and Diagnostic Tests

The athletic trainer who suspects that an athlete may have impetigo should remove the athlete from activity immediately to prevent spread of the infection to others and should refer the patient to a physician.[46] Diagnosis is mostly by clinical examination and history, but a culture may be obtained if the diagnosis is unclear.[44] In this case, the patient is treated for both impetigo and HSV until the cultures return.

Treatment and Return to Participation

Treatment for a small area of impetigo consists of a topical antibiotic, such as mupirocin (Bactroban), applied three times daily for 10 d or until the lesion has cleared. Larger areas of impetigo are generally treated with oral antibiotics that cover both *S. aureus* and *S. pyogenes*, such as clindamycin, erythromycin, cephalexin (Keflex), and dicloxacillin.[44,47]

The patient washes the area with soap and water three times daily, removes the crusts before application of a topical antibiotic, and is not allowed to participate in contact activity until the lesions have completely cleared.

The athlete may return to play on complete resolution of the crusted, infected, exposed areas. In wrestling, the NCAA and NFHS have very specific regulations (see the NCAA and NFHS Participation Regulations for Wrestlers With Bacterial Infections sidebar).

Prevention

Proper hygiene is paramount. The National Athletic Trainers' Association (NATA) and the NCAA are clear and consistent about preventing skin infections, and the key aspects of their message are presented in the Prevention Strategies for Infectious Dermatological Conditions in Athletes sidebar. When impetigo recurs multiple times, family members or close contacts may need to produce samples for nasopharyngeal culture because 30% to 40% may be asymptomatic carriers of the causative bacteria, such as *S. aureus*. A carrier who tests positive will need to apply mupirocin ointment to the nasal passages twice daily for 5 d.[44] Equipment that may have come in contact with athletes who have lesions must be sanitized daily to prevent the spread or recurrence of infection. In this case, equipment includes all mats, towels, protective gear, water bottles, clothing, and uniforms.[46]

Folliculitis

Folliculitis is another common bacterial skin infection. Two types of bacteria cause folliculitis: *S. aureus* and *Pseudomonas aeruginosa*. The latter is often associated with infections acquired in hot tubs.

Folliculitis is an inflammatory reaction in the hair follicles and most often occurs on the face, chest, axilla, buttocks, groin, and legs. The most common cause is shaving with a razor blade. When a razor blade nicks the skin, the opening allows bacteria to be introduced into the tissue (figure 16.13). Folliculitis may also be caused by friction from helmets, equipment padding, or straps.

The other common bacterial cause of folliculitis is *Pseudomonas* infection, which is commonly referred to as *hot tub folliculitis* (figure 16.14). This type usually appears 2 to 3 d after exposure to water contaminated with *P. aeruginosa*. The most common conduits are poorly maintained hot tubs, pools, baths, water slides, and contaminated waters. There does not appear to be any skin-to-skin transmission with *P. aeruginosa*.

Signs and Symptoms

Clinical presentation of folliculitis demonstrates small, tender, red papules or bumps in the hair follicles, with a hair shaft within the papule. These lesions tend to occur in multiples and are often pruritic.[46] The typical presentation of itchy red papules around hair follicles occurs in many

Prevention Strategies for Infectious Dermatological Conditions in Athletes

The National Athletic Trainers' Association and the National Collegiate Athletics Association have provided the following prevention strategies:

- Organizational support must be adequate to limit the spread of infectious agents.
- A clean environment must be maintained in the athletic training facility, locker rooms, and all athletic venues.
  - Clean and disinfect gym bags or travel bags and all protective gear on a regular basis.
  - Inspect playing fields for animal droppings that could cause bacterial infections of cuts or abrasions.
  - Sanitize athletic lockers between seasons.
  - Weight room equipment, including benches, handles, and bars, should be sanitized daily.
- Health care practitioners and athletes should follow good hand hygiene practices.
- Athletes must be encouraged to follow good overall hygiene practices.
- Athletes must be discouraged from sharing the following:
  - Towels
  - Athletic gear
  - Water bottles
  - Disposable razors
  - Hair clippers
- Athletes with open wounds, scrapes, or scratches must avoid whirlpools and common tubs.
- Athletes are encouraged to report all abrasions, cuts, and skin lesions and to seek attention from an athletic trainer for proper cleaning, treatment, and dressing.

Adapted from S.M. Zinder et al., "National Athletic Trainers' Position Statement: Skin Diseases." *Journal of Athletic Training* 45, no. 4 (2010): 411-428. This work is licensed under a Creative Commons Attribution 3.0 License.

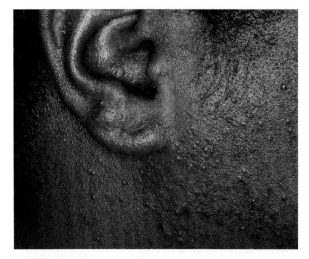

FIGURE 16.13 Folliculitis in a beard, characterized by superficial infection of hair follicles.

The Division of Dermatology at Brody School of Medicine, East Carolina University

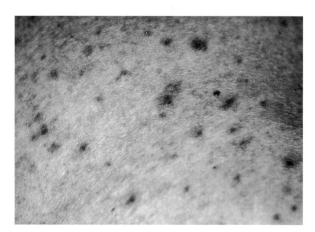

FIGURE 16.14 *Pseudomonas* folliculitis reaction resulting from exposure in a hot tub. The rash appears in areas covered by a swimsuit.

DermPics / Science Source

areas of the body but most commonly under areas covered by the swimsuit. Superficial folliculitis also presents with pruritus or mild pain, whereas patients with deep folliculitis can have pain and drainage. Recurrent folliculitis can result in scarring and/or hair loss.[48]

Differential diagnoses for folliculitis include *Pityrosporum* folliculitis, dermatophytic folliculitis, gram-negative folliculitis, HSV, acne, pityriasis rosea, molluscum contagiosum, fire ant bites, impetigo, and rosacea.[48]

Referral and Diagnostic Tests

The clinician refers patients who have persistent symptoms despite conservative treatment or those with an unusual presentation. Physician diagnosis is made based on clinical examination, but a Gram stain and culture may be obtained if the results of the examination are nonspecific or if the symptoms persist.

Treatment and Return to Participation

The use of antibacterial soap may resolve uncomplicated superficial folliculitis. For more inflamed folliculitis, warm saline compresses and a topical antimicrobial ointment, such as bacitracin, may also benefit the patient.[35] The treatment plan for deeper lesions includes topical or oral antibiotics that provide coverage for both *S. aureus* and *S. pyogenes*.[48] The athlete should follow the hygiene protocols outlined in the Prevention Strategies for Infectious Dermatological Conditions in Athletes sidebar. In cases of recurrent folliculitis, the patient may benefit from a nasal culture for *S. aureus*.[49] Sometimes antibiotic treatment is required. Treatment of *Pseudomonas* is not needed because this type of folliculitis usually resolves spontaneously in 7 to 10 d if there is no additional exposure. The patient may return to participation immediately and without restrictions.

An athlete may return to participation when lesions of folliculitis begin to heal. The amount of time it takes for these lesions to heal may depend on their location. Some areas, such as the beard, take much longer to heal, especially if the athlete wears headgear with a chin strap that may irritate the condition. The athlete with *Pseudomonas* may participate without restriction.

Furuncles and Carbuncles

Furunculosis is similar to folliculitis but occurs when lesions are deeper in the hair follicle cavity and contain pus. These lesions are also bacterial skin infections, and they are caused by *S. aureus* and include abscesses, furuncles, and carbuncles, which is a conglomeration of multiple furuncles. An **abscess** is a collection of pus that arises in a variety of locations. A **furuncle**, or boil, is a

walled-off abscess containing pus that usually develops in a preexisting site of folliculitis. Boils commonly occur at sites of trauma or friction, such as the beltline, waistline, axilla, groin, thighs, and buttocks; they are more common after puberty.[46]

A **carbuncle** is a collection of several coalescing furuncles. Carbuncles are common among wrestlers and readily transmitted by skin-to-skin contact. MRSA has become especially problematic in athletics when athletes are allowed to participate if they are receiving medical treatment. In response, the NFHS, the NATA, and other organizations have established policies on MRSA.[41,50-52] Resistant strains cause the athlete to sustain the effects of the infection for a longer period, allow more opportunity to spread the disease, and may result in severe systemic illness. (For a more detailed discussion of MRSA, please see chapter 14.)

Signs and Symptoms

The signs and symptoms of carbuncles or furuncles are a lesion that usually begins with a tender, deep, firm, erythematous papule that enlarges and becomes painful and fluctuant over a period of days (figure 16.15). The abscess remains deep, reabsorbs, or drains through the skin. Elevated temperatures and malaise are not uncommon.

Differential diagnoses include folliculitis, sebaceous cyst, skin cancer, severe HSV infection, **hidradenitis suppurativa** if located in the axilla or groin, and pilonidal cyst if the furuncle is located in the gluteal cleft.

Referral and Diagnostic Tests

The clinician refers to a physician any patient who presents with an elevated temperature, malaise, vomiting,

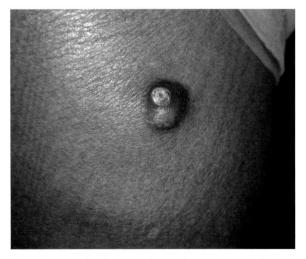

FIGURE 16.15 A furuncle, or boil, is an enlarged swollen purulent mass.

wirestock/iStock/Getty Images

MRSA

Methicillin-resistant Staphylococcus aureus (MRSA) was first observed in 1961. At the time, it was presumed to be associated only with nosocomial infections. However, in the decades that followed, MRSA has spread outside the hospital environment to pervade community settings. In particular, community-associated MRSA (CA-MRSA) has become a persistent and growing medical problem among the young and healthy population, including athletes. CA-MRSA epidemics have even been reported in entire communities. Because of its ubiquitous presence, it is important to recognize and treat CA-MRSA early to prevent its spread within the community, especially in young athletes participating in contact sports.[52]

Preventing MRSA involves following good hygiene practices in sport that are outlined in the Prevention Strategies for Infectious Dermatological Conditions in Athletes sidebar. For more on CA-MRSA, see chapter 14.

and persistence of furuncles after conservative treatment. Diagnostic tests include a Gram stain for gram-positive cocci and a culture to determine the organism involved; however, a culture is usually reserved for persistent infections that do not respond to treatment. A blood culture with antibiotic sensitivities may be obtained with symptoms of a systemic infection, such as fever and malaise.[46]

Treatment and Return to Participation

Treatment of furuncles consists of warm, moist compresses applied often throughout the day. If this fails, a physician incises and evacuates the abscess. Antibiotics are usually not effective once the abscess has developed, although they are still often prescribed.

A patient who often develops furuncles may need topical antibiotic ointment for the nasal passages to eradicate a carrier state, as happens with impetigo. Return to participation with protection is allowed when the infection begins to heal. In wrestling, however, the NCAA and the NFHS recommend that an athlete not return until there have been no new lesions for the last 48 h, among other criteria listed in the NCAA and NFHS Participation Regulations for Wrestlers With Bacterial Infections sidebar. As with the other bacterial infections, active lesions should not be covered to allow for participation.[53,54]

Prevention

Preventive measures include treating the athlete and close-contact members for *S. aureus* carrier states and recurrent infections. Other prevention techniques mentioned with folliculitis and impetigo will also help retard the spread of furuncles.

Acne

Acne is a common problem among adolescents, but very little information exists about acne and sport participation. Acne is a condition of the pilosebaceous unit and most commonly occurs where the concentration of sebaceous or sweat glands is the greatest, such as on the face, neck, chest, and back (figure 16.16). The condition is common in both males and females.

Signs and Symptoms

Acne consists of inflammatory and noninflammatory lesions. Inflammatory lesions are composed of erythem-

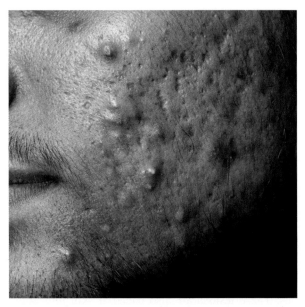

FIGURE 16.16 Acne is typical among athletes.
Science Photo Library / Science Source

atous papules, pustules, or deep cysts; noninflammatory lesions are made up of open and closed comedones. Open comedones are commonly referred to as *blackheads*, and closed comedones are commonly referred to as *whiteheads*.

The bacterium involved is *Propionibacterium acnes* and not *S. aureus* or *S. pyogenes*. The follicular shaft becomes plugged, and the proliferation of *P. acnes* secondarily increases keratin formation. This is known as a *noninflammatory reaction*, but when white blood cells are attracted to these lesions, the acne becomes inflammatory. Symptoms range from a few open or closed comedones on the face or another area to multiple comedones, pustules, and deep, large, painful cysts.[3]

The differential diagnoses for acne include bacterial folliculitis, *Pityrosporum* folliculitis, pseudofolliculitis, perioral dermatitis, human papillomavirus (HPV), HSV infections, and contact dermatitis.

Referral and Diagnostic Tests

Many people with simple episodic acne do not need referral. Typical over-the-counter treatments, such as antimicrobial soaps and washes, often contain benzoyl peroxide or retinoids focused on drying the skin, and they can be a great first-line treatment. These should be tried prior to referral if possible. Patients with acne are referred to a dermatologist if they have chronic or widespread acne. If personal hygiene is not the culprit, pharmaceutical intervention can help ameliorate most forms of acne.[55]

Treatment and Return to Participation

Depending on the type, acne responds well to a variety of agents. Noninflammatory acne responds well to topicals, including dapsone, adapalene (Differin), tretinoin (Retin-A, Avita), azelaic acid (Azelex, Finevin), and tazarotene (Tazorac). Benzoyl peroxide is an antibacterial agent but also works well for noninflammatory acne and is available over the counter in a variety of topical forms (gel, ointment lotions, washes, creams). Inflammatory acne responds well to topical benzoyl peroxide either alone or in combination with an antibiotic as well as topical and oral antibiotics. The primary treatment for moderate to severe acne is systemic antibiotics, with the tetracycline group having the most benefit and least side effects.[55] Oral antibiotics or hormonal therapy are usually prescribed, but steroid injection and chemical peels have also been used in some cases.[55]

The athletic trainer and the physician counsel athletes during acne treatment about the side effects of some acne medications. These medications may cause sensitivity to sunlight and, as a result, may increase the likelihood of sunburn.

Acne is not considered contagious or a limitation to activity, so athletes are allowed to participate without restrictions.

Paronychia or Onychia

Paronychia is an infection that affects the proximal or lateral nail fold that separates the skin from the nail, and **onychia** is an infection of the nail matrix. The infection may occur after manipulation, other infection, or trauma. The organism usually involved is *S. aureus*, but it can also be a fungal infection if the patient is immunocompromised. Other, more obscure causes include prolonged water exposure, HSV, or candidal vaginitis.[35]

Signs and Symptoms

A paronychia is a bright-red swelling of the folds of tissue surrounding a nail, which may show an accumulation of purulent material (figure 16.17). In contrast, an onychia is an infection of the nail bed. Differential diagnoses for paronychia include bacterial infections, fungal infections, *Pseudomonas*, and trauma.

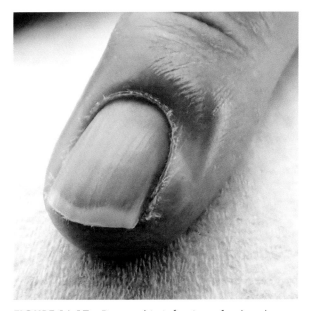

FIGURE 16.17 Paronychia infection of a thumb.
Tharlys Fabricio/iStock/Getty Images

Referral and Diagnostic Tests

Patients with infected nail beds are referred when conservative care is ineffective. Referral is also indicated for immunocompromised patients or those with persistent or worsening symptoms. If the patient is immunocompetent, no further diagnostic testing is needed unless the symptoms persist, and then a Gram stain, potassium hydroxide (KOH) preparation, and culture of the fluid are obtained.

Treatment and Return to Participation

Conservative treatment consists of warm to hot soaks and acetaminophen (Tylenol) for mild pain. If the infection is large, especially painful, or disabling, a small incision into the corresponding location will relieve the pressure by draining the infection. Sometimes antibiotics are needed if incision and drainage are inadequate. Prevention of paronychial or onychial infections consists of good nail and skin hygiene and limited manipulation with careful nail cutting. Keeping fingers and toes clean and dry will retard these infections.[3]

Participation is not restricted with a paronychial infection, and the prognosis after treatment is good. If the area was drained, the athletic trainer should follow basic wound care protocol to prevent further infection.

Viral Conditions

Viral infections are some of the most difficult and challenging problems in athletes, especially wrestlers. The viruses presented in this section include HSV, varicella-zoster virus, molluscum contagiosum, and HPV.

Herpes Simplex

HSV is also addressed in chapter 9. It is an extremely contagious viral infection and presents as cold sores or fever blisters, genital herpes, and **herpes gladiatorum**. There are more than 80 types of HSV, but the most common are HSV-1, which typically occurs above the waist, and HSV-2, which typically occurs below the waist. Both types, however, can be found in both areas, and typing may only be significant for predicting future outbreaks and responses to treatment.[56]

It is estimated that by age 30 yr, 50% of people in higher socioeconomic regions and 80% of those in lower socioeconomic areas test positive for HSV-1.[56] Not everyone develops symptoms once infected, and each person experiences a different rate of recurrence. HSV enters the skin through a site of previous injury (e.g., a cut or abrasion) or damage (e.g., eczema) and follows the nerve root to the dorsal root ganglion in the spinal cord.

Individuals may not develop symptoms or a rash during the primary infection. Subsequent HSV infections can be triggered by stress, sunburn, or even menstrual cycles.[56]

At various times, HSV will follow the nerves back to the skin and produce symptoms along the dermatomal distribution. HSV is never eradicated, but symptoms present in varying degrees. Approximately 70% of genital herpes is transmitted by asymptomatic shedding of the virus in people who report never having had the infection.[3]

When HSV occurs on the face and trunk, it is commonly known as *herpes gladiatorum*. The NFHS has established a position statement on this condition and has created a document that physicians can use in clearing high school wrestlers after infection.[41,54] Estimates indicate that 2.6% of high school wrestlers and 7.6% of collegiate wrestlers have been infected with HSV. In a 4 yr study on NCAA wrestlers, HSV infection led all other skin infections (43%), with fungal infections second (31%).[53] These numbers likely underestimate the problem because some lesions remain unrecognized. The infection typically spreads by direct skin-to-skin contact with an infected person. Outbreaks are usually found on the head and trunk but are not limited to these areas.

Complications of HSV are numerous and include chronic recurrences, skin lesions, possible scarring, eye or corneal scarring, and blindness. **Herpes keratoconjunctivitis** is a highly infectious condition of the cornea of the eye that may lead to corneal damage, scarring, or even blindness.[57] HSV keratoconjunctivitis is the leading infectious cause of blindness in the United States. The infection may occur either by direct contact or by reactivation of HSV through the ophthalmic branch of the trigeminal nerve.

So-called fever blisters or cold sores are also caused by HSV, and people with active lesions can transmit the virus to otherwise healthy body areas (figure 16.18). Cold sores, also known as *herpes labialis*, can be exacerbated by UV light from the sun, which is why wearing a lip balm with sunscreen is one good preventive idea.

Signs and Symptoms

Typical symptoms for the primary HSV infection mimic influenza and include fever, sore throat, lymphadenopathy, malaise, and vesicles on an erythematous base. Recurrent HSV infection symptoms include grouped vesicles of the same shape and age on an erythematous base. On occasion, tingling or pain precedes the outbreak.[56]

Outbreaks may present in many ways, however, and they do not always present as the typical vesicles on an erythematous base. In the early stages, they are often easily confused with ringworm, impetigo, acne, and eczema. Sometimes wrestlers break open the vesicles, cover the rash with makeup, sandpaper the rash, or even use bleach to alter the rash in order to continue to wrestle.[57,58] Obviously, diagnosis is then even more difficult, and the infection can spread more easily to others.

Differential diagnoses for HSV include bacterial infections such as impetigo, acne, various types of folliculitis, viral varicella-zoster, and fungal tinea infections.

Referral and Diagnostic Tests

The clinical diagnosis in many cases of HSV is made based on symptoms and exposure. The most definitive method of diagnosis is to unroof an intact moist vesicle and culture the base for HSV. This method may take 48 h to yield results; once a diagnosis is suspected, the athlete should be kept out of contact with other athletes.[56,59] The polymerase chain reaction test is accurate and fast, and it can also detect asymptomatic shedding. The direct fluorescent antigen test yields results in 2 to 3 h and, as with culturing, takes samples scraped from the ulcer base. Withholding an athlete from contact activity before a culture is taken and medications are started is critical to preventing disease spread.

Treatment and Return to Participation

Antiviral medications include acyclovir (Zovirax), valacyclovir (Valtrex), and famciclovir (Famvir) and have varying administration routes (oral, intravenous, and topical).[56] Doses differ depending on whether the condition is a primary or recurrent outbreak. For wrestlers, prophylactic medications should be continued after the outbreak for the remainder of the wrestling season. Prophylactic dosages are 400 mg of acyclovir two times

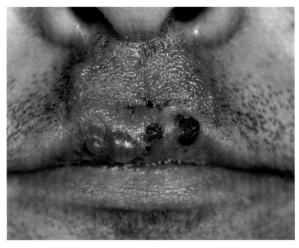

FIGURE 16.18 Herpes simplex, also called a *cold sore*, presents as tight vesicles that develop into pustules and ulcers.

daily or 500 mg of valacyclovir twice daily.[56] Since the 1940s, researchers have been trying to develop a vaccine to prevent both HSV-1 and HSV-2, but have fallen short. With the messenger RNA (mRNA) breakthrough research discovered during the COVID-19 pandemic, there is renewed hope for a mRNA vaccine for HSV, and robust clinical trials look promising.[60]

The patient with HSV must shower with antibacterial soap and launder all towels and uniforms daily. Although drug reactions with antiviral medications are rare, dehydration is a possible concern in wrestlers or in individuals with poor renal function and can lead to severe kidney problems.[47,59] Patients taking antiviral medications are encouraged to increase fluid intake for the duration of the medical course.

Current NCAA recommendations require that the athlete with HSV be withheld from contact sports until the athlete is asymptomatic.[53] The NFHS also provides recommendations for HSV and groups them with varicella and zoster. Primary outbreaks have a longer time requirement for oral antiviral medications before participation (10-14 d compared with 5 d required by the NCAA), but the NFHS aligns with collegiate wrestling rules in the case of recurrent infection (secondary outbreaks): Both require 120 h of antiviral medication use and 72 h with no new lesions.[40,42,53,54]

Varicella-Zoster

Varicella-zoster virus, otherwise known as *chicken pox* (for the initial infection with the varicella virus) and *shingles* (for reactivations with the herpes zoster virus), is another common viral infection.

As presented in chapter 14, chicken pox is a common childhood disease with some cases presenting in adolescence or adulthood. This infection is very contagious and is spread by respiratory droplets or direct skin-to-skin contact. Patients are contagious from about 2 d before rash onset until all lesions have crusted over.[47]

Herpes zoster, or shingles, is a reactivation of varicella-zoster virus involving the skin along its dermatomal distribution. It occurs at all ages but increases in frequency with advancing age. Reactivation may result from advancing age, immunosuppression, lymphoma, stress, and radiation therapy.[61,62] Shingles most commonly results from reactivation of a previous varicella-zoster virus infection, not from direct contact with someone with shingles.

Signs and Symptoms of Varicella

Symptoms of chicken pox are presented in chapter 14 and include low-grade fever, headache, and malaise before the rash begins; the patient will develop a papular or vesicular rash. The rash evolves in size and scope as it begins on the trunk, spreading to the extremities and face. Intense itching is often secondary to the rash.

Differential diagnoses for varicella include HSV, bullous impetigo, various types of folliculitis, and contact dermatitis.

Signs and Symptoms of Herpes Zoster

Typical symptoms of shingles include pain, tingling, burning, or itching before rash onset along a single dermatome. Symptoms may present along more than one dermatome or may cross the midline. The most common complication is postherpetic neuralgia (PHN), which may require strong analgesic medications to control the pain.[61,62]

Differential diagnoses for herpes zoster include migraine, acute dermatitis, spinal nerve compression, renal calculi, HSV infection, contact dermatitis, bullous impetigo, and conjunctivitis.[3]

Treatment and Return to Participation

Patients diagnosed with varicella are typically prescribed the antiviral medication acyclovir (800 mg four times per day for 5 d initially) to help prevent complications. Pediatric doses may vary depending on the patient's age and weight. These medications are used to help reduce the viral shedding, pain, and frequency of PHN. Symptomatic treatment also includes lotions and antihistamines to reduce itching. Sometimes prednisone is prescribed to

---

NCAA Participation Regulations for Wrestlers With Viral Infections

Primary HSV Infection
- Free of systemic symptoms such as fever and malaise
- No new lesions or blisters within the past 72 h
- No moist or exudative lesions, and all existing lesions must be dry with a firm, adherent crust
- Completion of at least 120 h (5 d) of an appropriate systemic antiviral therapy
- Active lesions *shall not* be covered to allow for participation

Secondary (Recurrent) HSV Infection
- No moist or exudative lesions, and all existing lesions must be dry with a firm, adherent crust
- Completion of at least 120 h (5 d) of an appropriate systemic antiviral therapy
- Active lesions *shall not* be covered to allow for participation

Molluscum Contagiosum
- All lesions must be removed (via cryotherapy or curetted) before participation.
- The only way that coverage assures prevention of transmission is if the molluscum is on the trunk or uppermost thighs which are assured of remaining covered with clothing; band aids are not sufficient.*
- Solitary or localized, clustered lesions can be covered with a gas impermeable dressing, prewrap and stretch tape that is appropriately anchored and cannot be dislodged.

*The NFHS does not mention the location of molluscum contagiosum in its infection guidelines.

*Verrucae (Warts)**
- Verrucae plana or vulgaris must be adequately covered for participation.
- Athletes with multiple facial verrucae digitata that cannot be adequately covered with a mask or curetted away may not participate.
- Solitary or scattered lesions may be curetted for participation but may not be seeping.
- Athletes with multiple verrucae plana or vulgaris must have the lesions adequately covered.

*The NFHS does not consider warts to be very contagious and requires no treatment or restrictions for high school athletes.

Adapted from NCAA (2019, 2022); National Federation of State High School Associations (2022).

reduce the chance of PHN. Narcotic analgesics are also used to help with pain control.

Prevention

The best prevention for chicken pox is administration of the varicella vaccine at age 12 to 23 mo, followed by a measles, mumps, rubella, and varicella vaccine at ages 4 to 6 yr (see chapter 14).[63] Limited exposure at a young age to known cases will prevent the individual from contracting the condition later in life when the disease presents more dramatically.

Molluscum Contagiosum

Molluscum contagiosum is a viral infection commonly found in children and in sexually active adults. It most commonly appears on the face, trunk, arms, legs, and genital areas. The palms and soles are usually not involved. It is easily spread via direct contact, such as children sharing a bath or athletes sharing equipment.[64] The disease is self-limited and typically resolves spontaneously after several months. It is caused by a virus in the *Poxviridae* family and is more common in swimmers, wrestlers, and gymnasts.[59]

Signs and Symptoms

Molluscum contagiosum presents as a small, skin-colored, sometimes erythematous, smooth, dome-shaped papule with a central punctum (figure 16.19). It is very contagious and is spread by **autoinoculation** and direct skin-to-skin contact. The lesions usually spontaneously resolve in 6 to 12 mo. Differential diagnoses include HPV, sebaceous hyperplasia, SCC, or BCC.[3]

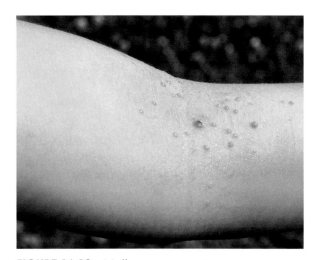

FIGURE 16.19 Molluscum contagiosum.
Robert Kirk/iStock/Getty Images

Treatment and Return to Participation

Conservative treatment of molluscum contagiosum is effective for most patients, but wrestlers and those in other contact sports may require aggressive therapy sooner. Lesions may be treated by freezing each one with liquid nitrogen or by curetting with a comedone extractor or small needle, although slight scarring is possible with these two procedures. After these treatments, the lesions are no longer contagious.

If the lesions are solitary or grouped, they can be covered with a gas-permeable membrane, such as OpSite (Smith & Nephew Healthcare), Tegaderm (3M), or Bioclusive (Johnson & Johnson), followed by prewrap and stretch tape so that participation can be allowed. If the lesions are too numerous or cannot be covered, then all lesions must be curetted or frozen before return is allowed.

Human Papillomavirus

Warts are caused by HPV and are most commonly found in children and young adults but may occur at any age. More than 100 types of HPV have been identified and can be seen any place on the skin. Some warts may spontaneously resolve in less than 2 yr, but others last a lifetime. Warts are spread by skin-to-skin contact and usually occur at sites of trauma, abrasion, or eczema, most commonly on the hands and feet. HPV is often associated with genital warts, which are addressed in chapter 9. Common warts (verruca vulgaris) are caused by five different types of HPV and are discussed here.[35]

Signs and Symptoms

The diagnostic feature of warts is their distortion or obscuring of the normal skin lines. Warts present as small, smooth, skin-colored papules that may progress to a rough surface, a flat-topped surface, or a deep, callus-like lesion (figure 16.20). Some warts have small black dots, which represent thrombosed capillaries. These dots are often considered a diagnostic sign of warts.

Differential diagnoses include molluscum contagiosum, seborrheic keratosis, actinic keratosis, SCC, BCC, corns, and calluses.

Referral and Diagnostic Tests

No specific tests are needed unless the diagnosis is atypical. In rare cases, a biopsy may aid in the diagnosis. Referral is indicated when conservative treatment has failed or when symptoms interfere with daily activities.

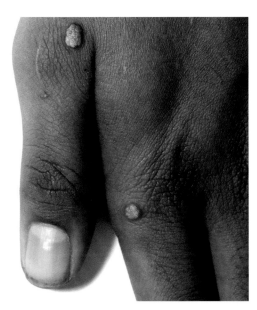

FIGURE 16.20 Warts, also called verruca vulgaris, can appear anywhere on the skin.

Science Photo Library / Science Source

Treatment and Return to Participation

The many treatments for warts include salicylic acid, liquid nitrogen, and podophyllin. Blunt dissection and laser treatment are reserved for resistant cases. Imiquimod (Aldara) has been approved for genital and perianal warts, and research shows that it may have some merit in treating common warts.[65] The NCAA will not permit wrestlers to participate if facial warts cannot be adequately covered with a mask. Furthermore, collegiate rules mandate that single or scattered verrucae be curetted before participation and cannot be seeping. In general, the NCAA mandates that verrucae be "adequately covered."[53] National high school rules do not provide treatment or restriction mandates.[54] Athletic trainers should check regional or state guidelines to be certain they are following local safety policies.

Prognosis is generally good because most lesions do eventually resolve spontaneously. Acid or freezing treatment of warts may result in a blood-tinged blister that eventually resolves into a scab. While the blister is present, it should be covered during participation. The best prevention for HPV is good skin hygiene that will help prevent transmission through damaged skin areas. There is currently a vaccine series (Gardasil 9) for males and females that prevents certain strains of HPV that can cause cervical cancer.[65] Chapter 14 provides the vaccine schedule for both children and adults.

Fungal Conditions

Fungal infections are extremely common in athletes, especially wrestlers, and the physically active. Fungal infections are often found on the skin, hair, and nails, with the most common infection sites being the scalp, face, extremities, trunk, groin, and feet. **Dermatophytes** are superficial fungal infections of the skin, and they are the most common infectious agents among humans.[66]

The dermatophytes discussed here are surface, or topical, fungal conditions and include tinea corporis, tinea cruris, tinea unguium, tinea pedis, tinea capitis, tinea barbae, and tinea versicolor. Tinea infections are named according to the affected body area. All are true fungal infections except for tinea versicolor, which is categorized as a yeast disorder. Table 16.2 lists the common tinea infections, their location on the body, and typical treatment. As a group, these conditions tend to be transmitted from person to person or from animal to person. Most respond well to topical antifungal ointments, but newer systemic oral medications have proven to be effective alternatives to their topical counterparts.[6]

Fungal infections are usually diagnosed based on appearance alone, but each can be distinguished by microscopic examination with a KOH stain. Patients who have recently used a topical over-the-counter antifungal medication may present with a false-negative KOH stain.[67] In general, medical treatment is continued for at least 2 wk after resolution of the lesions.[68]

Preventive measures for all fungal infections include keeping wet materials away from the body; fully drying clothing, towels, and uniforms before using them; and allowing light and air exposure to the skin as practical. Additional measures include good personal hygiene, as outlined in the Prevention Strategies for Infectious Dermatological Conditions in Athletes sidebar, including not sharing clothing, towels, or personal items such as grooming accessories and wearing foot protection when using common shower facilities. Showering with hot water and soap and washing hair with shampoo immediately after practices or athletic events helps prevent fungal and skin diseases in general.[46,57,58]

Unless specifically addressed in the categories that follow, unexposed (i.e., covered by a uniform or clothing) tinea infections have no restrictions, and the athlete can participate as tolerated. In both collegiate and high school wrestling, athletes with tinea infections require 72 h of medication treatment before returning to participation. When no longer contagious, these athletes should cover lesions with bio-occlusive dressings.[53,54] More specific guidelines are addressed in the NCAA

TABLE 16.2 **Comparison of the Tinea Fungi**

Name	Body part affected	Signs and symptoms	Treatment
Tinea corporis	Ringworm on the body	Scaling, deep erythema; well-defined margins; pruritic	Topical antifungal agents; difficult or recurrent cases may need griseofulvin or oral terbinafine
Tinea pedis	Athlete's foot	Within the interdigital web spaces; maceration, pruritic	Topical cream-based antifungals, such as tolnaftate (Tinactin) or terbinafine (Lamisil), are often used; oral antifungals may be necessary in difficult cases
Tinea unguium	Nails of the hands or feet	Nail thickening; multiple nails involved; hyperkeratosis	Griseofulvin, terbinafine, itraconazole (topical antifungal agents not effective)
Tinea capitis	Scalp	Scaly, patchy alopecia; pruritic	Oral antifungal agents; antibiotics if necessary; oral steroids to prevent scarring, hair loss
Tinea cruris	Jock itch, primarily in the groin	Scaly, erythematous rash; pruritic	Same as tinea corporis
Tinea barbae	Beard or base of neck	Inflammatory folliculitis on face; often scars	Oral terbinafine

and NFHS Participation Regulations for Wrestlers With Tinea Infections sidebar.

Tinea Corporis

Tinea corporis, otherwise known as *ringworm*, is caused by the *Trichophyton*, *Microsporum*, and *Epidermophyton* species. The organism most commonly identified is *T. rubrum*, which accounts for 47% of tinea corporis cases.[69]

Tinea corporis is common in wrestling and is spread mostly by skin-to-skin contact. Wrestlers develop mat burns, abrasions, and scrapes during competition that provide easy entry for fungal infection. Fungus also develops best in dark, damp, humid conditions. Sites inside shoes or in damp clothing that has not been properly laundered and is hung in a dark, enclosed locker are particularly favorable.[47]

Signs and Symptoms

The lesions of tinea corporis are erythematous, scaly areas of varying size and may have a clear area in the center (figure 16.21). The active areas of infection are at the border, and the central clearing develops as the fungus digests cells as it moves away from the center. Tinea corporis may be itchy or asymptomatic. It is important to also check the feet of a patient with tinea because this may be the original source.

Differential diagnoses for tinea corporis include contact dermatitis, psoriasis, atopic dermatitis, seborrheic

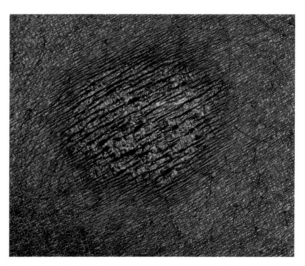

FIGURE 16.21 Tinea corporis, also called *ringworm*, presents with a red, scaly border.
Scott Camazine/Medical Images

dermatitis, pityriasis alba, pityriasis rosea, pityriasis versicolor, subacute lupus erythematosus, and erythema migrans.[3]

Referral and Diagnostic Tests

Diagnosis of tinea corporis is made by clinical and microscopic examination. The lesion is scraped onto a slide and examined with KOH staining under a microscope. Multiple hyphae (the branches of the fungus cell)

NCAA and NFHS Participation Regulations for Wrestlers With Tinea Infections

NCAA

- At least 72 h of oral or topical therapy for skin lesion must be completed. Over-the-counter medications are inappropriate for treatment.
- The NCAA Skin Evaluation and Participation Status form shall be provided at weigh-in and used to document the duration of therapy.
- If active lesions can be "adequately covered," a wrestler may participate. (There are specific instructions to be compliant with the "adequately covered" statement.)
- The physician or athletic trainer is responsible for completing skin checks and ensuring infections are adequately covered.
- On-site medical personnel will disqualify wrestlers with extensive, multiple lesions that are not under documented treatment following assessment.
- For diagnosed tinea capitis scalp lesions, at least 2 wk of prescription, oral systemic antifungal therapy must be completed.
- If active lesions cannot be adequately covered, the athlete may not participate.
- Final disposition of the student-athlete participation status may be decided on an individual basis by the on-site physician or certified athletic trainer.

NFHS

- Athletes with tinea infections cannot participate until they have been taking oral antifungal medication for 72 h and must wait a minimum of 1 wk after lesion resolution.
- Once the lesion is no longer infectious, it may be covered with a bio-occlusive dressing.
- The NFHS also adheres to the NCAA guideline on tinea capitis.

Adapted from NCAA (2019); National Federation of State High School Associations (2022)

are seen on active lesions. Patients with extensive skin involvement, persistence of symptoms despite treatment, and any lesions that are questionable should be referred to a physician.

Treatment and Return to Participation

Treatment employs topical or oral antifungal medications. Topical antifungal creams are the most commonly used. Typical treatment with topical antifungal medication for noninflammatory tinea corporis includes twice-daily treatment for 1 to 4 wk, depending on the type of cream. Each antifungal is different and is individually dose adjusted. On occasion, the lesions are too extensive for topical treatment, and oral medications such as terbinafine, itraconazole, and fluconazole are used. These medications must typically be taken for up to 4 wk to be fully effective.[35,69]

In addition, athletes should shower and clean the affected area daily. Clothing needs to be laundered after each practice or competition; sweaty clothes, elastic wraps, equipment, or towels should not be left in a closed locker.[67]

The prognosis for tinea corporis is good if the patient uses the treatment as directed. If infection recurs, then the fungus is resistant to the medication used, the treatment was not administered properly, or another source of infection exists that has not been detected. Athletes, especially wrestlers, may return to activity after 3 d of topical antifungal treatment for tinea corporis. Small local lesions are treated by washing with an antifungal shampoo (selenium sulfide or ketoconazole), applying a fungicidal cream (terbinafine or naftifine), covering with a semipermeable membrane (e.g., OpSite or Bioclusive), and wrapping with a prewrap followed by flexible tape. This process is repeated after each practice or match to allow the lesion to air dry.

Prevention

Many isolated cultures from the lesions are the same species as those cultured from the scalp. Therefore, it may be beneficial to have athletes, especially wrestlers, shampoo with an antifungal shampoo such as Head & Shoulders (Procter & Gamble) or Nizoral (Johnson & Johnson). Mats need to be cleaned daily and allowed to dry before storing.

Tinea Cruris

Tinea cruris, or *jock itch*, is another common fungal infection and usually occurs in the warm summer months. Although tinea cruris is more common in men, it also affects women. It affects the inner thigh, perineum, and perianal regions, with the scrotum, penis, and vagina typically not affected.[6] Most often, the culprits are tight-fitting clothing and humid conditions. Members of the military, athletes, and prison inmates have an increased risk of contracting tinea cruris because their clothing may be tight fitting and they may not be able to completely dry it out before rewearing it. Bathing suits that have not completely dried out can also cause tinea cruris.[70]

Signs and Symptoms

Signs and symptoms of tinea cruris are similar to those for other fungal infections. It presents with a well-demarcated, scaly, erythematous rash that tends to be pruritic.[70] As noted previously, tinea cruris is localized to the groin area. Patients who complain of symptoms from tinea cruris are referred to a physician if conservative over-the-counter treatment fails.

The differential diagnoses for tinea cruris include heat rash, candidiasis, erythrasma dermatitis from clothing or soap, or skin abrasion from clothing. If the lesions appear with a beefy red color and involvement of the scrotum, most likely the condition is candidiasis and not tinea cruris.

Treatment and Return to Participation

Antifungal agents are the treatment of choice for tinea cruris. Treatment includes completely drying off after showering and applying antifungal ointment. Loose-fitting clothing will promote healing, as will maintaining proper hygiene. Changing clothes often and laundering them in hot water also helps to break the cycle.[58,70] All areas of the body with an active tinea infection must be treated simultaneously to prevent recurrence.[68] Antifungal powders and sprays may help to prevent tinea cruris; however, creams are more effective.

Tinea Unguium

Tinea unguium is also known as *ringworm of the nails*. It is more common in the fingernails but can also occur in the toenails. Athletes who wear gloves to participate, such as goalkeepers, ice hockey, lacrosse, and football receivers, are more prone to this condition.

Signs and Symptoms

The most telling signs of tinea unguium are thickening and a lusterless, opaque coloring of the nail. As the condition progresses, the nail plate separates from the nail bed, and the nail itself may be destroyed. Patients who present with thickened, yellowish nails are referred to a physician for medication to treat the fungus causing the problem. The differential diagnosis for tinea unguium is injury to the nail.

Treatment and Return to Participation

Treatment of this condition is especially tedious and lengthy. Topical antifungal treatment is typically ineffective. Instead, oral systemic medication taken twice daily is required for up to 4 mo. Unlike antibiotics, this medication does not need to be taken until all signs of the fungus are gone. The systemic drugs bind to the nail plate and continue to work after oral administration is complete.[68]

As with many of the tinea infections, participation is not restricted for athletes with tinea unguium. Certain conditions, however, make athletes more prone to the condition. This includes wearing hand protection that covers their nails (e.g., soccer goalkeepers, hockey players). The dark, moist environment is an excellent place for this fungus to flourish. Equipment, especially equipment used in the summer or during twice-daily practices, is not always allowed to completely dry before reuse.[67]

Prevention

Using open-finger gloves, such as those used in cycling and weightlifting, is one way to reduce the risk of infection, but this is not possible in some sports. Athletes would be wise to avoid the warm, moist, dark conditions that encourage tinea infections, by keeping fingers and toes clean and dry; removing socks, shoes, and hand wear immediately after practice; allowing hand wear to completely dry before wearing again; and always wearing clean, dry socks.

Tinea Pedis

Tinea pedis, also known as *athlete's foot*, is the most common dermatophyte infection because shoes promote dark and moist conditions.

Signs and Symptoms

The most common sites for tinea pedis are between the toes and on the lateral areas of the feet and soles. The affected area between the toes is usually macerated and scaly (figure 16.22). The foot may also demonstrate the classic ringworm pattern of tinea corporis. The lateral edges and soles usually have dry, scaly, erythematous areas, and these lesions are usually, but not always, itchy.

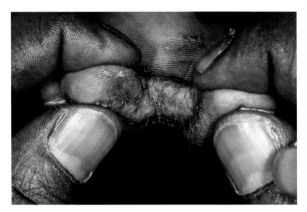

FIGURE 16.22 Tinea pedis starts in the moist areas between toes and is shown here spreading to the top of the foot.

Jack Jerjian/Medical Images

It is not uncommon for cracks or fissures to develop in the macerated skin.[71]

Referral and Diagnostic Tests

Diagnostic tests include scraping the scales for a microscopic evaluation with a KOH preparation. The patient is referred to a physician if symptoms persist despite treatment.

Differential diagnoses for tinea pedis include impetigo, erythrasma, pitted keratolysis, *P. aeruginosa* infection, psoriasis, allergic dermatitis, cutaneous candidiasis, dyshidrosis, and contact dermatitis.[71]

Treatment and Return to Participation

Treatment of tinea pedis consists of topical antifungal creams, first with application twice daily for 2 to 4 wk. If the infection does not respond, another antifungal drug family is tried.

People can help prevent tinea pedis fungal infections by wearing wicking socks, by wearing sandals, or by frequently removing their shoes to allow their feet to dry. Wearing sandals in public showering facilities also helps prevent transmission of the fungus.

Participation is not limited unless the athlete lets the condition go too far and develops secondary lymphangitis, cellulitis, or osteomyelitis. These dangerous sequelae must be managed before a full return to participation.[71]

Tinea Capitis

Tinea capitis, or *scalp ringworm*, occurs commonly in children and is spread by pets or other infected people. In addition to the scalp, tinea capitis can be found in the eyebrows and eyelashes. It has several varieties with slight differences in presentation.

In general, the infection starts in the scalp and moves into the hair shaft. Black dots on the scalp where the follicle has broken or small semibald patches surrounded by lusterless hairs may be present.[66] Often, there is a raised inflammatory response to the fungus resembling an abscess that quickly heals. The fungus may be limited to a small area in the hair, or it may persist, affecting the entire scalp.

Signs and Symptoms

The tinea capitis infection may be either inflammatory or noninflammatory. Most commonly, identifiable areas of hair loss, scales, and broken hair shafts are seen in the scalp (figure 16.23). Sometimes the infection causes an exaggerated inflammatory response and produces one or more inflamed, boggy, tender areas on the scalp called **kerions**. Because of this, the patient may present with low-grade but persistent inflammation.[47,68] The hair shafts are usually destroyed, and scarring is common after the kerion resolves.

The differential diagnoses for tinea capitis include **alopecia areata**, psoriasis, atopic dermatitis, and seborrheic dermatitis.

Referral and Diagnostic Tests

Individuals who experience patchy hair loss, who have been exposed to tinea capitis, or who have signs of tinea capitis are referred for medical treatment. Diagnosis is determined by clinical and microscopic examination. Hairs easily removed are examined with a KOH stain under a microscope. Multiple spores are seen either inside or outside infected hair shafts. A **Wood's lamp**, which provides UV light, demonstrates fluorescence in the case of some fungal infections, but it is not useful in identifying *Trichophyton tonsurans* (tinea corporis).

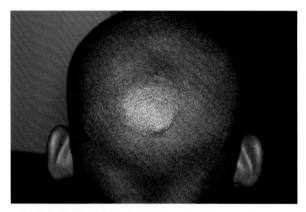

FIGURE 16.23 Tinea capitis is ringworm of the scalp, and it can lead to hair loss.

The Division of Dermatology at Brody School of Medicine, East Carolina University

Treatment and Return to Participation

Topical antifungal medications are not as effective with tinea capitis, and oral antifungal medications are often needed. Griseofulvin is the most common medication used in the treatment of tinea capitis. Treatment is continued until 2 wk after KOH preparations are negative. Prednisone and systemic antibiotics may also be used to treat tinea capitis.

The NCAA and the NFHS have specific regulations about unrestricted return to activity (see the NCAA and NFHS Participation Regulations for Wrestlers With Tinea Infections sidebar).[53,54] Return to participation is up to the discretion of the treating physician and may be less of an issue in noncontact sports or sports with helmets.

Because tinea capitis is easily transmitted on inanimate objects, all combs, brushes, hats, and other headgear used or worn by the athlete must be cleaned. Spores of tinea are shed into the air around infected persons and their clothing, so preventive measures must include laundering bed linens, towels, and clothing. Roommates or family members of affected athletes should also be examined for tinea capitis.[41,58,68]

Tinea Versicolor

Tinea versicolor is a common yeast infection seen in adolescents and young adults. This infection is not contagious and is common in high-humidity environments and sometimes in areas that feature prolonged use of topical corticosteroids. Tinea versicolor is marked by areas of hyper- or hypopigmentation. It may go unnoticed for months to years, and it usually produces very few symptoms, if any.[3]

This yeast is part of the normal skin flora, but it can produce an infection that is found mostly on the trunk, arms, neck, abdomen, and sometimes the groin. It is more common on the face and forehead in children but not in adults.

Signs and Symptoms

Tinea versicolor starts as multiple, small, round, scaly macules that enlarge radially. They may present as white, brown, or pink areas of the skin that increase, and they may or may not cause itching (figure 16.24). These areas typically will not tan when exposed to the sun or UV light.[68,78]

The differential diagnoses for versicolor include vitiligo, postinflammatory hypopigmentation, pityriasis alba, pityriasis rosea, nummular eczema, guttate psoriasis, seborrheic dermatitis, and tinea corporis.[72]

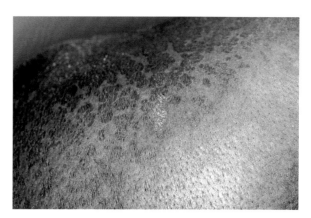

FIGURE 16.24   Tinea versicolor is often first noted as an area that does not tan.

The Division of Dermatology at Brody School of Medicine, East Carolina University

Referral and Diagnostic Tests

Patients who have patchy areas that do not tan, who have varying pigmentation, or who do not respond to conservative treatment are referred to a physician. The diagnosis is confirmed by scraping the scales onto a slide and examining them microscopically. Microscopic examination with KOH staining reveals a "spaghetti and meatballs" appearance. A Wood's lamp may demonstrate a pale-yellow, white, or even a blue-green fluorescence pattern.[49,67]

Treatment and Return to Participation

Tinea versicolor is treated in many ways. The most common treatment is with a selenium sulfide 2.5% lotion (Selsun Blue shampoo; Chattem), which is applied for 10 min and then washed off. Alternatively, the shampoo may be applied at bedtime to all body areas except the scrotum and washed off in the morning. The typical course of treatment is 7 d.[58]

Another treatment is ketoconazole cream or shampoo (Nizoral) applied once daily for 2 wk. For resistant cases, both cream and oral antifungal medication may be prescribed.

Prevention

Prevention of reinfection includes ketoconazole or selenium sulfide treatments once weekly or every other week. Using a salicylic acid, sulfur, or pyrithione zinc bar may also be helpful.

Parasitic Conditions and Bites

Parasitic infestations and insect bites are common causes of skin inflammation and infection. A wide range of insects can cause skin eruptions. The most common infections caused by parasites are pediculosis and scabies. **Pediculosis**, an infection caused by lice, occurs in three forms: head lice, body lice, and pubic lice. Lice feed on human blood after injecting their victim with saliva. In many, lice cause severe pruritus as a result of an allergic reaction to the parasite's saliva.[73,74] **Scabies** is caused by the mite *Sarcoptes scabiei*. Both are spread by person-to-person or person-to-object transmission. These parasites do not hop or fly; they move by crawling.

Head Lice

It is estimated that 6 to 12 million people are infested annually with head lice, also known as *Pediculus humanus capitis*.[75] The presence of head lice is not an indicator of a person's hygiene or environment. Lice occur most frequently in children ages 3 to 11 yr, and they are less common among African American individuals than among other races.[68,74] A single female louse lays three to six eggs (nits) per day that are glued to the base of hair shafts. The eggs hatch after 8 to 9 d. The hatched nymphs begin at 1 mm in length; they reach maturity in 9 to 12 d and can begin laying eggs.[74] When mature, these tiny insects are about 1/10 to 1/8 in. long and live on the human scalp while feeding on human blood. The lice themselves are hard to see, but the nits can be seen at the hairline behind the ears or on the base of the scalp (figure 16.25). Both forms of lice are transmitted by contact with a person who is already infested, through sharing personal items such as combs, towels, hats, helmets, or other clothing as well as bedding, carpet, couches, stuffed animals, or pillows.[74] Lice cannot survive without a human host for longer than 48 h.[74]

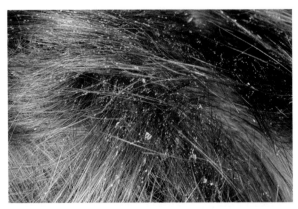

FIGURE 16.25 Pediculosis humanus capitis.

The Division of Dermatology at Brody School of Medicine, East Carolina University

Signs and Symptoms

Clinical presentation consists of intense itching of the scalp and the sighting of nits. The itching may not start until several weeks after infestation.

Referral and Diagnostic Tests

An individual who shows signs of lice is referred to a physician for confirmation of infestation. Nits that are attached more than 1/4 in. from the scalp are already hatched or dead, but the presence of dead nits may not be an indicator of a current infestation with head lice.[47,74] It is critical to continue to inspect for crawling nits, as they can be seen with the naked eye.

Treatment and Return to Participation

Treatment consists of the application of topical medications, including Nix, RID, malathion (Ovide), and lindane (Kwell). Nix (Insight Pharmaceuticals) and RID (Bayer HealthCare) are the initial treatments of choice because lindane has been associated with neurological toxicity in some cases. The lice are usually killed with one treatment, but a second treatment may be needed 7 to 10 d later. After the first treatment, a nit comb is used to remove the eggs. Any nits found more than 1/2 in. along the hair shaft are old and dead; nits less than 1/4 in. along the hair shaft 1 wk after treatment may be new and may necessitate retreatment. The person needs to be checked for lice every 2 or 3 d for 2 wk. Do not use a cream rinse, conditioner, or combination shampoo and conditioner before using medication because it will negate the effects of the treatment. The hair should not be rewashed for 1 to 2 d after treatment.[47,74,76]

It is also imperative to wash all bedding and recently worn clothing in hot water at a temperature greater than 54 °C (130 °F) and to dry them on a hot cycle for at least 20 min. Nonwashable clothing is dry-cleaned. Items that cannot be washed or dry-cleaned, such as helmets, headgear, and shoes, can be placed in a double plastic bag for 2 wk. Vacuuming the floor and furniture completes the extermination procedure. On occasion, fumigation or chemical dusting may be required of the living space.[74]

Athletes can resume normal activity levels when all lice and nits are confirmed gone. However, the NCAA recommends that athletes be treated with pediculicide and reexamined for complete extermination of lice before return to sport.[53] Avoiding exposure to infected people and their personal items is the best preemptive tool against lice infestation.

Body Lice

Body lice, or *Pediculus humanus corporis*, unlike head lice, do not live on the human body but in clothing. The nits are found in the seams of clothing and the bedding of infested humans or in body hair. The lice only leave clothing to feed on humans, typically at night.[74] Also, unlike head lice, female body lice lay 15 to 20 eggs per day in clothing or bedding, and the mature louse lives up to 30 d. Infestation usually occurs when poor hygiene and crowded environments necessitate frequent close contact with others. Homeless people without regular access to bathing facilities or clean clothes are particularly vulnerable. People who bathe regularly are seldom infested.[68]

The usual clinical presentation is itching and a rash, usually around the waist, groin, and thighs. Body lice are treated by changing clothes regularly, bathing regularly, washing all clothing in hot water at a temperature above 54 °C (130 °F), drying it in a hot dryer for at least 20 min, and using RID or Nix shampoo applied to the body.[35] Compared to other types of lice, body lice are more likely to require fumigation to eradicate.

Pubic Lice

Pubic lice, or *Pthirus pubis*, commonly referred to as *crabs*, are usually found in the genital area but may also be seen on the legs, axilla, mustache, beard, eyebrows, and eyelashes. These lice are usually spread through sexual contact rather than through contact with infested towels, clothing, or bedding. They typically live 2 wk, and females lay one or two eggs a day. Pubic lice can migrate from the pubis, crawling up to 10 cm per day.[74]

Clinical presentation is usually intense itching in the genital area. The lice and nits are much easier to identify than head or body lice. Treatment for crabs is with RID, Nix, or lindane shampoo, followed by removal of nits with fingernails or nit combs. Clothing is washed in hot water at a temperature greater than 54 °C (130 °F), dried in a hot dryer for at least 20 min, and changed regularly; sexual partners need to be informed and treated as well and sexual activity should be avoided until appropriate treatment has successfully eradicated the infestation.[6]

Scabies

The other common parasite associated with skin infection is the mite *S. scabiei*, which causes scabies. Worldwide, approximately 300 million cases of scabies are reported annually.[73] Mites burrow under the upper layer of the skin and lay their eggs, which cause a pimple-like lesion and intense itching. Spread is usually the result of direct contact, sexual contact, or sharing of infested clothes or bedding. Scabies is common in overcrowded areas such as prisons, nursing homes, and other close-quarter living arrangements. These mites can survive away from the host for 48 to 72 h and therefore can be more challenging to eradicate than lice.[75]

Signs and Symptoms

Intense itching that interferes with sleep is commonly associated with scabies. The wrists, fingers, and ankles are the most obvious sites, but the itching may occur anywhere on the body, with the head and neck usually spared. The patient develops small red bumps that may be arranged in a linear fashion after itching (figure 16.26).

Differential diagnoses for scabies include drug reactions, folliculitis, insect bites, lice, urticaria, and dermatographism.[73]

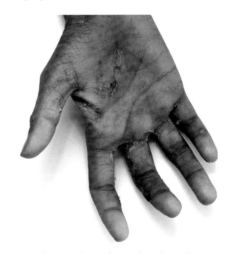

FIGURE 16.26   Palm infected with scabies.
Science Photo Library / Science Source

NCAA Participation Regulations for Wrestlers With Parasitic Conditions

The following regulations apply to participation with the parasitic conditions of pediculosis (lice) and scabies:

- Pediculosis must be treated with pediculicide and must show no infestation on reexamination.
- Athletes must have a negative scabies prep at the time of competition.

Adapted from NCAA (2019).

Referral and Diagnostic Tests

Diagnosis is usually made through clinical examination; however, finding a mite is extremely difficult and requires scraping the skin for a sample that is then examined under a microscope for a live mite. Sometimes a Burrow ink test is used for diagnosis. This test involves rubbing a washable felt marker across a suspected site, followed by removal of the ink with alcohol. The presence of scabies is confirmed when the ink penetrates the upper layer of the burrow, leaving a mark.[75] A diagnosis may also be confirmed microscopically via the presence of mite eggs or fecal matter (scybala).

Treatment and Return to Participation

Medications used to treat scabies (scabicides) are available only with a physician's prescription. Treatment is with 5% permethrin cream (Elimite) applied to the body from the neck down and washed off in 8 to 14 h, or 1% lindane per 1 oz of lotion, or 30 g of cream applied from the neck down and washed off after 8 h. Ivermectin taken orally is an alternative treatment.[73] The patient will likely need an antihistamine because itching may last for at least 2 wk after treatment begins. As with lice, all bedding and recently worn clothing need to be laundered in hot water above 54 °C (130 °F) and dried on a hot cycle for at least 20 min; nonwashable clothing needs to be dry-cleaned. Items that cannot be washed or dry-cleaned, such as helmets, headgear, and shoes, can be placed in a double plastic bag for 2 wk.[35] In addition, all floors and furniture must be vacuumed. The infected person needs to review close and sexual contacts within the past 30 d and notify those people for treatment as necessary.[77]

Insect Bites

Dermatological reaction to insect bites is extremely common. In the United States, 1 to 2 million people are severely allergic to insect venom. These bites also can lead to anaphylaxis, which causes 90 to 100 deaths in the United States each year.[78] These data may be underrepresented, as many deaths are attributed to heart attack or heatstroke. Exposure to insects becomes a possibility for physically active people during outdoor practice and events.

In addition to mosquitoes, covered in chapter 14, chiggers, ticks, wasps, bees, ants, and spiders can produce particularly bothersome reactions. Bites and stings can cause direct irritation from the insect's body parts or secretions, immediate or delayed-hypersensitivity responses, or specific effects from venoms, or they can serve as vectors for secondary invaders. Common reactions may be localized or spread across a larger part of the body and may include redness, pain, and swelling that may last as long as 10 d. Individuals with a prior history of allergic reaction to specific insect bites or stings can be extremely vulnerable and often carry an EpiPen (an epinephrine injection) when participating in outdoor activities.[79]

The brown recluse spider has received wide attention because of the possible dramatic reaction associated with its bites. Dermonecrotic arachnidism, described in the next section, is a condition that can result when this type of spider deposits venom within a host.[80] The brown recluse, also called the *fiddleback spider*, is very small at about 1.5 cm long and has a characteristic dark, violin-shaped marking on its dorsum with the broad base of the marking or "violin" located near the head and the narrow stem pointing toward the abdomen. The brown recluse spider is most prevalent in the southern half of the United States and prefers dark, quiet spaces under porches, woodpiles, and rocks or inside closets, barns, picture frames, and basements. It has also been found in dormitories, and it bites when a person is putting on clothing or rummaging through other materials where the spider resides.[81]

Signs and Symptoms

Insect bites can range from a nuisance to an emergency. Chigger bites can cause extreme discomfort for days and possibly lead to secondary lesions with bacterial infection as a result of scratching. Wasp and bee stings can be extremely dangerous when the person stung has an allergic reaction, which may quickly progress to anaphylaxis in sensitive individuals; therefore, first-aid kits should be equipped with EpiPens for emergencies. Symptoms resulting from tick bites, which can result in Rocky Mountain spotted fever or Lyme disease, do not develop immediately, often making diagnosis a challenge.[82]

A brown recluse spider bite can produce a dramatic and prolonged reaction called **dermonecrotic arachnidism**. The initial bite produces a bee sting–like pain and often only mild erythema and swelling, but these bites can create a severe reaction and may become necrotic within 6 h. In some cases, the wound begins to ache and becomes pruritic over the first 8 h, and subsequently a rapid blue-gray macular halo develops around the bite that represents local hemolysis. The area may become oblong or irregular and result in a sudden increase in pain. The macule then widens and sinks below the level of intact skin and may advance to necrosis, affecting the underlying muscle and broad areas of skin or even an entire extremity.[80] In such cases, when the dead tissue sloughs,

RED FLAGS FOR INSECT BITES

- Take the bites of any venomous insect seriously because the secretions, venom, and insect body parts can provoke dramatic or life-threatening reactions in sensitive individuals.
- Be aware of the insect varieties common to the geographical location.
- Recognize and refer individuals with signs and symptoms of anaphylaxis: agitation, chills, facial edema, swollen tongue, wheezing, difficulty breathing, flushing, generalized urticaria, hoarseness or difficulty talking, palpitations, near-syncopal or syncopal episodes, profuse sweating, palpitations, or cardiovascular collapse.
- Have epinephrine on hand for emergency use in the event of a severe reaction.

a large ulcer persists, resulting in significant scarring and prolonged healing. Systemically, patients with severe reactions often experience fever, chills, nausea, vomiting, myalgias, and weakness. These reactions are rare and generally limited to children.[79]

Referral and Diagnostic Tests

A patient who presents with a history of a bite with associated local severe reaction, fever, or systemic manifestations is referred to a physician immediately.

Treatment and Return to Participation

Insect bites usually are treated conservatively with ice and elevation of the affected extremity. Strenuous exercise, heat, and surgery are avoided.[82] Topical antibiotic ointment may be applied under a sterile dressing to retard infection. Antibiotics for *S. aureus* or *S. pyogenes* may be initiated, and a tetanus booster should be administered by a physician if the term of the vaccine has lapsed. Serious bites become evident in the first 24 to 48 h; in this event, the person is referred for medical treatment immediately.[81]

Prevention

Prevention of most insect bites involves avoiding the insects' habitat, including shrubs and wooded and bushy areas. Use chemical repellants properly by applying them over clothing. Use structural barriers, such as window screens, netting, and protective clothing, to prevent con-

tact with insects.[81,82] When putting on shoes, socks, and other apparel that have been left unattended outdoors, people must thoroughly shake them out. Exercise caution during storms and floods that may drive insects from their normal habitats.

Summary

This chapter introduces health care providers, educators, and students to the pathology of common skin conditions. Signs, symptoms, diagnostic tests, treatments, and suggestions for appropriate times to seek referral for dermatological disorders are discussed. A dermatological condition can be prevented from becoming more severe through early identification and referral for diagnosis and treatment. This chapter also presents the NCAA and NFHS guidelines for determining when wrestlers with various skin conditions may be allowed to participate. These regulations may differ or may vary from school district guidelines, amateur sport organization regulations, or the rules of other governing entities. Athletic trainers must become familiar with the rules for specific areas of athletic interest and must remain abreast of changes as they occur.

Clinical Tips
Proper Application of Insect Repellant

- Only use insect repellant approved by the U.S. Environmental Protection Agency (EPA).
- Do not use insect repellant on babies or pets.
- Repellant used on older children should have less than 10% DEET (*N*,*N*-diethyl-*m*-toluamide).
- Do not apply insect repellent to children's hands or faces.
- Spray repellant on clothing, hats, or skin but not on the face.
- Read the label to determine effectiveness time as well as specific insects the product deters.
- Completely wash hands with soap and water after application.

Adapted from "Tips to Prevent Mosquito Bites," Environmental Protection Agency, last modified July 6, 2023, https://www.epa.gov/insect-repellents/tips-prevent-mosquito-bites; M.R.M. da Silva and E. Ricci-Jnior, "An Approach to Natural Insect Repellent Formulations: From Basic Research to Technological Development," *Acta Tropica* 212 (2020): 105419.

Because these recommendations may be revised as research is conducted and made public, health care practitioners should continue to seek out new information as it becomes available. A prudent health care provider continues to educate patients about their personal responsibility for skin care, hygiene, and prevention regarding transmission of infectious skin disorders.

Apply It!

Go to HK*Propel* to complete the case studies for this chapter.

17

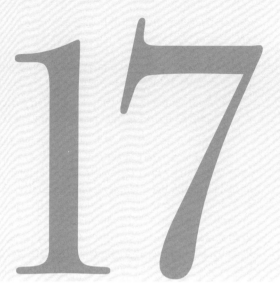

Psychological and Substance Use Disorders

Layne A. Prest

OBJECTIVES

At the completion of this chapter the reader should be able to do the following:

1. Recognize emotional and behavioral signs of common substance use disorders and psychological problems, including mood, anxiety, eating, and attention-deficit/hyperactivity disorders and suicidal ideation or risk of harm to self or others.

2. Intervene appropriately with the affected athlete through discussion, supportive confrontation, education, and referral.

3. Establish collaborative relationships with qualified physical and mental health professionals in the recognition and treatment process.

4. Identify a variety of educational and supportive resources (print, websites, and organizational materials) that are available to both professionals and patients affected by these disorders.

5. Educate patients about the effects, participation consequences, and risks of misuse and abuse of alcohol, tobacco, recreational drugs, performance-enhancing drugs, substances, and over-the-counter medications.

6. Develop and implement specific policies and procedures for the purposes of identifying and referring athletes in behavioral health crises to qualified providers.

The 21st century is supposed to be the era of healthier people, and, of course, athletes and physically active individuals usually are among the healthiest. Therein lies the main dilemma when assessing and intervening in potential mental health concerns of these individuals. Many people, perhaps athletes more than the average person, have been conditioned to minimize or even deny physical health problems, and they are even more inclined to do so with mental health issues. Being sick or disabled physically is one thing; being weak mentally or emotionally is quite another. Professionals working with athletes are becoming increasingly likely to have been educated about mental health issues or to know of someone who has struggled with emotional or behavioral problems. It is hoped that more open discussion about these disorders will increase the likelihood of early detection and appropriate intervention. This chapter describes the signs, symptoms, and prognoses of the most common mental health and substance use disorders. It is not intended to teach actual counseling techniques, which is beyond the scope of practice; rather, this chapter aims to help athletic trainers know when, and to whom, to refer patients. To that end, this chapter outlines the mental health problems most commonly experienced by athletes, discusses the frequent comorbidity among them, suggests red flags for early detection, and describes strategies for intervention.

According to the World Health Organization (WHO), the prevalence of mental health conditions is increasing worldwide, with a 13% rise in mental health conditions and substance use disorders since 2012.

- One in every eight people in the world live with a mental disorder.
- Twenty percent of the world's children and adolescents have a mental health condition.

- Suicide is the second leading cause of death among 15- to 29-year-olds.
- Approximately one in five people in postconflict settings have a mental health condition.[1]

The four leading causes of disability are several forms of depression, anxiety disorders, suicide or self-harm, and alcohol use. Other serious disorders include schizophrenia, bipolar disorder, dementia, obsessive–compulsive disorder, posttraumatic stress disorder, and panic disorder.[1] Problems with attention and concentration, disordered eating, personality issues, and other forms of substance abuse also contribute greatly to disease burden worldwide.[2] Some of these difficulties (chiefly depression, anxiety, and substance abuse problems) are ubiquitous and frequently co-occur in the United States. Others, including attention-deficit/hyperactivity disorder (ADHD), personality disorders, and disordered eating, are not as common. All can impair athletic performance and overall life adjustment. These conditions also can be difficult to treat, especially if allowed to escalate. Therefore, athletic trainers working with physically active people must be able to identify these potentially serious problems as early as possible. Following a description of typical physical and emotional symptoms, diagnostic criteria, and potential red flags, suggestions are made for initial intervention, referral, and treatment. The diagnostic criteria are taken from the fifth edition of the *Diagnostic and Statistical Manual of Mental Disorders* (*DSM-5*).[3]

Understanding the Role of Mental Health Professionals

At the outset, a full and comprehensive treatment plan must be developed in the context of the patient's relationship with a trusted, licensed mental health professional (MHP) operating within the scope of their professional practice. The athletic trainer, who may be among the first to detect a problem, can be instrumental in getting the patient needed help with an appropriate mental health provider. Athletic trainers need to be familiar with the professionals to whom they may refer someone for services. A reasonable place to start is with the patient's primary care physician.

The U.S. federal government identifies five disciplines as competent to provide mental health services: (1) psychiatry, (2) psychology, (3) marriage, couple, and family therapy, (4) social work, and (5) psychiatric nursing (table 17.1). Other professionals, besides primary caregivers, who provide mental health services include professional counselors and clergy members. Licensure and certification for most of these professionals are becoming standardized within each discipline, and boundaries are delineated between disciplines. Some overlap remains, however, and providers in any of these categories can potentially help with the clinical problems this chapter addresses. Referrals may be guided somewhat by the discipline of the professional but, more importantly, by the person's clinical specialty.

The training of psychiatrists and psychiatric nurse practitioners enables them to assess the patient from a medical point of view and to prescribe medicine to address the underlying physiological or chemical components of the problem. They may also provide supportive counseling, psychoeducation, or assistance in problem-solving. If a major mental disorder is suspected and medical intervention is needed, referral to one of these professionals would be appropriate.

The various types of psychologists—clinical, educational, and counseling—have different but overlapping training, experience, and areas of expertise. They can be trained at either the master's or doctoral level. Typically, psychologists are the professionals to contact if psychological or educational testing is needed. Psychologists also provide psychotherapy services.

Marriage, couple, and family therapists (MCFTs), especially medical family therapists, assess problems from the biopsychosocial point of view. Consequently, their clinical approach considers various aspects of the person's life. MCFTs work with typical mental health issues, such as depression, anxiety, eating disorders, and ADHD, but they will often do so by considering the sociocultural context and including part or all of the family in collaboration with a primary care provider.

TABLE 17.1 Disciplines Providing Mental Health Services

Discipline	Typical credentials	Approach
Psychiatry	MD, DO	Medical approach, including medication
Psychology	MS, PhD, PsyD, EdD	Psychological testing and psychotherapy; individual psychotherapy
Marriage, couple, and family therapy	MA, MS, PhD	Biopsychosocial assessment; family systems therapy
Social work	MSW	Holistic approach; social services
Psychiatric nursing	RN, APRN	Medical approach, including medication

Social workers usually specialize in addressing macro issues, such as housing, income, or food deficiencies and insurance needs, or micro issues, such as psychotherapy. Social work as a discipline also takes a holistic perspective on the client. Many social workers also provide psychotherapy services similar to those of other mental health providers.

MHPs increasingly are being called on to demonstrate the effectiveness of their work with clients. As a result, more attention is being focused on the development of evidence-based protocols. Therapy typically begins with an intake session, during which the professional gathers background information (e.g., family of origin details), a description of the problem and previous attempts to address it, and the client's goals. A contract governing the frequency and duration of sessions is negotiated, and parameters of confidentiality are discussed. If MHPs wish to contact other professionals, including the athletic trainer or family members working with the client, they will obtain a signed consent for release of information.

Overview of Mental Health Issues in the Athlete

Everyone has symptoms of some type of mental health and/or substance use issue at some time in life when one or several stressors overwhelm the person's ability to self-regulate. The symptoms are usually, and arbitrarily, labeled either physical or mental. This artificial dichotomy usually does not align with the affected person's reality. Rarely is an athlete with a strained hamstring not also worried about the injury or distressed by the pain. Similarly, the most common initial warning signs of depression or anxiety are the physical symptoms of tension, restlessness, and disturbed sleep, energy, and appetite. This is because the systems of the mind, body, spirit, and relationships overlap, and each is integrally connected to the others and located within sociocultural contexts that help give them meaning.[4] When the homeostasis of one or more systems is disrupted, people instinctively try to correct the problem regardless of its origin. In the mental health domain, signs of distress are emotional, mental, behavioral, and physical. The reported prevalence of mental health symptoms and disorders among current and former elite athletes has been reported from 19% for alcohol misuse to 34% for anxiety and/or depression.[5]

Framework for Understanding Mental Health

In almost all situations, a variety of overlapping factors contribute to symptom development. The **biopsychosocial–spiritual model (BPSS)** is a framework for understanding the person's responses in a given situation and the development of symptoms. Symptom etiology may

be conceptualized as a pie. Figure 17.1 shows how these various factors overlap and contribute to well-being. In a given person, the various pieces of the BPSS pie may be larger or smaller at any one time. The relative sizes of the pieces greatly influence the person's symptoms and ability to adapt.

For example, two runners may have identical injuries, but the effects of the injury and the course of rehabilitation in these two athletes will usually differ. The amount of pain they have, as well as the length of time until they are ready to compete again, will be influenced not only by the difference in respective levels of physical conditioning and injury history but also by other physical and emotional conditions, such as pain tolerance, attitude, perception of the problem, and its implications for life. The situation may also be affected by personality and temperament issues, variable resources for coping, and so on. Another example involves two wrestlers who seem to be equally competitive, but wrestler A, in a struggle to make or maintain weight, develops more obviously disordered eating patterns than wrestler B. Perhaps wrestler A has a family history of obesity and is genetically predisposed toward weight gain more than the other; temperamentally, wrestler A may tend to think more negatively about life challenges, become somewhat self-defeating in the face of adversity, and find emotional comfort in food and the process of eating. Often a variety of factors will help to explain the development of clinically significant problems.

This interplay of variables is the same for athletes as it is for others who are physically active, regardless of whether the symptoms of an injury or condition are

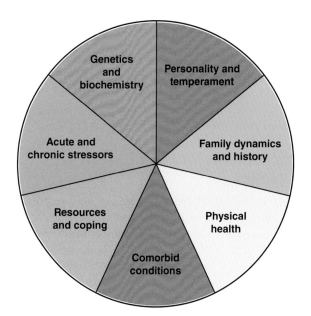

FIGURE 17.1 The biopsychosocial–spiritual model is a framework for understanding a person's responses in a given situation and the development of symptoms.

physical or emotional. Whereas one athlete may become depressed, another's symptoms may include anxiety or outbursts of anger and physical aggression. Sometimes one piece of the BPSS pie is so big that it seems to account for virtually the whole reason that someone is symptomatic (e.g., the chemical disequilibrium that comes with bipolar disorder). For this reason, it is a good practice to regularly consider the possibility that an organic cause may be the culprit and refer the person for a medical evaluation.

The treatments that have proven effective for the problems discussed in this chapter are based on the same BPSS approach as the assessment and diagnosis. Different strategies can be useful, depending on the bio-psychosocial–spiritual components that are implicated in the assessment process. Practitioners often recommend treatment plans based on their assessment and experience, and then these are negotiated with the patient or family members according to personal preferences. The treatment may be offered on either an inpatient or, more commonly, an outpatient basis.

Treatment may also involve the collaboration of a variety of treatment professionals. For example, eating disorder treatment often involves a physician, a registered dietitian, and a psychotherapist. This will be determined based on the severity of symptoms, the difficulty the patient has in making changes, the amount of support the patient has, and other resources that affect care, including financial concerns or insurance benefits. The important first step in treatment is accurate assessment, followed by clear and well-timed communication and education with the patient and family. The athletic trainer can play a valuable role here because people are much more likely to engage in treatment or some type of change process if they become convinced that there is a problem, they know what it is, and they know that something can be done about it. This is because most people will want to know what is going on with themselves, how they "got it," and what they can do to "get rid of it" or at least cope more effectively. Additional treatment recommendations specific to various clinical problems are listed in subsequent sections.

Implications for Participation in Athletics

Early identification and treatment are very helpful in preventing problems from worsening, but sometimes the stigma still associated with mental health conditions prevents people from recognizing these problems in themselves or others. In those cases, functioning in one or more areas of life can be affected, sometimes severely. Restricting participation in a sport, if necessary, will depend on the assessment of the athlete's level of functioning by the athlete, the coach, and the athletic trainer. For example, while a medication dosage is initially being adjusted, the athlete could experience adverse effects that could affect participation or performance, such as nausea, headache, sedation, disturbed balance, or overstimulation. It is important for the physician and the athletic trainer to work closely together to understand how various medications might affect the athlete's performance. The National Collegiate Athletics Association has no restrictions on the medications typically used to treat these conditions except for stimulants such as pemoline, a medication prescribed to treat ADHD.[6]

The last general point to be made is that some people experiencing psychological and/or substance use disorders may consider suicide, self-harm, or become threatening to others and even homicidal. Most health care professionals or other professionals are required by law or by a professional code of ethics (e.g., the American Association for Marriage and Family Therapy Code of Ethics[70]) to report to the authorities if a patient is a danger to themself or others. Athletic trainers, too, may encounter an athlete with depression, panic disorder, or substance abuse who is considering suicide or harming someone else. The athletic trainer must seek immediate consultation if in doubt about the need to report. An assessment of whether one is considering or intent on harming self or others includes determining whether the person has a specific plan, the means to carry it out, the intention to carry it out, and how lethal the plan is. Those with a personal or family history of this type of ideation or action or whose judgment is impaired, perhaps through substance use, are more at risk of following through.

Role of Stress in Psychological and Substance Use Disorders

A related topic for the health care professional to consider is the role of stress in the patient's life. Determining how much stress an individual is experiencing, and how well they are coping, is an important part of assessing the overall level of functioning. First, what is stress? Stress is alternately considered bad, normal, healthy in moderation, or an inescapable fact of life. In fact, all of these are true. *Stress* is the term used for the effects that physical, emotional, psychological, and social experiences have on individuals. Athletes, like all human beings, experience stress just by living life, and because of the demands that training places on them, athletes have additional stress with which to contend. But stress is a two-sided coin. Individuals need the stimulation, challenge, and motivation that come from being stressed. Because individuals are stressed, they strive to meet basic survival needs for themselves and their loved ones. Being stressed is what helps individuals push toward a goal and rise to the occasion in competitions. But too much stress can be debilitating. Ineffective stress management contributes to the psychological and substance use disorders described in this chapter. When overloaded with demands, athletes and physically active individuals can begin to decompensate, becoming less effective and ultimately failing in their pursuits. The discussion of stress for the last several decades has focused on both sides of the coin. Research and clinical experiences suggest that individuals should strive for a balance between rest and activity, pushing for improvement and adjusting to limitations, and between a goal-directed orientation and being in the experience. Athletic trainers should help the athletes and patients with whom they work to pause and reflect on the amount of stress they are under and whether the effects are helpful and motivational or undermining and disabling.

There are a variety of tools for measuring stress—some adapted for specific populations. One that has been used in studying athletes in a variety of sports is the COPE Inventory (full and brief versions are available online). By having an athlete complete this inventory, the athletic trainer can get a clearer sense about the patient's coping strategies and the degree to which the patient is coping successfully and constructively.

Anxiety Disorders

Anxiety is one of the most common human experiences despite some cross-cultural differences.[7] For example, most people have experienced a momentary sensation of "butterflies" in the stomach. In fact, the ability to respond with anxiety is considered normal and even desirable, and anxiety is what helps individuals "get their game face on." However, given the right set of factors—physiology, central nervous system sensitivity, perceptual filters, belief system, coping, and support system—people may respond to one or more acute or chronic stressors by developing anxiety serious enough to be considered a disorder. This is a case of too much of a good or necessary thing. The individual is wracked with very serious and debilitating apprehension, excessive and ongoing worry, overwhelming fears, panic attacks, or compulsive behaviors. Slightly more than 18% of the American population experiences one of the more debilitating forms of anxiety and has been diagnosed with an anxiety disorder.[7] Another study indicates that 31.9% of adolescents suffer from serious anxiety.[8]

Red flags for problems with anxiety include outbursts of irritability or anger, substance abuse, changes in athletic performance, or other behaviors that are uncharacteristic for the athlete or patient. Anxiety symptoms include both somatic–behavioral and emotional–cognitive disturbances.[7] The presence of some or all of these symptoms may signal an anxiety problem or even an anxiety disorder:

- Difficulty getting to sleep
- Shortness of breath
- Dizziness, lightheadedness
- Sweating
- Feeling of choking
- Impairment of performance
- Feelings of unreality
- Worry, nervousness
- Appetite disturbance
- Paresthesias
- Chills or hot flashes
- Gastritis, nausea
- Psychomotor agitation
- Irritability
- Fear of losing control
- Feelings of going crazy or dying

People can be screened for anxiety disorders using a variety of standardized measures, such as the Generalized Anxiety Disorder-7 (GAD-7) available from the Anxiety and Depression Association of America website.[9]

Generalized Anxiety Disorder

Generalized anxiety disorder (GAD) is a condition in which the person is worried or nervous about many or most things in life. The person may complain on a regular basis of one or more of the anxiety symptoms listed previously. Criteria for diagnosing generalized anxiety are as follows:

- excessive daily anxiety or worry for 6 mo;
- difficulty controlling the worry;
- three or more anxiety symptoms; and
- impairment in social, academic or occupational, or relational functioning because of the anxiety.

It has been estimated that 6.8 million people, or 3.1% of the U.S. population, have this disorder in a 12 mo period. Women are twice as likely as men to report generalized anxiety.[7] Consistent with the prevalence in general population, GAD symptom ratings tend to be higher for female athletes than male athletes.[10-12] Adolescents and young adults into their 20s are prone to develop anxiety as well.[8] Consistent with the BPSS model described previously, the causes of GAD and other anxiety problems are varied. Fortunately, a few effective treatment approaches and self-help measures are available.[13]

Panic Attacks

Among the 6 million people (2.7% of the U.S. population) who experience panic attacks, some say that these episodes seem to come out of nowhere when, in fact, they are probably in response to an accumulation of stressors.

At other times, the attacks may be stimulated by an identifiable, acutely stressful event.[14,15] Symptoms that seem to be cardiovascular, such as chest pain or shortness of breath, are especially striking during these episodes. The attacks can be so overwhelming and can produce such fear (e.g., of dying) and intense anxiety that the affected person may begin avoiding stressful situations and other stimuli perceived as triggers. As a result, the panic attacks may become **panic disorder**. In some situations, this experience can also include agoraphobia, avoiding open spaces or public places. Panic disorder can be so severe and distressing that some victims might consider suicide as the only way out; in fact, up to 20% of those affected consider this step. Women experience panic attacks at twice the rate of men.[12,16]

Posttraumatic Stress Reactions

Similar to the intense responses involved in panic attacks are varying degrees of posttraumatic stress reactions, such as **acute stress disorder (ASD)** and **posttraumatic stress disorder (PTSD)**, experienced by approximately 7.7 million Americans.[17,18] An estimated 7 to 8 out of 100 people will experience PTSD at some point in their life.[19,20] These reactions are in response to exposure to life-threatening events or other situations outside the normal range of human experience (e.g., war, serious physical or sexual assault, motor vehicle accident). ASD and PTSD result because the survivors have witnessed or experienced events that include serious injury, life-threatening trauma, or death. Examples of situations that have caused some of those involved to develop PTSD are the various domestic terrorism-related assaults, school shootings, and other killings that have occurred in the last few decades. People can be so overwhelmed by the event or series of events that they will go to great lengths to avoid similar situations, as well as the thoughts or feelings associated with the original experience, because their responses involved intense fear, helplessness, or horror.

Often, people will replay or reexperience the traumatic event in the form of recurrent or intrusive and distressing recollections, images, thoughts, perceptions, dreams, illusions, or hallucinations. They often have strong physiological reactions to these experiences and, therefore, try to avoid stimuli and to numb their responses. This leads them to avoid thoughts, feelings, conversations, activities, places, and people they associate with the traumatic event. At times, this process of compartmentalization can be so severe that it leads to an inability to recall important aspects of the event, marked **anhedonia**, detachment or estrangement, restricted range of affect, and a sense of a foreshortened future. Without intervention to help survivors deal with what they have experienced, PTSD can develop and cause many physical, emotional, and social difficulties for years to come.[3]

Obsessive–Compulsive Disorder

Approximately 19 million people, or 8.7% of the U.S. population, display characteristics of anxiety in a more circumscribed manner by developing phobias to specific triggers or fears about specific issues. These include abnormal anxiety about being in social situations, fear of public speaking, fear of flying, or preoccupations with germs or disease.[3,7] These manifestations of anxiety can be manageable if the person can avoid the stimuli without compromising normal activities, but otherwise they can be quite disruptive. Some aspects of anxiety can be useful. For example, attention to detail and the ability to be thorough can be valuable in environments such as athletic competition, where excellent performance is rewarded. However, taken or driven to the extreme, these impulses can be debilitating.

Obsessive–compulsive disorder (OCD) is a condition that affects approximately 2.2 million people in the United States and is equally common among men and women. The basis for OCD is persistent thoughts, impulses, or images about exaggerated or imaginary circumstances.[1,21] The thoughts the person has are experienced as intrusive or inappropriate to the situation. Compulsive or repetitive behaviors are paired with the obsessions, with the goal of eliminating, reducing, or ignoring the resultant anxiety. As with the obsessions, the person often recognizes that the compulsive behaviors are, to some degree, excessive or unreasonable, especially if they impede the person's performance, routine, or social activities. The most common obsessive thoughts are those concerning contamination, doubts, loss of order, horrible trauma, and sexuality. Table 17.2 summarizes common compulsive behaviors.

Clinical Tips

Diagnostic Criteria for Obsessive–Compulsive Disorder

- Obsessions or recurrent and persistent thoughts, impulses, or images that are not simply about life problems
- Attempts to suppress or neutralize such thoughts with other thoughts or actions while recognizing they are a product of the person's own mind
- Compulsive thoughts or actions engaged in accordance to rigid rules even though they may not be rationally connected to the intrusive thoughts

Treatment of Anxiety Disorders

Treatment plans for anxiety disorders are often recommended by the practitioner on the basis of assessment and experience, and then negotiated with the individual or family members according to personal preferences. The treatment plan for anxiety can include one or all of a group of evidence-based interventions.[22]

When there is a strong family history of anxiety problems, there is likely a biological or physiological predisposition that can be managed with medication. One class of **psychotropic medications** often used includes those that act on the serotonin system: selective serotonin reuptake inhibitors (SSRIs). Examples of SSRIs include fluoxetine (Prozac), sertraline (Zoloft), paroxetine (Paxil), and escitalopram (Lexapro). When anxiety coexists with depression, medications that affect dopamine (e.g., bupropion [Wellbutrin]) or norepinephrine (e.g., venlafaxine [Effexor] and mirtazapine [Remeron]) may be used. **Benzodiazepines** have been used for many years to treat anxiety and are well known. These medications include clonazepam (Klonopin), diazepam (Valium), lorazepam (Ativan), and alprazolam (Xanax). Benzodiazepines are not the first choice for use with athletes, because they impair performance.[23]

Antianxiety drugs are prescribed according to their rate of onset, effects, and adverse effect profiles. Medication can be used from the outset or added after treatment begins. It is usually recommended that the person continue on the medication for 9 to 12 mo or until symptoms are fully resolved. The dosage may need to be adjusted, or a different type or class of medication altogether may be needed. In the case of first or second episodes of anxiety, medication can be discontinued after the person has developed healthy coping strategies. If the anxiety recurs, then the person may need to take the medication for the duration.

Other important steps to take to reduce anxiety on a physical level are to exercise regularly and to regulate sleep. Exercise, especially aerobic exercise, has been shown to significantly reduce levels of anxiety. This may be a moot point for those who are already physically active, but, at times, people will stop exercising if they are distressed enough. For the injured athlete, maintaining aerobic conditioning during rehabilitation is important for mental as well as physical well-being. Most people should be encouraged to slowly reestablish healthy patterns of physical activity. Similarly, good sleep hygiene addresses the basic human need for restful sleep, which in turn supports well-being and stable functioning:

- Establish regular times for going to bed and awakening.

TABLE 17.2   **Common Compulsive Thoughts and Behaviors Associated With Obsessive–Compulsive Disorder**

Worrisome thoughts	Compensatory behaviors
Contamination or infection	Washing of hands Excessive cleaning
Doubts	Requesting or demanding assurance
Loss of order	Ritualized behaviors Certain order to getting dressed
Personal safety	Making sure doors are locked Checking to make sure appliances are turned off (e.g., stove and coffee maker)
Sexuality	Religious or psychological correction Self-flagellation Defense

Considerations for Psychiatric Medication Use in Athletes

There may be the potential for the following:[24]

- Negative effect on athletic performance
- Therapeutic performance-enhancing effects (owing to improvement in the patient's condition)
- Nontherapeutic performance-enhancing (ergogenic) effects
- Safety risks

- Minimize distractions and noises.
- Avoid stimulating activity or substances before bedtime (e.g., exercise, caffeine).

Negative patterns of thought or behavior can exacerbate anxiety. Therefore, cognitive–behavioral psychotherapy is used to help people recognize automatic thoughts and reflexive behaviors and replace them with more constructive ones. On a related note, minimizing stress and distinguishing controllable from uncontrollable events are important to addressing anxiety problems. Stress management strategies include breathing exercises, progressive muscle relaxation, guided imagery, meditation, and prayer. Problem-solving and conflict resolution skills can be learned. Developing social support systems is also helpful.

GAD, OCD, and panic attacks are often treated through a combination of medication and support techniques. These include stress management, conflict resolution, problem-solving, supportive relationships with others, exercise, and good sleep hygiene. In addition, psychotherapy emphasizing cognitive–behavioral and interpersonal therapy is important. Individuals with ASD or PTSD often benefit from group therapy because this process helps to normalize the sense of unreality or disconnection that victims of trauma often experience. People with phobias do not usually respond to the use of medication; instead, a process of systematic desensitization helps to lessen or even eliminate their phobic responses.[25,26]

Mood Disorders

Transient feelings of sadness or depressed mood are normal in response to life's ups and downs. At the other end of the spectrum, however, depression can be so severe that people experience psychotic symptoms. Like anxiety, depression can appear as changes in physical, mental, emotional, relational, or spiritual well-being. Depression can be mild, moderate, or severe, and it can be situational or global. The incidence of depression is highest in middle-aged people. According to the WHO, depression accounts for the heaviest burden of disability among mental and emotional disorders, and it is among the most devastating of all health problems (second only to heart disease).[27,28]

Depression can affect people at any time of life. The reported prevalence of depressive symptoms in college students during COVID-19 was 34%.[29] The prevalence of depressive symptoms in elite athletes and the general population appears to be similar.[30] However, elite athletes may not recognize or acknowledge depressive symptoms or may not seek support in part related to stigma.[31] In addition, comorbidity between anxiety and mood disor-

> ### Clinical Tips
> ## Stressors That Sometimes Lead to Depression in Athletes
>
> *Situational Stressors*
> - Not meeting performance expectations of self or others
> - Change in playing status, coaches, teams, or partners
> - Death or serious illness in a family member
> - Relationship breakup
>
> *Developmental Stressors*
> - Major life transitions (e.g., move, change of schools)
> - Birth of a baby in the family

ders is high.[32] Some people become depressed in response to situational stressors (e.g., a change in performance or playing status, a move, illness in a family member) or developmental stressors (e.g., the transition from high school to college, birth of a baby in the family). In most cases, depression will come and go within a limited time.

Persistent symptoms, however, may be a sign of a more serious problem. Among individuals who develop more serious forms of depression that are not treated adequately, 35% will experience relapse within 2 years and 60% will experience relapse within 12 years.[1,27] As with the other conditions discussed in this chapter, the development, progression, and recovery or relapse of depression are affected by many things, which again reflect the pieces of the BPSS pie.[27,33] In more serious forms of depression, the person demonstrates both depressed mood and diminished interest in daily activities.

Typical physical symptoms include both somatic–behavioral and emotional–cognitive disturbances. Individuals may experience changes in sleeping patterns, such as waking very early and being unable to return to

 RED FLAGS FOR DEPRESSION

- Depressed mood
- Diminished interest in usual activities
- Irritability or anger
- Diminished performance
- Substance abuse
- Social withdrawal or isolation
- Preoccupation with escape or death

a restful sleep or wanting to sleep all the time. The prevalence of sleep concerns is high in the athletic population, with 49% of Olympic athletes classifying themselves as poor sleepers.[34] Some of these sleep concerns may be attributable to disruption of the normal circadian rhythm as a result of travel or training.[34] Approximately 64% of Olympic athletes reported significant symptoms of insomnia, which has been shown to exacerbate depressive symptoms.[35] Other symptoms include either loss of appetite or eating more than usual, loss of energy, and concentration difficulties.[3]

A depressed athlete is also very likely to complain of various somatic pains or irregularities, such as muscle aches, bowel problems, or headaches. A depressed person is often sad, can become self-critical, and feels out of control, despair, and hopeless, even to the point of being suicidal.[3,27]

The minor form of a mood disorder is called an *adjustment disorder*. The *DSM-5* guidelines, although somewhat arbitrary, suggest that an adjustment disorder is two to four symptoms with onset within 3 mo and resolution within 6 mo of termination of the stressor. If the symptoms are more severe in number or quality, an even more significant problem may have developed. This more serious form, major depressive episode, involves a greater number and more severe depressive symptoms for at least 2 wk.[3] Criteria for a major depressive episode are as follows:

At least 2 wk of the following:

- Lack of interest in usual activities
- Depressed mood

Plus four or more of the following:

- Appetite change along with weight gain or loss
- Insomnia or hypersomnia
- Psychomotor agitation or retardation
- Fatigue
- Worthlessness or guilt
- Difficulty concentrating or indecisiveness
- Recurrent thoughts of death or suicide

Mood disorders, such as major depression, can be assessed according to the diagnostic criteria listed, but the busy practitioner or athletic trainer who is not an expert in this area can use one or more screening instruments to measure the level of impairment.

- *Patient Health Questionnaire-9 (PHQ-9):* This questionnaire is frequently used in primary care settings in the United States. The PHQ-9 is used as an initial assessment and to track symptoms over time to see if an individual is responding to treatment.[36,37]

- *Center for Epidemiological Studies Depression Scale (CES-D):* The National Institute of Mental Health (NIMH) publishes the CES-D, and it is free to use and is available at the NIMH website.[27]

- *Baron Depression Screener for Athletes (BDSA):* The BDSA is the only depression screening tool specifically developed for use with athletes. Although the validity and reliability of the BDSA have not been studied, it holds promise because its items pertain to the athlete's experience.[38]

Even depressed people can have periods from days to weeks or even months during which they do not feel so bad and can rally to perform well. Some people have cyclical fluctuations in mood, energy, and appetite. Not surprisingly, one mood disorder is termed **cyclothymia**. In this case, the athlete may perform well in practice or competitions for several days or weeks but then inexplicably hit a slump. Another form of fluctuating depression, **seasonal affective disorder (SAD)**, is tied to exposure to changing amounts of sunlight. The prevailing theory is that sunlight, by way of the optic nerve, stimulates the brain to produce melatonin, which is a chemical related to serotonin. The hormone serotonin helps to regulate mood, appetite, activity level, and the wake–sleep cycle. When there is relatively less exposure to sunlight, less of this chemical is being produced, which in turn leads to depression.[3] These cycles are often tied to the changing of the seasons. Therefore, the changes in mood, energy, and performance may take place over longer periods.

The most debilitating mood disorder, **bipolar disorder** (formerly manic depression), is associated with significant fluctuations of symptoms. In this condition, people may experience periods of depression (mild to severe), mania (hypomania), or both. Mania and hypomania are on a continuum with a normal sense of well-being and the depression previously described. Mania is characterized by extremes of energy, euphoria, irritability, frustration, and rapid or grandiose thinking, speaking, and acting. In more moderate circumstances, patients with bipolar disorder can be very productive and creative; in extreme situations, they can be driven to put themselves and others at risk because of impulsivity, poor judgment, and lack of focus and concentration. Mania is also characterized by thrill seeking, such as engaging in risky sexual behavior, substance use, impulsive travel, or buying sprees.

Treatment of depression is similar to that of anxiety problems because the biopsychosocial–spiritual issues underlying these disorders overlap and, as stated earlier, they frequently occur in a comorbid fashion. Therefore, the interventions are those mentioned previously: medication (summarized in table 17.3), psychotherapy, sleep hygiene, exercise, skill building, stress management, and social–spiritual support.

Research has shown that in cases of adjustment disorders and even mild or moderate depression, medication is usually not needed.[39,40] People tend to heal with time, reassurance, supportive relationships with others, exercise, good sleep hygiene, and sometimes a short course of psychotherapy, either cognitive–behavioral or interpersonal therapy. When the depression is more serious, research-based practice indicates that psychotherapy and medication can both be helpful.[40] Whereas medication is more effective in the short term, therapy tends to be more helpful over longer periods. Severe depression requires aggressive treatment with both medication and psychotherapy. The other strategies are helpful additions to the treatment plan in both moderate and severe depression.[39]

Eating Disorders

It is estimated that eating disorders affect 8.5% of women and 2.5% of men and that nearly 30 million people in the United States have an eating disorder.[41] Perhaps this is because Americans have a love-hate relationship with food and their bodies. They are surrounded by cheap, high-calorie foods that contain generous amounts of fat and sugar. A growing focus on fitness and healthy lifestyles is paired incongruously with record levels of obesity and related health problems, such as diabetes, coronary artery disease, and stroke. The resulting disordered patterns of eating often have their onset in childhood and early adolescence.[42] This is a time when individuals becoming increasingly aware of themselves and attuned to peer group messages about acceptability, attraction, and competence.

Even though athletes are usually more physically active and fit than the average person, the demands of performance, such as maintaining a certain body weight or proportions, can strongly affect their approach to food. Wrestlers, gymnasts, dancers, and swimmers are especially prone to developing problems with food and weight. The estimated prevalence of eating disorders among athletes is up to 45% in women and up to 19% in men. This is considerably higher than in nonathletes, especially within the "lean sport" types.[43-45]

Like the other issues discussed in this chapter, disordered eating can be viewed on a spectrum of severity. People with these problems often do not fit into clear-cut categories.

Anorexia Nervosa

Anorexia nervosa is a potentially life-threatening condition with long-term mortality rates approaching 20%.[46] Anorexia develops when the person restricts or otherwise compensates for eating to the point that the person drops below 85% of ideal body weight.[3] An important point for athletic trainers to consider is that overtraining is a common compensatory behavior.

TABLE 17.3   **Uses and Side Effects of Medications Commonly Used for Treatment of Mood Disorders**

Medication category (examples)	Used for	Common side effects	Clinical tips
Benzodiazepines, such as alprazolam (Xanax), lorazepam (Ativan), and clonazepam (Klonopin)	Severe anxiety Situational (flying, performance anxiety)	Sedation Decreased appetite	High abuse potential Usually short-term use Not used with alcohol or other drugs
SSRIs, such as fluoxetine (Prozac), citalopram (Celexa), and sertraline (Zoloft)	Depression Premenstrual syndrome Anxiety Panic Bulimia PTSD	Insomnia Gastrointestinal problems Sexual problems	Most effective in moderate to severe symptoms Best in combination with psychotherapy Frequently discontinued by patients because of side effects or misinformation
SNRIs, such as venlafaxine (Effexor) and duloxetine (Cymbalta)	Depression Generalized anxiety	Insomnia Gastrointestinal problems Sexual problems	Most effective in moderate to severe symptoms Best in combination with psychotherapy Frequently discontinued by patients because of side effects or misinformation

Note: PTSD = posttraumatic stress disorder; SNRI = serotonin and norepinephrine reuptake inhibitor; SSRI = selective serotonin reuptake inhibitor.

RED FLAGS FOR EATING DISORDERS

- Frequent comments about feeling fat or overweight
- Fluctuations or other changes in weight
- Secretive, peculiar, or ritualized eating habits
- Avoidance of social situations involving food
- Mood changes
- A history of weight problems
- Excessive training regimen
- Gastrointestinal problems
- Dizziness
- Dental or oral problems
- Ability to recall specific details about food portions
- Wearing baggy clothing

Anorexia is a relatively rare condition, with about 5 to 10 new cases per 100,000 people each year and a prevalence of 0.5%. Most cases of anorexia are found in females, but approximately 10% to 15% of cases occur in males.[46] Anorexia occurs more often in industrialized than in nonindustrialized societies. The two subtypes of anorexia are the restricting type and the binge eating–purging type. Individual patient behaviors may vary from time to time.[42]

The possible physical sequelae include gastrointestinal problems (stomachache, diarrhea, constipation, heartburn), amenorrhea or other menstrual irregularities, dehydration, electrolyte imbalance, bradycardia, hypotension, decreased muscle mass and body fat, musculoskeletal injuries, lowered core body temperature, development of **lanugo** hair on the body, and fatigue and weakness.[42] Emotionally and mentally, people develop a distorted

Clinical Tips
Criteria for Anorexia Nervosa

- Refusal to maintain weight at a minimum of 85% of expected
- Intense fear of gaining weight or being fat
- Disturbed perception of body weight or body image
- Absence of at least three consecutive menstrual cycles

body image, emotional lability, cognitive rigidity, perfectionist attitudes, social isolation, an intense fear of becoming fat, and eventual impairment of mental functions.[3] Concomitant psychiatric diagnoses are significantly more common in persons diagnosed with anorexia nervosa.[47]

Bulimia

Bulimia is another type of eating disorder that affects athletes and physically active individuals and is more common than anorexia. Even though the athlete is often at or slightly above normal weight, bulimia can also be life-threatening. It is characterized by binge eating followed by an inappropriate compensatory act designed to prevent weight gain and, perhaps more importantly, to combat the person's sense of being out of control.[3,46] These compensatory acts include restricting food (dieting or fasting), vomiting, laxative or diuretic use, and exercise. A stereotypical binge involves eating large amounts in secret in a short period of time. In fact, people may or may not be especially secretive, and the amount of food constituting a binge is a matter of perception. People with bulimia who believe they have eaten too much may see even one too many cookies or slices of pizza as a binge. In response, they engage in one or more compensatory behaviors.

The results of this behavior include fluid and electrolyte imbalance, gastrointestinal difficulties, inflammation of the esophagus and parotid glands, dental conditions, visual disturbances, muscle weakness, and menstrual irregularities. Vomiting, laxatives, or diuretics usually are what cause the problems. From psychological and behavioral points of view, people with bulimia often exhibit excessive concern about body weight and shape,

Clinical Tips
Criteria for Diagnosing Bulimia

- Recurrent eating of a larger amount of food than normal in a discrete amount of time and in an out-of-control manner
- Recurrent, inappropriate compensatory behavior, such as vomiting or laxative or diuretic abuse
- Compensatory excessive exercise
- Behavior happens regularly over at least 3 mo
- Behavior influenced by perceptions of body weight or image
- Excessive dental caries resulting from frequent vomiting or malnutrition

irritability, social withdrawal, depression, and impulsive behavior.[3,46]

Binge Eating Disorder

A third category is **binge eating disorder**.[3] Considered to be the most common eating disorder, it is characterized by eating in binges that result in emotional or physical discomfort similar to bulimia but without the obvious compensatory behaviors mentioned previously.[48]

Treatment of Eating Disorders

Eating disorders of all types require a thorough assessment and interprofessional treatment. This treatment can be done on an outpatient basis, but inpatient stabilization may be needed for more serious problems that create life-threatening electrolyte imbalances or starvation. The athletic trainer should have an identified team in place for expediated referral and patient-centered treatment. The most effective treatment teams include medical, nutritional, and mental health practitioners. The antianxiety and depression medications described previously are used to treat underlying or comorbid conditions (see table 17.3 on medications). These medications are especially useful in treating the dysphoria associated with low self-esteem and disturbed identity, the anxiety that comes with changed eating behaviors (e.g., eating but not purging, fear of gaining weight), and the obsessive–compulsive nature of the disorder.[49,50]

Group therapy—or more generally, milieu therapy—can help the patient to confront unrealistic expectations, maladaptive behaviors, and distorted thinking. Nutritionists work with patients with eating disorders to help them gain a more realistic understanding of the body's physiology and nutritional needs and to establish expectations about diet and exercise. Individual and family therapy is especially helpful with children and adolescents, and it addresses dysfunctional social, cultural, and family dynamics within which eating behaviors are often embedded.[49]

Substance Use and Dependence

As with eating and weight issues, social messages around drug and alcohol use seem to conflict and to exacerbate substance problems. On one hand, alcohol use in the United States is legal and normative for individuals age 18 to 21 yr, depending on state laws. On the other hand, millions of dollars are spent on alcohol and drug awareness programs for school children to combat the problems associated with their use. Peer pressure among younger adolescents often encourages alcohol use. The use of mind- or mood-altering substances takes many forms, including use, misuse, abuse, and dependence.[3,51]

It can be difficult to draw the line among appropriate use, misuse, abuse, and dependence. But from a health care professional's point of view, the lines might be defined by the effects of the use on patient health and well-being, including athletic performance.

Drug or alcohol use involves using the substance without meaningful impairment. Substance misuse includes occasional use of an illegal substance or use of a legal substance to excess, resulting in impairment of one's ability to function. Substance abuse is a maladaptive pattern of substance use occurring within a 12 mo period that causes impairment in social or occupational functioning. A substance abuser will continue this pattern of use despite its ongoing or increasingly negative consequences. Substance dependence or addiction is a maladaptive pattern of substance abuse occurring within a 12 mo period that leads to significant impairment or distress and is characterized by either tolerance—the need for markedly increased amounts of the substance or markedly diminished effects from continued use of the same amounts—or withdrawal, even if withdrawal does not happen because the patient uses a substance to relieve or avoid withdrawal symptoms.[3]

Alcohol, illegal street drugs (e.g., cocaine, methamphetamine, ecstasy), and other substances (e.g., inhalants

---

CONDITION HIGHLIGHT

Alcohol Abuse

Depression gets a lot of press. Anxiety is the most common disorder afflicting average Americans, including athletes. But the behavior that is associated with more risk-taking and results in the most injuries and fatalities is the abuse of alcohol. The top three contributors to morbidity and mortality among people age 16 to 24 yr are homicide, accidents, and suicide, all three of which are more likely to occur when people overuse alcohol.[28] Young adults (athletes alike) are more likely to be victims of physical or sexual assault when alcohol and other drugs are being consumed.[28] Alcohol is often used by individuals with mood and anxiety disorders to self-medicate, exacerbating the underlying mental health condition. Therefore, athletic trainers must be careful not to normalize the consumption of alcohol or to ignore the effects that it can have on well-being and performance.

such as glue, gasoline, propellants) can be used for their intoxicating effects. There are historically high rates of use of methamphetamines, opioids like oxycontin and fentanyl, and "party drugs" such as MDMA or ecstasy,[52] especially among older adolescents and younger adults. One stark indicator of this trend is the 4% increase in age-adjusted overdose deaths between 2018 and 2019 in the United States.[53] The highest rates of inhalant use are found among children age 8 to 12 yr.[27] The highest rates of illicit drug use, at 36%, are found in 16- to 20-year-olds, with alcohol and marijuana being the most used drugs.[54] Binge drinking prevalence (28.2%) and intensity (9.3 drinks) were reported to be highest among people age 18 to 24 yr and is nearly twice as common among men than women. Among high school students who binge drink, 44% consumed eight or more drinks in a row.[54,55]

Alcohol is the third leading cause of preventable mortality, contributing to 100,000 deaths each year, and nearly 92,000 people in the U.S. died in 2020 from a drug-involved overdose, including from illicit drugs and prescription opioids. Overdose from opioids (prescription, natural, and synthetic) has continuously risen from 2017 to 2022.[56] Increasingly, prescription drugs are being obtained by deception or theft and used or distributed to others, including in schools and universities. An estimated 20% of people in the United States (including 15% of high school seniors) have used prescription drugs for nonmedical reasons.[57] The types of drugs most often misused and abused include narcotic painkillers (e.g., oxycodone, hydrocodone), sedatives and tranquilizers (e.g., alprazolam, diazepam, zolpidem [Ambien]), and stimulants (e.g., methylphenidate [Ritalin], modafinil [Provigil]).[56] Over-the-counter drugs, such as no-sleep or diet aids (for stimulative effects) and cough syrups (containing dextromethorphan and used for sedative effects), can also be misused, abused, or part of a person's dependence.[57]

The misuse of substances can be found in families of all socioeconomic, racial, and ethnic backgrounds, and it negatively affects the lives of family members at many levels because of the potential relational, social, and legal difficulties. Paradoxically, substance abusers are often enabled by family members who may cover for such compulsive or addictive behavior patterns. The effect of substance abuse on the user and the family depends on the type of drug, length of use, amount being used, and any comorbid conditions. In cases in which athletes are having training- or performance-related difficulties, the athletic trainer should consider substance abuse as a potential contributor. A simple set of screening questions is represented by the mnemonic CAGE:

C: Have you ever tried to cut down on your (substance) use?

A: Have you ever felt angry or annoyed when someone asks or confronts you about your substance use?

G: Have you ever felt guilty about your substance use?

E: Have you ever used an eye-opener (used your substance of choice first thing in the morning to get going)?

Denial is often a complicating factor when working with these individuals and their families. Often, they will not want to acknowledge or discuss substance abuse problems. Because of the possibility of denial, the athletic trainer must be alert for simple clues such as performance problems, absenteeism, marital discord, or vehicular and everyday accidents. It also helps if the athletic trainer can provide a safe, nonjudgmental environment within which patients can share personal struggles. Successful intervention is based on the person's desire to stop, willingness to find alternative coping strategies, and, when indicated, effective detoxification, treatment of dual diagnoses, or relapse prevention through individual or family treatment or participation with groups such as Alcoholics Anonymous or Narcotics Anonymous.

Substance abuse is associated with many possible comorbid conditions that either contribute to or result from the substance abuse itself.[58,59] Comorbid conditions associated with substance abuse include the following:

- Mood and anxiety disorders
- Marital or family dysfunction
- Partner or child abuse
- Physical injury to self
- Engaging in dangerous behaviors
- Driving while intoxicated
- Falls (especially in older adults)
- Overdosing
- Physical complaints
- Gastrointestinal problems
- Malnutrition
- Numbness
- Weakness and fatigue
- Hypertension

Many people with comorbid problems self-medicate with alcohol or other drugs to correct or compensate for the difficulty with mood, anxiety, or concentration.

The first step in substance abuse intervention is usually assessment by a qualified professional, such as a certified drug and alcohol abuse counselor, mental health practitioner, or physician trained in addictions. If the person is determined to be dependent on alcohol or other drugs, inpatient or outpatient detoxification may be necessary. This person needs to be educated and even confronted about the effects of the substance abuse. Treatment options include referral to a 12-step group (e.g., Alcoholics Anonymous, Narcotics Anonymous), an alternative treatment method (e.g., Rational Recovery [RR], Moderation Management), outpatient individual or group psychotherapy, or inpatient treatment and aftercare follow-up. RR is an alternative to the 12-step model and is based on a perspective of substance use as a pattern of problematic behavior and thinking but not a lifelong addictive disease. RR is not a group-based approach; rather, the organization provides information and training on their alternative to AA.

Relapse is a normal part of the change process with most lifestyle, behavioral, or addiction problems. This is obviously the case with substance abuse. In addition to education and referral, the athletic trainer can play an important role in offering ongoing support for the person to stay with the behavior change and recovery process.

Attention-Deficit/Hyperactivity Disorder

Attention-deficit/hyperactivity disorder (ADHD) is a neurobehavioral condition that impairs a person's ability to sustain attention or to control activity and impulses in at least two settings, such as home and school or work.[3] As with the other conditions discussed in this chapter, ADHD can be mild, moderate, or severe in its effects on one's ability to function. It is often first detected in childhood, especially when children enter school; however, ADHD in adulthood is a focus of clinical concern. An estimated 4% to 12% of children are affected by ADHD; it appears to affect boys more than girls by a ratio of 3:1. Girls are more likely to manifest the inattentive type, and boys generally display the hyperactive or combined type.[60] Differences in socialization may account for some of this discrepancy.

ADHD among adults is gaining more attention because of its long-term consequences if unrecognized and untreated.[61,62] Initially, the athlete with ADHD is much less likely than the student with ADHD to come to the attention of teachers or other concerned adults. This is because the athlete may just seem to have more energy than peers, but eventually coaches and even teammates may become irritated or frustrated with the athlete's inability to sit still, listen to directions, or follow through on plans.

ADHD is seen in several forms: primarily hyperactive, primarily inattentive, or mixed.[3] People with primarily hyperactive ADHD can be very easy to detect because they are "wound up like a top." Those with primarily inattentive disorder may be more difficult to detect because they fade into the academic woodwork. Most people with ADHD have elements of hyperactivity, impulsivity, and inattention. Typical symptoms of hyperactivity, impulsivity, and inattention are as follows:

Hyperactivity and Impulsivity

- Difficulty unwinding
- Restless, fidgety, or always "on the go"
- Talking excessively or interrupting
- Difficulty remaining still when required (e.g., waiting turns)
- Difficulty engaging in quiet activities
- Irritability
- Impulsive behavior (e.g., clowning around, unnecessarily touching others)

Inattention

- Difficulty paying attention, especially to details
- Problems concentrating on instructions
- Failure to follow directions
- Difficulty following through to a goal
- Making careless mistakes
- Distractibility
- Memory problems (e.g., appointments, deadlines)

In general, people with ADHD do not perform as well academically as they should according to their standardized test scores. If ADHD is suspected in an athlete, questions about classroom performance and standardized tests can be helpful. It is also useful to understand the diagnostic criteria for ADHD.

There is high comorbidity among ADHD, substance abuse, mood and anxiety disorders, and other mental health and behavioral problems.[61,63] In fact, people with untreated ADHD are almost twice as likely as those who are treated with medication to develop substance abuse problems.[63] Many professionals believe that people with ADHD who also use or abuse substances are, at least in part, self-medicating the underlying problem. Therefore, treatment needs to address the medical, behavioral, family, and psychoeducational needs of the patient with respect to ADHD and these comorbid conditions.

The clinical practice guidelines of the American Academy of Pediatrics recommend that assessment begin with an interview, a medical checkup, and administration of checklists.[61] To be diagnosed with ADHD, a person must, for at least 6 mo, experience inattention, including the following:

- Problems attending to details or making careless mistakes
- Difficulty sustaining attention
- Appearance of not listening
- Difficulty with follow-through on tasks or instructions

- Difficulty with organization
- Avoidance or dislike of tasks requiring sustained mental effort
- Problems losing things
- Distraction occurs easily
- Forgetfulness

In the athlete with ADHD, psychosocial interventions should be used and can be as effective as stimulant medication in athletes with mild functional impairment.[62] From a medical standpoint, first-line ADHD treatment includes the use of stimulant medication, such as methylphenidate in its various forms. Stimulants may be ergogenic and are often misused because of the perception of performance enhancement. Stimulants are prohibited by the World Anti-Doping Agency in competition,[64] so athletes taking them for medical purposes must obtain a therapeutic use exemption. Some α-2a blockers typically used for blood pressure control (e.g., guanfacine [Intuniv]) have an endorsement from the Food and Drug Administration for use alone or in combination with stimulant medications. Older tricyclic antidepressants such as imipramine, newer dopaminergic agents such as bupropion, or drugs that block norepinephrine reuptake such as atomoxetine (Strattera) are also being used. Bupropion is indicated for the treatment of ADHD in adults, and atomoxetine is useful for people with comorbid ADHD and depression because of its norepinephrine effects. Other treatment options for ADHD are as follows:

Mild

- Educate patient and family about the disorder.
- Develop adaptive strategies that increase organizational skills and concentration.

Moderate to Severe

- Add medication.
- Use individual therapy to problem-solve.
- Add family therapy.
- Reinforce adaptive strategies.
- Address problematic interpersonal dynamics.

Children, adolescents, and adults with ADHD all benefit from education about the nature of the disorder. Those with ADHD also benefit from coaching to reinforce coping strategies that address the problematic behavior and thought processes, such as eliminating distraction, setting short-term goals, and seeking frequent feedback on performance. Family sessions can help others develop realistic expectations for the person and can open communication about what may have been a very painful and disruptive set of behaviors. Similar communication with teachers, coaches, or work supervisors can be valuable as well.[61]

Frequently clinicians need to consider differentials in assessing and diagnosing the patients' health status. It is helpful to keep in mind the variety of conditions that might be causing the alterations in patient behavior and function. A more recent issue that can produce issues similar to ADHD in many people is the influence of technology in the modern world. The *DSM-5* identifies *Internet gaming disorder* as a diagnosable condition developed by people who become nearly completely immersed in the world of technology.[3] They become preoccupied with games (and/or social media), experience withdrawal symptoms if access is taken away, develop tolerance requiring increasing time spent, have unsuccessful attempts to change their behavior, lose interest in other activities and relationships, continue with the behavior despite negative consequences, and use the technology to escape negative moods.[3] As a result, the athletic trainer's discussions with individuals experiencing mood, anxiety, performance, and other issues should inquire about their use of Internet games and social media to not miss a "modern" contribution to the development of emotional or mental distress and disorders.

In the Time of Pandemic

As discussed earlier, mental health and substance use issues occur in the context of the social and cultural webs in which individuals live. Phenomena that take place throughout neighborhoods, states and provinces, countries, and continents of course tend to have relatively universal effects. COVID-19 is a poignant example. The health, political, relational, and emotional stress related to this pandemic has contributed to an overall increase in the reported experience of stress and distress in the general populations of countries throughout the world.[65] One in three high school students report having "poor mental health" because of the pandemic; the incidence is increased in LGBTQIA+ populations.[53] And one need only look as far as the 2022 Olympics for an example of effects on athletes and their ability to participate in their chosen sports. The pandemic is a reminder that athletic trainers should consider such contextual variables when assessing patient well-being.

Stages of Readiness

The concerned athletic trainer will routinely screen troubled patients for one or more of the problems described in this chapter. The athletic trainer who finds a problem that needs to be addressed will be able to educate the patient about the problem and to discuss options. The screening process should include an assessment of the individual's readiness to recognize that a problem exists and a desire to do something about it. Prochaska and DiClemente developed a useful framework for this step in 1983 that is still used today.[66-68] It involves assessing the athlete's readiness for change.[66] People in need of change can be in one of five different stages of the change process:

1. *Precontemplation stage:* The individual has not considered that there might be a problem with substance use, eating habits, or mood. This person needs to be educated and encouraged to consider the presence of a problem.

2. *Contemplation stage:* The individual has begun to think about the problem and has wondered whether it is time to change—that is, to stop using the substance or to seek medical treatment. This should be encouraged, and an athletic trainer can help the athlete to look honestly at the effect of the condition on performance, satisfaction, or general life circumstances.

3. *Preparation stage:* Once the individual has decided to change or seek help, there needs to be a plan. The athletic trainer can help by brainstorming possible components of an effective plan for change.

4. *Action stage:* The individual has begun making behavioral, situational, or attitudinal changes, including seeking professional help. Referrals from the athletic trainer can be very important now.

5. *Follow-up or relapse prevention stage:* This involves continued implementation or changes to the plan despite possible setbacks. The athletic trainer can use contacts with the individual on the field or in the office to support the individual's decision to address the problem, to support progress, or to confront relapse.

It will not be a productive use of time or relationship capital for the athletic trainer to try to get the patient to do something the patient is not ready to do. Athletic trainers cannot persuade individuals to develop a plan of action or even take steps to correct a problem when they are still in denial about it. Athletic trainers will be more effective by first assessing and asking good questions, providing support, and offering educational input. When the patient moves from precontemplation to contemplation and preparation, then it is time for the patient and the athletic trainer to partner in developing a plan.

What to Do in a Crisis

Even during the best of times, individuals can become overwhelmed by feelings, psychological tensions, or interpersonal conflicts. An acute stressor (e.g., a lost match, relationship breakup, or conflict with teammates or coach) can precipitate strong emotional responses. There may be preexisting problems with depression or anxiety, or the reaction may seem to come out of the blue. In these situations, the athletic trainer may be called on to help defuse the crisis and arrange for acute follow-up care. This is especially important when the athletic trainer can identify certain factors that indicate the likelihood of heightened risk for the athlete or others:[69]

- Inconsolable emotion (e.g., sobbing, rage)
- Drastic change in typical behavior
- Use of alcohol or drugs
- Suicidal or homicidal ideation, threats, or plans
- History of suicidal or homicidal ideation

The most important goal is to help the person to deescalate and see through the emotion to a more hopeful or less distressing future. The following are some strategies for doing so:

- Engagement with the athlete should be by someone who is skilled *and* likely to be trusted.
- Speak in a calm, soothing tone without being patronizing. (Clinicians should avoid making statements such as "I know how you feel" unless they have that life experience.)
- Ask open-ended questions to encourage the person to talk and allow sufficient time to talk things out (e.g., "I can see you are upset. I'd like to help if I can. Can you tell me what's going on?").
- Reassure the athlete that, unless there is a legal exception, revealing the source of the crisis will not be held against them.
- Help the person to verbalize feelings and validate them (e.g., "You look mad. Could it be that you are feeling guilty about how you did today? Are you afraid the team is mad at you?" [If there is an affirmative response] "That makes a lot of sense. I can see why you might feel that way.").
- Then move on to help the athlete begin to rationalize and think things through. (e.g., "Have you

ever been through something like this before? What happened then? Did you feel the same way? How did you get past it that time? What do you think you need now? Is there something you think would help?")

At times, even the most highly trained mental health practitioner may not be able to help someone calm down and begin to cope effectively. In these circumstances, other steps need to be taken:

- When possible, ensure that the person is not in immediate jeopardy or a threat to others (e.g., remove objects or weapons with which the person might cause injury, prevent the person from driving).
- Call 911 or campus security.
- Take the person to the nearest emergency department.

It is important to involve a MHP as part of the sports medicine team. The ability to recognize when an athlete may be in trouble and to refer that athlete for professional help before the situation escalates to a dangerous level may help to defuse a difficult situation.

Summary

The athletic trainer attends to the patient as a whole person and not just to their physical health and performance. This is because performance, physical health, mental health, behaviors, and life situation affect each other. This chapter highlights the most common mental health conditions of athletes that clinicians need to recognize. Based on this chapter and continuing education, athletic trainers should be able to identify emotional and behavioral signs of common mental health issues, including ADHD and anxiety, mood, eating, and substance use disorders.

Informed athletic trainers will be equipped to intervene with affected athletes through discussion, supportive confrontation, and referral. This involves knowing when and to whom to refer for qualified professional services and knowing potential effects on performance for various medical treatments of mental health issues. This chapter also mentions educational and supportive resources, such as organizational procedures, printed materials, and website resources, that are available to both professionals and patients affected by these disorders.

Apply It!   Go to HK*Propel* to complete the case studies for this chapter.

18

Working With Special Populations

OBJECTIVES

At the completion of this chapter the reader should be able to do the following:

1. Discuss aspects of the medical history as needed when assessing people with selected disabilities.

2. Recognize the importance of the preparticipation physical examination in identifying baseline norms in the athlete with a disability.

3. Relay typical symptoms and clinical signs of pathological conditions seen in individuals with selected disabilities.

4. Apply typical treatment and prevention measures for pathological conditions seen in people with selected disabilities.

5. Explain how common medical conditions can have devastating consequences to a person with a disability.

6. Communicate effectively with individuals with selected disabilities.

Participation in organized sports and recreation by individuals with disabilities has increased significantly, with more than 3 million participating in the United States alone. This has created a deeper field of competition, requiring athletes to train and compete at higher levels to attain success. Athletes who use a wheelchair have broken the four-minute mile and have completed marathons in less than 90 min. Alan Oliveira has run the 100 m on two prosthetic legs in 10.77 s. In January 2015, the Eastern College Athletic Conference became the first NCAA-sanctioned conference to adopt an inclusive strategy to provide new athletic opportunities for student-athletes with a variety of disabilities at the collegiate level. War also has affected participation in athletics by people with disabilities. A combined 48 active-duty service members and veterans represented the United States in the 2020 Tokyo Olympic Games and the 2022 Beijing Olympic and Paralympic Games.[1,2] In Europe, the Duke of Sussex founded the Invictus Games for servicemembers suffering life-changing injuries, visible or otherwise. As of 2018, these games are held annually and supported by different countries, with 450 to 550 athletes competing each year.[3] The popular television show *Dancing With the Stars* hosted the first Deaf competitor, Marlee Matlin, in 2008, and its first blind competitor, Paralympian Danelle Umstead, in 2018. Several other warriors and athletes with physical disabilities have also successfully participated in the series, including Nyle DiMarco, the first Deaf cast member who won the famed mirror ball trophy. This seasonal television series has been praised for its inclusivity in competitors. With millions watching athletic events (and TV competitions), active people with disabilities have been displayed as strong individuals who do not allow any disability to get in the way of activity, even on the world class levels.

In the United States, special education programs make school attendance possible for more than 7.2 million children with disabilities.[4] Adapted physical education provides opportunities to participate in sports and recreation through training in physical conditioning, noncompetitive and competitive sports, outdoor physical activities, and health centers. Quality sports medicine care is as important for special populations as for other populations.

Risks of injury and illness are inherent in all physical activity and injury rates for individuals with disabilities approximate those of individuals without disabilities.[5] However, athletes with disabilities have some unique challenges. Ferrara and Buckley developed the first disability register for athletes with disabilities, and they found that musculoskeletal injuries accounted for 79.7% of reported injuries.[6] General medical problems (i.e., illness or disability related) accounted for 20.3% of those athletes who were unable to participate.[6] Athletic trainers working with world-class athletes will note that Paralympians file more therapeutic use exemptions with the governing bodies than do their Olympic counterparts, which is attributable to the more complex nature of their medical conditions.

Person-first terminology should be used to refer to individuals with disabilities. Person-first terminology recognizes the individual before the disability.[7] For example, the health care provider identifies the patient as a person with spina bifida or a person with a visual impairment, rather than a disabled or blind person. Using appropriate terminology reflects an overall philosophy of the person being first and the disability being second. It also supports a social model of disability in which the focus is on changing attitudes, facilities, structures, and policies to promote participation rather than the medical model of disability, in which the focus is on the limitations, abnormalities, and impairments of the individual. The social model is preferred by persons with disabilities.

This chapter focuses on issues related to general medical concerns for the active person with a disability. The disabilities covered are traumatic tetraplegia and paraplegia, spina bifida, poliomyelitis, cerebral palsy (CP), amputations, sensory disabilities, and intellectual disabilities.

Preparticipation Examination for Athletes With Disabilities

Individuals with disabilities must complete a thorough preparticipation physical examination (PPE) so baseline norms can be established. The general approach of this PPE is similar to that for individuals without disabilities. However, often the focus is on the primary condition or disability, and the athletic trainer and other members of the sports medicine team may overlook other medical issues. This is known as **diagnostic overshadowing**.[8,9] Patel and Greydanus stressed the importance of obtaining a detailed history, and they suggest that the PPE be completed by a sports medicine team that is involved in the patient's long-term care and is familiar with their baseline functioning.[18] Another suggestion is to avoid the mass or station method of conducting PPEs with individuals with disabilities,[9] because decreased mobility makes the method impractical. Specific recommendations include talking at eye level with individuals who use a wheelchair, asking them what movement patterns are possible and which parts of the body have normal sensation, and being aware of skin conditions and pressure sores. Patients with a history of seizures have two and a half times more injuries than those without seizures.[10,11] This further necessitates a careful PPE during which the clinician obtains information on seizure history and documentation of antiseizure medication, including type, dose, frequency of use, and performance-related side effects.

Many individuals with spinal cord disabilities have constant or residual pain, and they may not be able to distinguish whether the pain is from a sports injury or the disability. Having a baseline appreciation of a patient's condition helps with the assessment process should a general medical condition arise later. Another part of the examination includes ensuring proper fit and adequacy of any prostheses, orthoses, sports wheelchairs, or other assistive devices.[12,13] Stump care in individuals with amputations and bowel and bladder habits in individuals with spinal cord injury (SCI) will also be in the athletic trainer's purview during the PPE. Having a parent or guardian present may help in obtaining an accurate history for a patient with an intellectual disability. Athletic trainers should seek assistance from professionals with expertise in the specific area of disability.

To identify medical problems, collect baseline data and identify training goals. Jacob and Hutzler developed the Sports-Medical Assessment Protocol (SMAP), which is a tool for the evaluation of athletes with neurological disabilities.[14] The SMAP includes a clinical interview, cardiopulmonary testing, and physical and functional assessments.[14] Concerning participation guidelines, the American Academy of Orthopaedic Surgeons developed a sport participation possibility chart designed to provide initial guidance for the patient and sports medicine team about which sports are appropriate. Factors in matching patients to sports include psychological maturity, adaptive and protective equipment, modification of the sport, patient and parent understanding of the risks of injury, current health condition, and level of competition and position played.[9]

Preparticipation Physical Examination

Additional points to consider during the PPE for an individual with a disability including the following:[13]

- Inspect all braces, orthoses, wheelchairs, and other assistive devices.
- Make sure braces are clean and free of rough areas.
- Ensure a proper fit of all braces for the patient.
- Obtain a resting blood pressure in at least two positions: supine and sitting or standing.
- Inquire about bladder and bowel habits.
- Ask about the patient's management plan.
- Determine the method of voiding and evacuating (e.g., catheter, bag).
- Inquire about a history of autonomic dysreflexia and the offending agent.
- Inquire about a history of heat-related illnesses.
- Inquire about experiences with stimuli that cause spasms.
- Note the history and frequency of urinary tract or bladder infections.
- Note the history of spina bifida.
- Note the presence of a cerebral shunt.
- Note the history of latex allergy.
- Note the history of poliomyelitis.
- Note the history of seizures and the management plan (medications, last seizure, type of seizure).
- Note the history of visual impairment (age at onset, cause, protective lenses).
- Note history of hearing impairment (age of onset, assistive devices, communication preference [sign language, reading, lipreading, translator]).

Siow and colleagues suggest that the following questions be asked during the PPE for individuals with particular disabilities:[8,13]

- Does the patient have a history of seizures, hearing loss, or vision loss? Are the seizures controlled? Seizures are commonly seen in Special Olympics athletes. Uncontrolled seizures often require consultation with a neurologist and delay in clearing the patient for sports participation.
- Does the patient have a history of cardiopulmonary disease? Congenital cardiac disorders, including heart murmurs, ventricular septal defects, and endocardial cushion defects, are more common in people with Down syndrome.
- Does the patient have a history of renal disease or a unilateral kidney? Various renal anomalies, such as hypoplasia, dysplasia, and obstruction, are more common in people with Down syndrome.
- Does the patient have a history of atlantoaxial instability? Spontaneous or traumatic subluxation of the cervical spine is a potential risk in individuals with Down syndrome.
- Has the patient had heatstroke or heat exhaustion? Thermoregulation in individuals with SCI is impaired because of skeletal muscular paralysis and loss of autonomic nervous system control. Medications used for pain and bladder dysfunction can interfere with the normal sweat response.
- Has the patient had any fractures or dislocations? Ligamentous laxity and joint hypermobility are prominent features in individuals with Down syndrome.
- What prosthetic devices or special equipment does the patient use during sport participation? Health care providers need to be aware of a patient's need for adaptive equipment and regulations concerning its use in different sports.
- Does the patient use an indwelling urinary catheter or require intermittent catheterization of the bladder? Individuals with SCI or other neurologic disorders often have bladder dysfunction or a neurogenic bladder.
- Does the patient have a history of pressure sores or ulcers? Individuals who use a wheelchair are prone to pressure ulcers at the sacrum and ischial tuberosities, and those who use prostheses are prone to pressure ulcers at prosthetic sites.

> continued

Preparticipation Physical Examination *continued*

- At what levels of competition has the individual previously participated?
- What is the patient's level of independence for mobility and self-care?
- What medications is the patient taking?
- Is the patient adhering to a special diet?
- Does the patient have a history of autonomic dysreflexia? This is an acute, potentially life-threatening syndrome of excessive, uncontrolled sympathetic output that can occur in individuals with SCIs at or above the sixth thoracic spinal cord level.

Overview of Anatomy and Physiology

The anatomy and physiology pertinent to traumatic SCI is also pertinent to spina bifida, poliomyelitis, and CP. Chapters 10 through 12 discuss anatomy and physiology related to intellectual and sensory disabilities and amputation. Recall from chapter 10 that the spinal cord is a cylindrical mass of nerve tissue that consists of 31 pairs of spinal nerves and extends from the medulla to the first or second lumbar vertebra (figure 18.1a). The

spinal cord is protected by the vertebral column, which consists of 7 cervical, 12 thoracic, 5 lumbar, 5 fused sacral, and 4 or more fused coccygeal vertebrae (figure 18.1b). The lumbar and sacral roots of the spinal cord fan out like a horse's tail at L1 to L2, giving rise to the term **cauda equina**.

Nerve impulses are conducted by the spinal cord and nerves between the brain and other parts of the body, and trauma to the spine can severely affect these intricate processes. In addition, the nervous system has other, nonmotor functions. The autonomic nervous system consists

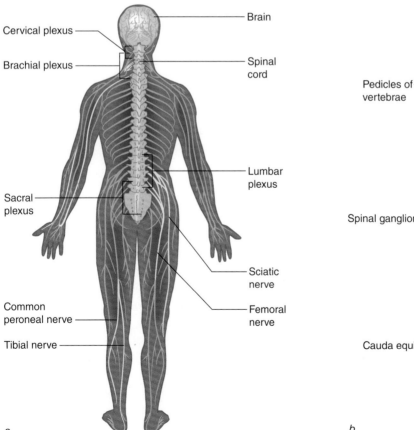

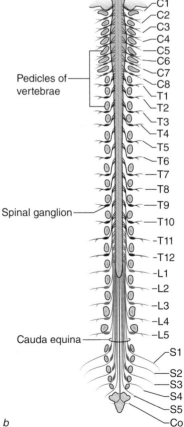

FIGURE 18.1   The spinal cord has 31 pairs of nerves that interpret sensory and motor stimuli and allow movement to occur. The level of a lesion to the cord is associated with the type of disability, typically sensory and motor, and will affect all areas distal to the lesion.

of the sympathetic and parasympathetic systems. The sympathetic system controls increases in heart rate, blood pressure, and temperature, whereas the parasympathetic system controls decreases in heart rate, blood pressure, and temperature.

Pathological Conditions

Spinal cord disability results from some form of injury or disease to the vertebrae or the nerves of the spinal column. Some degree of paralysis usually accompanies the disability. The degree of paralysis is a function of the location of the injury on the spinal column and the number of neural fibers destroyed by the injury. The level of function for an individual with a spinal cord disability depends on the level of lesion. The lower the level of lesion on the spinal cord, the greater the person's functional ability. Table 18.1 provides a summary of the relationship between level of lesion and functional ability. Note that a person with lesions above S2 will experience bowel and bladder concerns. It is appropriate for the clinician to discreetly ask the individual how bowel and bladder issues are controlled.

The pathological conditions associated with SCI, whether tetraplegia or paraplegia, spina bifida, or poliomyelitis, are often seen in CP as well. Sequelae unique to specific conditions are discussed here.

Pathological conditions associated with amputations, sensory disabilities, and intellectual disabilities are also covered in this chapter.

Traumatic Tetraplegia and Paraplegia

The extent of an SCI is generally described by means of a 5-point grading system. The American Spinal Injury Association (ASIA) advocates an impairment scale according to which a patient is classified as one of the following:[15,16]

ASIA A: complete

ASIA B: incomplete with sensation only

ASIA C: incomplete with nonfunctional motor ability

ASIA D: incomplete with motor function

ASIA E: normal motor and sensory function

A full explanation of this impairment scale can be found in figure 18.2. An individual with complete **tetraplegia** (formerly called *quadriplegia*) has a lesion above T1 that involves the cervical spine and affects all four limbs, has no trunk control or sitting balance, and usually uses a high-backed sports wheelchair. This individual will also be strapped into the wheelchair for safety during activity. An individual with complete **paraplegia** has a lesion below T1 that affects the lower extremities, has full use of the upper extremities, and may or may not have trunk control and sitting balance. A training apparatus is available to encourage correct movement. Updates to this classification include documentation from non-SCI impairments (peripheral nerve dysfunction, pain) and an updated definition of the zone of partial preservation.[55]

TABLE 18.1   Level of Spinal Cord Lesion Related to Functional Ability

Level of lesion	Functional abilities
C4	Has use of neck and diaphragm Needs total assistance for transfers Has limited respiratory endurance Controls electronic wheelchair by mouth-operated joystick
C7	Can extend elbow and flex and extend fingers Uses wheelchair independently Transfers to some extent independently Has a weak grasp
T1-T9	Can use upper extremities Has little or no use of lower extremities Lower-level injury: has some control of upper back, abdominal, and rib muscles; may ambulate with braces
T10-T12	Has complete control of upper back, abdominal, and rib muscles Ambulates mainly with use of long leg braces or crutches Uses a wheelchair for convenience; wheelchair sport possible
L1-L3	Has hip joint flexibility and ability to flex hip Ambulates independently with short leg braces, a cane, or crutches
S1	Can flex knees and lift feet Ambulates without crutches but may need ankle braces or orthopedic shoes

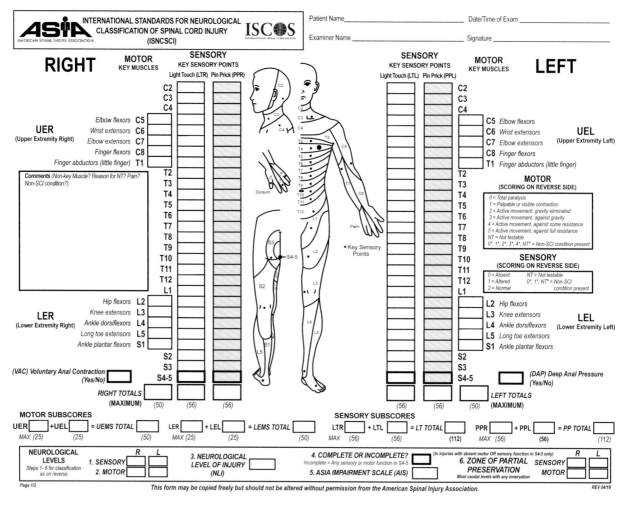

FIGURE 18.2 American Spinal Injury Association standard neurological classification of spinal cord injury.

American Spinal Injury Association: International Standards for Neurological Classification of Spinal Cord Injury, revised 2019; Richmond, VA.

> continued

Individuals with incomplete spinal lesions will have varied and unpredictable responses to many neurological tests. For example, a wheelchair basketball player with a T10 incomplete lesion may respond within normal limits to dermatome testing below T10.

Individuals with SCI have a higher resting heart rate and lower blood pressure than their counterparts without SCI. The higher heart rate is attributable primarily to the smaller venous return from the nonworking muscles in the lower extremities. To maintain cardiac output when stroke volume is reduced, the heart compensates by increasing its rate. In turn, the blood pressure lowers to accommodate a decreased perfusion need in the nonworking limbs. Clinicians know that the baseline blood pressure for adults with tetraplegia may be as low as 90/60 mmHg and that peak heart rates for persons with tetraplegia typically do not exceed 130 beats/min. As part of the PPE, blood pressure should be obtained in two of three positions: supine and sitting or standing, as applicable.[17-19] A change of less than 10 mmHg between positions is acceptable. Resting pulse is checked, as tachycardia (heart rate >120 beats/min) may be the only sign of pneumonia or pulmonary embolus in a patient with a high-level SCI.

Autonomic Dysreflexia

Autonomic dysreflexia (AD), also known as *hyperreflexia*, is a clinical phenomenon unique to people with SCI above the major sympathetic nervous system outflow tract. It is a potentially life-threatening complication of SCI, particularly among patients with lesions above T6, although attacks are possible in individuals with lesions to T10. With AD, blood pressure rises to dangerous levels (systolic blood pressure can reach 300 mmHg)[20] and can lead to stroke or death if not treated. In a clinical context, AD is defined as a sudden rise in systolic blood pressure of more than 20 mmHg above baseline.[20-22] Thus, the importance of obtaining a baseline blood pressure cannot

Muscle Function Grading

0 = Total paralysis

1 = Palpable or visible contraction

2 = Active movement, full range of motion (ROM) with gravity eliminated

3 = Active movement, full ROM against gravity

4 = Active movement, full ROM against gravity and moderate resistance in a muscle specific position

5 = (Normal) active movement, full ROM against gravity and full resistance in a functional muscle position expected from an otherwise unimpaired person

NT = Not testable (i.e. due to immobilization, severe pain such that the patient cannot be graded, amputation of limb, or contracture of > 50% of the normal ROM)

0*, 1*, 2*, 3*, 4*, NT* = Non-SCI condition present [a]

Sensory Grading

0 = Absent   **1** = Altered, either decreased/impaired sensation or hypersensitivity

2 = Normal   **NT** = Not testable

0*, 1*, NT* = Non-SCI condition present [a]

[a] Note: Abnormal motor and sensory scores should be tagged with a '*' to indicate an impairment due to a non-SCI condition. The non-SCI condition should be explained in the comments box together with information about how the score is rated for classification purposes (at least normal / not normal for classification).

When to Test Non-Key Muscles:

In a patient with an apparent AIS B classification, non-key muscle functions more than 3 levels below the motor level on each side should be tested to most accurately classify the injury (differentiate between AIS B and C).

Movement	Root level
Shoulder: Flexion, extension, adbuction, adduction, internal and external rotation **Elbow:** Supination	C5
Elbow: Pronation **Wrist:** Flexion	C6
Finger: Flexion at proximal joint, extension **Thumb:** Flexion, extension and abduction in plane of thumb	C7
Finger: Flexion at MCP joint **Thumb:** Opposition, adduction and abduction perpendicular to palm	C8
Finger: Abduction of the index finger	T1
Hip: Adduction	L2
Hip: External rotation	L3
Hip: Extension, abduction, internal rotation **Knee:** Flexion **Ankle:** Inversion and eversion **Toe:** MP and IP extension	L4
Hallux and Toe: DIP and PIP flexion and abduction	L5
Hallux: Adduction	S1

ASIA Impairment Scale (AIS)

A = Complete. No sensory or motor function is preserved in the sacral segments S4-5.

B = Sensory Incomplete. Sensory but not motor function is preserved below the neurological level and includes the sacral segments S4-5 (light touch or pin prick at S4-5 or deep anal pressure) AND no motor function is preserved more than three levels below the motor level on either side of the body.

C = Motor Incomplete. Motor function is preserved at the most caudal sacral segments for voluntary anal contraction (VAC) OR the patient meets the criteria for sensory incomplete status (sensory function preserved at the most caudal sacral segments S4-5 by LT, PP or DAP), and has some sparing of motor function more than three levels below the ipsilateral motor level on either side of the body. (This includes key or non-key muscle functions to determine motor incomplete status.) For AIS C – less than half of key muscle functions below the single NLI have a muscle grade ≥ 3.

D = Motor Incomplete. Motor incomplete status as defined above, with at least half (half or more) of key muscle functions below the single NLI having a muscle grade ≥ 3.

E = Normal. If sensation and motor function as tested with the ISNCSCI are graded as normal in all segments, and the patient had prior deficits, then the AIS grade is E. Someone without an initial SCI does not receive an AIS grade.

Using ND: To document the sensory, motor and NLI levels, the ASIA Impairment Scale grade, and/or the zone of partial preservation (ZPP) when they are unable to be determined based on the examination results.

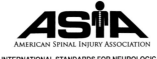

AMERICAN SPINAL INJURY ASSOCIATION

INTERNATIONAL STANDARDS FOR NEUROLOGICAL CLASSIFICATION OF SPINAL CORD INJURY

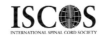

INTERNATIONAL SPINAL CORD SOCIETY

Page 2/2

Steps in Classification

The following order is recommended for determining the classification of individuals with SCI.

1. Determine sensory levels for right and left sides.
The sensory level is the most caudal, intact dermatome for both pin prick and light touch sensation.

2. Determine motor levels for right and left sides.
Defined by the lowest key muscle function that has a grade of at least 3 (on supine testing), providing the key muscle functions represented by segments above that level are judged to be intact (graded as a 5).
Note: in regions where there is no myotome to test, the motor level is presumed to be the same as the sensory level, if testable motor function above that level is also normal.

3. Determine the neurological level of injury (NLI).
This refers to the most caudal segment of the cord with intact sensation and antigravity (3 or more) muscle function strength, provided that there is normal (intact) sensory and motor function rostrally respectively.
The NLI is the most cephalad of the sensory and motor levels determined in steps 1 and 2.

4. Determine whether the injury is Complete or Incomplete.
(i.e. absence or presence of sacral sparing)
*If voluntary anal contraction = **No** AND all S4-5 sensory scores = **0** AND deep anal pressure = **No**, then injury is **Complete**.*
*Otherwise, injury is **Incomplete**.*

5. Determine ASIA Impairment Scale (AIS) Grade.
Is injury <u>Complete</u>? If YES, AIS=A

NO ↓

Is injury <u>Motor Complete</u>? If YES, AIS=B

NO ↓   (No=voluntary anal contraction OR motor function more than three levels below the <u>motor level</u> on a given side, if the patient has sensory incomplete classification)

Are <u>at least</u> half (half or more) of the key muscles below the <u>neurological level of injury</u> graded 3 or better?

NO ↓   YES ↓

AIS=C   AIS=D

If sensation and motor function is normal in all segments, AIS=E
Note: AIS E is used in follow-up testing when an individual with a documented SCI has recovered normal function. If at initial testing no deficits are found, the individual is neurologically intact and the ASIA Impairment Scale does not apply.

6. Determine the zone of partial preservation (ZPP).
The ZPP is used only in injuries with absent motor (no VAC) OR sensory function (no DAP, no LT and no PP sensation) in the lowest sacral segments S4-5, and refers to those dermatomes and myotomes caudal to the sensory and motor levels that remain partially innervated. With sacral sparing of sensory function, the sensory ZPP is not applicable and therefore "NA" is recorded in the block of the worksheet. Accordingly, if VAC is present, the motor ZPP is not applicable and is noted as "NA".

FIGURE 18.2   *> continued*

be overstated: Patients with a cervical SCI have a lower resting blood pressure than those with lower SCI, and they may present with a relatively "normal" blood pressure while experiencing AD.

AD is an imbalanced reflex sympathetic discharge that occurs when there is a painful, irritating, or even strong stimulus below the level of injury, such as an insect bite, bone fracture, or distended bowel or bladder. Other physiological causes of AD include urinary tract infection, epididymitis or scrotal compression, menstruation, gastritis or gastric ulcers, bowel impaction, or appendicitis. External causes of AD can include constricting clothing, uniforms, shoes, or equipment or blisters, sunburn, ingrown toenails, or contact with sharp objects. Finally, the environment can play a role, because temperature fluctuations can trigger AD. Intact peripheral sensory nerves transmit impulses that stimulate sympathetic neurons in the spinal cord below the level of lesion. The inhibitory outflow above the SCI is increased, but it cannot pass below the SCI. The large sympathetic outflow causes the release of various neurotransmitters,

such as norepinephrine and dopamine, resulting in systemic vasoconstriction and a sudden increase in blood pressure. Vasomotor brainstem reflexes try to lower blood pressure by increasing parasympathetic stimulation to the heart through stimulation of the vagus nerve, resulting in bradycardia. Because messages from the parasympathetic system cannot pass through the SCI, the blood pressure remains elevated. The most common cause of AD is impairment in the urinary system (bladder distension or urinary tract infection). Everyday training and rehabilitation sessions can provoke AD.

Signs and Symptoms

AD is characterized by sudden-onset high blood pressure and slowed heart rate, profuse sweating above the level of lesion, piloerection (goose bumps), flushing of the skin above the level of lesion, headache, and nasal congestion.[23] It is possible for signs or symptoms to be absent despite the elevated blood pressure. It is critical to take a blood pressure reading when AD is suspected. Special

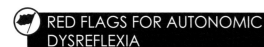

RED FLAGS FOR AUTONOMIC DYSREFLEXIA

Immediately examine a patient who presents with the following signs or symptoms of AD, and treat by removing the offending stimulus:

- Sudden onset of elevated blood pressure
- Accompanying lowered heart rate
- Profuse sweating above the level of impairment
- Piloerection
- Flushing of the skin above the level of impairment
- Headache
- Nasal congestion

attention is paid to any blood pressure reading more than 20 to 40 mmHg above the reference range for systole. To detect this, the athletic trainer must know the patient's normal blood pressure. Because bowel impaction and bladder distension can lead to AD, the clinician should also inquire about the patient's bowel and bladder habits.

Treatment and Return to Participation

The response to AD must be quick and thorough. First, the offending stimulus must be removed. The patient should be in a sitting position because sitting leads to pooling of blood in the lower extremities and may aid in reducing blood pressure. Clothing is loosened, as is protective equipment. A thorough examination should begin with the urinary system. Indwelling catheters are checked along the entire length of the system for constrictions, obstructions, or kinks. Health care providers must be familiar with the mechanism of these catheters because they are commonly used by many individuals with SCI. The bladder should be drained; fecal matter is evacuated. If neither the bladder nor colon is full, the clinician checks for other causes, such as sunburn, pressure sores, ingrown toenails, and insect bites. A physician may administer sublingual nifedipine to lower arterial blood pressure while the causes of AD are being determined. Caution is recommended when using antihypertensive agents with older adults or those with coronary artery disease. Most individuals who are susceptible to AD—that is, those with lesions above T6—typically have received extensive education from an SCI therapist on the hazards of the condition. However, the athletic trainer should never assume that the patient is fully aware of the causes or the signs and symptoms.

It is essential that the underlying causal agent be found and ameliorated. If symptoms do not seem to resolve immediately or if the cause of the AD has not been identified, emergency medical services should be summoned. Return to play should be based on physician clearance. The patient's symptoms and blood pressure are monitored for at least 2 h after resolution of the episode to ensure that AD does not reoccur.

Prevention

Prevention is key with AD. Because most episodes result from forgetfulness or carelessness about urine needs,[58] patients should inspect the catheter and void the bladder before activity. Patients must be asked about the type of bowel and bladder management program they maintain. They should avoid the risk of sunburn by using sunscreen, wearing a hat or visor, seeking shade during nonactivity, and covering susceptible areas. To prevent episodes of AD, the individual and the athletic trainer should perform a careful inspection after training or competition for contributors such as blisters, sunburn, pressure sores, and constricting clothing or equipment. To date, no specific relationship between AD and age has been documented. Because more males sustain SCI, AD is primarily a male phenomenon.

Boosting

Boosting is a dangerous technique used by some athletes with SCI to gain an advantage over an opponent or to improve race times. Bhambhani and colleagues reported that 66% of respondents surveyed at the 2008 Paralympic Games had experienced AD, and 16.7% had intentionally boosted.[25] Boosting is the intentional induction of AD for the purpose of enhancing performance through increased blood circulation. Athletes with SCI can induce AD by holding their urine or clamping their catheter before an event, sitting on a sharp object, sitting for a prolonged period, strapping their legs very tightly, or aggressively pinching or striking themselves. Self-induced lower leg fractures have also been reported.[18]

Boosting has been attributed to improvements of approximately 10% in track and swimming times as reported in athletes with disabilities who used this tactic.[25,26] This would be equivalent to reducing the able-bodied 26-mile marathon record by 12 min! However, this practice is, at the very least, unethical and must be prevented at all costs. The International Paralympic Committee (IPC) bans boosting as a method of doping and sees it as a safety risk. The athletic trainer must know that boosting is extremely risky and must strongly discourage the behavior. Athletes may think they are only receiving a catecholamine response and heart rate reserve that could normally be attained if uninjured. However, the significant rise in blood pressure that occurs with AD cannot be controlled by the body's autonomic nervous system. Other factors, such as inadequate hydration, fatigue, thermal stress, illness, or anxiety, can add to the AD and push the athlete to the point of autonomic shutdown, which can lead to death.[23]

Athletes anecdotally report that boosting is obvious when watching competitors at the starting line.[60] Athletes who have boosted typically present at the starting line with profuse sweating, goose flesh, and significant leg spasms. These athletes should be immediately suspected. The athlete's blood pressure is monitored, and those with elevated measurements (the IPC uses 180 mmHg systole as a cut point) are given 10 min to bring them down; if a diagnosis of AD, whether intentional or not, is confirmed, the competitor is withdrawn from the event.

Thermoregulation Concerns

Evaporative cooling is the most effective heat loss mechanism for the body, providing more than 80% of heat loss in the able-bodied athlete. Individuals with SCI cannot depend on the autonomic nervous system to lower their core temperature by regulating blood flow. In addition, sweating is often impaired below the level of spinal cord lesion, requiring the body to rely on less surface area for evaporative cooling.[27,28] Therefore, individuals with SCI are at increased risk of heat illness, and the athletic trainer must keep careful watch over athletes during high-energy sports that raise their core temperature. Individuals with tetraplegia and those with lesions above T6 are especially vulnerable to heat illness because they cannot increase the heart rate to sustain cardiac output when blood must flow to both the muscle and the skin.[28]

Likewise, individuals with SCI may lack normal warming mechanisms, such as piloerection, shivering, and circulatory shunting, in cold conditions. A lack of working muscle mass below the level of lesion contributes to temperature regulation problems. Even temperatures around 10 °C (50 °F) may pose problems for an individual with a cervical or high thoracic lesion. Impaired or absent sensation intensifies the risk of **hypothermia** because these individuals may be unaware of the loss of body heat.

CONDITION HIGHLIGHT

Hyperthermia

Hyperthermia occurs when the body temperature rises and remains above the normal 37 °C (98.6 °F) because of the body's failure to thermoregulate. Athletic trainers need to alert all patients to factors that can contribute to temperature-related illnesses. Health care providers must also be able to recognize conditions that put the physically active at risk of hyperthermia and understand that these factors may occur in combination to create a risky environment. These factors contribute to heat-related illness:

- Hot, humid conditions
- Recent illness
- Inability to sweat
- Lack of acclimation to temperature
- High-intensity workout
- Dehydration
- Dark-colored clothing
- Use of medications or dietary supplements
- Lack of fitness
- Excessive motivation
- Behavior risks (e.g., lack of sleep, alcohol intake)
- Amount and type of clothing or equipment causing impaired evaporation

The most severe form of hyperthermia is *heatstroke*. Heatstroke is a life-threatening emergency characterized by a core temperature over 40.5 °C (105 °F)[30,31] and a rapid increase in pulse (160-180 beats/min). The chief symptom of heatstroke is central nervous system dysfunction. Other symptoms are similar to those associated with concussion: namely, confusion, agitation, inappropriate behavior or language, apathy, vacillating emotions, stupor, and coma or death if untreated.

Individuals with SCI are particularly susceptible to cold. The athlete, athletic trainer, coaches, and other team members need to be sensitive to not only the environmental conditions but also inadequate clothing, prolonged levels of inactivity during competition, improper warm-up, and dehydration.

Signs and Symptoms

Recognizing the early warning signs and symptoms of dehydration in the athlete with SCI is crucial in preventing severe complications from heat stress. Signs and symptoms include thirst, irritability, fatigue, headache, weakness, dizziness, decreased performance, erratic wheelchair propulsion, flushed skin, head or neck heat sensations, vomiting or nausea, and general discomfort. Although chills and muscle cramps are common in athletes, such signs may not be present in athletes with SCI if piloerection is impaired. Cramping of the gastrocnemius and abdominal muscles is common, but these muscles are often nonworking in athletes with SCI.

Dehydration can also occur in hyperthermal situations during cold weather or when hypothermia also exists. Dehydration causes reduced blood volume, resulting in less fluid available to cool or warm tissues. Low temperatures accentuated by wind and dampness can pose a major threat to any individual but especially to the athlete with SCI, who may lack the normative mechanisms for warming.[29]

Referral and Diagnostic Tests

Thermoregulatory problems are often incorrectly attributed to fatigue, illness, hypoglycemic reactions, concussion, or head injury.[32] To determine hyperthermia, the clinician checks a distressed athlete for hot skin. Because the person with SCI has a diminished ability to regulate blood flow beneath the lesion, rectal temperatures may not provide accurate readings of core temperature; studies have been successfully completed using esophageal temperatures to better determine core temperature.[31,56,57] In addition, when the thermoregulatory system is impaired, typical signs such as shivering might not be observable. It is critical that the health care provider be able to review a thorough patient medication and nutritional supplement history that includes prescriptions and over-the-counter products. Sympathomimetics and anticholinergics affect thermoregulation, as do diuretics and excessive caffeine intake.[18] Emergency referral is warranted if the athlete is not responding to treatment or if heatstroke is suspected.

Treatment and Return to Participation

Treating thermoregulatory problems in patients with a spinal cord disability is similar to that for the general population. For hyperthermia, the patient is moved to a shaded or cooled area, clothing is loosened, equipment is removed, oral fluids are administered, and cooling is accomplished with cold water. Intravenous fluids are administered if the patient is not coherent. If heatstroke is suspected, emergency measures to reduce the patient's temperature (e.g., sponge application of cool water, fanning the body with a towel) are performed first; then the individual must be transported to an advanced emergency care facility.[30,31] Although immersion in an ice bath has been recommended, this treatment should be used with caution for individuals with SCI, especially those with a complete, high level of lesion: Their thermoregulatory system is impaired, and cooling may occur too rapidly. To date, research in this area for individuals with SCI is incomplete. Therefore, the patient's physician should discuss indications and contraindications before the patient exercises in the heat.

Treating hypothermia involves administering warm fluids, transporting the patient to a warm environment, and removing wet clothing immediately and replacing it with warm, dry clothing. Heat applied to areas without sensation is contraindicated, so use of heating pads or hot water bottles on paralyzed areas should be avoided.

The National Athletic Trainers' Association established an Inter-Association Task Force that created a statement on exertional heat illness containing return-to-activity guidelines.[30] In general, these guidelines include physician clearance and gradual and monitored return to activity, and they may be used with patients with SCI as well.

Prevention

Heat-related illnesses are entirely preventable. Hyperthermia can be prevented by ensuring availability of proper hydration and rehydration techniques, appropriately adapting to environmental conditions, wearing appropriate clothing, and screening for a prior history of heat-related illnesses. Individuals who use a wheelchair should attach to the chair a water bottle for drinking and a spray bottle for surface cooling. A tented area adjacent to the competition should be established to provide ready access to shade. Medications should be monitored, because some nutritional supplements and prescription, over-the-counter, and recreational drugs can adversely affect heat production and heat loss. The risk of heat illness is much greater for individuals who use these agents, so it stands to reason that some medications could influence similar mechanisms in individuals with SCI. Certain medications may also predispose individuals to temperature regulation problems in the cold.

Prevention of hypothermia includes encouraging individuals to drink plenty of fluids, warm up properly, wear adequate layers of clothing, change wet clothing immediately after exercise, and wear a hat. Athletic trainers should screen participants for a history of hypothermia.

Special Concerns in the Adolescent and Mature Individual

Athletic trainers should also closely monitor youth or master-level athletes for thermoregulatory issues.[30] Children tend to absorb more heat from their surroundings, have a lower sweating capacity, and produce more metabolic heat per mass unit than adults. Therefore, exercise time and intensity are reduced when environmental conditions are extreme. In addition, athletic trainers should make sure that children have 10 to 14 d of acclimatization. Older adults may have decreased fitness levels, decreased lean body mass, and chronic diseases and may use prescription medications, all of which may affect their reaction to the environment. Athletic trainers should check for fitness, acclimatization, and frequent fluid intake, and they should consult with the patient's physician about medications.

Skin Breakdown and Pressure Sores

Individuals with complete SCI are unable to feel sensations, which makes them susceptible to skin breakdown. Wrinkled socks, poorly fitted shoes, or orthoses can create blisters that become infected. Inattention to personal hygiene may also cause skin breakdown.[58] Circulatory problems related to paralysis increase the risk of infection and slow healing. Pressure sores, or decubitus ulcers, result in a loss of training and competition time and may lead to bed rest, hospitalization, or death in extreme cases. Skin over bony prominences is at greatest risk (e.g., sacrum, buttocks, and ankles). Athletes with pressure sores should not be allowed to compete.

Sports wheelchairs are designed so that the athlete's knees are at a higher level than the buttocks. This position increases pressure over the sacrum and ischial tuberosities. Body weight creates shear and compressive forces when combined with moisture created by competitive activity. Impaired circulation is exacerbated by perspiration and friction with the chair. Athletes who use a wheelchair and train without or in a perspiration-soaked shirt, such as tennis and basketball players, may experience breakdown of skin on their upper back from contact with the wheelchair back.

Signs and Symptoms

Skin appearance will vary with breakdown severity (figure 18.3).

- Stage I: The sore is red or discolored, but the skin is not broken. The discoloration or redness does not disappear within 30 min of pressure being removed from the site.
- Stage II: There is partial-thickness skin loss; the epidermis or top layer is broken, creating a shallow, open sore, but drainage may or may not be present.
- Stage III: The break in the skin has extended deep through the dermis or second layer into the subcutaneous and fat tissue, creating a full-thickness tear, and drainage is present.
- Stage IV: The breakage is more severe and extends into the muscle tissue and possibly down to the bone, and extensive tissue necrosis and drainage are present.

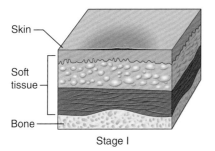
Stage I

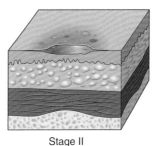
Stage II

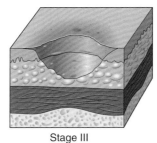
Stage III

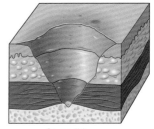
Stage IV

Skin — Soft tissue — Bone —

FIGURE 18.3 Staging of pressure sores.

Signs and symptoms that indicate further complication of a pressure sore include fever, black areas around the sore, greenish drainage, and odor.

Referral and Diagnostic Tests

Sores are typically overlooked because an athletic trainer or other health care provider may not inspect for them, or they are dismissed as abrasions or contusions from equipment. The athletic trainer and the athlete should thoroughly inspect the skin over at-risk body parts. Young athletes need special reminders to make this inspection a habit. When a pressure sore is discovered, the offending pressure must be removed (e.g., the athlete transfers from the wheelchair to a treatment table or the athlete stops lying or sitting on that skin area). If the discoloration or redness does not disappear within 30 min, the location and color should be noted, along with any drainage, in the medical file. If drainage is present, the health care provider inspects, monitors, and notes the color and odor and refers the patient to a physician.

Treatment and Return to Participation

Treatment begins with keeping pressure off the sore. If this is not possible during athletic activity and the sore is not severe enough to warrant restriction from activity, the individual must relieve pressure from the area when not participating in athletics. These sores must be cleaned and treated as potential infections. Appropriate hygiene and sanitation must be maintained and medicated dressing applied if necessary. Treatment for pressure sores is stage dependent as follows:

Stage I

- Remove pressure
- Practice proper hygiene (avoid vigorous scrubbing; pat dry)
- Evaluate diet for nutritional deficits
- Evaluate mattress use, wheelchair cushions, and transfer techniques
- Apply Tegaderm (3M) or similar dressing to prevent friction
- Refer if the sore persists 3 to 5 d

Stage II

- Complete stage I plan
- Cleanse with saline and pat dry
- Apply dressing such as Tegaderm or DuoDERM (ConvaTec)
- Refer if sign of infection

Stage III

- Complete stage I and II plans except for dressing
- Use a pressure-relieving mattress (physician can authorize)
- Apply advanced wound care for cleansing, debriding, and packing; most likely will need referral
- Administer oral or topical antibiotics
- Refer if sign of infection

Stage IV

- Consult with physician immediately
- Undergo surgery, as is often required

Only when a pressure sore is completely healed can the area receive pressure. The epidermis should not be broken and there should not be any redness or discoloration. One recommendation for determining whether a sore is completely healed is to gradually allow pressure to be accepted by the area again. For example, 15 min of pressure could be allowed, followed by 15 min of waiting for the redness to subside. If the discoloration does not subside, the area is not ready to accept pressure. If the redness subsides, the procedure can be repeated in 1 h. After three successful and consecutive 30 min trials, the area is usually ready to accept pressure. Athletes with pressure sores should not be allowed to compete.

Prevention

Prevention of pressure sores and skin breakdown includes regular skin inspection, use of seat cushions in the everyday wheelchair, frequent position changes, proper transferring mechanics to avoid shear, good hygiene, adequate nutrition, and keeping the skin dry. Athletes should promptly towel dry to remove perspiration after heavy exercise, swimming, and bathing or showering.

Children especially need to be reminded of preventive measures to avoid skin breakdown, such as proper hygiene, adequate nutrition, and routine visual inspections.[18] Because the skin of physically active older adults is more inclined to break down, it is paramount that preventive measures be stressed with these participants as well.

Spasms

Spasms can occur in individuals with spinal cord lesions above L1. Spasms are caused by excessive reflex activity below the level of lesion and appear as the sudden, involuntary jerk of a body part. The brain coordinates reflex activity; in spinal paralysis, impulse transmission is impaired. A spasm in a muscle group can be strong enough to launch an individual out of a wheelchair. Although spasms are frustrating for individuals, they are considered good for the circulation, especially among those who use a wheelchair.[33] Some evidence indicates that athletes with SCIs report higher levels of spasticity at lower temperatures, indicating that sports in cooler weathers may provoke spasms.[34] Most people who use a wheelchair experience spasms, although ambulatory people with incomplete SCI can have them, too.

The stimuli that provoke spasms differ from one person to another. Three main stimuli are responsible:

1. Sensory input, generally from touching hot or cold items
2. Pathology, such as bladder infections or skin breakdowns
3. Menstrual period

Spasms are not inherently negative, and they may not be preventable because they are associated with the reflex activity in spinal cord lesions above L1. However, because bladder infections may contribute to spasm intensity and frequency, avoiding such infections is critical.

Signs and Symptoms

A spasm may vary in duration and intensity but is most often a sudden, rapid, involuntary jerking of the paralyzed limb. The strength, frequency, and duration of the spasms should be noted and compared with the patient's norm; this information will vary from individual to individual. Spasms can be confused with seizure disorders or spasticity.

Referral and Diagnostic Tests

Clinicians must obtain a history of spasms during the PPE in order to have comparison data. During the general medical assessment, questions about stimuli that can cause spasms are also noted. Again, having a record of the patient's baseline when problems arise is the reason why a complete history is essential. For example, an individual who reports severe or more frequent spasms might be asked about a possible bladder infection. When bladder infection is suspected, the patient is referred to a physician for a complete urinalysis. In addition, the athlete is always referred to a physician if conservative measures do not alleviate the spasms and improve the condition.

Treatment and Return to Participation

Typically, no treatment is necessary for spasms, especially once the cause is addressed. However, when spasms are severe, treatments such as stretching, medication (e.g.,

baclofen, dantrolene, or diazepam [Valium]), nerve blocks, and surgery are options.

Individuals usually do not need to be restricted from activity because of spasms. If the spasms are excessive, then the underlying cause must be addressed. Otherwise, spasms usually pose no medical threat to participation.

Bladder Dysfunction

Athletes with SCI have a neurogenic bladder, meaning that the bladder does not always empty properly or completely. This can lead to infections, kidney stones, and obstructions.

The health care provider must inquire about the patient's bladder management plan. Ideally, this is discussed during the PPE. The patient may use an indwelling catheter to drain the bladder. These patients usually have frequent, if not constant, bacteria in their urine.[33,35,36] Bacteria in the bladder can spread to the kidneys and bloodstream and cause further illness and even death. Individuals who use intermittent catheterization, such as self-catheterization only when the urge to urinate is sensed, are also at risk of bladder infections, although to a lesser degree than those who use indwelling catheters. The clinician should be aware if timely access to appropriate facilities is a problem. These factors, as well as inadequate hydration, lead to increased risk of urinary tract infection among individuals with SCI.

Individuals with SCI also have problems with constipation and stool retention, which require that they regularly follow a bowel regimen.

Signs and Symptoms

Patients with SCI do not sense symptoms of pain and burning. Other signs and symptoms include bacteria in the urine, discolored urine, and fever. As stated previously, a bladder problem is the most common cause of AD, which can cause death. Differential diagnoses for bladder dysfunction include kidney infection, kidney stones, bladder infection, urinary tract infection, urethritis, cystitis, and contusion to the ureter, bladder, or urethra.

 RED FLAGS FOR BLADDER DYSFUNCTION

Identify and immediately treat patients with SCI who have bladder dysfunction because this condition can lead to autonomic dysreflexia (AD). When untreated, AD can cause death because of the combination of high blood pressure and lowered heart rate.

Referral and Diagnostic Tests

A proper assessment includes asking patients in-depth questions about their bowel and bladder routine (e.g., type, frequency, hygiene) and hydration history and performing a catheter inspection, urinalysis, and body temperature assessment. The athletic trainer should be aware that athletes have often been known to withhold hydration while on road trips; they avoid the perceived hassle of bladder voiding, but arrive at competition in a less than hydrated condition. Chapter 2 provides a description of how to take a dipstick reading for an on-site evaluation for many properties of the urine; table 2.3 lists the normal values for urine.

Treatment and Return to Participation

Antibiotics are the typical treatment for bladder infections. Athletes must refrain from training and competition for at least 8 h after initiating antibiotic treatment, in addition to being fever free for at least 24 h.

Prevention

Athletes and physically active individuals need to drink at least 2 L of water a day in order to regularly flush the bladder. They should be advised to use sterile voiding techniques in order to avoid contamination during catheterization and urinary drainage. In addition, the athletic trainer creates and promotes an environment in which patients do not feel self-conscious about taking care of their bowel and bladder needs.

Children need education and encouragement about independent care of bowel and bladder habits. Young athletes may be embarrassed by different routines (e.g., new environment, school), accidents, and odor.[9] They may also be too preoccupied with the sporting activity to adhere to a prescribed routine. This adds to the risk of infection and to embarrassment should an accident occur.

Spina Bifida

Spina bifida is a congenital spinal cord disability in which the neural tube fails to close completely during the first 4 to 6 wk of fetal development. Subsequently, the posterior arch of one or more vertebrae does not develop properly, leaving an opening in the posterior bony aspect of the spinal column. Spina bifida occurs most often in the low back and is more prevalent in females than in males. It causes muscular weakness or paralysis below the deficit. From least to most severe, the types of spina bifida are (1) occulta, (2) meningocele, and (3) meningomyelocele.

- *Spina bifida occulta* is so named because the defect is hidden under the skin (*occult* meaning hidden or secret). This mild form of spina bifida does not cause paralysis or muscle weakness. However, it is associated with low back pain in adults. In some people with spina bifida occulta, a birthmark, dimple, or a tuft of hair will mark the occulta. Usually, diagnosis is obtained incidentally by radiographs for other problems.

- *Meningocele* is characterized by the protruding of the meninges, the spinal cord covering, through a vertebral cleft into a sac, resulting in weakness in the lower extremities (figure 18.4).

- The most common type of spina bifida is *meningomyelocele*, also termed *myelomeningocele* (figure 18.5). In this condition, the spinal cord and nerve roots exit through a vertebral cleft and fill a tumorous sac, causing a significant deficit below the lesion.

The latter two conditions require surgical correction for spinal cord fluid leakage into the sac. Spina bifida is nonprogressive; the defect at the spine will not become worse with time.

Individuals with spina bifida experience many problems common to all forms of spinal paralysis, including bladder and bowel dysfunction, spasms, and skin lesions. However, these problems are greater for children.[37] Without sensation in the lower extremities, children with meningomyelocele might not notice and report skin lesions until serious infection occurs. This is attributable to children's proclivity to play with abandon, disregarding seemingly mild contusions and abrasions. Children are also more likely to be wearing splints and braces than adults. The health care provider needs to be diligent in the visual inspection of areas covered by assistive devices. Proper fitting of assistive devices must be ensured to avoid skin problems.

In addition, people with spina bifida often have a heightened **gag reflex**, which is related to the vagus nerve.[38] This exaggerated gag reflex may make swallowing pills, having the throat examined, or having a complete cranial nerve assessment more difficult.

Cerebral Shunts

Individuals with spina bifida may have an implanted cerebral shunt to control cerebrospinal fluid that backs up into the ventricles of the brain. The shunt relieves **hydrocephalus**—that is, the buildup of cerebrospinal fluid in the ventricles. One end of a tube, which has a one-way valve for outflow of fluid, is inserted into the ventricles; the other end is threaded just under the skin down to the abdomen, where fluid is then reabsorbed by blood vessels in the membranes surrounding internal organs.[39] During the PPE, athletic trainers should be sure

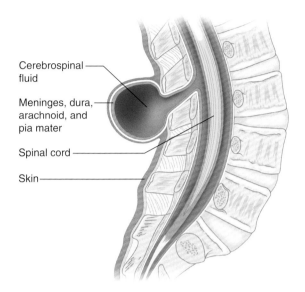

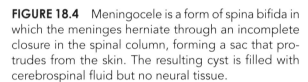

Labels (left figure): Cerebrospinal fluid; Meninges, dura, arachnoid, and pia mater; Spinal cord; Skin

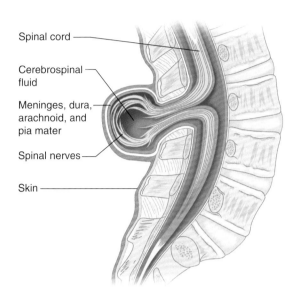

Labels (right figure): Spinal cord; Cerebrospinal fluid; Meninges, dura, arachnoid, and pia mater; Spinal nerves; Skin

FIGURE 18.4   Meningocele is a form of spina bifida in which the meninges herniate through an incomplete closure in the spinal column, forming a sac that protrudes from the skin. The resulting cyst is filled with cerebrospinal fluid but no neural tissue.

FIGURE 18.5   Meningomyelocele, or myelomeningocele, is a form of spina bifida that is apparent at birth. The herniation contains cerebrospinal fluid and a portion of the spinal cord.

to inquire about shunts. Shunts typically pose no restrictions on activity except avoidance of head trauma, such as that experienced in soccer heading. Some athletes wear an appropriate helmet or headgear for protection. A small scar may be noticed behind the ear of an individual with spina bifida who has a shunt. The athlete with suspected shunt problems should be referred to a physician. Clinical features of shunt malfunction include headache, thoracic pain, vomiting, drowsiness, and **papilledema**. If an athlete sustains an impact sufficient to cause a laceration to the skin overlying the shunt, referral to a neurosurgeon should occur immediately.[39]

Latex Allergy

Individuals with spina bifida have a higher incidence of latex allergy. Latex products such as gloves, stretch bands or rubber tubing, adhesive bandages and tape, and rescue breathing masks should never come into contact with athletes with spina bifida. The clinician must have nonlatex substitutes available when working with these patients, and it is wise to have substitutes on hand for the athletic and patient populations in general. Although most reactions to latex are mild, some may be life-threatening.

Treatment for severe reactions includes administration of epinephrine, such as with an epinephrine-injecting pen (EpiPen; see chapter 3). Because the best method is prevention, the use of nonlatex products with individuals known to have this allergy is crucial. An allergist can conduct testing to confirm the allergy.

RED FLAGS FOR LATEX ALLERGY

Note: Individuals with spina bifida may have a higher incidence of latex allergy. Signs and symptoms of latex allergy include the following:

- Sneezing or runny nose
- Itchy, red, watery eyes
- Coughing
- Rash or hives
- Shock
- Chest tightness and shortness of breath
- Change in voice or hoarseness
- Difficulty breathing

Poliomyelitis

Poliomyelitis, or polio, is a form of paralysis caused by a viral infection that affects motor cells of the spinal cord. Sensation, as well as bowel and bladder control, is not affected. The severity and degree of paralysis depends on the number and location of motor cells destroyed by the virus. Because of widespread use of the Salk vaccine, developed in the 1950s, polio is rare in school-aged athletes. However, in countries such as Nigeria, India, and Pakistan, polio continues to cause paralysis.

Many people who previously had polio have experienced symptom recurrence years after the initial attack. These symptoms include new muscle and joint pain, muscle weakness at old and new sites, severe fatigue, muscle atrophy, and new respiratory problems.[40] This combination of symptoms is known as **post-polio syndrome**. According to the National Institutes of Health National Institute of Neurological Disorders and Stroke, post-polio syndrome can occur 15 to 40 yr after polio onset. The syndrome is not infectious but can affect activities of daily living. Signs and symptoms of post-polio syndrome include muscular weakness and atrophy, joint pain, scoliosis, and fatigue.[41]

Polio is similar to SCI and spina bifida, in that muscles are paralyzed. However, because polio does not attack sensory nerve fibers, sensation is intact. Paralysis is often incomplete, which makes judging the level of lesion difficult.[40] Therefore, a complete assessment of functional abilities should be conducted during the PPE.

Other than the possible presence of post-polio syndrome, few general medical conditions are unique to these individuals. The overall general medical assessment process is facilitated in this group because they have sensation and can detect pain.

Cerebral Palsy

Cerebral palsy (CP) is a chronic neurological disorder caused by a lesion in the brain that affects movement and posture. CP occurs before, at, or soon after birth and is not hereditary or progressive. CP affects the ability to move and maintain balance and posture because of damage to areas of the brain that control muscle tone and spinal reflexes. The disorder varies from mild, evidenced by general clumsiness and a slight limp, to severe, in which the individual is dominated by reflexes, unable to ambulate without a motorized chair, and nonverbal.

The United States Cerebral Palsy Athletic Association uses a classification system based on an athlete's functional ability. This system also includes athletes with other conditions characterized by nonprogressive brain lesions. Neurotrauma, such as stroke and traumatic brain injury, are included in the classification because many Paralympic sports use a functional classification system across disabilities rather than isolated competition within disabilities. The system is controversial but was designed to allow for the grouping of athletes with similar abilities to compete within specific categories.

Some individuals with CP may have associated conditions such as deafness, vision disturbances, impaired hand–eye coordination, intellectual disabilities, and seizures. Seizure conditions are common in athletes with disabilities. However, athletic trainers should know that exercise decreases the incidence of seizures, and individuals with CP should not be discouraged from participation

based on seizure history. These factors influence the risk of injury but not necessarily illness. Because the disorder can be complicated by other impairments, communication with patients with CP is critical.

CP is characterized by **spasticity**, **athetosis**, or ataxia. Individuals with CP may be further grouped according to how many limbs are affected and their functional ability. They may present with decreased musculotendinous flexibility, decreased strength, and considerable muscle imbalance. Flexibility is the most important fitness goal in athletes and physically active individuals with CP.

Spastic Cerebral Palsy

Spastic CP, the most common type, is characterized by hypertonic muscle tone during voluntary movement. Typically, the flexor muscles are stronger than the extensor muscles. An exaggerated myotatic reflex is associated with spasticity. This reflex normally serves as a protective mechanism. However, in athletes with an exaggerated myotatic reflex (i.e., a reflex reaction in response to stretching a muscle), mild stretching may evoke a heightened response varying from a mild recoil to a violent withdrawal of the limb. In some individuals, this reflex is so disruptive that they strap their limbs down. Athletes with CP should start stretching after a warm-up period. This stretching is slow and sustained to prevent activation of the myotatic reflex.

Individuals who are ambulatory may walk with a scissors gait, which is characterized by a pigeon-toed walk caused by extreme tightness of the hip flexors, adductors, and internal rotators. The knee flexors and ankle plantar flexors are also abnormally tight, which causes the athlete to bend their knees when walking and

---

Clinical Tips

Communication Considerations: Individuals With Cerebral Palsy

- Be patient and allow the individual enough time to communicate; speech may be very slow or difficult to understand.

- Position the athlete carefully during assessment, because incorrect positioning on a treatment table can elicit abnormal reflexes that will interfere with movement.

- Use word boards or other visual aids related to the general medical condition.

- Avoid ballistic movements during assessment; move the patient's body parts slowly to avoid increased muscle tone or abnormal reflexive responses.

to walk on their toes. The health care provider needs to be aware that spasticity increases with stress and fatigue.

Athetoid Cerebral Palsy

Athetoid CP, the second most common type, is characterized by constant, purposeless, and unpredictable movement that is caused by fluctuating muscle tone. Fluctuating muscle tone occurs when muscles are **hypertonic** and are then periodically **hypotonic**. This causes characteristics of drooling, lack of head control, and trouble with speaking, eating, and writing. Most people with athetosis are tetraplegic; some use a wheelchair and others walk with an unsteady gait. Signs and symptoms of athetosis increase with stress and fatigue.

Ataxic Cerebral Palsy

Ataxic CP, the least common type, can result from disorders of the spinal cord and brain. It varies from mild to severe and occurs in approximately 10% of people with CP. Ataxic CP is diagnosed only in persons who can walk unaided. Athletes with ataxia have balance and coordination disturbances. They can usually maintain balance when their eyes are open but not when they are closed. Walking on uneven ground, managing stairs, and stepping over objects pose problems for individuals with CP.

Pathological Reflexes

In infants, involuntary, predictable muscle and postural tone shifts are normal and considered important for development. However, reflexes that are not integrated at the developmentally appropriate times become pathological and affect the smoothness and coordination of movement. These reflexes can be elicited spontaneously or by an external stimulus.

Patients with CP often exhibit these pathological reflexes. During the assessment, the athletic trainer should be aware of reflexes that the patient has not integrated so they can be positioned such that those reflexes are not elicited and do not interfere with the examination. Although a comprehensive discussion of the more than 25 primitive reflexes that might be present in this population is beyond the scope of this chapter, some must be mentioned. The following four problematic reflexes can manifest in individuals with CP, and they are considered troublesome because they are initiated by head movements.

- *Prone tonic labyrinthine reflex:* The TLR-prone reflex is characterized by increased flexor tone elicited by a change in head position. When gravity pulls the head downward and the body responds by assuming a flexion posture, this indicates the TLR-prone reflex.

- *Supine tonic labyrinthine reflex:* The TLR-supine reflex is characterized by increased extensor tone in response to any change in head position. If the head is thrown backward and the body responds in an extension posture, this is evidence of the TLR-supine reflex.

- *Asymmetrical tonic neck reflex:* The ATNR is also known as the *fencing reflex* because, when activated, the upper extremities assume the en garde position of fencers. Rotation or lateral flexion of the neck causes obligatory extension of the arm on the face side and simultaneous flexion on the nonface side. Taking a position in front of the athlete or patient before addressing them (to avoid head turning) reduces the chance of eliciting this reflex.

- *Symmetrical tonic neck reflex:* The STNR is characterized by bilateral arm and leg responses to up-and-down head movements. Head flexion causes flexor tone of the upper body and extensor tone of the lower body; head extension elicits the opposite. Positioning at eye level with the athlete or patient will help to reduce the chance of eliciting this reflex.

Health care providers need to remember that these reflexes are involuntary motions or postures, and although they are not painful, they can compromise certain body positions. Communication with athletes and patients can be enhanced by understanding the reflexes and working around the stimuli that elicit them.

Seizures

Seizures have many causes, with epilepsy being one, but they are also common in individuals with CP. For more information on epilepsy, review that section in chapter 10. Seizures should be identified at the PPE and then carefully monitored on an ongoing basis. The sports medicine team should be especially familiar with the different options available for antiseizure medication as well as potential side effects. Side effects include impaired attention span, ataxia, nystagmus, strabismus, and cognitive impairment. Seizure medications are chosen for an individual based on the seizure type. Because no single drug controls all types of seizures, individuals with CP may take various medications, and some may require a combination of seizure medications to achieve good seizure control. Carbamazepine is often recommended with caution for this athletic population, because it has been known to cause **hyponatremia**.[59] Seizures during aerobic activity are rare, but that does not preclude the need for caution. Compliance with medication is extremely important. Therefore, medications are kept on the athlete's person

Clinical Tips

Athlete Medication Challenges When Traveling

- Special attention must be given to patients taking prescribed medications when competition travels to a different time zone.
- Unless there are special circumstances, athletes should have ready access to their own prescribed medications.
- A plan must be activated to maintain sustained medication levels in the athlete.
- Consult with the provider to determine the best method of maintaining therapeutic levels of prescribed medications when traveling across time zones.

so that doses are not missed. During competition that involves travel, athletic trainers need to prompt athletes to take medications at the correct times. Travel often disrupts routines, making many athletes more likely to forget doses. The health care provider should know when athletes have had their antiseizure medications adjusted. The athlete, physician, and athletic trainer work together to set up the most appropriate seizure control plan.

Amputations

Congenital or acquired disorders may necessitate limb amputation. Common indications for amputation include a necrotic extremity associated with peripheral vascular disease or diabetes; life-threatening emergency conditions related to cancer or infection; and congenital deformity or injuries to the brachial plexus, which cause the arm to be hypersensitive, such that it is sometimes deemed a "nuisance extremity."[42] War and terrorist attacks have affected the emergence and development of sports participation among individuals with disabilities as well. Young, physically active men and women who have been injured during armed conflicts still want a competitive or fitness outlet, such as the Invictus Games mentioned earlier in this chapter.

People who have had an amputation can continue to participate in sporting events despite the loss of one or both of the upper or lower extremities. Track and field and swimming events are the most popular for athletes with amputations. Athletes with double amputations compete in wheelchair tennis or basketball events. In track and field, the rules for individual events are the same as for all competitors; athletes may use prostheses, but no other assistive device is allowed. Prosthesis use is

optional in most events, but it is not permitted in the high jump. Balance may be adversely affected in athletes with amputation because of changes in their center of gravity.

Sport governing bodies have rules that allow or disallow participation with prosthetic devices. In the United States, the National Federation of State High School Associations does not prohibit prostheses and leaves the decision to each state association.[43] The National Collegiate Athletics Association has guidelines and standards regulating the use of artificial limbs in sports in its *Sports Medicine Handbook*.[44] Factors considered include the type of amputation and prosthesis, the potential harm to other players, and the question of an unfair advantage for the athlete because of the prosthetic device. Extremity prostheses can give an athlete full range of motion for competitive success in a variety of sports, including basketball and throwing sports.

Amputations are categorized by location (AE, above the elbow; AK, above the knee; BE, below the elbow; BK, below the knee) and number for identification in sport classifications:

A1: AK double

A2: AK single

A3: BK double

A4: BK single

A5: AE double

A6: AE single

A7: BE double

A8: BE single

A9: Combined lower and upper limbs

Skin breakdown and **phantom leg pain** are the primary medical problems seen in athletes who have had amputations.

Skin Breakdown

In a previous study, Anderson and colleagues found that individuals who use a wheelchair may have greater risk of skin breakdown than those who do not.[45] Individuals with an amputation are generally aware of skin irritation or breakdown when it begins. Prevention includes ensuring that the prosthesis fits properly. An excessively loose or tight fit increases stress at the junction. Prostheses can increase local skin pressure and contribute to abrasions, blisters, and rashes. Other skin disorders affecting individuals with an amputation include contact dermatitis (e.g., from cleaning agents, ointments, lotions, or perfumed powders), cysts, folliculitis, fungal infections, adherent scars, and eczema. Various materials, such as gels, silicone, soft materials, and foam padding, have been used between the skin and the socket to reduce stress from vigorous athletic activity. It is necessary to clean and thoroughly dry the stump and to change any padding that has become moist from perspiration. Morning washes are not advised unless a stump sock is worn, because the damp skin can swell inside the prosthetic socket. A fragrance-free soap or antiseptic cleaner should be used, and the skin should be dried thoroughly. The socket of the prosthetic should also be cleaned and dried often. Talcum powder and roll-on or solid antiperspirants are commonly used to control perspiration buildup in the socket. If the skin breakdown is advanced, the individual may have to temporarily discontinue use of the prosthesis and reduce athletic participation; many times, stump rest is the best prescription. An athlete participating in wheelchair sports does not have to discontinue play. For minor skin irritations, lotions, such as silicone-based ALPS skin lotion (Alps South) or Derma Prevent (Ottobock Healthcare), or a film-like OpSite (Smith & Nephew Healthcare) can be used. If a minor abrasion is present, medicated lotions, such as those with zinc oxide, are helpful.

Younger athletes with amputations have special needs because the appliances are small and require frequent adjustments to accommodate growth. However, skin breakdown is less frequent at younger ages.

An athletic trainer may be required to assist in or perform wrapping of the stump. Although therapists may have subtle differences in the way they wrap, the basic technique for providing edema control and support without restricting circulation is the same:

- Apply the bandage with the limb extended to prevent contractures.
- All turns of the bandage should be diagonal, versus circular, to promote circulation.
- Wrap the bandage less firmly in the distal to proximal direction on the stump. No skin should be showing except for the joint itself, which usually is not bandaged at all.
- Wrap right up to the crease of the buttocks and around the waist (similar to the common hip spica wrapping technique) of an athlete with an above-the-knee amputation.
- No pain should be associated with the wrapping.

Encourage athletes to wash their bandages by hand and squeeze rather than wring out the water. Spread bandages out on a flat surface to dry; never put them in a dryer. Some individuals may use **shrinkers**, which are elastic compression "socks" that are pulled over the stump. They are not as effective as wraps in controlling edema, but they are easier to use. The shrinker should fit tightly but not be painful or restrict blood flow. Avoid allowing athletes to roll or fold down the top of the shrinker, as this compromises its effectiveness.

Abnormal Sensation and Phantom Pain Syndrome

Abnormal sensations can be felt from the amputated body part, ranging from mild to severe. These include feelings of size, position, movement, itchiness, heat, cold, and touch. In some people with amputations, the abnormal sensation is pain. This is known as *phantom pain syndrome* and is more common in adults than children. It can also range from mild to severe. For severe pain, antidepressants have been used to provide relief. In the nonathletic population, narcotics have also been prescribed. Any person using narcotics for phantom pain needs to consult a physician before entering an exercise program.[46]

Sensory Disabilities

Individuals with sensory disabilities make up a unique segment of the athletic population. General treatment of illness and sport-related injuries is similar, but individuals with sensory disabilities may require other communication approaches.[42] The medical team should be prepared to find alternative ways to deliver and obtain information. In each of the following sections, recommendations for communication are presented. In this chapter, the term *sensory disability* refers to visual impairments and blindness as well as deafness and hardness of hearing.

Visual Impairments and Blindness

Individuals with visual impairments have visual acuity that ranges from legal blindness with partial sight to total blindness. Athletes with visual impairments compete and excel in a variety of sports, such as track and field, wrestling, swimming, tandem cycling, power lifting, goal ball, judo, gymnastics, skiing, baseball, and golf. Participation may be facilitated by the use of assistive technology, such as a joint optical reflective display (JORDY) system, sighted guides, step or stroke counting, a tether or guide wire, or a sound source, depending on the degree of visual impairment. Table 18.2 lists the classification system for sport competition used by the United States Association of Blind Athletes.

The cause of blindness should be noted. Blindness can be caused by birth defects, including congenital cataracts and optic nerve disease. Excessive oxygen in incubation in babies born in the 1950s was a common cause but has decreased. Other causes include tumors, albinism, injuries, and infectious diseases. In older people, common causes of blindness are diabetes, macular degeneration, glaucoma, and cataracts.

During the PPE, the useful vision of the patient is determined. About 80% to 90% of people who are blind have some **residual vision**.[46] Residual vision can be

TABLE 18.2 **United States Association of Blind Athletes Visual Classification System for Sport Competition**

Level	Characteristics
B1	From no light perception in either eye up to light perception, but inability to recognize the shape of a hand at any distance or in any direction
B2	From ability to recognize the shape of a hand up to visual acuity of 20/600* and a monocular visual field of less than 5° in the best eye with the best practical eye correction
B3	From visual acuity above 20/600 and up to visual acuity of 20/200 and a monocular visual field of less than 20° and more than 5° in the best eye with the best practical eye correction

*See chapter 11 for a discussion of visual acuity as expressed according to Snellen eye chart numbers.

Adapted by permission from U.S. Association of Blind Athletes: U.S. Association of Blind Athletes (USABA) visual classification. Available: http://usaba.org/index.php/membership/visual-classifications/.

ascertained by questioning patients about what they see, in addition to conducting a visual acuity examination. The health care provider must also be sensitive to the fact that lighting in the clinic or athletic training facility may affect the patient's ability to see. The athletic trainer should determine at what age the patient became visually impaired and if loss of sight was congenital or occurred later in life.

Overall, there are few special concerns in sports medicine regarding the athlete with visual impairment. First and foremost is the issue of communication. It is up to the athletic trainer to effectively communicate information to the athlete, especially because so much of the general assessment is gained through the preparticipation history. Thorough documentation will help the athletic trainer and coach provide a positive athletic experience and can be obtained through a variety of communication modes.

Some people who are blind often exhibit **blindisms**—that is, repetitive movements such as rocking, hand waving, finger flicking, or digging the fingers into the eyes. There is no inherent harm in displaying blindisms other than social stigma. Many parents, teachers, and coaches have worked with children who are blind to stop these movements in certain situations. Postural deviations, such as a forward head and slumping, may also be prevalent, especially in those who are congenitally blind and have never seen others sit, stand, and move. Most experienced adult athletes develop proper posture through cueing and physical activity. Some novice athletes with visual impairments may exhibit poor balance, fewer social skills, and low cardiovascular fitness.

Documentation of illness and other general medical conditions in athletes who are visually impaired is extremely limited. Musculoskeletal injury data show that these athletes have a high proportion of lower extremity injuries. Athletes with visual impairments expend more energy than matched sighted athletes and therefore are more likely to fatigue quickly. This could be an important consideration when determining return-to-play guidelines after illness.

Albinism

Albinism is characterized by a lack of pigment in the iris and throughout the body. The eyes of individuals with albinism are sensitive to light. Therefore, they may need to wear tinted glasses inside and outside to help reduce glare. Nystagmus may also be present and should be noted in the PPE. Because individuals with albinism are more susceptible to sunburn, the athlete who exercises outdoors, even in overcast or cool weather, should generously and repetitively use sunscreen. Wearing of hats or visors and long-sleeved shirts is also advised.

Glaucoma

Glaucoma is an increase in pressure in the globe of the eye, caused by inability of the intraocular fluid to drain properly. This excess pressure damages the optic nerve. Visual loss may be gradual, sudden, or present at birth. Glaucoma typically appears after age 40 yr, and most commonly among people in their sixth decade of life. Although evidence confirms that physical activity lessens the chances of developing glaucoma, athletes with this condition do participate in competitive sport.[47] A patient reporting that lights appear to have halos around them may be experiencing the early stages of glaucoma. Individuals with glaucoma must avoid isometric activities, swimming underwater, inverted body positions, excess fluid intake, antihistamine use, and other practices that could increase eye pressure.[46,47] Individuals with glaucoma may also need to use moistening eyedrops.

Deafness and Hardness of Hearing

In the United States, people who are Deaf do not consider themselves disabled but rather members of a subculture of American society. Person-first terminology, discussed at the beginning of this chapter, is not supported by these athletes. The preferred term is *Deaf*, with an uppercase D. **Hearing loss** is a general term that describes people who are hard of hearing or Deaf. **Hardness of hearing** (previously described as *hearing impaired*) is defined as a condition that makes understanding speech difficult through use of the ears alone, with or without a hearing aid. Deafness is a condition in which a person is unable to understand speech using the ears alone, with or without a hearing aid. Hearing loss can range from mild to profound and is classified as one of three types: conductive, sensorineural, and mixed.

Conductive hearing loss is mechanically caused; sound does not pass through the external and middle ear to reach the inner ear (analogous to a radio with the volume on low).[48] A buildup of impacted wax, injury, or infection in the external ear can cause conductive loss. Individuals with conductive hearing loss typically have intelligible speech and may wear hearing aids to increase the volume. See chapter 12 for other conditions related to temporary hearing loss.

Sensorineural hearing loss is more serious and involves the inner ear, where sensory receptors convert sound waves into neural impulses that are transmitted to the brain for translation. Most people who are born Deaf have this type of loss (analogous to a radio that is not well tuned). Causes of this type of loss are generally idiopathic. Others identified include hereditary factors, meningitis, measles, scarlet fever, mumps, and encephalitis. The speech of people with sensorineural loss may be difficult to understand. Those with more loss will most likely use sign language to communicate. Balance problems sometimes accompany this type of loss.

The mixed type of hearing loss is a combination of conductive and sensorineural losses. It is more common in older adults and might not be seen as often in the athletic population as the other types of losses.

Communication is the primary concern in the care of Deaf individuals, and it needs to be addressed during the PPE. In addition to the standard preparticipation examination, ask the following questions of patients who are hard of hearing or Deaf:

- Has the hearing loss progressed? Has it worsened, stayed the same, or improved with aids?

- At what age did the loss occur?

- What method of communication does the patient prefer (e.g., sign language, speech reading)?

- Does the patient use hearing aids or have cochlear implants?

- Does the patient use earplugs during swimming and water activities?

- Does the patient have a history of ear infections?

- Is the hearing loss related to or accompanied by balance problems or vertigo?

It is up to the practitioner to find alternative ways to communicate. One method of communication that is relatively easy for medical personnel to learn is American Sign Language (ASL). Although there are shortcuts to certain words and phrases, the simple alphabet can be articulated by hand signs; it is depicted in figure 18.6.

Hearing Aids and Implants

A variety of hearing aids exist for the Deaf. Hearing aids do not clarify or make speech sound clearer; they simply amplify sound. The four basic types of hearing aids are (1) on the chest or body, (2) behind the ear, (3) in the ear, and (4) on the eyeglasses.

Cochlear implants are recommended for individuals for whom a hearing aid is not helpful. The implants are surgically placed in the inner ear and are activated by an external speech processor worn on a belt or in a pocket. A microphone is worn as a headpiece externally behind the ear. Sound is translated by the speech processor into distinctive electrical signals that travel up a thin cable to the headpiece and are transmitted across the skin via radio waves to the implanted electrodes in the cochlea. The auditory nerve is stimulated, and information is transmitted to the brain, where it is interpreted (figure 18.7). Some models do not have external wires. Although the National Association of the Deaf does not promote cochlear implants, they are being increasingly implanted in children with sensorineural loss,[48] and their use and usefulness has been internationally supported with evidence-based rationale.[49] The external apparatus should be removed during exercise to reduce the chance of electrostatic discharge.[46] People with cochlear implants must also stay away from plastic or rubber mats, balls, and equipment to avoid exposure to electrostatic discharge that can damage the electrodes.

Once communication barriers, type and care of hearing aids or implants, and any related conditions (e.g., balance problems, ear infections) have been addressed, the general medical assessment is the same as that for individuals who are not Deaf or hard of hearing.

Intellectual Disabilities

In October 2010, U.S. President Barack Obama signed a bill called "Rosa's Law," which promoted the term *intellectual disability* and mandated that federal statutes would no longer use the terms *mental retardation* and *mentally retarded*. Intellectual disabilities are among the best known because of the visibility they receive from the Special Olympics. Athletes with intellectual disabilities compete in more than 30 individual and team sports, such as aquatics, basketball, gymnastics, figure skating,

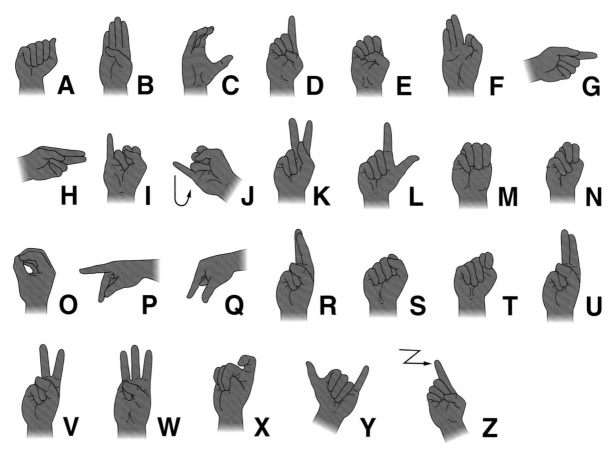

FIGURE 18.6 The ASL alphabet can be used to communicate effectively with Deaf athletes. ASL has shortcuts and abbreviations for words or phrases that facilitate communication, but this alphabet shows the basis for the language.

Clinical Tips

Communication Considerations: Individuals With Visual Impairment

- The examiner should always start an interaction by stating their name; for example, "Jordan, hi. It's Tamika, and I'm going to discuss your symptoms with you." They should not expect the patient to recognize the sound of their voice.

- Ask the patient if they need assistance with mobility. Do not grab the patient's arm; rather, offer an upper arm and allow the patient to grasp it.

- Provide the patient with verbal cues that indicate changes in surface, location of the examining table, doors to be opened in or out, and steps up or down.

- Use tactile sense when performing an assessment; the examiner should allow the athlete to follow their hands through the evaluation.

- Demonstrate a maneuver within the patient's field of vision.

- Conduct the assessment in a brightly lit area and use colored instruments or materials that contrast with the background (e.g., brightly colored stethoscopes and reflex hammers, colored tape around edges of furniture or doorways).

- Understand that individuals with albinism and glaucoma can better distinguish solid-colored objects under nonglare lights and away from the glare from sunlight.

- Ask the patient how they prefer to receive written materials (e.g., large print, Braille, audio clips, computer software–based files), such as treatment instructions or medical staff contact information.

- Keep the examination and treatment areas free of clutter and low-hanging objects.

Clinical Tips

Communication Considerations: Deaf Athletes

- Speak directly to the patient and not to a guest or interpreter who might be present.
- Maintain eye contact and face the patient in order to facilitate speech or lipreading; even the best speech readers will understand only about 30% of what is said.
- Speak normally if the patient uses a hearing aid.
- Use facial expressions, body language, gestures, and common signs, such as thumbs up and down for "okay" and "not okay."
- Demonstrate any technique before performing it on a patient.
- Use video, computer movie files, or other visual media as another form of demonstration.
- Use visual and tactile cues.
- Learn basic American Sign Language.
- Orient the patient to all aspects of the facility, with special attention to exits and fire evacuation procedures.
- Do not pretend to understand the patient if speech is unclear to you; instead, ask for repeats.
- Use instant messaging, email, or other similar electronic methods to communicate.
- Use strobe fire alarms or other visual alerting devices in the facility so the patient is notified in an emergency; point out these systems to the patient.
- Avoid loud or constant music or background noise, even at low levels; it reduces hearing aid effectiveness and may even cause the patient to develop headaches.
- Avoid "visual noise" such as extra physical or visual movements behind a person who is speaking.

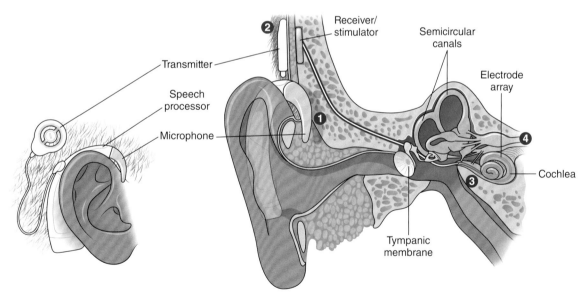

❶ Sounds are picked up by and enter the system through a microphone.

❷ The sound is transferred through the coil to the implant just under the skin to the receiver.

❸ The implant sends a pattern of electrical pulses to the electrodes in the cochlea.

❹ The auditory nerve (CN VIII) picks up the electrical pulses and sends them to the brain. The brain receives the signals and CN VIII interprets them as sound.

FIGURE 18.7   A cochlear implant can restore hearing through electronic assistive devices.

and alpine skiing. Eunice Kennedy Shriver established the Special Olympics in 1968 as a means for awareness, attitude change, and equal opportunity, and it is the premier sport event for persons with intellectual disabilities.

The American Psychiatric Association identifies intellectual disabilities by noting insufficiencies in multiple mental faculties, such as problem-solving, reasoning, judgment, planning, academic learning, abstract thinking, and learning from experience.[50] Inability to adequately function in the aforementioned areas can affect communication, social interaction, personal independence, work or academic ability, and social responsibility. Diagnosis of intellectual disabilities requires three specific criteria established in the fifth edition of the *Diagnostic and Statistical Manual of Mental Disorders*, and severity is determined as mild, moderate, severe, or profound.[50]

Athletic trainers will most likely serve individuals with mild intellectual disability. In general, these individuals attain reading and math skills equivalent to grade levels 3 through 6.[51] During the assessment of athletes with intellectual disabilities, the terminology used and directions provided must be clear and concise. Athletic trainers should provide ample time for patients to become familiar with the treatment or athletic training facility. Demonstrating the task first is best accompanied by simple, one-step instructions reinforced to the patient verbally and continually. Patients should be asked to repeat instructions to ensure that they understand.

Down syndrome is the most common chromosomal abnormality that causes intellectual disability. It is an autosomal chromosomal condition that results in a host of medical concerns in addition to those seen in other athletes with intellectual disabilities. Medical conditions associated with Down syndrome include atlantoaxial instability, balance deficits, obesity, poor hand–eye coordination, postural or orthopedic posture problems (e.g., kyphosis, club foot, lordosis), vision concerns (e.g., strabismus, nystagmus, cataracts), and cardiac issues (e.g., ventricular septal defect, atrioventricular canal defect, mitral valve prolapse).

Generalizations are difficult for people with intellectual disabilities because their abilities and medical concerns vary widely. Assessment during the PPE is the best method of determining normative values for each athlete. In addition to a thorough history and physical examination, echocardiograms may be indicated to screen for cardiac defects such as atrioventricular septal defects, ventricular septal defects, and atrial septal defects.[52] Maximal heart rates of persons with intellectual disabilities are 8% to 20% lower than expected. For example, they exhibit maximal heart rates of 10 to 15 contractions/min below expected levels, and people with Down syndrome have even lower maximal heart rates (e.g., approximately 30-35 contractions/min below expected levels). In the general

RED FLAGS FOR DETERMINING PAIN

Individuals with an intellectual disability may be insensitive or indifferent to pain, or they may not be able to articulate the severity of pain they are experiencing. It is essential that the athletic trainer thoroughly evaluate for signs of trauma or illness if there is cause to believe something is wrong.

population, people with cognitive disorders have lower fitness levels than those without intellectual disabilities.

Associated Medical Concerns

Documented medical concerns associated with intellectual disabilities include seizures, pain insensitivity, and medication use. Seizures occur in approximately 20% of individuals with mild intellectual disabilities. The PPE should include inquiries about seizure control methods and medications. Approximately 25% of people with intellectual disabilities show signs of pain insensitivity or indifference that place them at serious medical risk.[51,53] Reports have documented individuals with intellectual disabilities who died from appendicitis and bowel obstruction that went undiagnosed because they did not report pain.[24] The health care provider needs to carefully check for signs of trauma and must not rely exclusively on what the patient reports. Anticonvulsive, hypnotic, neuroleptic, and antidepressant medications are commonly used in this population. Hypothyroidism is common in persons with Down syndrome, and many may be receiving thyroxine replacement therapy. Side effects of some of these hypothyroidism medications can cause angina until a stable dose has been determined.[46] Vision problems are common in people with intellectual disabilities, necessitating a careful visual examination during the PPE.

Atlantoaxial Instability

Atlantoaxial instability is used to describe laxity of the ligaments and muscles that surround the first and second cervical vertebrae. Approximately 17% of people with Down syndrome have atlantoaxial instability.[54] The Special Olympics requires radiographic results to confirm the condition prior to participation.

Full participation of the medical team in completing a thorough PPE that screens for the previously described health problems is paramount. An athlete with Down syndrome should have the presence of atlantoaxial instability ruled out before unrestricted participation in sport is approved. Without medical clearance on file, athletes with Down syndrome are restricted from participating in judo, equestrian sports, snowboarding, alpine skiing, squat lifting, gymnastics, some swimming activities (e.g., butterfly stroke events, flip turns, and diving), high jump, pentathlon events, soccer, and warm-up exercises that place pressure on the head and neck muscles.[54] This restriction can be waived if signed acknowledgment of the risks is obtained from the adult athlete, or from a parent or guardian if the athlete is a minor or not able to give informed consent, and written certifications from two physicians, excluding the examining physician on record.[53]

Summary

Although people with disabilities do not have a higher incidence of general medical conditions than the general population, they do present with some unique conditions that the athletic trainer must be prepared to recognize through assessment. Individuals with SCI are susceptible to AD, thermoregulatory problems, bowel and bladder complications, spasms, and skin breakdown. In addition, people with spina bifida may have latex allergies.

The athletic and medical teams need to be creative and committed when communicating with athletes and patients who are sensory impaired, whether they are visually impaired, blind, Deaf, or hard of hearing. Knowing the common limitations associated with each disability can enable the athletic trainer to be prepared to provide quality care to these patients.

Appreciating the critical importance of a thorough PPE enables the clinician to discover possible future problems and address them before they arise. The PPE is the most powerful tool team members have for managing the sports health care of people with a disability. Each patient presents with unique characteristics, and baseline measurements are imperative.

Apply It!

Go to HK*Propel* to complete the case studies for this chapter.

GLOSSARY

abdominal aortic aneurysm (AAA)—Enlargement of the lower part of the aorta.

abscess—A cavity containing pus and surrounded by inflamed tissue, formed as a result of suppuration in a localized infection.

absorption—The process of getting drugs into the body through a variety of routes, including oral, rectal, vaginal, intravenous, intramuscular, inhalation, and topical application to the skin.

acne—A disease of the skin common where sebaceous glands are numerous.

actinic dermatitis—An inflammation of the skin from exposure to sunlight or another irritating light source.

actinic keratoses—Rough, slightly raised areas of skin due to prolonged sun exposure. It is a precursor to skin cancers.

acute pancreatitis—A sudden inflammation of the pancreas.

acute stress disorder (ASD)—Dissociative symptoms following a traumatic event; these symptoms are characterized by a decrease in emotional responsiveness, difficulty concentrating, and a feeling of detachment.

adenoids—Pharyngeal tonsils.

adenoma—A tumor of glandular epithelium, in which the cells of the tumor are arranged in a recognizable glandular structure.

administration—The direct application of a single dose of a drug.

adnexal—In relation to accessory organs.

adventitious breath sounds—Abnormal breath sounds superimposed over normal breath sounds: crackles, rhonchi, wheezes, pleural friction rubs.

afebrile—Without fever; apyretic.

afferent pupillary defect—When pupils react differently to light shown in one pupil at a time.

agonist—A drug that exerts its effect by attaching to cellular receptors in the body, causing stimulation of the receptor.

alopecia areata—A disease of unknown cause in which well-defined bald patches occur.

ambient temperature—The encompassing prevailing temperature.

amblyopia—A condition resulting from no apparent pathology in which vision is reduced or dimmed; also known as *lazy eye.*

amyloidosis—A disease in which a waxy, starch-like glycoprotein (amyloid) accumulates in tissues and organs, impairing their function.

anaphylactic shock—A severe, sometimes fatal systemic hypersensitivity reaction to a sensitizing substance, such as a drug, vaccine, food, serum, allergen extract, insect venom, or chemical.

anastomosis—A connection between two vessels, or a surgical connection between two vessels, ducts, or intestine.

anemia—A decreased number of red blood cells or a decreased hemoglobin concentration in the blood.

aneurysm—A sac filled with fluid or clotted blood that results from dilation of the wall and that can cause stenosis of the coronary artery.

angina—Pain or pressure in the chest.

angioedema—An acute, painless dermal, subcutaneous, or submucosal swelling of short duration. It involves the face, neck, lips, larynx, hands, feet, genitalia, or viscera.

angiotensin-converting enzyme (ACE) inhibitor—A protease inhibitor found in serum that promotes vasodilation by blocking the formation of angiotensin II and slowing the degradation of bradykinin and other kinins.

anhedonia—Inability to experience pleasure in acts that are typically pleasurable.

anisocoria—Unequal pupil sizes commonly associated with head trauma.

anorexia nervosa—Eating disorder that results in loss of weight, emaciation, intense fear of weight gain, and distorted body image; characterized by stringent diet restrictions, refusal to eat, or purging of ingested food.

antagonist—A drug that exerts its effect by binding to a cellular receptor but does not cause stimulation of the receptor.

antiemetic agent—A medication used to alleviate symptoms of nausea or vomiting.

antiphospholipid antibodies—Associated with immune-mediated illnesses, syphilis, and stroke; thought to result from a hypercoagulable disorder.

antipyretic—A medication to reduce fever, or an agent used to stop itching.

aortic dissection—Occurs when the innermost layer of the aorta tears, allowing inner and middle layers to separate as a result of blood flow into the area. If the blood-filled area ruptures through the outside aortic wall, it is usually fatal.

aortic stenosis—Narrowing or structure of the aortic valve.

AP view—Positioning depicted on a radiograph from front (anterior) to back (posterior), most commonly associated with the direction of an X-ray beam.

apical systolic murmur—A cardiac murmur occurring during systole that is heard over the apex of the heart.

aplastic anemia—A deficiency of all the formed elements of blood representing a failure to the cell-generating capacity of bone marrow.

apnea—Absence of spontaneous respiration.

appendicitis—Inflammation of the vermiform appendix.

arboviruses—A large group of viruses recovered largely from bats, rodents, and arthropods (e.g., insects and crustaceans).

arrhythmogenic right ventricular dysplasia (ARVD)—A rare cardiomyopathy in which fat or fibrous tissue replaces the normal muscle properties of the right ventricle.

arthrocentesis—Aspiration of a joint.

asepsis—Absence of infectious organisms.

aseptic technique—Technique to prevent transfer of microorganisms.

Asherman's syndrome—Adhesions or scars within the uterus.

ataxia—An abnormal condition characterized by impaired ability to coordinate movement.

athetosis—A condition in which involuntary, slow, irregular, twisting movements occur in the extremities, especially in the hands and fingers.

athlete's heart—An enlarged but otherwise normal heart of an athlete trained for endurance.

athletic amenorrhea—A condition where a female does not have a period because of high exercise levels and low body fat percentage.

atrioventricular (AV) block—A disorder of cardiac impulse transmission that reflects prolonged, intermittent, or absent conduction of impulses between the atria and ventricles.

atropine—A drug used to dilate the pupils or relax muscles.

attention deficit hyperactivity disorder (ADHD)—Neurobehavioral condition that impairs the person's ability to maintain attention.

autoinoculation—The inoculation of a microorganism obtained by contact with a lesion on one's own body, producing a secondary infection.

autonomic dysreflexia (AD)—A potentially life-threatening condition characterized by the sudden onset of excessively high blood pressure in persons with lesions at or above the sixth thoracic nerve; also known as *hyperreflexia*.

bacterial vaginosis—A bacterial infection of the vagina.

bactericidal—Causing bacterial cell death.

bacteriostatic—Inhibiting further replication of bacteria but not causing cell death.

bacteriuria—Bacteria in the urine.

balanitis—Inflammation of the foreskin of the penis.

bell clapper deformity—Failure of the testes to be secured to the scrotum, leaving them free, much like a clapper within a bell.

benzodiazepine—A psychotropic medication used to alleviate anxiety.

bifid—Cleft, or split into two parts, or branches.

biguanides—A member of the class of oral antihyperglycemic (a substance that prevents or counteracts high blood levels of glucose) agents that works by limiting glucose production and glucose absorption.

biliary colic—Painful contraction of the gallbladder that results from a gallstone that had obstructed the cystic duct.

binge eating disorder—Eating in binges that results in emotional or physical discomfort similar to bulimia but without the compensatory behaviors of bulimia.

biopsychosocial–spiritual model (BPSS)—Framework for understanding a person's response in a given situation.

bipolar disorder—Mental disorder marked by episodes of mania and depression.

bisferiens pulse—An arterial pulse that has two palpable peaks, the second of which is slightly weaker than the first.

bleb—Accumulation of fluid under the skin.

blepharospasm—Squeezing of the eyelid.

blindisms—Repetitive movements such as rocking, hand waving, finger flicking, or digging the fingers into the eyes.

boosting—The intentional induction of autonomic dysreflexia for the purpose of enhancing performance through increased blood circulation.

bradypnea—Abnormally low rate of breathing.

bronchial breath sound—A loud, high-pitched, and predominantly expiratory sound that represents air moving through large airways; normally heard only over the trachea in the anterior chest midline.

bronchophony—Increased intensity and clarity of vocal resonance caused by increased density of lung tissue.

bronchovesicular breath sounds—Heard when air moves through medium-sized airways, such as the main stem bronchi; can be heard both anteriorly and posteriorly, toward the center of the thorax. These sounds are of medium pitch and moderate intensity. Inspiratory and expiratory phases are approximately equal.

Brudzinski's sign—An involuntary flexion of the arm, hip, and knee when the neck is passively flexed. It occurs in patients with meningitis.

bruit—An abnormal blowing or swishing sound or murmur heard while auscultating a carotid artery, the aorta, an organ, or a gland, such as the liver or thyroid, and resulting from blood flowing through a narrow or partially occluded artery.

bulbar conjunctiva—Conjunctiva overlying the sclera.

bulimia—Eating disorder characterized by repeated incidences of binge eating and self-induced vomiting, diarrhea, or excessive exercise.

bulla—Air- or fluid-filled sac in the chest.

candidiasis—An infection caused by a species of *Candida* found most often in skin folds, the rectum, and nails. Oral candidiasis is also possible and is known as *thrush*.

carbuncle—A large site of staphylococcal infection containing purulent matter in deep, interconnecting subcutaneous pockets.

cardiac event monitor—Device worn over a period of time to capture prolonged electrocardiograph recordings; formerly called a *Holter monitor*.

cardiac stress test—A graded test, typically on a stationary bicycle or treadmill, that challenges the heart activity.

cardioangiography—The process of producing a radiograph of the heart and its great vessels.

cataract—Clouding of the lens of the eye.

cauda equina—The terminal portion of the spinal cord and the spinal nerves below the first lumbar nerve.

cephalocaudal—In the case of an examination, covering all areas from head to toe.

cerebral palsy (CP)—A chronic neurological disorder caused by a lesion in the brain that affects movement and posture.

cerebrovascular accident (CVA)—Cerebral vascular hemorrhage in the brain, resulting in ischemia of brain tissues normally perfused by the damaged vessels.

cerumen—The wax-like substance normally found in the external canal of the ear; earwax.

cheerleader's nodules—Laryngitis caused by excessive use of the voice.

chemoprophylaxis—Antimicrobial medication that prevents the spread of pathogens from one area of the body to another.

Cheyne-Stokes respiration—Breathing pattern characterized by periods of apnea.

choanae—The posterior openings in the nasal cavity that connect the nasal cavity with the nasopharynx, allowing the inhalation and expiration of air.

cholecystitis—Acute or chronic inflammation of the gallbladder.

cholelithiasis—Gallstones.

cholinergic—An agent that stimulates the elaboration of acetylcholine at the myoneural junction.

cholinergic urticaria—Skin condition, which results in hives, caused by sweat.

choriocapillaris—Vascular tissue between the retina and the sclera.

chronic fatigue syndrome (CFS)—A condition characterized by disabling fatigue accompanied by symptoms such as muscle pain, multijoint pain, and headache.

claudication—Cramp-like pains in the calves caused by poor circulation of blood to the leg muscles.

clearance—The measure of the body's ability to eliminate a drug.

cold urticaria—Reactive disorder that manifests as hives after exposure to cold.

colonoscopy—A process of viewing into the colon of the digestive tract with a colonoscope.

comedones—A blackhead; the basic lesion of acne vulgaris, caused by an accumulation of keratin and sebum within the opening of a hair follicle.

commotio cordis—Damage to the heart, frequently fatal, resulting from a forceful nonpenetrating blow to the adjacent body surface.

comorbid—Two or more medical conditions that exist at the same time but that may be unrelated.

complete blood count (CBC)—A blood test looking at the major components of the blood under a microscope to determine whether each component is within the usual range or value.

computed tomography (CT) scan—Computerized diagnostic imaging technique using electromagnetic radiation in a 360° motion around the patient to create an image of the body in cross-sectional slices for examination.

conductive hearing loss—A hearing loss caused by a mechanical deviation whereby sound does not pass through the external and middle ear to reach the inner ear.

congenital aortic valve stenosis (AS)—Narrowing or stricture of the aortic valve present at birth.

congestive heart failure (CHF)—An abnormal condition that reflects impaired cardiac pumping and the inability to maintain the metabolic needs of the body.

conjunctivitis—Inflammation of the vascular tissue covering the anterior sclera and the posterior surface of the eyelids; commonly caused by bacteria, allergies, or viral infection.

contact dermatitis—An inflammation of the skin caused by direct contact with a specific allergen.

contraindication—Situation in which a drug or treatment should be avoided.

contrast venography—The use of dye to detect the actions elicited in a vein.

cosmesis—The appearance of a patient or wound. Wound closure methods are intended to improve the cosmesis of the wound.

crackles—Adventitious sounds that occur as a result of disruption of airflow in the smaller airways, usually by fluid; also known as *rales*.

CREST syndrome—A syndrome consisting of *c*alcinosis cutis, *R*aynaud's phenomenon, *e*sophageal dysfunction, *s*clerodactyly, *t*elangiectasia, as well as scleroderma, carpal tunnel syndrome, and Buerger's disease.

cribriform plate—A perforated structure in the posterior portion of the ethmoid bone.

Crohn's disease—A chronic inflammatory bowel disease (IBD) characterized by inflammation of the gastrointestinal tract.

croup—Acute viral infection of the upper and lower respiratory tracts.

cyclothymia—A form of seasonal affective disorder where the athlete may perform well in practice or competitions for several days or weeks but then inexplicably hit a slump.

cystoscopy—The process of examining the lining of the bladder and the urethra.

deep vein thrombosis (DVT)—A disorder involving a thrombus (blood clot) in one of the deep veins of the body, most commonly the iliac or femoral vein.

dehiscence—Splitting open, separation of the layers of a surgical wound.

déjà vu—The sensation or illusion that one has encountered an experience or place before.

dermatitis—An inflammatory condition of the skin. Various cutaneous eruptions occur and may be unique to a particular allergen, disease, or infection. The condition may be chronic or acute; treatment is specific to the cause.

dermatographism—An urticaria due to physical allergy in which a pale, raised welt or wheal with a red flare on each side is elicited by stroking or scratching the skin with a dull instrument.

dermatophyte—Any of several fungi that cause parasitic skin disease in humans.

dermonecrotic arachnidism—Tissue destruction caused by spider venom.

diabetic ketoacidosis (DKA)—Diabetic coma; a life-threatening condition in uncontrolled diabetes mellitus.

diagnostic imaging—The use of radiographic, sonographic, nuclear, and other technologies to create visual representations for medical analysis and evaluation.

diagnostic overshadowing—The tendency for clinicians to attribute all signs and symptoms to the major condition (disability), leaving other coexisting conditions undiagnosed.

diagnostic testing—Process of using diagnostic imaging and procedures to identify a condition or disease.

dilutional pseudoanemia—"Anemia" not attributable to a low red blood cell count but to increased blood volume; not a true anemia.

diplopia—Condition in which the patient sees two of a single object; also known as *double vision.*

dispensing—The act of delivering a medication to an ultimate user pursuant to a medical order issued by a practitioner authorized to prescribe.

distribution—The process of getting drugs delivered throughout the tissues and fluids of the body.

dysautonomic cephalgia—A dysfunction in the autonomic system causing headaches in the back of the head.

dysdiadochokinesia—An inability to perform rapid alternating movements.

dyshidrosis—Any disorder of eccrine sweat glands.

dysmenorrhea—Abnormally painful or irregular menstruation.

dysmetria—Uncontrolled movements in a specific muscle group.

dyspareunia—Pain during sexual intercourse that is not normal.

dysphagia—Difficulty swallowing.

dysplastic nevi—An atypical mole or freckle.

dyspnea—Labored or difficult breathing.

egophony—Altered voice sound in a patient with pleural effusion.

electrocardiogram (ECG)—A graphic recording of the heart's electrical activity in the form of a PQRST wave.

electrocardiography—The process of having an electrocardiograph performed on a person.

electroencephalogram (EEG)—Electrodes placed on scalp that detect the electric potential produced by brain cells. The record of this test is the *gram* aspect of this test, whereas electroencephalography is the process of the recording.

electromyogram (EMG)—Process of applying electrodes to skeletal muscle to measure the electrical activity during muscle contraction.

electromyography—Record of the electrical activity in skeletal muscle.

elimination—Process of getting a drug out of the body.

encephalitis—An inflammatory condition of the brain, usually caused by an infection.

endocrine glands—Glands that secrete hormones directly into the bloodstream, allowing specific body functions to occur.

endoscopy—A procedure using an instrument to view internal structures of the body, typically the gastrointestinal system.

enophthalmos—Recession of the eyeball deeper into the orbit.

enterovirus—A group of RNA viruses that can cause diseases in humans, typically found in the respiratory secretions and stools of infected people.

epidermis—The superficial avascular layers of the skin made up of an outer dead, cornified part and a deeper living, cellular part.

epidermoid cysts—A painless, slow-growing cyst that is noncancerous and arises from the upper layers of the skin.

erythema migrans—A skin lesion that begins as a small papule and spreads peripherally. It is sometimes associated with Lyme disease.

eustachian tube—A mucous membrane–lined tube that joins the nasopharynx and the middle ear cavity; opened during yawning, chewing, and swallowing to allow for equalization of air pressure.

exercise-induced laryngeal obstruction (EILO)—Wheezing and dyspnea caused by transient obstruction of the upper airways during exercise.

exophthalmos—An abnormal condition characterized by a marked protrusion of the eyeballs.

factor V Leiden anticoagulant gene mutation—A genetic mutation of factor V that causes venous thrombosis (blood clots).

fibromyalgia—A form of nonarticular rheumatism characterized by musculoskeletal pain, spasm and stiffness, fatigue, and sleep disturbances.

fluoroscopy—A diagnostic imaging device creating immediate radiographic imaging on a fluorescent screen for visual examination in real time.

folliculitis—Inflammation of the hair follicles.

fornices—The loose arching folds connecting the conjunctival membranes on the inside of the eyelid and those covering the eyeball.

furuncle—A localized suppurative staphylococcal skin infection originating in a gland or hair follicle and characterized by pain, redness, and swelling.

furunculosis—An acute skin disease characterized by boils or successive crops of boils that are caused by staphylococci or streptococci.

gag reflex—A reflex contraction of the muscles of the throat elicited by touching the soft palate or posterior pharynx.

gastritis—Diffuse inflammation of the lining of the stomach.

gastroenteritis—Inflammatory condition of the stomach and intestines that is usually caused by bacteria or a virus.

gastroesophageal reflux disease (GERD)—Condition in which stomach acid travels up through the lower esophageal sphincter into the esophagus or even into the back of the throat.

generalized anxiety disorder (GAD)—Disorder marked by worry over or nervousness about many or most things in life.

gingiva, gingivae—The gum tissue of the mouth that encircles the necks of the teeth.

gingivitis—An inflammation of the gingivae in which the margins close to the teeth are red, swollen, and bleeding.

glaucoma—Group of eye diseases characterized by increased intraocular pressure.

goiter—A visible swelling on the anterior neck due to an enlarged thyroid gland.

gonorrhea—A common sexually transmitted infection that affects the genitourinary system and often the rectum and pharynx.

Graves' disease—The common name for hyperthyroidism.

gustatory hallucinations—A false taste sensation of either food or beverage.

hairy leukoplakia—A white plaque visible on the surface of the tongue that is most often associated with severe immunodeficiency.

half-life—The length of time that it takes for blood or tissue levels of a drug to decrease by one-half.

hardness of hearing—A condition that makes understanding speech difficult through the use of the ears alone, with or without a hearing aid.

hearing loss—A general term that describes people who are hard of hearing or Deaf.

heatstroke—A life-threatening emergency characterized in the able-bodied population as having a core temperature over 40.5 °C (105 °F).

heliotrope rash—An upper eyelid rash that is red to purple and indicative of dermatomyositis.

hemoglobin electrophoresis—A blood test used to differentiate different forms of hemoglobin.

hemoglobinuria—Abnormal presence in the urine of hemoglobin that is not attached to red blood cells.

hemolysis—The breakdown of red blood cells and the release of hemoglobin that occur normally at the end of the life span of a red blood cell.

hemolytic anemia—A disorder characterized by acute or chronic premature destruction of red blood cells.

hemoptysis—Productive cough of sputum that may contain blood.

hemothorax—Collection of the blood in the pleural cavity of the thorax.

hepatomegaly—An abnormal enlargement of the liver that is usually the sign of a disease.

hepatosplenomegaly—Enlargement of the spleen and liver.

herpes gladiatorum—Herpes simplex virus (HSV) found on the trunk that is typically transmitted via skin-to-skin contact, such as in the sport of wrestling.

herpes keratoconjunctivitis—A highly contagious form of herpes simplex that affects the cornea of the eye.

herpes zoster—An acute infection caused by reactivation of the latent varicella-zoster virus, which mainly affects adults.

hidradenitis suppurativa—An infection or inflammation of the sweat glands.

hirsutism—Excessive body hair in a masculine distribution pattern as a result of heredity, hormonal dysfunction, porphyria, or medication.

Hodgkin's lymphoma—A malignant condition of lymphoreticular origin; different from Non-Hodgkin's lymphoma because of the presence of Reed-Sternberg cells.

homatropine—A drug used to dilate the pupils; less potent than atropine.

Horner's syndrome—A condition caused by damaged sympathetic trunk nerves.

hot spots—Locations on a nuclear diagnostic image that illuminate due to higher levels of detected radiation as a result of increased absorption of radionuclide.

hydrocephalus—The accumulation of cerebrospinal fluid in the ventricles of the brain.

hydronephrosis—Swelling of one kidney due to the failure of normal drainage of urine from the kidney to the bladder.

hydrophilicity—The degree to which a compound is soluble in water.

hyperandrogenism—A condition in which there are excessive levels of androgens in the body.

hyperemia—An increase in blood flow to a body part; characterized by reddening of the skin.

hyperglycemia—An excess of glucose in the blood caused by ineffective use of insulin, specifically in diabetic patients. Untreated, coma or death can occur.

hyperinsulinemia—An excessive amount of insulin in the body.

hyperlipidemia—An excess of lipids, including glycolipids, lipoproteins, and phospholipids, in the plasma.

hyperopia—Farsightedness, in which a person can see objects in the distance clearly, but closer objects are out of focus.

hyperpnea—Rapid breathing with very large breaths; >24 breaths/min.

hyperthyroidism—An abnormal endocrine condition characterized by hyperactivity of any of the four parathyroid glands with excessive secretion of the parathyroid hormone (PTH).

hypertonic—Increased muscle tension whereby muscle tone is abnormally rigid and range of motion may be hampered.

hypertrophic cardiomyopathy (HCM)—An abnormal condition characterized by gross hypertrophy of a ventricle of the heart, but having a normal chamber size.

hyperuricemia—Results from either the increased production of uric acid or the decreased elimination of uric acid by the kidneys.

hyphema—Blood in the anterior chamber of the eye.

hypoglycemia—A lower than normal amount of glucose in the blood (less than 60 mg/dL) that can lead to death if not rectified.

hypogonadism—Deficiency in the activity of the gonads; testes for males, ovaries for females.

hyponatremia—A condition where the level of sodium in the blood is drastically depleted, which can lead to coma and death. Overhydrating can cause this.

hypopnea—Shallow, slow breathing.

hypothermia—A potentially life-threatening emergency characterized in the able-bodied population as having a core body temperature under 35 °C (95 °F).

hypotonic—Diminished or flaccid muscle tone whereby muscle contraction speed is slow and strength is impaired.

immunosuppressed patient—A patient who has a condition that produces an inhibited ability to respond to antigenic stimuli.

impetigo—A streptococcal, staphylococcal, or combined infection of the skin beginning as focal erythema and progressing to pruritic vesicles, erosions, and honey-colored crusts.

in situ—The natural or original position or place.

indication—Condition for which a drug has been found to have a therapeutic effect.

infectious mononucleosis—Disease caused by the Epstein-Barr virus; associated with symptoms of fatigue, pharyngitis, fever, and lymphadenopathy; also known as the *kissing disease.*

inflammatory bowel disease (IBD)—A group of intestinal disorders that cause prolonged inflammation of the digestive tract.

international normalized ratio (INR)—A standardized measure of time it takes for blood to clot.

intravenous pyelogram (IVP)—A specific type of X-ray that shows images of the kidneys, the bladder, the ureters, and the urethra.

ipsilateral miosis—Ipsilateral pertains to the same side of the body, and miosis is a constricted pupil. Together this means only one pupil (of the eye) is constricted.

irritable bowel syndrome (IBS)—Disorder of gastrointestinal motility with abnormal cycles of muscle contraction and relaxation.

islets of Langerhans—Clusters of cells within the pancreas that produce insulin, glucagon, and pancreatic polypeptide. They are important regulators of carbohydrate metabolism.

jamais vu—A sensation of being a stranger to a previously known place or person.

Kaposi's sarcoma—A malignant condition beginning with dark papules on the feet or hard palate of the mouth that metastasizes to lymph nodes or other organs. It is associated with autoimmune or immunodeficiency conditions as well as with lymphomas.

Kawasaki's disease—Rare, inflammatory condition of unknown origin that usually occurs in young childhood.

keratinous cysts—An epithelial cyst containing keratin.

kerions—An inflamed, boggy granuloma that develops as an immune reaction to a superficial fungus infection, generally in association with tinea capitis of the scalp.

Kernig's signs—A diagnostic sign for meningitis that occurs when the patient cannot straighten the leg when it is fully flexed at the knee and hip.

Kiesselbach's plexus—An area of small, fragile arteries and veins located in the nasal septum; the root of most nosebleeds.

Korotkoff sounds—A series of sounds produced by distention of an artery by the blood pressure cuff; the level at which the sound disappears is the diastolic pressure, often referred to as the *fifth or last Korotkoff sound.*

Kussmaul breathing—Deep, rapid, sighing breaths characterized by diabetic ketoacidosis.

labial agglutination—When the labia majora stick together.

lactic acidosis—A disorder characterized by an accumulation of lactic acid in the blood, resulting in a lowered pH in muscle and serum.

lagophthalmos—Inability to close the eyelids completely, usually the result of a severe subconjunctival hemorrhage.

lanugo—Fine, downy hair covering the body.

laparoscopic—Surgical procedure in which a laparoscope is used to examine the abdominal cavity through one or two small incisions in the abdominal wall.

laparoscopy—A process of viewing within a body cavity with a laparoscope.

laryngitis—Inflammation of the larynx.

lateral view—Positioning on a radiograph taken from the outermost side, most commonly associated with the direction of an X-ray beam.

lesion—A wound, injury, or pathological change in body tissue. Any visible, local abnormality of the tissues of the skin, such as a wound, sore, rash, or boil. A lesion may be described as benign, cancerous, gross, occult, or primary.

leukemias—Uncontrolled proliferation of white blood cells in the bone marrow, which accumulate and replace normal blood cells in the marrow.

leukocytosis—An abnormal increase in the amount of circulating white blood cells.

leukopenia—An abnormal decrease in the number of white blood cells, fewer than 5,000 cells per cubic centimeter.

leukoplakia—White plaque found on the lateral borders of the tongue that may be folded or smooth in appearance; associated with severe immunodeficiency.

lipophilicity—The degree to which a compound is soluble in fat.

long QT syndrome (LQTS)—An inherited cardiac disorder characterized by prolongation of the QT interval.

lymphadenopathy—A condition where either a lymph node is diseased or a disease of the lymph nodes.

lymphocytosis—A proliferation of lymphocytes, as occurs in certain chronic diseases.

lymphoreticular system—A system composed of the primary lymphoid organs, such as bone marrow or the thymus, which serve to produce lymphocytes.

lymphosarcoma—Any of a heterogeneous group of malignant tumors involving lymphoid tissue.

maculopapular rash—A skin eruption characterized by distinctive macules or papules.

Marfan syndrome—An autosomal dominant, heritable disorder of connective tissue.

mastication—Chewing, tearing, or grinding food with teeth while it becomes mixed with saliva.

melanin—A black or dark brown pigment that occurs naturally in hair, skin, and the iris and choroid of the eye.

melanocyte—A body cell capable of producing melanin.

melanoma—Any group of malignant neoplasms that originate in the skin and are composed of melanocytes.

meningitis—Any infection or inflammation of the membranes covering the brain and spinal cord.

meningoencephalitis—An inflammation of both the brain and meninges, usually caused by a bacterial infection.

metabolism—In pharmacology, the process by which a drug is changed into one or more chemical entities.

metastasis—A process that occurs when cancerous cells establish a remote colony of cancerous cells from the original cancer.

metastatic—The process of tumor cells spreading from an initial disease site to another area of the body.

methicillin-resistant *Staphylococcus aureus* (MRSA)—An infection caused by a strain of staphylococcus (staph) bacteria that is resistant to many medications used to treat other staph infections.

microcytic anemias—Include iron deficiency, thalassemia, lead poisoning, and sideroblastic anemia.

mitral regurgitation—A backflow of blood from the left ventricle into the left atrium in systole across a diseased mitral valve.

mittelschmerz—Abdominal pain mid-way through the menstrual cycle associated with the release of the ovum (ovulation).

molluscum contagiosum—A viral disease of the skin and mucous membranes caused by a poxvirus that involves nodules that are small, smooth, painless, and have a pink coloration. When the area is compressed, a milky fluid is produced.

mononucleosis (mono)—An abnormal amount of mononuclear leukocytes in the blood; represented by swollen glands and chronic fatigue.

MRI (magnetic resonance imaging) scan—Diagnostic imaging technique using radiofrequency pulses from a powerful magnetic field to produce high-resolution images of organs, soft-tissue structures, and bone.

Murphy's sign—Sudden cessation of inspiration during deep palpation over the liver when the patient takes a deep breath; may be a result of gallstones.

myocardial bridging—Strands of myocardial fibers lying over the coronary arteries. If long or deep enough, they may cause asystole, myocardial infarction, or necrosis of the affected tissue.

myocarditis—An inflammatory process of the cardiac myocytes.

myocytes—Muscle cells.

myopia—Nearsightedness, in which patients can see objects up close clearly, but objects in the distance are out of focus.

nares—The pair of openings in the front and back of the nasal cavity that allow air to pass to the pharynx.

nasopharynx—The uppermost portion of the three regions of the throat (pharynx), extending from the posterior nares to the level of the soft palate.

nebulizer—A machine that uses compressed air to cause aerosolization of a liquid drug, which is then inhaled through a mask or a mouthpiece.

necrotizing fasciitis—A rapid tissue death that results from a bacterial infection.

nerve conduction study (NCS)—An electrodiagnostic test that involves placing an electrical stimulator over a nerve and measuring the time required for an impulse to travel over a measured segment of the nerve. It is used to test the integrity of peripheral nerves.

nerve conduction velocity (NCV)—An electrodiagnostic test of the integrity of the peripheral nerves.

neuropathy—Inflammation or disease of the nerves.

nongonococcal urethritis (NGU)—An infection of the urethra in males that is characterized by mild dysuria and penile discharge. The discharge may be white or clear, thin or thick.

nonspecific urethritis (NSU)—Inflammation of the urethra not caused by a specific organism. Symptoms are often related to sexual intercourse. Symptoms include urethral discharge in males and reddening of the urethra mucosa in females.

nonsuppurative—Pertaining to inflammation without forming pus.

nosocomial infection—Infection that is acquired at a hospital after the patient is admitted for hospital care for something other than the infection.

nuchal rigidity—A resistance to flexion in the neck, usually seen with patients with meningitis.

nuclear stress test—A diagnostic test using a radioactive tracer to measure the blood flow to the heart at rest and in stress. It can illuminate areas of ischemic heart tissue.

obsessive–compulsive disorder (OCD)—Anxiety disorder characterized by persistent behaviors that markedly impair the person's functioning.

oligomenorrhea—Abnormally light menstruation or reduction in menstruation.

onychia—Inflammation of the nail bed.

oophoritis—The process of inflammation involving the ovaries.

open globe—Eyeball that has been ruptured after blunt trauma, allowing leakage of intraocular fluid or extrusion of intraocular tissue.

orbital emphysema—"Crunchy" sensation under the skin associated with an orbital fracture; results from air from the sinuses being trapped under the skin.

orchitis—Inflammation of one or both testes.

orthopnea—Shortness of breath while lying down.

orthostatic hypotension—Abnormally low blood pressure that occurs when an individual suddenly assumes the standing position.

orthostatic syncope—Brief lapse in consciousness while moving from a lying or sitting to a standing position.

otalgia—Pain in the ear.

otolaryngologist—A physician who specializes in the treatment and evaluation of the ears, nose, and throat.

otorrhea—Any discharge from the external ear.

oxygenation—In respiration, the exchange of gases in the alveolar–capillary beds.

PA view—Positioning depicted on a radiograph from back (posterior) to front (anterior), most commonly associated with the direction of an X-ray beam.

palliative therapy—Therapy designed to relieve the intensity of symptoms and support the patient; does not produce a cure.

palpebral conjunctiva—The part of the conjunctiva lining the eyelids.

palpitations—A pounding or racing of the heart.

panic disorder—Anxiety disorder marked by an acute period of intense fear or anxiety.

papilledema—Swelling of the optic disk in the eye usually caused by pressure in the brain or intracranial pressure.

paraplegia—Impairment in motor or sensory function of the legs and possibly the trunk, caused by a lesion below the first thoracic nerve or a congenital condition affecting the neural elements of the spinal cord.

parenchyma—Functional tissue or cells of an organ.

paronychia—An infection of the fold of skin at the margin of a nail.

parotitis—Inflammation of the parotid salivary glands.

paroxysmal nocturnal dyspnea—Disorder characterized by sudden attacks of respiratory distress that awaken a person after a few hours of sleeping in a reclining position.

pectus deformity—A chest deformity normally resulting in convex or concave abnormalities.

pediculosis—An infestation with blood-sucking lice.

peptic ulcer disease (PUD)—Ulcer found in the stomach or duodenum.

pericarditis—An inflammation of the sac surrounding the epicardium of the heart.

periodontitis—An inflammation or infection of the supporting structures of the teeth.

peripheral arterial disease (PAD)—Also referred to as *peripheral vascular disease*, a condition caused primarily by atherosclerosis.

perirenal fat—Accumulation of fat outside of the peritoneal cavity surrounding the kidney.

person-first terminology—An example of disability etiquette that places the individual (e.g., athlete) before the descriptive phase (e.g., with a disability) thereby focusing on the person rather than the disability.

petechiae—Tiny purple or red spots appearing on the skin as a result of tiny hemorrhages within the dermal or submucosal layers.

phantom leg pain—Also known as *phantom limb pain.* Sensations, such as tingling, numbness, pain, heat, or cold, that are perceived by people with amputated limb(s).

pharmacodynamics—Study of the actions of a drug on the body, including mechanism of action and medicinal effect.

pharmacokinetics—Study of how the body acts on a drug, including the absorption, distribution, metabolism, and elimination of the drug.

photophobia—Pain occurring when light is shone into the eye.

photopsia—Sensation of flashes of light.

pilonidal cyst—A cyst that often develops in the sacral region of the skin.

pleural rubs—Sounds that occur outside the respiratory tree and result from friction between visceral and parietal pleura.

pleurisy—Inflammation of the lining of the lungs.

pneumothorax—Presence of air or gas in the pleural space, causing the lung to collapse.

polycystic ovarian disease—An endocrine disorder that can result in hirsutism, and a lack of ovulation, menstruation, and fertility.

polycythemia—An increase in red blood cell count and circulating red blood cell mass that may be primary or secondary to pulmonary disease, heart disease, or prolonged exposure to high altitudes.

polydipsia—A feeling of excessive thirst.

polymenorrhea—A condition in which the menstrual cycle is abnormally recurrent; more than one cycle per month.

polyuria—A condition of increased urination.

positron emission tomography (PET) scan—Computerized radiographic technique that requires ingestion or injection of a biochemically radioactive substance that is used to measure metabolic activity in the desired body structure with color-coded images.

posterior vitreous detachment (PVD)—When the vitreous liquefies and peels away from the retina, resulting in "floaters" in the field of vision.

postphlebitic syndrome—A condition that occurs when valves of veins become damaged, allowing fluid to pool distally from the weakened valve.

post-polio syndrome—A neurological disorder characterized by new and progressive muscular weakness, pain, and fatigue that affects polio survivors years after recovery from the initial infection of the poliomyelitis virus.

posttraumatic stress disorder (PTSD)—Psychiatric disorder in response to a traumatic event, resulting in intense psychological distress.

potassium hydroxide (KOH) preparation—Using a surface scraping of the affected tissue, a KOH solution is added to the scraping and viewed under a microscope. The results determine whether a skin condition is present.

preauricular lymphadenopathy—Small, tender lymph node located just in front of the tragus of the ear and commonly associated with conjunctivitis.

premature atrial contraction (PAC)—An atrial depolarization that occurs earlier than expected; an early P wave.

premature ventricular contraction (PVC)—A ventricular depolarization that occurs earlier than expected, portrayed as an early and wide QRS complex without a preceding related P wave.

presbycusis—Hearing loss due to aging.

presbyopia—Loss of flexibility of the crystalline lens inside the eye, resulting in an inability to focus on near objects.

prodromal—Pertaining to early symptoms that may mark the onset of a disease.

prophylaxis—Using preventative measures to avoid disease or illness.

proptosis—Downward or forward displacement of the eyeball as a result of swelling; also referred to as *exophthalmos.*

prostate-specific antigen (PSA)—A protein produced by the prostate that is abnormally high in patients with cancer or other disease involving the prostate.

prostatic calculi—Calcifications formed within the prostate.

prostatic tuberculosis—Tuberculosis of the prostate caused by bacteria.

prothrombin time (PT)—Test used to time clot formation; can detect defects in the ability of the blood to coagulate, which are usually caused by a deficiency of factor V, VII, or X (normal PT, 11–12.5 s).

pruritic—The symptom of itching, an uncomfortable sensation leading to the urge to scratch.

pruritus—A condition of itching.

psoriasis—A common chronic skin disorder characterized by circumscribed red patches covered by thick, dry, silvery adherent scales that are a result of excessive development of epithelial cells.

psychotropic medication—A medication that alters a person's psychic function or behavior.

ptosis—Drooping of upper eyelid.

pulmonary embolism—A blockage of the pulmonary artery by fat, air, tumor tissue, or a thrombus that usually arises from a peripheral vein (most frequently one of the deep veins of the legs).

purulent—Producing or containing pus.

pyelonephritis—A bacterial infection that causes inflammation to the kidney.

radiofrequency catheter ablation—Unmodulated high-frequency alternating current flow that is applied to the heart tissue to raise its temperature and injure cells for the purpose of destroying the ectopic foci and accessory pathways.

radionuclide bone scan—Noninvasive injection of a radioactive substance for visualization of a bone with an image produced by the emission of radioactive particles.

Raynaud's disease—Intermittent attacks of ischemia in the extremities of the body, especially the fingers, toes, ears, and nose, caused by exposure to cold or emotional stimuli.

Raynaud's phenomenon—Vasospasm of the arteries caused by an underlying issue.

Reed-Sternberg cells—Large, abnormal, multinucleated cells found in Hodgkin's disease.

renin–angiotensin system—The regulation of sodium balance, fluid volume, and blood pressure.

residual vision—The remaining vision the person has; what the individual can see.

retractions—Visible sinking in of the soft tissue of the chest.

Reye's syndrome—A combination of acute encephalopathy and fatty infiltration of the internal organs that may follow viral infections.

rhabdomyolysis—A potentially fatal syndrome caused by the breakdown of skeletal muscle fibers.

rhinitis—Inflammation of the mucous membranes of the nose, typically accompanied by swelling of the mucosa and nasal discharge.

rhinoplasty—A procedure in which the structure of the nose is altered by plastic surgery.

rhinorrhea—Thin, watery discharge from the nose or flowing of cerebrospinal fluid from the nose after injury to the head.

rhinovirus—Ribonucleic acid–based virus that causes acute respiratory illness.

rhonchus, rhonchi—Low-pitched, sonorous wheeze.

rubella—Another term for *German measles*, which is a viral disease that can cause a low fever, swollen glands, joint pain, and a fine red rash on the skin.

rubeola—Another term for measles, also called *red measles*, which is a virus that causes a skin rash.

salpingitis—The process of inflammation involving the fallopian tubes.

scabies—A contagious disease caused by *Sarcoptes scabiei*, the itch mite, characterized by intense itching of the skin and excoriation from scratching.

scleroderma—Chronic hardening and thickening of the skin caused by new collagen formation.

seasonal affective disorder (SAD)—Mood disorder characterized by lethargy and depression as a result of shorter exposure to daylight and longer exposure to darkness during the fall and winter.

sebaceous cysts—A misnomer for epidermoid, epidermal, or pilar cysts. Sebaceous cysts arise from the oil glands in the skin.

seminoma—A tumor on the testis.

sensorineural hearing loss—Hearing loss involving the inner ear, where sensory receptors convert sound waves into neural impulses that are transmitted to the brain for translation. Most people who are born Deaf have this type of loss.

serology—Test that identifies specific antibodies in the blood.

shrinker—An elastic sock pulled over the stump of an amputated limb that is designed to control edema, promote healing, and assist in shaping the stump.

sickle cell anemia—A severe, chronic, hereditary disease that causes red blood cells to be misshapen (sickle-shaped), leading to blockages that cause damage to areas distal from the blockage.

sideroblastic anemia—A form of anemia in which the bone marrow does not produce healthy red blood cells but rather ringed sideroblasts (abnormal immature red blood cells) that cannot transform readily available iron sources into hemoglobin.

sinusitis—Acute or chronic inflammation of the sinus with or without purulent drainage.

Sjogren's syndrome—A disorder of the immune system marked by inefficient production of certain glands (e.g., salivary, lacrimal) resulting in dryness.

slit-lamp—An instrument equipped with a high-intensity light source that can be focused to shine as a slit; used to examine structures at the front of the eye for any existing pathologies.

solar urticaria—Wheals caused by exposure to the sun.

spasticity—Motor disorder characterized by involuntary, sudden movement or muscle contraction, increased muscle tone, and exaggerated tendon jerks.

splenomegaly—An enlarged spleen.

Stevens-Johnson syndrome—Severe form of erythema multiforme caused by a dermatological reaction to antibiotics; characterized by malaise, headache, fever, and arthralgia.

stridor—High-pitched sound caused by obstruction in the larynx or trachea.

subconjunctival hemorrhage—Bright-red blood appearing in a sector of the eye under the clear conjunctiva.

sulfonylureas—An oral antibiotic that increases insulin production in the pancreas.

suppurative—To form pus.

syncope—A brief lapse in consciousness caused by transient cerebral hypoxia (fainting).

syphilis—A sexually transmitted infection that has distinct stages that cover years; can affect almost any body organ.

T1—In the case of MRI scans, T1 is a technical term that allows certain structures to be lighter or darker on imaging. In terms of the vertebrae, T1 is the first thoracic vertebra.

T2—In the case of MRI scans, T2 provides more intensity (lightness) for fat, water, and fluid. In terms of the vertebrae, T2 is the second thoracic vertebra.

tachypnea—Rapid breathing; >24 breaths/min.

tactile fremitus—Palpable vibration generated from the larynx and transmitted through the bronchi and lungs to the chest wall.

tension pneumothorax—Air in the pleural space caused by a rupture through the chest wall.

tetraplegia—Impairment in motor or sensory function of all four extremities, usually caused by a lesion of the cervical spinal cord; also known as *quadriplegia*.

thalassemia—Production and hemolytic anemia characterized by microcytic, hypochromic red blood cells.

thoracentesis—Surgical procedure that perforates the chest wall or pleural space to aspirate fluid for diagnosis or treatment purposes.

thrombocytopenia—Any disorder of the blood coagulation mechanism caused by an abnormality or dysfunction of platelets.

thrombophlebitis—Inflammation of a vein accompanied by the formation of a clot.

thrush—White patches on the tongue caused by *Candida*; typically benign in children, but it can be caused by an immunodeficiency condition.

thyroid gland—A gland in the anterior throat that secretes hormones that regulate growth and metabolism.

tinea corporis—A superficial fungal infection of the non-hairy skin of the body, most prevalent in hot, humid climates and usually caused by species *Trichophyton* or *Microsporum*.

tinea versicolor—A fungal infection of the skin caused by *Malassezia furfur* and characterized by finely desquamating, pale tan patches on the upper trunk and upper arms that may itch and do not tan.

tinnitus—The sensation of ringing in the ears.

tonic–clonic seizure—Convulsive seizure that affects the entire brain.

torsades de pointes—An extremely rapid ventricular tachycardia determined by a changing QRS complex as seen on an electrocardiogram (ECG); may be self-limited or may progress to ventricular fibrillation.

traumatic iritis—Inflammation of the iris secondary to blunt trauma.

traumatic mydriasis—Condition in which one pupil is dilated; usually associated with traumatic iritis.

trephination—A technique where a burr hole is drilled into a hard surface such as a nail or a flat bone.

trichomoniasis—Infection of the vagina caused by *Trichomonas vaginalis*. Symptoms include itching, burning, and frothy, light-yellow discharge.

triphasic—Having three phases.

Turner's syndrome—An abnormality in females marked by the absence of one X chromosome.

tympanogram—A test providing graphic representation of the acoustic impedance and air pressure in the middle ear, as well as the mobility of the tympanic membrane.

ultrasound—Imaging technique projecting high-frequency sound waves into the body, producing a real-time image of internal structures from the reflective properties of sound waves.

urinalysis (UA)—A process of analyzing urine for certain attributes or components.

urticaria—A group of distinct skin conditions characterized by itchy, wheal-and-flare skin reactions, commonly known as *hives*.

uterine synechiae—Scars or adhesions on the uterus.

vector—An organism that carries and transmits a disease, usually from one species to another.

venous puncture—Poking a hole into a vein for the purpose of extracting blood, injecting a substance, or inserting an intravenous line.

ventilation—In respiration, the process by which air moves through the respiratory tract.

ventilation–perfusion scan—A scan to determine whether one or more areas of the lungs are getting air but not blood or blood but no air.

vesicular breath sounds—Normal sound of rustling or swishing that represents air moving into the smaller airways.

Wernicke's aphasia—A type of aphasia that involves impairment in the comprehension of written and spoken words.

Western blot—A blood test used to determine whether specific antibodies are present.

wheezes—Adventitious breath sounds that represent airway obstruction by mucus, spasm, or even a foreign body.

whispered pectoriloquy—Whispered speech heard clearly through the stethoscope.

Wolff-Parkinson-White (WPW) syndrome—A disorder of atrioventricular conduction involving an accessory pathway. This syndrome is often identified by a characteristic delta wave seen on an ECG at the beginning of the QRS complex.

Wood's lamp—An illuminating device with a nickel oxide filter that holds back all light except for a few violet rays of the visible spectrum and ultraviolet wavelengths of about 365 nm.

X-ray—Electromagnetic radiation at a shorter wavelength than visible light, transmitted through the body to investigate the integrity of underlying structures, particularly bone.

REFERENCES

Chapter 1

1. Jameson L, Fauci A, Kasper D, Hauser S, Longo D, Loscalzo J. *Harrison's Manual of Medicine*. 20th ed. McGraw Hill; 2020.

2. Ball J, Dains J, Flynn J, Solomon BS, Stewart RW. *Seidel's Guide to Physical Examination: An Interprofessional Approach*. 10th ed. Elsevier; 2022.

3. Jarvis C. *Physical Examination & Health Assessment*. 8th ed. Elsevier; 2019.

4. Belval LN, Hosokawa Y, Casa DJ, et al. Practical hydration solutions for sports. *Nutrients*. 2019;11(7):1550.

5. Bickley L, Szilagyi P, Hoffman R. *Bates' Guide to Physical Examination and History Taking*. 13th ed. Wolters Kluwer; 2021.

6. Rakel R, Rakel D. *Textbook of Family Medicine*. 9th ed. Elsevier/Saunders; 2015.

7. Ferri FF. *Ferri's Clinical Advisor 2022*. Elsevier; 2022.

8. Miller KC, Adams WM. Common body temperature sites provide invalid measures of body core temperature in hyperthermic humans wearing American football uniforms. *Temperature (Austin)*. 2021;8(2):166-175.

9. Mogensen CB, Wittenhoff L, Fruerhøj G, Hansen S. Forehead or ear temperature measurement cannot replace rectal measurements, except for screening purposes. *BMC Pediatr*. 2018;18(1):15.

10. Casa DJ. *Preventing Sudden Death in Sport and Physical Activity*. Jones and Bartlett; 2011.

11. Casa DJ, Guskiewicz KM, Anderson SL. National Athletic Trainers' Association position statement: Preventing sudden death in sports. *J Athl Train*. 2012;47(1):96-118.

12. Dante A, Franconi I, Marucci AR, Alfes CM, Lancia L. Evaluating the interchangeability of forehead, tympanic, and axillary thermometers in Italian paediatric clinical settings: Results of a multicentre observational study. *J Pediatr Nursing*. 2020;52:e21-e25.

13. Perry A, Potter P, Ostendorf W, Laplante N. *Clinical Nursing Skills & Techniques*. 10th ed. Elsevier; 2021.

14. American Academy of Family Physicians, American Academy of Pediatrics, American College of Sports Medicine, American Medical Society for Sports Medicine, American Orthopaedic Society for Sports Medicine, American Osteopathic Academy of Sports Medicine. *Preparticipation Physical Evaluation*. 5th ed. American Academy of Pediatrics; 2019.

15. Leggit JC, Wise S. Preparticipation physical evaluation: AAFP and others update recommendations. *Am Fam Physician*. 2020;101(11):692-694.

16. Parsons JT. *2014-15 NCAA Sports Medicine Handbook*. 25th ed. National Collegiate Athletics Association; 2014.

Chapter 2

1. Radiological Society of North America. Contrast materials. Updated March 16, 2016. Accessed April 24, 2016. www.radiologyinfo.org/en/info.cfm?pg=safety-contrast

2. Johns Hopkins Medicine. Bone scan. 2022. Accessed June 15, 2022. www.hopkinsmedicine.org/healthlibrary/test_procedures/orthopaedic/bone_scan_92,p07663/

3. Taylor CR. Abdominal computed tomography scanning medication. Medscape. September 13, 2017. Accessed June 15, 2022. https://emedicine.medscape.com/article/2114236-medication

4. Radiological Society of North America. PET/CT. Updated February 8, 2021. Accessed June 15, 2022. www.radiologyinfo.org/en/info.cfm?pg=pet

5. National Institute of Biomedical Imaging and Bioengineering. Magnetic resonance imaging (MRI). 2022. Accessed June 18, 2022. www.nibib.nih.gov/science-education/science-topics/magnetic-resonance-imaging-mri

6. Ball JW, Dains JE, Flynn JA, Solomon BS, Stewart RW. *Seidel's Guide to Physical Examination: An Interprofessional Approach*. 10th ed. Elsevier; 2022.

7. Akinpelu D. Treadmill stress testing. Updated November 21, 2018. Accessed October 18, 2023. https://emedicine.medscape.com/article/1827089-overview

Chapter 3

1. Health Canada. Drugs and health products. Updated August 12, 2022. Accessed August 18, 2022. www.canada.ca/en/health-canada/services/drugs-health-products.html

2. Food and Drug Administration. List of controlled substances. Accessed August 18, 2022. www.deadiversion.usdoj.gov/schedules

3. Food and Drug Administration. What we do: FDA mission. Accessed August 18, 2022. www.fda.gov/AboutFDA/WhatWeDo/default.htm

4. Chang CJ, Weston T, Higgs JD, et al. Inter-association consensus statement: The management of medications by the sports medicine team. *J Athl Train*. 2018;53(11):1103-

1112.

5. Drug Enforcement Administration. Diversion Control Division Registration. Accessed August 18, 2022. www.deadiversion.usdoj.gov/drugreg/index.html

6. Young CC, Higgs JD, Chang CJ. Managing medications in the training room and on the sidelines. *Curr Sports Med Rep.* 2020;19(7):249-250.

7. Hoffman M, Murphy M, Koester MC, Norcross EC, Johnson ST. Use of lifesaving medications by athletic trainers. *J Athl Train.* 2022;57(7):613-620.

8. Commission on Accreditation of Athletic Training Education. *Pursuing and Maintaining Accreditation of Professional Programs in Athletic Training.* CAATE; 2021.

9. Brunton LL, Hilal-Dandan R, Knollman BC. *Goodman & Gilman's: The Pharmacological Basis of Therapeutics.* 13th ed. McGraw Hill; 2018.

10. Clinical Pharmacology. Clinical Pharmacology Gold Standard. Accessed August 2022. www.clinicalkey.com/pharmacology/login

11. Rao R, Mahant S, Chhabra L, Nanda S. Transdermal innovations in diabetes management. *Curr Diabetes Rev.* 2014;10(6):343-359.

12. Murthy SN. Approaches for delivery of drugs topically. *AAPS PharmSciTech.* 2020;21:30.

13. Rigby JH, Draper DO, Johnson AW, Myrer JW, Eggett DL, Mack GW. The time course of dexamethasone delivery using iontophoresis through human skin, measured via microdialysis. *J Orthop Sports Phys Ther.* 2015;45(3):190-197.

14. Jeong WY, Kwon M, Choi HE, Kim KS. Recent advances in transdermal drug delivery systems: A review. *Biomater Res.* 2021;25(1):24.

15. Epocrates. Epocrates Drug Database. 2022. Accessed August 22, 2022. https://online.epocrates.com/drugs

16. Bindu S, Mazumder S, Bandyopadhyay U. Non-steroidal anti-inflammatory drugs (NSAIDs) and organ damage: A current perspective. *Biochem Pharmacol.* 2020;180:114147.

17. Bavry AA, Thomas F, Allison M, et al. Nonsteroidal anti-inflammatory drugs and cardiovascular outcomes in women: Results from the Women's Health Initiative. *Circ Cardiovasc Qual Outcomes.* 2014;7(4):603-610.

18. Ross JS, Krumholz HM. Bringing Vioxx back to market. *BMJ.* 2018;360:k242.

19. Lexicomp Online. Clinical Drug Information Facts & Comparisons. Accessed September 2022. www.wolterskluwercdi.com/facts-comparisons-online

20. U.S. Anti-Doping Agency. USADA's anti-doping programs. Accessed September 2022. www.usada.org/about/programs

21. World Anti-Doping Agency. Therapeutic use exemptions (TUEs). Accessed April 20, 2022. www.wada-ama.org/en/athletes-support-personnel/therapeutic-use-exemptions-tues

22. National Collegiate Athletics Association. NCAA Banned

Substances. Updated 2022. Accessed July 20, 2022. www.ncaa.org/2015-16-ncaa-banned-drugs

23. Lang P, McGuine T, Mack L, et al. Prevalence of over the counter pain medication use among high school volleyball players. *Orthop J Sports Med.* 2020;8(4 suppl 3):2325967120S00250.

24. Omeragic E, Marjanovic A, Djedjibegovic J, et al. Prevalence of use of permitted pharmacological substances for recovery among athletes. *Pharmacia.* 2021;68(1):35-42.

25. Trinh KV, Kim J, Ritsma A. Effect of pseudoephedrine in sport: A systematic review. *BMJ Open Sport Exerc Med.* 2015;1(1):e000066.

26. Buell JL, Franks R, Ransone J, et al. National Athletic Trainers' Association position statement: Evaluation of dietary supplements for performance nutrition. *J Athl Train.* 2013;48(1):124-136.

Chapter 4

1. Soriano-Maldonado A, Klokker L, Bartholdy C, et al. Intra-articular corticosteroids in addition to exercise for reducing pain sensitivity in knee osteoarthritis: Exploratory outcome from a randomized controlled trial. *PLoS One.* 2016;11(2):e0149168.

2. Lin C-Y, Huang S-C, Tzou S-J, et al. A positive correlation between steroid injections and cuff tendon tears: A cohort study using a clinical database. *Int J Environ Res Public Health.* 2022;19(8):4520.

3. van Vollenhoven RF, Petri M, Wallace DJ, et al. Cumulative corticosteroids over 52 weeks in patients with systemic lupus erythematosus: Pooled analyses from the phase III belimumab trials. *Arthritis Rheumatol.* 2016;68(9):2184-2192.

4. Valenzuela CV, Liu JC, Vila PM, Simon L, Doering M, Lieu JE. Intranasal corticosteroids do not lead to ocular changes: A systematic review and meta-analysis. *Laryngoscope.* 2019;129(1):6-12.

5. Zhang M, Ni J-Z, Cheng L. Safety of intranasal corticosteroids for allergic rhinitis in children. *Expert Opin Drug Saf.* 2022;21(7):931-938.

6. Rigby JH, Draper DO, Johnson AW, Myrer JW, Eggett DL, Mack GW. The time course of dexamethasone delivery using iontophoresis through human skin, measured via microdialysis. *J Orthop Sports Phys Ther.* 2015;45(3):190-197.

7. Baktir S, Ozdincler AR, Mutlu EK, Bilsel K. The short-term effectiveness of low-level laser, phonophoresis, and iontophoresis in patients with lateral epicondylosis. *J Hand Ther.* 2019;32(4):417-425.

8. Lexicomp Online. Clinical Drug Information Facts and Comparisons. Accessed September 2022. www.wolterskluwercdi.com/facts-comparisons-online

9. Dieu-Donne O, Theodore O, Joelle Z, et al. An open randomized trial comparing the effects of oral NSAIDs versus steroid intra-articular infiltration in congestive osteoarthritis of the knee. *Open Rheumatol J.* 2016;10:8-12.

10. Domper Arnal MJ, Hijos-Mallada G, Lanas A. Gastroin-

testinal and cardiovascular adverse events associated with NSAIDs. *Expert Opin Drug Saf.* 2022;21(3):373-384.

11. Hamilton K, Davis C, Falk J, Singer A, Bugden S. High risk use of OTC NSAIDs and ASA in family medicine: A retrospective chart review. *Int J Risk Saf Med.* 2015;27(4):191-199.

12. Bhosale UA, Quraishi N, Yegnanarayan R, Devasthale D. A comparative study to evaluate the cardiovascular risk of selective and nonselective cyclooxygenase inhibitors (COX-Is) in arthritic patients. *J Basic Clin Physiol Pharmacol.* 2015;26(1):73-79.

13. Schmidt M, Sørensen HT, Pedersen L. Cardiovascular risks of diclofenac versus other older COX-2 inhibitors (meloxicam and etodolac) and newer COX-2 inhibitors (celecoxib and etoricoxib): A series of nationwide emulated trials. *Drug Safety.* 2022;45(9):983-994.

14. Tscholl PM, Vaso M, Weber A, Dvorak J. High prevalence of medication use in professional football tournaments including the World Cups between 2002 and 2014: A narrative review with a focus on NSAIDs. *Br J Sports Med.* 2015;49(9):580-582.

15. Ussai S, Miceli L, Pisa FE, et al. Impact of potential inappropriate NSAIDs use in chronic pain. *Drug Des Devel Ther.* 2015;9:2073-2077.

16. National Collegiate Athletics Association. NCAA Banned Substances. Updated 2022. Accessed July 20, 2022. www.ncaa.org/2015-16-ncaa-banned-drugs

17. U.S. Anti-Doping Agency. USADA anti-doping programs. Accessed September 2022. www.usada.org/about/programs

18. World Anti-Doping Agency. Therapeutic use exemptions (TUEs). Accessed April 20, 2022. www.wada-ama.org/en/athletes-support-personnel/therapeutic-use-exemptions-tues

19. Clinical Pharmacology. Clinical Pharmacology Gold Standard. Accessed August 2022. www.clinicalkey.com/pharmacology/login

20. Reurink G, Goudswaard GJ, Moen MH, Weir A, Verhaar JA, Tol JL. Myotoxicity of injections for acute muscle injuries: A systematic review. *Sports Med.* 2014;44(7):943-956.

21. Schrock JB, Carver TJ, Kraeutler MJ, McCarty EC. Evolving treatment patterns of NFL players by orthopaedic team physicians over the past decade, 2008-2016. *Sports Health.* 2018;10(5):453-461.

22. Gultekin S, Jomaa MC, Jenkin R, Orchard JW. Use and outcome of local anesthetic painkilling injections in athletes: A systematic review. *Clin J Sport Med.* 2021;31(1):78-85.

23. Anderson LA. Antibiotic resistance: The top 10 list. Drugs.com. Accessed January 4, 2023. www.drugs.com/article/antibiotic-resistance.html

24. Ferri FF. *Ferri's Clinical Advisor 2022.* Elsevier; 2022.

25. Chinen T, Sasabuchi Y, Matsui H, Yasunaga H. Association between third-generation fluoroquinolones and Achilles tendon rupture: A self-controlled case series analysis. *Ann Fam Med.* 2021;19(3):212-216.

26. Kermani F, Moosazadeh M, Hosseini SA, Bandalizadeh Z, Barzegari S, Shokohi T. Tinea gladiatorum and dermatophyte contamination among wrestlers and in wrestling halls: A systematic review and meta-analysis. *Curr Microbiol.* 2020;77(4):602-611.

27. Olson JM, Troxell T. Griseofulvin. In: *StatPearls.* StatPearls Publishing; 2023.

28. Svetaz LA, Postigo A, Butassi E, Zacchino SA, Sortino MA. Antifungal drugs combinations: A patient review 2000-2015. *Expert Opin Ther Pat.* 2016;26(4):439-453.

29. Payares-Salamanca L, Contreras-Arrieta S, Florez-García V, Barrios-Sanjuanelo A, Stand-Niño I, Rodriguez-Martinez CE. Metered-dose inhalers versus nebulization for the delivery of albuterol for acute exacerbations of wheezing or asthma in children: A systematic review with meta-analysis. *Pediatr Pulmonol.* 2020;55(12):3268-3278.

30. Drugs.com. Xopenex. Accessed January 4, 2023. www.drugs.com/xopenex.html

31. Boulet LP, Turmel J. Cough in exercise and athletes. *Pulm Pharmacol Ther.* 2019;55:67-74.

32. Epocrates. Epocrates Drug Database. 2022. Accessed August 22, 2022. https://online.epocrates.com/drugs

33. Katzung B, Trevor A. *Basic and Clinical Pharmacology.* 13th ed. McGraw Hill; 2014.

34. American Hospital Formulary Service. *American Hospital Formulary Service Drug Information.* American Society of Health-System Pharmacists; 2016.

35. Pasquel FJ, Klein R, Adigweme A, et al. Metformin-associated lactic acidosis. *Am J Med Sci.* 2015;349(3):263-267.

36. Lee B. What are biologics? 5 examples of biological drugs you may already be taking. GoodRx Health. Accessed January 10, 2023. www.goodrx.com/healthcare-access/medication-education/biologics-biological-drugs-examples

Chapter 5

1. Board of Certification for the Athletic Trainer. State regulation. October 23, 2022. Accessed October 24, 2022. https://bocatc.org/state-regulation/state-regulation

2. Centers for Disease Control and Prevention. Update: Universal precautions for prevention of transmission of human immunodeficiency virus, hepatitis B virus, and other bloodborne pathogens in health-care settings. *MMWR Morb Mortal Wkly Rep.* 1988;37(24):377-382, 387-388.

3. Phan TMD, Nguyen NMT. *The Practices of Aseptic Technique of Perioperative Nurses in Operation Room to Prevent Surgical Site Infection: Integrative Literature Review.* Thesis. LAB University of Applied Sciences; 2021.

4. Perry A, Potter P, Ostendorf W, Laplante N. *Clinical Nursing Skills & Techniques.* 10th ed. Elsevier; 2021.

5. Potter P, Perry A, Stockert P, Hall H. *Basic Nursing: Essentials for Practice.* 11th ed. Elsevier; 2022.

6. Rothrock J. *Alexander's Care of the Patient in Surgery.* 14th ed. Mosby; 2016.

7. Roberts J. *Roberts and Hedges' Clinical Procedures in Emergency Medicine and Acute Care.* 7th ed. Elsevier;

2022.

8. Bal-Ozturk A, Cecen B, Avci-Adali M, et al. Tissue adhesives: From research to clinical translation. *Nano Today*. 2021;36:101049.

9. Smith TO, Sexton D, Mann C, Simon D. Sutures versus staples for skin closure in orthopaedic surgery: Meta-analysis. *BMJ*. 2010;340:c1199.

10. Liu Z, Liu B, Yang H, Zhao L. Staples versus sutures for skin closure in hip arthroplasty: A meta-analysis and systematic review. *J Orthop Surg Res*. 2021;16(1):735.

Chapter 6

1. Ball J, Dains J, Flynn J, Solomon BS, Stewart RW. *Seidel's Guide to Physical Examination: An Interprofessional Approach*. 10th ed. Elsevier; 2022.

2. Clemm HH, Olin JT, McIntosh C, et al. Exercise-induced laryngeal obstruction (EILO) in athletes: A narrative review by a subgroup of the IOC Consensus on "acute respiratory illness in the athlete." *Br J Sports Med*. 2022;56(11):622-629.

3. Hamdan A-L, Sataloff RT, Hawkshaw MJ. Exercise-induced laryngeal obstruction (EILO) in athletes. In: *Voice Disorders in Athletes, Coaches and Other Sports Professionals*. Springer; 2021:155-182.

4. Bickley L, Szilagyi P, Hoffman R. *Bates' Guide to Physical Examination and History-Taking*. 13th ed. Wolters Kluwer; 2021.

5. Jarvis C. *Physical Examination & Health Assessment*. 8th ed. Elsevier; 2019:896.

6. Del Giacco S, Couto M, Firinu D, Garcia-Larsen V. Management of intermittent and persistent asthma in adolescent and high school athletes. *J Allergy Clin Immunol Pract*. 2020;8(7):2166-2181.

7. Simpson AJ, Romer LM, Kippelen P. Self-reported symptoms after induced and inhibited bronchoconstriction in athletes. *Med Sci Sports Exerc*. 2015;47(10):2005-2013.

8. Krafczyk MA, Asplund CA. Exercise-induced bronchoconstriction: Diagnosis and management. *Am Fam Physician*. 2011;84(4):427-434.

9. Carey DG, Aase KA, Pliego GJ. The acute effect of cold air exercise in determination of exercise-induced bronchospasm in apparently healthy athletes. *J Strength Cond Res*. 2010;24(8):2172-2178.

10. Boulet L-P, Turmel J. Cough in exercise and athletes. *Pulm Pharmacol Ther*. 2019;55:67-74.

11. Nielsen EW, Hull J, Back V. High prevalence of exercise-induced laryngeal obstruction in athletes. *Med Sci Sports Exerc*. 2013;45(11):2030-2035.

12. Backer V. Not all who wheeze have asthma. *Breathe*. 2010;7(1):16-22.

13. Zeiger JS, Weiler JM. Special considerations and perspectives for exercise-induced bronchoconstriction (EIB) in Olympic and other elite athletes. *J Allergy Clin Immunol Pract*. 2020;8(7):2194-2201.

14. Bonini M, Cilluffo G, La Grutta S, et al. Anti-muscarinic drugs as preventive treatment of exercise-induced bronchoconstriction (EIB) in children and adults. *Respir Med*. 2020;172:106128.

15. Parsons JP, Cosmar D, Phillips G, Kaeding C, Best TM, Mastronarde JG. Screening for exercise-induced bronchoconstriction in college athletes. *J Asthma*. 2012;49(2):153-157.

16. Aggarwal B, Mulgirigama A, Berend N. Exercise-induced bronchoconstriction: Prevalence, pathophysiology, patient impact, diagnosis and management. *NPJ Prim Care Respir Med*. 2018;28(1):31.

17. Boulet L-P, Hancox RJ, Fitch KD. Exercise and asthma: β_2-Agonists and the competitive athlete. *Breathe*. 2010;7(1):65-71.

18. Allen H, Price OJ, Hull JH, Backhouse SH. Asthma medication in athletes: A qualitative investigation of adherence, avoidance and misuse in competitive sport. *J Asthma*. 2022;59(4):811-822.

19. Backer V, Mastronarde J. Pharmacologic strategies for exercise-induced bronchospasm with a focus on athletes. *Immunol Allergy Clin North Am*. 2018;38(2):231-243.

20. Atchley TJ, Smith DM. Exercise-induced bronchoconstriction in elite or endurance athletes: Pathogenesis and diagnostic considerations. *Ann Allergy Asthma Immunol*. 2020;125(1):47-54.

21. Hull JH, Godbout K, Boulet LP. Exercise-associated dyspnea and stridor: Thinking beyond asthma. *J Allergy Clin Immunol Pract*. 2020;8(7):2202-2208.

22. Rodriguez Bauza DE, Silveyra P. Sex differences in exercise-induced bronchoconstriction in athletes: A systematic review and meta-analysis. *Int J Environ Res Public Health*. 2020;17(19):7270.

23. Mahase E. Winter pressure: RSV, flu, and COVID-19 could push NHS to breaking point, report warns. *BMJ*. 2021;374:n1802.

24. Shah SJ, Barish PN, Prasad PA, et al. Clinical features, diagnostics, and outcomes of patients presenting with acute respiratory illness: A retrospective cohort study of patients with and without COVID-19. *EClinicalMedicine*. 2020;27:100518.

25. Havers F, Flannery B, Clippard JR, et al. Use of influenza antiviral medications among outpatients at high risk for influenza-associated complications during the 2013-2014 influenza season. *Clin Infect Dis*. 2015;60(11):1677-1680. doi:10.1093/cid/civ146

26. US Centers for Disease Control and Prevention. About flu. December 27, 2022. Accessed October 18, 2023. www.cdc.gov/flu/about/index.html

27. Hull JH, Loosemore M, Schwellnus M. Respiratory health in athletes: Facing the COVID-19 challenge. *Lancet Respir Med*. 2020;8(6):557-558.

28. Boulet L-P. Cough and upper airway disorders in elite athletes: A critical review. *Br J Sports Med*. 2012;46(6):417-421.

29. Pagels CM, Dilworth TJ, Fehrenbacher L, Singh M, Brummitt CF. Impact of an electronic best-practice advisory in combination with prescriber education on antibiotic prescribing for ambulatory adults with acute, uncomplicated bronchitis within a large integrated health system. *Infect Control Hosp Epidemiol.* 2019;40(12):1348-1355.

30. Mirza S, Clay RD, Koslow MA, Scanlon PD. COPD guidelines: A review of the 2018 GOLD report. *Mayo Clin Proc.* 2018;93(10):1488-1502.

31. Vogelmeier CF, Román-Rodríguez M, Singh D, Han MK, Rodríguez-Roisin R, Ferguson GT. Goals of COPD treatment: Focus on symptoms and exacerbations. *Respir Med.* 2020;166:105938.

32. Holland AE, Hill CJ, Jones AY, McDonald CF. Breathing exercises for chronic obstructive pulmonary diseases. *Cochrane Database Syst Rev.* 2012;10:CD008250.

33. Spielmanns M, Fuchs-Bergsma C, Winkler A, Fox G, Kuruger S, Baum K. Effects of oxygen supply during training on subjects with COPD who are normoxemic at rest and during exercise: A blinded randomized controlled trial. *Respir Care.* 2015;60(4):540-548. doi:10.4187/respcare.03647

34. Klign P, Van Keimpema A, Legemaat M, Gosselink R, Van Stel H. Prescribing exercise in advanced COPD: Training smart, not just hard! *Eur Respir J.* 2012;40(suppl 56):P1900.

35. Smoot MK, Hosey RG. Pulmonary infections in the athlete. *Curr Sports Med Rep.* 2009;8(2):71-75.

36. Domino FJ, Baldor RA, Barry KA, Golding J, Stephens MB. *The 5-Minute Clinical Consult Premium 2022.* 30th ed. Wolters Kluwer; 2021.

37. Plojoux J, Froudarakis M, Janssens JP, Soccal PM, Tschopp JM. New insights and improved strategies for the management of primary spontaneous pneumothorax. *Clin Respir J.* 2019;13(4):195-201.

38. Feden JP. Closed lung trauma. *Clin Sports Med.* 2013;32(2):255-265.

39. Rahman NM. Pneumothorax. In: *Merck Manual.* Revised August 2023. Accessed August 22, 2023. www.merck-manuals.com/professional/pulmonary-disorders/mediastinal-and-pleural-disorders/pneumothorax

40. Asli RH, Aghajanzadeh M, Asli HH. Evaluation of the relationship between primary spontaneous pneumothorax and exercise and patient return to previous activities in patients after treatment. *GSC Adv Res Rev.* 2021;9(2):008-014.

41. U.S. Centers for Disease Control and Prevention. Tuberculosis. Accessed November 7, 2022. www.cdc.gov/tb/default.htm

42. Furin J, Cox H, Pai M. Tuberculosis. *Lancet.* 2019;393(10181):1642-1656.

43. Suárez I, Fünger SM, Kröger S, Rademacher J, Fätkenheuer G, Rybniker J. The diagnosis and treatment of tuberculosis. *Dtsch Arztebl Int.* 2019;116(43):729-735.

44. Quist M, Langer SW, Lillelund C, et al. Effects of an exercise intervention for patients with advanced inoperable lung cancer undergoing chemotherapy: A randomized clinical trial. *Lung Cancer.* 2020;145:76-82.

45. Cabry R Jr, Ballyamanda S, Kraft M, Hong E. Understanding paraneoplastic syndromes in athletes. *Curr Sports Med Rep.* 2013;12(1):33-40.

Chapter 7

1. O'Toole MT. *Mosby's Dictionary of Medicine, Nursing & Health Professions.* Elsevier Health Sciences; 2015.

2. Flack JM, Adekola B. Blood pressure and the new ACC/AHA hypertension guidelines. *Trends Cardiovasc Med.* 2020;30(3):160-164.

3. Ball JW, Dains JE, Flynn JA, et al. *Seidel's Guide to Physical Examination E-Book: An Interprofessional Approach.* Elsevier Health Sciences 2021.

4. Booher MA, Smith BW. Physiological effects of exercise on the cardiopulmonary system. *Clin Sports Med.* 2003;22(1):1-21.

5. Lavie CJ, Arena R, Swift DL, et al. Exercise and the cardiovascular system: Clinical science and cardiovascular outcomes. *Cir Res.* 2015;117(2):207-219.

6. Li G, Li J, Gao F. Exercise and cardiovascular protection. In: Xiao J, ed. *Physical Exercise for Human Health.* Springer; 2020:205-216.

7. George K, Whyte GP, Green DJ, et al. The endurance athlete's heart: Acute stress and chronic adaptation. *Br J Sports Med.* 2012;46(suppl 1):i29-i36.

8. Nagashima J, Musha H, Takada H, Murayama M. New upper limit of physiologic cardiac hypertrophy in Japanese participants in the 100-km ultramarathon. *J Am Coll Cardiol.* 2003;42(9):1617-1623.

9. Asif IM. The cardiovascular preparticipation evaluation (PPE) for the primary care and sports medicine physician, part I. *Curr Sports Med Rep.* 2015;14(3):246.

10. Palermi S, Serio A, Vecchiato M, et al. Potential role of an athlete-focused echocardiogram in sports eligibility. *World J Cardiol.* 2021;13(8):271-297.

11. Maron BJ, Levine BD, Washington RL, et al. Eligibility and disqualification recommendations for competitive athletes with cardiovascular abnormalities: Task Force 2: Preparticipation screening for cardiovascular disease in competitive athletes: A scientific statement from the American Heart Association and American College of Cardiology. *J Am Coll Cardiol.* 2015;66(21):2356-2361.

12. Yousaf R, Marwat DMK. Impact of aerobic exercise on resting heart rate and cardiovascular endurance in non-athlete students. *Int J Comput Intelligence Control.* 2022;14(1):133-142.

13. Casa DJ, Guskiewicz KM, Anderson SA, et al. National Athletic Trainers' Association position statement: Preventing sudden death in sports. *J Athl Train.* 2012;47(1):96-118.

14. Kucera KL, Klossner D, Colgate B, Cantu R. *Annual Survey of Football Injury Research: 1931-2021.* University of North Carolina, Chapel Hill National Center for Catastrophic Sport Injury Research; 2022.

15. Kucera KL, Cantu RC. *Catastrophic Sports Injury Research, Thirty-Eighth Annual Report: Fall 1982 to Spring 2020*. National Center for Catastrophic Sport Injury Research: University of North Carolina at Chapel Hill; 2020.

16. Wasfy MM, Hutter AM, Weiner RB. Sudden cardiac death in athletes. *Methodist Debakey Cardiovasc J*. 2016;12(2):76-80.

17. Peterson DF, Kucera K, Thomas LC, et al. Aetiology and incidence of sudden cardiac arrest and death in young competitive athletes in the USA: A 4-year prospective study. *Br J Sports Med*. 2021;55(21):1196-1203.

18. Maron BJ, Udelson JE, Bonow RO, et al. Eligibility and disqualification recommendations for competitive athletes with cardiovascular abnormalities: Task Force 3: Hypertrophic cardiomyopathy, arrhythmogenic right ventricular cardiomyopathy and other cardiomyopathies, and myocarditis: A scientific statement from the American Heart Association and American College of Cardiology. *Circulation*. 2015;132(22):e273-e280.

19. Ackerman MJ, Zipes DP, Kovacs RJ, et al. Eligibility and disqualification recommendations for competitive athletes with cardiovascular abnormalities: Task Force 10: The cardiac channelopathies: A scientific statement from the American Heart Association and American College of Cardiology. *Circulation*. 2015;132(22):e326-e329.

20. Link MS, Estes NA III, Maron BJ, et al. Eligibility and disqualification recommendations for competitive athletes with cardiovascular abnormalities: Task Force 13: Commotio cordis: A scientific statement from the American Heart Association and American College of Cardiology. *Circulation*. 2015;132(22):e339-e342.

21. Singh M, Link MS. Commotio cordis in athletes. In: *Sports Cardiology*. Springer; 2021:375-381.

22. De Gregorio C, Magaudda L. Blunt thoracic trauma and cardiac injury in the athlete: Contemporary management. *J Sports Med Phys Fitness*. 2018;58(5):721-726.

23. Lucas JF. Sudden cardiac death in school aged athletes. *J S C Med Assoc*. 2016;112(2):185-189.

24. School CPR. States where CPR is mandatory for coaches. 2022. Accessed October 1, 2022. https://schoolcpr.com/requirements/coaches/

25. Narayanan K, Bougouin W, Sharifzadehgan A, et al. Sudden cardiac death during sports activities in the general population. *Card Electrophysiol Clin*. 2017;9(4):559-567.

26. Maron BJ, Maron MS. Hypertrophic cardiomyopathy. *Lancet* 2013;381(9862):242-255. doi:10.1016/S0140-6736(12)60397-3

27. Zorzi A, Brunetti G, Corrado D. Differential diagnosis between athlete's heart and hypertrophic cardiomyopathy: New pieces of the puzzle. *Int J Cardiol*. 2022;353:77-79.

28. Bakogiannis C, Mouselimis D, Tsarouchas A, Papatheodorou E, Vassilikos VP, Androulakis E. Hypertrophic cardiomyopathy or athlete's heart? A systematic review of novel cardiovascular magnetic resonance imaging parameters. *Eur J Sport Sci*. 2023;23(1):143-154.

29. Malek LA, Milosz-Wieczorek B, Marczak M. Diagnostic yield of cardiac magnetic resonance in athletes with and without features of the athlete's heart and suspected structural heart disease. *Int J Environ Res Public Health*. 2022;19(8):4829.

30. Maron BJ, Bonow RO, Cannon RO III, Leon MB, Epstein SE. Hypertrophic cardiomyopathy. *New Engl J Med*. 1987;316(14):844-852.

31. Rowin EJ, Maron MS, Adler A, et al. Importance of newer cardiac magnetic resonance-based risk markers for sudden death prevention in hypertrophic cardiomyopathy: An international multicenter study. *Heart Rhythm*. 2022;19(5):782-789.

32. Miller SM, Peterson AR. The sports preparticipation evaluation. *Pediatr Rev*. 2019;40(3):108-128.

33. Maron BJ. Clinical course and management of hypertrophic cardiomyopathy. *New Engl J Med*. 2018;379(7):655-668.

34. Pelliccia A, Borjesson M, Villiger B, Di Paolo F, Schmied C. Incidence and etiology of sudden cardiac death in young athletes. *Schweizerische Zeitschrift fur Sportmedizin und Sporttraumatologie*. 2011;59:74-78.

35. Levine BD, Baggish AL, Kovacs RJ, et al. Eligibility and disqualification recommendations for competitive athletes with cardiovascular abnormalities: Task Force 1: Classification of sports: Dynamic, static, and impact: A scientific statement from the American Heart Association and American College of Cardiology. *J Am Coll Cardiol*. 2015;66(21):2350-2355.

36. Albaeni A, Davis JW, Ahmad M. Echocardiographic evaluation of the athlete's heart. *Echocardiography*. 2021;38(6):1002-1016.

37. Gräni C, Kaufmann PA, Windecker S, Buechel RR. Diagnosis and management of anomalous coronary arteries with a malignant course. *Interv Cardiol*. 2019;14(2):83-88.

38. Maron BJ, Shirani J, Poliac LC, Mathenge R, Roberts WC, Mueller FO. Sudden death in young competitive athletes: Clinical, demographic, and pathological profiles. *JAMA*. 1996;276(3):199-204.

39. Chappex N, Schlaepfer J, Fellmann F, Bhuiyan ZA, Wilhelm M, Michaud K. Sudden cardiac death among general population and sport related population in forensic experience. *J Forensic Leg Med*. 2015;35:62-68.

40. Toukola T, Hookana E, Junttila J, et al. Sudden cardiac death during physical exercise: Characteristics of victims and autopsy findings. *Ann Med*. 2015;47(3):262-267.

41. Thompson PD, Myerburg RJ, Levine BD, et al. Eligibility and disqualification recommendations for competitive athletes with cardiovascular abnormalities: Task Force 8: Coronary artery disease: A scientific statement from the American Heart Association and American College of Cardiology. *Circulation*. 2015;132(22):e310-e314.

42. Betriu A, Tubau J, Sanz G, Magriña J, Navarro-Lopez F. Relief of angina by periarterial muscle resection of myocardial bridges. *Am Heart J*. 1980;100(2):223-226.

43. Van Hare GF, Ackerman MJ, Evangelista JA, et al. Eligibility and disqualification recommendations for competitive athletes with cardiovascular abnormalities: Task Force 4: Congenital heart disease: A scientific statement from the American Heart Association and American College of Cardiology. *Circulation.* 2015;132(22):e281-e291.

44. Braverman AC, Harris KM, Kovacs RJ, et al. Eligibility and disqualification recommendations for competitive athletes with cardiovascular abnormalities: Task Force 7: Aortic diseases, including Marfan syndrome: A scientific statement from the American Heart Association and American College of Cardiology. *J Am Coll Cardiol.* 2015;66(21):2398-2405.

45. Inna P. Marfan syndrome (MFS). Medscape. Updated August 24, 2022. Accessed October 2, 2022. https://emedicine.medscape.com/article/1258926-overview

46. Donaldson RM, Emanuel RW, Olsen EG, Ross DN. Management of cardiovascular complications in Marfan syndrome. *Lancet.* 1980;316(8205):1178-1181.

47. El Habbal MH. Cardiovascular manifestations of Marfan's syndrome in the young. *Am Heart J.* 1992;123(3):752-757.

48. Gerry J Jr, Morris L, Pyeritz R. Clinical management of the cardiovascular complications of the Marfan syndrome. *J La State Med Soc.* 1991;143(3):43-51.

49. Marsalese DL, Moodie DS, Vacante M, et al. Marfan's syndrome: Natural history and long-term follow-up of cardiovascular involvement. *J Am Coll Cardiol.* 1989;14(2):422-428.

50. Salchow DJ, Gehle P. Ocular manifestations of Marfan syndrome in children and adolescents. *Eur J Ophthalmol.* 2019;29(1):38-43.

51. Pugh A, Bourke JP, Kunadian V. Sudden cardiac death among competitive adult athletes: A review. *Postgrad Med J.* 2012;88(1041):382-390.

52. Tang WHW. Myocarditis clinical presentation. Medscape. Updated December 28, 2021. Accessed October 3, 2022. https://emedicine.medscape.com/article/156330-clinical

53. Daniels CJ, Rajpal S, Greenshields JT, et al. Prevalence of clinical and subclinical myocarditis in competitive athletes with recent SARS-CoV-2 infection: Results from the Big Ten COVID-19 Cardiac Registry. *JAMA Cardiol.* 2021;6(9):1078-1087.

54. Le Vu S, Bertrand M, Jabagi MJ, et al. Age and sex-specific risks of myocarditis and pericarditis following Covid-19 messenger RNA vaccines. *Nat Commun.* 2022;13(1):3633.

55. Modica G, Bianco M, Sollazzo F, et al. Myocarditis in athletes recovering from COVID-19: A systematic review and meta-analysis. *Int J Environ Res Public Health.* 2022;19(7):4279.

56. Kim JH, Levine BD, Phelan D, et al. Coronavirus disease 2019 and the athletic heart: Emerging perspectives on pathology, risks, and return to play. *JAMA Cardiol.* 2021;6(2):219-227.

57. Martinez MW, Tucker AM, Bloom OJ, et al. Prevalence of inflammatory heart disease among professional athletes with prior COVID-19 infection who received systematic return-to-play cardiac screening. *JAMA Cardiol.* 2021;6(7):745-752.

58. Zipes DP, Link MS, Ackerman MJ, et al. Eligibility and disqualification recommendations for competitive athletes with cardiovascular abnormalities: Task Force 9: Arrhythmias and conduction defects: A scientific statement from the American Heart Association and American College of Cardiology. *Circulation.* 2015;132(22):e315-e325.

59. Bonow RO, Nishimura RA, Thompson PD, et al. Eligibility and disqualification recommendations for competitive athletes with cardiovascular abnormalities: Task Force 5: Valvular heart disease: A scientific statement from the American Heart Association and American College of Cardiology. *J Am Coll Cardiol.* 2015;66(21):2385-2392.

60. Jelani Q. Mitral valve prolapse. Medscape. Updated March 23, 2022. Accessed October 3, 2022. https://emedicine.medscape.com/article/155494-overview

61. Levine BD, Baggish AL, Kovacs RJ, et al. Eligibility and disqualification recommendations for competitive athletes with cardiovascular abnormalities: Task Force 1: Classification of sports: Dynamic, static, and impact: A scientific statement from the American Heart Association and American College of Cardiology. *Circulation.* 2015;132(22):e262-e266.

62. Ellis CR. Wolff-Parkinson-White syndrome. Medscape. Updated January 8, 2017. Accessed October 3, 2022. https://emedicine.medscape.com/article/159222-overview

63. Sovari AA. Long QT syndrome. Medscape. Updated November 29, 2017. Accessed October 3, 2022. https://emedicine.medscape.com/article/157826-overview

64. Moss AJ, Robinson J. Clinical features of the idiopathic long QT syndrome. *Circulation.* 1992;85(1 suppl):I140-I144.

65. Johnson JN, Ackerman MJ. Return to play? Athletes with congenital long QT syndrome. *Br J Sports Med.* 2013;47(1):28-33.

66. Harmon KG, Asif IM, Maleszewski JJ, et al. Incidence, cause, and comparative frequency of sudden cardiac death in National Collegiate Athletic Association athletes: A decade in review. *Circulation.* 2015;132(1):10-19.

67. Vettor G, Zorzi A, Basso C, Thiene G, Corrado D. Syncope as a warning symptom of sudden cardiac death in athletes. *Cardiol Clin.* 2015;33(3):423-432.

68. Dreisbach AW. Epidemiology of hypertension. Medscape. Updated December 30, 2020. Accessed October 3, 2022. https://emedicine.medscape.com/article/1928048-overview#a3

69. Rosendorff C, Lackland DT, Allison M, et al. Treatment of hypertension in patients with coronary artery disease: A scientific statement from the American Heart Association, American College of Cardiology, and American Society of Hypertension. *Circulation.* 2015;131(19):e435-e470.

70. Black HR, Sica D, Ferdinand K, et al. Eligibility and disqualification recommendations for competitive athletes with cardiovascular abnormalities: Task Force 6: Hypertension: A scientific statement from the American Heart Association and the American College of Cardiology. *Circulation.* 2015;132(22):e298-e302.

71. American Heart Association. High blood pressure. 2022. Accessed October 31, 2022. www.heart.org/en/health-topics/high-blood-pressure

72. Parsons JT. *2014-15 NCAA Sports Medicine Handbook.* 25th ed. National Collegiate Athletics Association; 2014.

73. Brooks M. Diet change tops for reducing CVD risk in stage 1 hypertension. Medscape. Updated September 9, 2022. Accessed October 1, 2022. www.medscape.com/viewarticle/980522#vp_2

74. Hurley WL, Comins SA, Green RM, Canizzaro J. Atraumatic subclavian vein thrombosis in a collegiate baseball player: A case report. *J Athl Train.* 2006;41(2):198-200.

75. National Heart, Lung, and Blood Institute. What is venous thromboembolism? Updated March 24, 2022. Accessed October 3, 2022. www.nhlbi.nih.gov/health/venous-thromboembolism

76. Patel KK. Deep vein thrombosis (DVT). Medscape. Updated June 5, 2019. Accessed October 3, 2022. https://emedicine.medscape.com/article/1911303-overview

77. Ageno W, Squizzato A, Garcia D, Imberti D. Epidemiology and risk factors of venous thromboembolism. *Semin Thromb Hemost.* 2006;32(7):651-658.

78. Wells PS, Anderson DR, Bormanis J, et al. Value of assessment of pretest probability of deep-vein thrombosis in clinical management. *Lancet* 1997;350(9094):1795-1798.

79. Modi S, Deisler R, Gozel K, et al. Wells criteria for DVT is a reliable clinical tool to assess the risk of deep venous thrombosis in trauma patients. *World J Emerg Surg.* 2016;11:24.

80. Schreiber D. Anticoagulation in deep venous thrombosis. Medscape. Updated October 30, 2020. Accessed October 31, 2022. http://emedicine.medscape.com/article/1926110-overview

81. Coleman JJ, Zarzaur BL, Katona CW, et al. Factors associated with pulmonary embolism within 72 hours of admission after trauma: A multicenter study. *J Am Coll Surg.* 2015;220(4):731-736.

82. Casals M, Martinez JA, Cayla JA, Martin V. Do basketball players have a high risk of pulmonary embolism? A scoping review. *Med Sci Sports Exerc.* 2016;48(3):466-471.

83. Bushnell BD, Anz AW, Dugger K, Sakryd GA, Noonan TJ. Effort thrombosis presenting as pulmonary embolism in a professional baseball pitcher. *Sports Health.* 2009;1(6):493-499.

84. McDonald LS, Maher PL, McDonald VS, Chin C, Dines JS. Pulmonary embolism in a baseball pitcher following open shoulder capsular repair. *HSS J.* 2016;12(1):81-84.

85. Kahanov L, Daly T. Bilateral pulmonary emboli in a collegiate gymnast: A case report. *J Athl Train.* 2009;44(6):666-671.

86. Devilbiss Z, O'Connor F. Pulmonary embolism in a collegiate softball athlete: A case report. *Curr Sports Med Rep.* 2020;19(2):53-57.

87. Dominguez JA. Peripheral arterial occlusive disease. Medscape. Updated July 29, 2022. Accessed October 3, 2022. https://emedicine.medscape.com/article/460178-overview

88. Alahdab F, Wang AT, Elraiyah TA, et al. A systematic review for the screening for peripheral arterial disease in asymptomatic patients. *J Vasc Surg.* 2015;61(3):42S-53S.

89. Curry SJ, Krist AH, Owens DK, et al.; US Preventive Services Task Force. Screening for peripheral artery disease and cardiovascular disease risk assessment with the ankle-brachial index: US Preventive Services Task Force recommendation statement. *JAMA.* 2018;320(2):177-183.

90. Eichner ER. Anemia in athletes, news on iron therapy, and community care during marathons. *Curr Sports Med Rep.* 2018;17(1):2-3.

91. Capanema FD, Lamounier JA, Ribeiro JGL, et al. Anemia and nutritional aspects in adolescent athletes: A cross-sectional study in a reference sport organization. *Rev Paul Pediatr.* 2021;40:e2020350.

92. Braden CD. Chronic anemia. Medscape. Updated January 22, 2020. Accessed October 2, 2022. https://emedicine.medscape.com/article/780176-overview

93. Moretti D, Goede JS, Zeder C, et al. Oral iron supplements increase hepcidin and decrease iron absorption from daily or twice-daily doses in iron-depleted young women. *Blood.* 2015;126:1981-1989.

94. Nagalla S. Hemolytic anemia. Medscape. Updated February 19, 2022. Accessed October 3, 2022. https://emedicine.medscape.com/article/201066-overview

95. Anderson S, Eichner ER. Exertional sickling in football players with sickle cell trait. In: Farmer KW, ed. *Football Injuries.* Springer; 2021:311-322.

96. Tufano L, Hochstetler J, Seminerio T, Lopez RM. Exercise and the effects of hydration on blood viscosity in sickle cell trait carriers: A critically appraised topic. *Int J Athl Ther Train.* 2022;27(2):59-64.

97. Maakaron JE. Sickle cell disease (SCD). Medscape. November 2, 2021. Accessed October 4, 2022. https://emedicine.medscape.com/article/205926-overview

98. Payne AB, Mehal JM, Chapman C, et al. Trends in sickle cell disease-related mortality in the United States, 1979 to 2017. *Ann Emerg Med.* 2020;76(3S):S28-S36.

99. Liem RI. Balancing exercise risk and benefits: Lessons learned from sickle cell trait and sickle cell anemia. *Hematology Am Soc Hematol Educ Program.* 2018;2018(1):418-425.

100. Maron BJ, Harris KM, Thompson PD, et al. Eligibility and disqualification recommendations for competitive athletes with cardiovascular abnormalities: Task Force 14: Sickle cell trait: A scientific statement from the American Heart Association and American College of Cardiology. *J Am Coll Cardiol.* 2015;66(21):2444-2446.

101. Al-Rimawi H, Jallad S. Sport participation in adolescents with sickle cell disease. *Pediatr Endocrinol Rev.* 2008;6(suppl 1):214-216.

102. Gati S, Malhotra A, Sedgwick C, et al. Prevalence and progression of aortic root dilatation in highly trained young athletes. *Heart.* 2019;105:920-925.

103. Gurevitz M, Weinberger A, Miller D. Aortic root aneurysm in an extreme athlete. *Cureus.* 2022;14(7):e26661.

104. Schnell F, Behar N, Carré F. Long-QT syndrome and competitive sports. *Arrhythm Electrophysiol Rev.* 2018;7(3):187-192.

105. Gomez AT, Prutkin JM, Rao AL. Evaluation and management of athletes with long QT syndrome. *Sports Health.* 2016;8(6):527-535.

106. Tsao CW, Aday AW, Almarzooq ZI, et al. Heart disease and stroke statistics—2022 update: A report from the American Heart Association. *Circulation.* 2022;145(8):e153-e639.

107. Sosa TA. Kawasaki disease. Medscape. Updated June 7, 2022. Accessed October 19, 2023. https://emedicine.medscape.com/article/965367-overview

Chapter 8

1. Ball J, Dains J, Flynn J, Solomon BS, Stewart RW. *Seidel's Guide to Physical Examination: An Interprofessional Approach.* 10th ed. Elsevier; 2022.

2. Viljoen CT, Janse van Rensburg DC, Verhagen E, et al. Correction to: Epidemiology of injury and illness among trail runners: A systematic review. *Sports Med.* 2022;52(1):191-192.

3. Waterman JJ, Kapur R. Upper gastrointestinal issues in athletes. *Curr Sports Med Rep.* 2012;11(2):99-104.

4. Bickley L, Szilagyi P, Hoffman R. *Bates' Guide to Physical Examination and History-Taking.* 13th ed. Wolters Kluwer; 2021.

5. De Oliveria EP, Burini R, Jeukendrup A. Gastrointestinal complaints during exercise: Prevalence, etiology, and nutritional recommendations. *Sports Med.* 2014;44(suppl 1):79-85.

6. Morton D, Callister R. Exercise-related transient abdominal pain (ETAP). *Sports Med.* 2015;45(1):23-35.

7. Gannon EH, Howard T. Splenic injuries in athletes: A review. *Curr Sports Med Rep.* 2010;9(2):111-114.

8. Jaworski CA, Rygiel V. Acute illness in the athlete. *Clin Sports Med.* 2019;38(4):577-595.

9. Barr W, Smith A. Acute diarrhea. *Am Fam Physician.* 2015;89(3):180-189.

10. Ferri FF. *Ferri's Clinical Advisor 2022.* Elsevier; 2022.

11. Domino F, Barry K, Baldor RA, Golding J, Stephens MB. *The 5-Minute Clinical Consult: Premium 2022.* Wolters Kluwer; 2021.

12. Wilson PB. "I think I'm gonna hurl": A narrative review of the causes of nausea and vomiting in sport. *Sports (Basel).* 2019;7(7):162.

13. Parnell JA, Wagner-Jones K, Madden RF, Erdman KA. Dietary restrictions in endurance runners to mitigate exercise-induced gastrointestinal symptoms. *J Int Soc Sports Nutr.* 2020;17(1):32.

14. Gillani SMB, Ahmed SI, Ali B. Nutritional supplements & athletes: An analysis of potential side effects. *SKY-Int J Phys Ed Sports Sci.* 2020;(1):94-100.

15. Erdman KA, Jones KW, Madden RF, Gammack N, Parnell JA. Dietary patterns in runners with gastrointestinal disorders. *Nutrients.* 2021;13(2):448.

16. Hamdan A-L, Sataloff RT, Hawkshaw MJ. Exercise-induced laryngeal obstruction (EILO) in athletes. In: *Voice Disorders in Athletes, Coaches and Other Sports Professionals.* Springer; 2021:155-182.

17. Lanas-Gimeno A, Hijos G, Lanas Á. Proton pump inhibitors, adverse events and increased risk of mortality. *Expert Opin Drug Saf.* 2019;18(11):1043-1053.

18. Leggit JC. Evaluation and treatment of GERD and upper GI complaints in athletes. *Curr Sports Med Rep.* 2011;10(2):109-114.

19. Wilkins T, Pepitone C, Alex B, Schade R. Diagnosis and management of IBS in adults. *Am Fam Physician.* 2012;86(5):419-426.

20. Killian LA, Lee S-Y. Irritable bowel syndrome is underdiagnosed and ineffectively managed among endurance athletes. *Appl Physiol Nutr Metab.* 2019;44(12):1329-1338.

21. Brandt LJ, Chey WD, Foxx-Orenstein AE, et al.; American College of Gastroenterology Task Force on Irritable Bowel Syndrome. An evidence-based position statement on the management of irritable bowel syndrome. *American Journal of Gastroenterology.* 2009;104(suppl 1):S1-S35.

22. Carter D, Lang A, Eliakim R. Endoscopy in inflammatory bowel disease. *Minerva Gastroenterol Dietol.* 2013;59(3):273-284.

23. Lebwohl B, Rubio-Tapia A. Epidemiology, presentation, and diagnosis of celiac disease. *Gastroenterology.* 2021;160(1):63-75.

24. Caio G, Volta U, Sapone A, et al. Celiac disease: A comprehensive current review. *BMC Med.* 2019;17(1):142.

25. Volta U, Caio G, Giancola F, et al. Features and progression of potential celiac disease in adults. *Clin Gastroenterol Hepatol.* 2016;14(5):686-693.

26. Vivas S, Vaquero L, Rodriguez-Martin L, Caminero A. Age-related differences in celiac disease: Specific characteristics of adult presentation. *World J Gastrointest Pharmacol Ther.* 2015;6(4):207-212.

27. Byrne G, Feighery CF. Celiac disease: Diagnosis. *Methods Mol Biol.* 2015;1326:15-22.

28. Mancini LA, Trojian T, Mancini AC. Celiac disease and the athlete. *Curr Sports Med Rep.* 2011;10(2):105-108.

29. Sapone A, Bai JC, Ciacci C, et al. Spectrum of gluten-related disorders: Consensus on new nomenclature and classification. *BMC Med.* 2012;10(1):13.

30. Cohen DL, Shirin H. Inflammatory bowel disease: Its effects on physical activity, sports participation, and athletes. *Curr Sports Med Rep.* 2021;20(7):359-365.

31. Trivedi I, Keefer L. The emerging adult with inflammatory bowel disease: Challenges and recommendations for the adult gastroenterologist. *Gastroenterol Res Pract.* 2015;2015:260807.

32. Papadimitriou K. The influence of aerobic type exercise on active Crohn's disease patients: The incidence of an elite athlete. *Healthcare (Basel).* 2022;10(4):713.

33. Steinberg JM, Charabaty A. The management approach to the adolescent IBD patient: Health maintenance and medication considerations. *Curr Gastroenterol Rep.* 2020;22(1):5.

34. Di Saverio S, Podda M, De Simone B, et al. Diagnosis and treatment of acute appendicitis: 2020 update of the WSES Jerusalem guidelines. *World J Emerg Surg.* 2020;15(1):27.

35. DeFilippis EM, Callahan LM. Atypical presentation of appendicitis in an adolescent cheerleader. *Clin J Sport Med.* 2013;23(6):494-495.

36. Moris D, Paulson EK, Pappas TN. Diagnosis and management of acute appendicitis in adults: A review. *JAMA.* 2021;326(22):2299-2311.

37. Littlefield A, Lenahan C. Cholelithiasis: Presentation and management. *J Midwifery Womens Health.* 2019;64(3):289-297.

38. American Cancer Society. Key statistics for colorectal cancer. Accessed September 28, 2022. www.cancer.org/cancer/colon-rectal-cancer/about/key-statistics.html

39. Moghadamyeghaneh Z, Alizadeh RF, Phelan M, et al. Trends in colorectal cancer admissions and stage at presentation: Impact of screening. *Surg Endosc.* 2016;30(8):3604-3610.

40. Jensen LF, Hvidberg L, Pedersen AF, Vedsted P. Symptom attributions in patients with colorectal cancer. *BMC Fam Pract.* 2015;16:115.

Chapter 9

1. Perales M, Santos-Lozano A, Sanchis-Gomar F, et al. Maternal cardiac adaptations to a physical exercise program during pregnancy. *Med Sci Sports Exerc.* 2016;48(5):896-906.

2. Ferri FF. *Ferri's Clinical Advisor 2023.* Elsevier; 2023.

3. Qaseem A, Dallas P, Forciea MA, et al. Dietary and pharmacologic management to prevent recurrent nephrolithiasis in adults: A clinical practice guideline from the American College of Physicians. *Ann Intern Med.* 2014;161(9):659-667.

4. Favus MJ, Feingold KR. Kidney stone emergencies. In: Feingold KR, Anawalt B, Blackman MR, et al., eds. *Endotext.* MDText.com, Inc.; 2000. Accessed September 19, 2022. https://www.ncbi.nlm.nih.gov/books/NBK278956/

5. Dave CN. Nephrolithiasis. Medscape. Updated September 16, 2021. Accessed November 17, 2022. https://emedicine.medscape.com/article/437096-overview

6. Fontenelle LF, Sarti TD. Kidney stones: Treatment and prevention. *Am Fam Physician.* 2019;99(8):490-496.

7. Gendreau-Webb R. Is it a kidney stone or abdominal aortic aneurysm? *Nursing 2020.* 2006;36(5):22-24.

8. Borrero E, Queral LA. Symptomatic abdominal aortic aneurysm misdiagnosed as nephroureterolithiasis. *Ann Vasc Surg.* 1988;2(2):145-149.

9. Cheungpasitporn W, Rossetti S, Friend K, et al. Treatment effect, adherence, and safety of high fluid intake for the prevention of incident and recurrent kidney stones: A systematic review and meta-analysis. *J Nephrol.* 2016;29(2):211-219.

10. Lippi G, Sanchis-Gomar F. Exertional hematuria: Definition, epidemiology, diagnostic and clinical considerations. *Clin Chem Lab Med.* 2019;57(12):1818-1828.

11. Varma P, Sengupta P, Nair R. Post exertional hematuria. *Ren Fail.* 2014;36(5):701-703.

12. Albersen M, Mortelmans LJ, Baert JA. Mountainbiker's hematuria: A case report. *Eur J Emerg Med.* 2006;13(4):236-237.

13. Bernard JJ. Renal trauma: Evaluation, management, and return to play. *Curr Sports Med Rep.* 2009;8(2):98-103.

14. Gulati S. Hematuria. Medscape. Updated May 10, 2020. Accessed November 17, 2022. https://emedicine.medscape.com/article/981898-overview

15. Brusch JL. Urinary tract infection (UTI) and cystitis (bladder infection) in females. Medscape. Updated January 2, 2020. Accessed November 17, 2022. https://emedicine.medscape.com/article/233101-overview

16. Rizvi RM, Siddiqui KM. Recurrent urinary tract infections in females. *J Pak Med Assoc.* 2010;60(1):55-59.

17. Brusch JL. Urinary tract infection (UTI) in males. Medscape. Updated January 2, 2020. Accessed November 17, 2022. https://emedicine.medscape.com/article/231574-overview

18. Fiore DC, Fox C-L. Urology and nephrology update: Recurrent urinary tract infection. *FP Essent.* 2014;416:30-37.

19. Guay DR. Cranberry and urinary tract infections. *Drugs.* 2009;69(7):775-807.

20. González de Llano D, Moreno-Arribas MV, Bartolomé B. Cranberry polyphenols and prevention against urinary tract infections: Relevant considerations. *Molecules.* 2020;25(15):3523.

21. Centers for Disease Control and Prevention. Chlamydia. Updated April 12, 2022. Accessed November 15, 2022. www.cdc.gov/std/chlamydia/default.htm

22. Porter RE, ed. *The Merck Manual of Diagnosis and Therapy.* 20th ed. Merck, Sharp & Dohme; 2018.

23. Whitaker DL. Urethritis. Medscape. 2022. Accessed November 18, 2022. https://emedicine.medscape.com/article/438091-overview

24. Centers for Disease Control and Prevention. STI treatment guidelines. Updated July 21, 2021. Accessed November 18, 2022. www.cdc.gov/std/treatment-guidelines/default.htm

25. Centers for Disease Control and Prevention. Pelvic inflammatory disease (PID). Updated April 18, 2022. Accessed November 16, 2022. www.cdc.gov/std/PID/STDFact-PID.htm

26. Ayoade FO. Herpes simplex. Medscape. Updated May 24, 2021. Accessed November 11, 2022. http://emedicine.medscape.com/article/218580-overview

27. Gilroy SA. HIV infection and AIDS. Medscape. Updated December 10, 2021. Accessed November 15, 2022. http://emedicine.medscape.com/article/211316-overview

28. Centers for Disease Control and Prevention. HIV Statistics Center. Updated August 9, 2021. Accessed November 15, 2022. www.cdc.gov/hiv/statistics/

29. American College of Obstetricians and Gynecologists. Labor and delivery management of women with human immunodeficiency virus infection. Updated March 2022. Accessed November 15, 2022. www.acog.org/Patients/FAQs/Exercise-During-Pregnancy

30. Koay WLA, Zhang J, Manepalli KV, et al. Prevention of perinatal HIV transmission in an area of high HIV prevalence in the United States. *J Pediatr.* 2021;228:101-109.

31. World Health Organization. World Health Statistics for 2022: World Health Organization. Updated May 19, 2022. www.who.int/data/gho/publications/world-health-statistics accessed November 5, 2022.

32. Parsons JT. *2014-15 NCAA Sports Medicine Handbook.* 25th ed. National Collegiate Athletics Association; 2014.

33. Gearhart PA. Human papillomavirus (HPV). Medscape. Updated February 20, 2020. Accessed November 9, 2022. http://emedicine.medscape.com/article/219110-overview

34. Centers for Disease Control and Prevention. Syphilis. Updated February 10, 2022. Accessed November 15, 2022. www.cdc.gov/std/syphilis/stdfact-syphilis.htm

35. Chandrasekar PH. Syphilis. Medscape. Updated July 11, 2017. Accessed November 15, 2022. http://emedicine.medscape.com/article/229461-clinical

36. Centers for Disease Control and Prevention. Sexually transmitted disease surveillance, 2020. Updated April 12, 2022. Accessed November 18, 2022. www.cdc.gov/std/statistics/2020/overview.htm#Syphilis

37. Centers for Disease Control and Prevention. Gonorrhea Statistics. Updated September 1, 2022. Accessed November 15, 2022. www.cdc.gov/std/gonorrhea/stats.htm

38. Qureshi A. Gonorrhea. Medscape. Updated June 15, 2021. Accessed November 14, 2022. http://emedicine.medscape.com/article/218059-overview

39. Qureshi A. Chlamydia (chlamydial genitourinary infections). Medscape. Updated March 9, 2021. Accessed November 14, 2022. http://emedicine.medscape.com/article/214823-overview

40. Hyun GS. Testicular torsion. *Rev Urol.* 2018;20(2):104-106.

41. Nassiri N, Zhu T, Asanad K, et al. Testicular torsion from bell-clapper deformity. *Urology.* 2021;147:275.

42. Caesar RE, Kaplan GW. Incidence of the bell-clapper deformity in an autopsy series. *Urology.* 1994;44(1):114-116.

43. Karakan T, Bagcioglu M, Özcan S, et al. Seasonal preponderance in testicular torsion: Is it a myth? *Arch Esp Urol.* 2015;68(10):750-754.

44. de Oliveira Gomes D, Vidal RR, Foeppel BF, et al. Cold weather is a predisposing factor for testicular torsion in a tropical country. A retrospective study. *Sao Paulo Med J.* 2015;133(3):187-90.

45. Rupp T. Testicular torsion in emergency medicine. Medscape. Updated October 22, 2019. Accessed November 14, 2022. http://emedicine.medscape.com/article/778086-overview

46. Laher A, Ragavan S, Mehta P, et al. Testicular torsion in the emergency room: A review of detection and management strategies. *Open Access Emerg Med.* 2020;12:237-246.

47. Bourke MM, Silverberg JZ. Acute scrotal emergencies. *Emerg Med Clin North Am.* 2019;37(4):593-610.

48. Ong CYG, Low HM, Chinchure D. Scrotal emergencies: An imaging perspective. *Med J Malaysia.* 2018;73(6):445-451.

49. Rudkin SE. Hydrocele in emergency medicine. Medscape. Updated November 5, 2021. Accessed November 18, 2022. https://emedicine.medscape.com/article/777386-overview

50. Parke JC. Hydrocele. Medscape. Updated July 5, 2022. Accessed November 18. 2022. https://emedicine.medscape.com/article/438724-overview

51. White WM. Varicocele. Medscape. Updated April 9, 2021. Accessed November 14, 2022. http://emedicine.medscape.com/article/438591-overview

52. Su JS, Farber NJ, Vij SC. Pathophysiology and treatment options of varicocele: An overview. *Andrologia.* 2021;53(1):e13576.

53. Roque M, Esteves SC. A systematic review of clinical practice guidelines and best practice statements for the diagnosis and management of varicocele in children and adolescents. *Asian J Androl.* 2016;18(2):262-268.

54. National Cancer Institute. Cancer Stat Facts: Testicular cancer. 2020. Accessed November 14, 2022. https://seer.cancer.gov/statfacts/html/testis.html

55. Sachdeva K. Testicular cancer. Medscape. Updated August 17, 2021. Accessed November 20, 2022. https://emedicine.medscape.com/article/279007-overview

56. Martin FC, Conduit C, Loveland KL, et al. Genetics of testicular cancer: A review. *CurrO pin Urol.* 2022;32(5):481-487.

57. Gilligan T, Lin DW, Aggarwal R, et al. Testicular cancer, version 2.2020, NCCN clinical practice guidelines in oncology. *J Natl Compr Canc Netw.* 2019;17(12):1529-1554.

58. Saab MM, Landers M, Hegarty J. Testicular cancer awareness and screening practices: A systematic review. *Oncol Nurs Forum.* 2016;43(1):E8-E23.

59. Fadich A, Giorgianni SJ, Rovito MJ, et al. USPSTF testicular examination nomination—self-examinations and examinations in a clinical setting. *Am J Mens Health.* 2018;12(5):1510-1516.

60. Centers for Disease Control and Prevention. Prostate cancer. Updated August 25, 2022. Accessed November 15, 2022. www.cdc.gov/cancer/prostate/

61. Plym A, Penney KL, Kraft P, et al. Evaluation of a multiethnic polygenic risk score model for prostate cancer. *J Natl Cancer Inst.* 2022;114(5):771-774.

62. U.S. Preventive Services Task Force. Final Recommendation Statement. Prostate Cancer: Screening. 2018. Accessed November 17, 2022. www.uspreventiveservicestaskforce. org/uspstf/document/RecommendationStatementFinal/ prostate-cancer-screening

63. Tracy CR. Prostate cancer workup. Medscape. Updated April 28, 2022. Accessed November 20, 2022. https://emedicine.medscape.com/article/1967731-workup#showall

64. Tough DeSapri KA. Pelvic inflammatory disease. Medscape. Updated August 16, 2021. Accessed November 20, 2022. https://emedicine.medscape.com/article/256448-overview

65. American College of Obstetricians and Gynecologists. Pelvic inflammatory disease. Updated June 2022. Accessed November 15, 2022. www.acog.org/womens-health/faqs/ pelvic-inflammatory-disease

66. Kho KA, Shields JK. Diagnosis and management of primary dysmenorrhea. *JAMA.* 2020;323(3):268-269.

67. Martire FG, Lazzeri L, Conway F, et al. Adolescence and endometriosis: Symptoms, ultrasound signs and early diagnosis. *Fertil Steril.* 2020;114(5):1049-1057.

68. Zannoni L, Giorgi M, Spagnolo E, et al. Dysmenorrhea, absenteeism from school, and symptoms suspicious for endometriosis in adolescents. *J Pediatr Adolesc Gynecol.* 2014;27(5):258-265.

69. McKenna KA, Fogleman CD. Dysmenorrhea. *Am Fam Physician.* 2021;104(2):164-170.

70. Hewitt G. Dysmenorrhea and endometriosis: Diagnosis and management in adolescents. *Clin Obstet Gynecol.* 2020;63(3):536-543.

71. Apostolopoulos NV, Alexandraki KI, Gorry A, et al. Association between chronic pelvic pain symptoms and the presence of endometriosis. *Arch Gynecol Obstet.* 2016;293(2):439-445.

72. Dong A. Dysmenorrhea. Medscape. Updated November 15, 2021. Accessed November 20, 2022. https://emedicine. medscape.com/article/253812-overview

73. Ji L-W, Jing C-X, Zhuang S-L, et al. Effect of age at first use of oral contraceptives on breast cancer risk: An updated meta-analysis. *Medicine (Baltimore).* 2019;98(36):e15719.

74. Tough DeSapri KA. Amenorrhea. Medscape. 2019. Accessed November 20, 2022. https://emedicine.medscape. com/article/252928-overview

75. Barrack MT, Van Loan MD, Rauh M, et al. Disordered eating, development of menstrual irregularity, and reduced bone mass change after a 3-year follow-up in female adolescent endurance runners. *Int J Sport Nutr Exerc Metab.* 2021;31(4):337-344.

76. Mountjoy M, Sundgot-Borgen J, Burke L, et al. The IOC consensus statement: Beyond the female athlete triad—relative energy deficiency in sport (RED-S). *Br J Sports Med.* 2014;48(7):491-497.

77. Holtzman B, Popp KL, Tenforde AS, et al. Low energy availability surrogates associated with lower bone mineral density and bone stress injury site. *PM R.* 2022;14(5):587-596.

78. Bonci CM, Bonci LJ, Granger LR, et al. National Athletic Trainers' Association position statement: Preventing, detecting, and managing disordered eating in athletes. *J Athl Train.* 2008;43(1):80-108.

79. Turocy PS, DePalma BF, Horswill CA, et al. National Athletic Trainers' Association position statement: Safe weight loss and maintenance practices in sport and exercise. *J Athl Train.* 2011;46(3):322-36.

80. Kontele I, Vassilakou T. Nutritional risks among adolescent athletes with disordered eating. *Children (Basel).* 2021;8(8):715.

81. O'Toole MT. *Mosby's Dictionary of Medicine, Nursing & Health Professions.* Elsevier Health Sciences; 2015.

82. Sudha SG. Mittelschmerz. *Int J Adv Nurs Manage.* 2020;8(1):103-104.

83. American Cancer Society. Cancer facts and statistics. Updated 2022. Accessed November 10, 2022. www.cancer. org/research/cancerfactsstatistics/cancerfactsfigures

84. American Cancer Society. Cervical cancer. 2022. Accessed November 15, 2022. www.cancer.org/cancer/cervicalcancer/index

85. Chan CK, Aimagambetova G, Ukybassova T, et al. Human papillomavirus infection and cervical cancer: Epidemiology, screening, and vaccination—review of current perspectives. *J Oncol.* 2019;2019:3257939

86. Boardman CH. Cervical cancer. Medscape. Updated May 13, 2022. Accessed November 15, 2022. http://emedicine. medscape.com/article/2500003-overview

87. Centers for Disease Control and Prevention. Adult immunization schedule. Updated February 17, 2022. Accessed October 21, 2022. www.cdc.gov/vaccines/schedules/hcp/ imz/adult.html

88. Centers for Disease Control and Prevention. Child and adolescent immunization schedule. Updated February 17, 2022. Accessed Oct 21, 2022. www.cdc.gov/vaccines/ schedules/hcp/imz/child-adolescent.html

89. Centers for Disease Control and Prevention. Breast cancer statistics. Updated June 6, 2022. Accessed November 15, 2022. www.cdc.gov/cancer/breast/statistics/

90. American Cancer Society. Breast cancer. Updated 2022. Accessed November 15, 2022. www.cancer.org/cancer/ breastcancer/index

91. Chalasani P. Breast cancer. Medscape. Updated September 19, 2022. Accessed November 20, 2022. https://emedicine. medscape.com/article/1947145-overview

92. May LE, Scholtz SA, Suminski R, et al. Aerobic exercise during pregnancy influences infant heart rate variability at one month of age. *Early Hum Dev.* 2014;90(1):33-38.

93. Bø K, Artal R, Barakat R, et al. Exercise and pregnancy in recreational and elite athletes: 2016 evidence summary from the IOC expert group meeting, Lausanne. Part 2—the effect of exercise on the fetus, labour and birth. *Br J Sports Med.* 2016;50(21):1297-1305.

94. American College of Obstetricians and Gynecologists. Exercise during pregnancy. Updated March 2022. Accessed November 15, 2022. www.acog.org/Patients/FAQs/Exercise-During-Pregnancy

95. Hendriks E, Rosenberg R, Prine L. Ectopic pregnancy: Diagnosis and management. *Am Fam Physician.* 2020;101(10):599-606.

96. American College of Obstetricians and Gynecologists. Tubal ectopic pregnancy. Updated March 2018. Accessed November 25, 2022. www.acog.org/clinical/clinical-guidance/practice-bulletin/articles/2018/03/tubal-ectopic-pregnancy

97. Gilroy SA. HIV Infection and AIDs. January 2023. Accessed May 16, 2023. https://emedicine.medscape.com/article/211316-overview

98. Ellis R. Moderna launches clinical trial for HIV vaccine. Medscape. January 28, 2022. Accessed May 16, 2023. www.medscape.com/viewarticle/967491

99. O'Mary L. Highly anticipated HIV vaccine fails in large trail. Medscape. January 19, 2023. Accessed May 16, 2023. www.medscape.com/viewarticle/987208

100. Murphy SE, Johnston CA, Strom C, et al. Influence of exercise type on maternal blood pressure adaptation throughout pregnancy. *AJOG Glob Rep.* 2021;2(1):100023.

101. Romero-Gallard L, Roldan-Reoyo O, Castro- Piñero J, et al. Physical fitness assessment during pregnancy *ACSM Health Fit J.* 2022;26(5):84-90.

Chapter 10

1. Baugh CM, Kroshus E, Bourlas AP, et al. Requiring athletes to acknowledge receipt of concussion-related information and responsibility to report symptoms: A study of the prevalence, variation, and possible improvements. *J Law Med Ethics.* 2014;42(3):297-313.

2. Zuckerman SL, Kerr ZY, Yengo-Kahn A, et al. Epidemiology of sports-related concussion in NCAA athletes from 2009-2010 to 2013-2014: Incidence, recurrence, and mechanisms. *Am J Sports Med.* 2015;43(11):2654-2662.

3. Bryan MA, Rowhani-Rahbar A, Comstock RD, et al. Sports- and recreation-related concussions in US youth. *Pediatrics.* 2016;138(1):e20154635.

4. Guskiewicz KM, Register-Mihalik J, McCrory P, et al. Evidence-based approach to revising the SCAT2: Introducing the SCAT3. *Br J Sports Med.* 2013;47(5):289-293.

5. Gessel LM, Fields SK, Collins CL, et al. Concussions among United States high school and collegiate athletes. *J Athl Train.* 2007;42(4):495-503.

6. McCrory P, Meeuwisse W, Dvorak J, et al. Consensus statement on concussion in sport—The 5th International Conference on Concussion in Sport held in Berlin, October 2016. *Br J Sports Med.* 2017;51(11):838-847.

7. Kontos AP, Elbin RJ, Trbovich A, et al. Concussion Clinical Profiles Screening (CP Screen) Tool: Preliminary evidence to inform a multidisciplinary approach. *Neurosurgery.* 2020;87(2):348-356.

8. McCrea M, Broglio S, McAllister T, et al. Return to play and risk of repeat concussion in collegiate football players: Comparative analysis from the NCAA Concussion Study (1999-2001) and CARE Consortium (2014-2017). *Br J Sports Med.* 2020;54(2):102-109.

9. Thomas DJ, Coxe K, Li H, et al. Length of recovery from sports-related concussions in pediatric patients treated at concussion clinics. *Clin J Sport Med.* 2018;28(1):56-63.

10. Broglio SP, Cantu RC, Gioia GA, et al. National Athletic Trainers' Association position statement: Management of sport concussion. *J Athl Train.* 2014;49(2):245-265.

11. Harmon KG, Clugston JR, Dec K, et al. American Medical Society for Sports Medicine position statement on concussion in sport. *Br J Sports Med.* 2019;53(4):213-225.

12. Broglio SP, Harezlak J, Katz B, et al. Acute sport concussion assessment optimization: A prospective assessment from the CARE Consortium. *Sports Med.* 2019;49(12):1977-1987.

13. Giza CC, Kutcher JS, Ashwal S, et al. Summary of evidence-based guideline update: Evaluation and management of concussion in sports: Report of the Guideline Development Subcommittee of the American Academy of Neurology. *Neurology.* 2013;80(24):2250-2257.

14. Harvey HH. Reducing traumatic brain injuries in youth sports: Youth sports traumatic brain injury state laws, January 2009-December 2012. *Am J Public Health.* 2013;103(7):1249-1254.

15. Chrisman SP, Schiff MA, Chung SK, et al. Implementation of concussion legislation and extent of concussion education for athletes, parents, and coaches in Washington State. *Am J Sports Med.* 2014;42(5):1190-1196.

16. Shenouda C, Hendrickson P, Davenport K, et al. The effects of concussion legislation one year later—What have we learned: A descriptive pilot survey of youth soccer player associates. *PM R.* 2012;4(6):427-435.

17. Bompadre V, Jinguji TM, Yanez ND, et al. Washington State's Lystedt law in concussion documentation in Seattle public high schools. *J Athl Train.* 2014;49(4):486-492.

18. Gibson TB, Herring SA, Kutcher JS, et al. Analyzing the effect of state legislation on health care utilization for children with concussion. *JAMA Pediatr.* 2015;169(2):163-168.

19. Mackenzie B, Vivier P, Reinert S, et al. Impact of a state concussion law on pediatric emergency department visits. *Pediatr Emerg Care.* 2015;31(1):25-30.

20. Pop Warner. Pop Warner Concussion Policy. 2015. Accessed 14, 2015. www.popwarner.com/safety/concussionpolicy.htm

21. Preparticipation Physical Evaluation Working Group. *Preparticipation Physical Evaluation.* 4th ed. American Academy of Pediatrics; 2020.

22. Scopaz KA, Hatzenbuehler JR. Risk modifiers for concussion and prolonged recovery. *Sports Health.* 2013;5(6):537-541.

23. Gioia GA, Schneider JC, Vaughan CG, et al. Which symptom assessments and approaches are uniquely appropriate for paediatric concussion? *Br J Sports Med.* 2009;43(suppl 1):i13-i22.

24. Echemendia RJ, Meeuwisse W, McCrory P, et al. The Sport Concussion Assessment Tool, 5th edition (SCAT5): Background and rationale. *Br J Sports Med.* 2017;51(11):848-850.

25. Broglio SP, Puetz TW. The effect of sport concussion on neurocognitive function, self-report symptoms and postural control: A meta-analysis. *Sports Med.* 2008;38(1):53-67.

26. Barr WB. Methodologic issues in neuropsychological testing. *J Athl Train.* 2001;36(3):297-302.

27. Maddocks DL, Dicker GD, Saling MM. The assessment of orientation following concussion in athletes. *Clin J Sports Med.* 1995;5:32-35.

28. Young C, Jacobs B, Clavette K, et al. Serial sevens: Not the most effective test of mental status in high school athletes. *Clin J Sports Med.* 1997;7:196-198.

29. McCrea M. Standardized mental status testing on the sideline after sport-related concussion. *J Athl Train.* 2001;36(3):274-279.

30. McCrea M, Kelly JP, Randolph C. *The Standardized Assessment of Concussion: Manual for Administration, Scoring, and Interpretation.* 2nd ed. Brain Injury Association; 2000.

31. McCrea M, Kelly JP, Randolph C, et al. Immediate neurocognitive effects of concussion. *Neurosurgery.* 2002;50(5):1032-1042.

32. McCrea M, Guskiewicz KM, Marshall SW, et al. Acute effects and recovery time following concussion in collegiate football players: The NCAA Concussion Study. *JAMA.* 2003;290(19):2556-2563.

33. McCrea M, Barr W, Guskiewicz K, et al. Standard regression-based methods for measuring recovery after sport-related concussion. *J Int Neuropsychol Soc.* 2005;11:58-69.

34. Barr WB, McCrea M. Sensitivity and specificity of standardized neurocognitive testing immediately following sports concussion. *J Int Neuropsychol Soc.* 2001;7:693-702.

35. Valovich McLeod TC, Perrin DH, Guskiewicz KM, et al. Serial administration of clinical concussion assessments and learning effects in healthy youth sports participants. *Clin J Sport Med.* 2004;14(5):287-295.

36. Grindel SH, Lovell MR, Collins MW. The assessment of sport-related concussion: The evidence behind neuropsychological testing and management. *Clin J Sport Med.* 2001;11:134-143.

37. Belanger HG, Vanderploeg RD. The neuropsychological impact of sports-related concussion: A meta-analysis. *J Intl Neuropsychol Soc.* 2005;11:345-357.

38. Guskiewicz KM. Postural stability assessment following concussion: One piece of the puzzle. *Clin J Sports Med.* 2001;11:182-189.

39. Riemann BL, Guskiewicz KM. Effects of mild head injury on postural stability as measured through clinical balance testing. *J Athl Train.* 2000;35(1):19-25.

40. Howell DR, Osternig LR, Chou LS. Single-task and dual-task tandem gait test performance after concussion. *J Sci Med Sport.* 2017;20(7):622-626.

41. Valovich McLeod TC, Hale TD. Vestibular and balance issues following sport-related concussion. *Brain Inj.* 2015;29(2):175-184.

42. Mucha A, Collins MW, Elbin RJ, et al. A Brief Vestibular/Ocular Motor Screening (VOMS) assessment to evaluate concussions: Preliminary findings. *Am J Sports Med.* 2014;42(10):2479-2486.

43. Galetta KM, Brandes LE, Maki K, et al. The King-Devick test and sports-related concussion: Study of a rapid visual screening tool in a collegiate cohort. *J Neurol Sci.* 2011;309(1-2):34-39.

44. Galetta KM, Morganroth J, Moehringer N, et al. Adding vision to concussion testing: A prospective study of sideline testing in youth and collegiate athletes. *J Neuroophthalmol.* 2015;35(3):235-241.

45. McCrory P, Meeuwisse W, Aubry M, et al. Consensus statement on concussion in sport—the 4th International Conference on Concussion in Sport held in Zurich, November 2012. *Clin J Sport Med.* 2013;23(2):89-117.

46. Van Kampen DA, Lovell MR, Pardini JE, et al. The "value added" of neurocognitive testing after sports-related concussion. *Am J Sports Med.* 2006;34(10):1630-1635.

47. Broglio SP, Macciocchi SN, Ferrara MS. Sensitivity of the concussion assessment battery. *Neurosurgery.* 2007;60:1050-1058.

48. Leddy JJ, Master CL, Mannix R, et al. Early targeted heart rate aerobic exercise versus placebo stretching for sport-related concussion in adolescents: A randomised controlled trial. *Lancet Child Adolesc Health.* 2021;5(11):792-99.

49. Haider MN, Herget L, Zafonte RD, et al. Rehabilitation of sport-related concussion. *Clin Sports Med.* 2021;40(1):93-109.

50. Lumba-Brown A, Teramoto M, Bloom OJ, et al. Concussion guidelines step 2: Evidence for subtype classification. *Neurosurgery.* 2020;86(1):2-13.

51. Kontos AP, Sufrinko A, Sandel N, et al. Sport-related concussion clinical profiles: Clinical characteristics, targeted treatments, and preliminary evidence. *Curr Sports Med Rep.* 2019;18(3):82-92.

52. Valovich McLeod TC, Gioia GA. Cognitive rest: The often neglected aspect of concussion management. *Athl Ther Today.* 2010;15(2):1-3.

53. Thomas DG, Apps JN, Hoffmann RG, et al. Benefits of strict rest after acute concussion: A randomized controlled trial. *Pediatrics.* 2015;135(2):213-223.

54. Halstead ME, McAvoy K, Devore CD, et al. Returning to learning following a concussion. *Pediatrics.* 2013;132(5):948-957.

55. Sady MD, Vaughan CG, Gioia GA. School and the concussed youth: Recommendations for concussion education and management. *Phys Med Rehabil Clin N Am.* 2011;22(4):701-719, ix.

56. McAvoy K, Eagan-Johnson B, Halstead M. Return to learn: Transitioning to school and through ascending levels of academic support for students following a concussion. *NeuroRehabilitation.* 2018;42(3):325-330.

57. Gioia GA. Multimodal evaluation and management of children with concussion: Using our heads and available evidence. *Brain Inj.* 2015;29(2):195-206.

58. DeMatteo C, Stazyk K, Giglia L, et al. A balanced protocol for return to school for children and youth following concussive injury. *Clin Pediatr (Phila).* 2015;54(8):783-792.

59. D'Silva L, Devos H, Hunt SL, et al. Concussion symptoms experienced during driving may influence driving habits. *Brain Inj.* 2021;35(1):59-64.

60. Schmidt JD, Hoffman NL, Ranchet M, et al. Driving after concussion: Is it safe to drive after symptoms resolve? *J Neurotrauma.* 2017;34(8):1571-1578.

61. Schmidt JD, Lynall RC, Lempke LB, et al. Post-concussion driving behaviors and opinions: A survey of collegiate student-athletes. *J Neurotrauma.* 2018;35(20):2418-2424.

62. Schmidt JD, Lempke LB, Devos H, et al. Post-concussion driving management among athletic trainers. *Brain Inj.* 2019;33(13-14):1652-1659.

63. Lempke LB, Lynall RC, Hoffman NL, et al. Slowed driving-reaction time following concussion-symptom resolution. *J Sport Health Sci.* 2021;10(2):145-153.

64. Christensen J, McGrew CA. When is it safe to drive after mild traumatic brain injury/sports-related concussion? *Curr Sports Med Rep.* 2019;18(1):17-19.

65. Ritter K MA, Robinson K, Mistry DJ, Choe MC, McLeod TV. Concussion Management among National Collegiate Athletics Association swim programs. *Int J Athl Ther Train.* 2022;1(aop):1-5.

66. May KH, Marshall DL, Burns TG, et al. Pediatric sports specific return to play guidelines following concussion. *Int J Sports Phys Ther.* 2014;9(2):242-255.

67. Makdissi M, Schneider KJ, Feddermann-Demont N, et al. Approach to investigation and treatment of persistent symptoms following sport-related concussion: A systematic review. *Br J Sports Med.* 2017;51(12):958-968.

68. Fehr SD, Nelson LD, Scharer KR, et al. Risk factors for prolonged symptoms of mild traumatic brain injury: A pediatric sports concussion clinic cohort. *Clin J Sport Med.* 2019;29(1):11-17.

69. Meehan WP III, Mannix R, Monuteaux MC, et al. Early symptom burden predicts recovery after sport-related concussion. *Neurology.* 2014;83(24):2204-2210.

70. Meehan WP III, O'Brien MJ, Geminiani E, et al. Initial symptom burden predicts duration of symptoms after concussion. *J Sci Med Sport.* 2016;19(9):722-725.

71. Barnhart M, Bay RC, Valovich McLeod TC. The influence of timing of reporting and clinic presentation on concussion recovery outcomes: A systematic review and meta-analysis. *Sports Med.* 2021;51(7):1491-1508.

72. Zemek R, Barrowman N, Freedman SB, et al. Clinical risk score for persistent postconcussion symptoms among children with acute concussion in the ED. *JAMA.* 2016;315(10):1014-1025.

73. Howell DR, Zemek R, Brilliant AN, et al. Identifying persistent postconcussion symptom risk in a pediatric sports medicine clinic. *Am J Sports Med.* 2018;46(13):3254-3261.

74. Root JM, Gai J, Sady MD, Vaughan CG, Madati PJ. Identifying risks for persistent postconcussive symptoms in a pediatric emergency department: An examination of a clinical risk score. *Arch Clin Neuropsychol.* 2022;37(1):30-39.

75. Benson BW, Hamilton GM, Meeuwisse WH, et al. Is protective equipment useful in preventing concussion? A systematic review of the literature. *Br J Sports Med.* 2009;43(suppl 1):i56-i67.

76. Benson BW, McIntosh AS, Maddocks D, et al. What are the most effective risk-reduction strategies in sport concussion? *Br J Sports Med.* 2013;47(5):321-326.

77. Emery CA, Black AM, Kolstad A, et al. What strategies can be used to effectively reduce the risk of concussion in sport? A systematic review. *Br J Sports Med.* 2017;51(12):978-984.

78. Chisholm DA, Black AM, Palacios-Derflingher L, et al. Mouthguard use in youth ice hockey and the risk of concussion: Nested case-control study of 315 cases. *Br J Sports Med.* 2020;54(14):866-870.

79. Van Pelt KL, Caccese JB, Eckner JT, et al. Detailed description of Division I ice hockey concussions: Findings from the NCAA and Department of Defense CARE Consortium. *J Sport Health Sci.* 2021;10(2):162-171.

80. Black AM, Macpherson AK, Hagel BE, et al. Policy change eliminating body checking in non-elite ice hockey leads to a threefold reduction in injury and concussion risk in 11- and 12-year-old players. *Br J Sports Med.* 2016;50(1):55-61.

81. Emery C, Palacios-Derflingher L, Black AM, et al. Does disallowing body checking in non-elite 13- to 14-year-old ice hockey leagues reduce rates of injury and concussion? A cohort study in two Canadian provinces. *Br J Sports Med.* 2020;54(7):414-420.

82. Wiebe DJ, D'Alonzo BA, Harris R, et al. Association between the experimental kickoff rule and concussion rates in Ivy League Football. *JAMA.* 2018;320(19):2035-2036.

83. Shanley E, Thigpen C, Kissenberth M, et al. Heads up football training decreases concussion rates in high school football players. *Clin J Sport Med.* 2021;31(2):120-126.

84. Sarmiento K, Mitchko J, Klein C, et al. Evaluation of the Centers for Disease Control and Prevention's concussion initiative for high school coaches: "Heads Up: Concussion in High School Sports". *J Sch Health.* 2010;80(3):112-118.

85. Williamson RW, Gerhardstein D, Cardenas J, et al. Concussion 101: The current state of concussion education programs. *Neurosurgery.* 2014;75(suppl 4):S131-S135.

86. Tsao CW, Aday AW, Almarzooq ZI, et al. Heart disease and stroke statistics—2022 update: A report from the American Heart Association. *Circulation.* 2022;145(8):e153-e639.

87. Ji R, Schwamm LH, Pervez MA, et al. Ischemic stroke and transient ischemic attack in young adults: Risk factors, diagnostic yield, neuroimaging, and thrombolysis. *JAMA Neurol.* 2013;70(1):51-57.

88. Putaala J. Ischemic stroke in young adults. *Cerebrosvascular Dis.* 2020;26(2):386-414.

89. VanWie C, Casiero D. Acute ischemic stroke in a male collegiate football athlete. *Athl Train Sports Health Care.* 2021;13(4):e247-e251.

90. James SD. Pediatric stroke often misdiagnoses, treatment delayed. ABC News. 2013. Accessed November, 2021. https://abcnews.go.com/Health/pediatric-stroke-misdiagnosed-treatment-delayed/story?id=18444256

91. Tanner J. Bouncing back. *The Leader.* November 23, 2016.

92. Doyle-Baker PK, Mitchell T, Hayden KA. Stroke and athletes: A scoping review. *Int J Environ Res Public Health.* 2021;18(19):10047.

93. Aroor S, Singh R, Goldstein LB. BE-FAST (Balance, Eyes, Face, Arm, Speech, Time) reducing the proportion of strokes missed using the FAST Mnemonic. *Stroke.* 2017;48(2):479-481.

94. Papadakis MA, McPhee SJ, Rabow MW, McQuaid KR. *Current Diagnosis & Treatment.* 62nd ed. McGraw Hill; 2023.

95. Ferri FF. *Ferri's Clinical Advisor 2023.* Elsevier; 2023.

96. Jauch EC. Acute management of stroke. Medscape. Updated September 8, 2017. Accessed November 5, 2022. http://emedicine.medscape.com/article/1159752-overview

97. McDonald MW, Black SE, Copland DA, et al. Cognition in stroke rehabilitation and recovery research: Consensus-based core recommendations from the second Stroke Recovery and Rehabilitation Roundtable. *Int J Stroke.* 2019;14(8):774-782.

98. Bernhardt J, Borschmann KN, Kwakkel G, et al. Setting the scene for the second Stroke Recovery and Rehabilitation Roundtable. *Int J Stroke.* 2019;14(5):450-456.

99. Centers for Disease Control and Prevention. Leading Causes of Death. Updated September 6, 2022. Accessed November 5, 2022. www.cdc.gov/nchs/fastats/leading-causes-of-death.htm

100. American Heart Association. High blood pressure. 2022. Accessed October 31, 2022. www.heart.org/en/health-topics/high-blood-pressure

101. Olesen J. International classification of headache disorders. *Lancet Neurol.* 2018;17(5):396-397.

102. Chawla J. Migraine headache. Medscape; 2021. Updated October 1, 2021. Accessed Nov 6, 2022. https://emedicine.medscape.com/article/1142556-overview

103. Flynn O, Fullen BM, Blake C. Migraine in university students: A systematic review and meta-analysis. *Eur J Pain.* 2022;27(1):14-43.

104. Porter RE. *The Merck Manual of Diagnosis and Therapy.* 20th ed. Merck, Sharp & Dohme Corp; 2018.

105. National Institute of Neurological Disorders and Stroke. Migraine. Updated 2022. Accessed November 6, 2022. www.ninds.nih.gov/health-information/disorders/migraine?search-term=headache

106. Kinart CM, Cuppett MM, Berg K. Prevalence of migraines in NCAA Division I male and female basketball players. *Headache.* 2002;42(7):620-629.

107. Blanda M. Cluster headache. Medscape; 2021. Accessed November 6, 2022. https://emedicine.medscape.com/article/1142459-overview

108. Smith ED, Swartzon M, McGrew CA. Headaches in athletes. *Curr Sports Med Rep.* 2014;13(1):27-32.

109. Ali M, Asghar N, Hannah T, et al. A multicenter, longitudinal survey of chronic headaches and concussions among youth athletes in the United States from 2009 to 2019. *J Headache Pain.* 2023;24(1):6.

110. Tsuha M, Liu M, Hori K, et al. Prevalence of concussions and chronic headaches in female collegiate athletes. *J Womens Sports Med.* 2022;2(1):30-40.

111. Blanda M. Tension headache. Medscape. Updated November 21, 2017. Accessed November 6, 2022. https://emedicine.medscape.com/article/792384-overview

112. Ko DY. Epilepsy and seizures. Medscape. Updated July 26, 2022. Accessed November 6, 2022. https://emedicine.medscape.com/article/1184846-overview

113. Beghi E. The epidemiology of epilepsy. *Neuroepidemiology.* 2020;54(2):185-191.

114. Segan S. Absence seizures. Medscape. September 25, 2018. Accessed November 6, 2022. https://reference.medscape.com/article/1183858-overview

115. Casa DJ, DeMartini JK, Bergeron MF, et al. National Athletic Trainers' Association position statement: Exertional heat illnesses. *J Athl Train.* 2015;50(9):986-1000.

116. Beitchman JA, Burg BA, Sabb DM, et al. The pentagram of concussion: An observational analysis that describes five overt indicators of head trauma. *BMC Sports Sci Med Rehabil.* 2022;14(1):39.

117. Ko DY. Epilepsy and seizures. Medscape. Updated July 26, 2022. Accessed November 6, 2022. https://emedicine.medscape.com/article/1184846-overview

118. Pagura JR, Alessi R. Epilepsy and seizures. In: *The Sports Medicine Physician.* Springer; 2019:235-240.

119. Melinosky C. Epilepsy drugs to treat seizures. WebMD. Updated February 2, 2022. Accessed November 7, 2022. www.webmd.com/epilepsy/medications-treat-seizures

120. Capovilla G, Kaufman KR, Perucca E, et al. Epilepsy, seizures, physical exercise, and sports: A report from the ILAE Task Force on Sports and Epilepsy. *Epilepsia.* 2016;57(1):6-12.

121. Manuel C FR. Sports participation for young athletes with medical conditions: Seizure disorder, infections and single organs. *Curr Probl Pediatr Adolesc Health Care.* 2018;48(5-6):161-171.

122. Carter JM, McGrew C. Seizure disorders and exercise/sports participation. *Curr Sports Med Rep.* 2021;20(1):26-30.

123. DerSarkissian C. If I have epilespy, can I drive? WedMD. Updated January 23, 2022. Accessed Nov 7, 2022. www.webmd.com/epilepsy/guide/seizures-driving

124. Epilepsy Foundation. Driving and transportation. 2013. Accessed November 7, 2022. www.epilepsy.com/lifestyle/driving-and-transportation

125. O'Toole MT. *Mosby's Dictionary of Medicine, Nursing & Health Professions*. Elsevier Health Sciences; 2015.

126. Taylor DC. What Can Trigger Vertigo? MedicineNet. Updated April 21, 2022. Accessed November 7, 2022. www.medicinenet.com/vertigo_overview/article.htm

127. Li JC. Benign paroxysmal positional vertigo. Medscape. Updated January 14, 2022. Accessed November 7, 2022. https://emedicine.medscape.com/article/884261-overview

128. AlGarni MA, Mirza AA, Althobaiti AA, et al. Association of benign paroxysmal positional vertigo with vitamin D deficiency: A systematic review and meta-analysis. *Eur Arch Otorhinolaryngol*. 2018;275(11):2705-2711.

129. Suh K OS, Chae H, Lee S, Chang M, Mun S. Can osteopenia induce residual dizziness after treatment of benign paroxysmal positional vertigo? *Otol Neurotol*. 2020;41(5):e603-e606.

130. Rabie AN. Canalith-repositioning maneuvers. Medscape. Updated August 19, 2021. Accessed November 7, 2022. https://emedicine.medscape.com/article/82945-overview

131. NATA Research and Educational Foundation. Symptoms & treatment of benign paroxysmal positional vertigo (BPPV). 2016. Accessed November 30, 2022. www.natafoundation.org/wp-content/uploads/NATA_BPPVInfogfxR4-WEB.pdf

132. Mehta P, Raymond J, Punjani R, et al. Prevalence of amyotrophic lateral sclerosis in the United States using established and novel methodologies, 2017. *Amyotroph Lateral Scler Frontotemporal Degener*. 2023;24(1-2):108-116.

133. Armon C. Amyotrophic lateral sclerosis. Medscape. Updated June 14, 2018. Accessed November 7, 2022. https://emedicine.medscape.com/article/1170097-overview

134. Berdyński M, Miszta P, Safranow K, et al. SOD1 mutations associated with amyotrophic lateral sclerosis analysis of variant severity. *Sci Rep*. 2022;12(1):103.

135. Ilieva H, Polymenidou M, Cleveland DW. Non–cell autonomous toxicity in neurodegenerative disorders: ALS and beyond. *J Cell Biol*. 2009;187(6):761-772.

136. Farace C, Fenu G, Lintas S, et al. Amyotrophic lateral sclerosis and lead: A systematic update. *Neurotoxicology*. 2020;81:80-88.

137. Mitsumoto H, Garofalo DC, Gilmore M, et al. Case-control study in ALS using the National ALS Registry: Lead and agricultural chemicals are potential risk factors. *Amyotroph Lateral Scler Frontotemporal Degener*. 2022;23(3-4):190-202.

138. McKay KA, Smith KA, Smertinaite L, et al. Military service and related risk factors for amyotrophic lateral sclerosis. *Acta Neurol Scand*. 2021;143(1):39-50.

139. National Institute of Neurological Disorders and Stroke. Amyotrophic Lateral Sclerosis. Updated July 25, 2022. Accessed November 7, 2022. www.ninds.nih.gov/amyotrophic-lateral-sclerosis-als-fact-sheet

140. Gompf SG. Rabies. Medscape. Updated April 26, 2022. Accessed November 7, 2022. https://emedicine.medscape.com/article/220967-overview

141. Gupta G. Complex regional pain syndromes. Medscape. Updated June 20, 2018. Accessed November 8, 2022. https://emedicine.medscape.com/article/1145318-overview

142. Rao TPS. Complex regional pain syndrome type 1 (reflex sympathetic dystrophy). Medscape. Updated Mar 9, 2021. Accessed November 8, 2022. https://emedicine.medscape.com/article/334377-overview

143. Johnson S, Cowell F, Gillespie S, et al. Complex regional pain syndrome what is the outcome? A systematic review of the course and impact of CRPS at 12 months from symptom onset and beyond. *Eur J Pain*. 2022;26(6):1203-1220.

144. Harden RN, Bruehl S, Stanton-Hicks M, et al. Proposed new diagnostic criteria for complex regional pain syndrome. *Pain Med*. 2007;8(4):326-331.

145. Goebel A, Birklein F, Brunner F, et al. The Valencia consensus-based adaptation of the IASP complex regional pain syndrome diagnostic criteria. *Pain*. 2021;162(9):2346.

146. Rao J. Acne vulgaris. Medscape. Updated August 27, 2020. Accessed November 12, 2022. http://emedicine.medscape.com/article/1069804-overview

147. Kessler A, Yoo M, Calisoff R. Complex regional pain syndrome: An updated comprehensive review. *NeuroRehabilitation*. 2020;47(3):253-264.

148. Hosseini AH, Lifshitz J. Brain injury forces of moderate magnitude elicit the fencing response. *Med Sci Sports Exerc*. 2009;41(9):1687-1697.

149. Beitchman JA, Burg BA, Sabb DM, Hosseini AH, Lifshitz J. The pentagram of concussion: An observational analysis that describes five overt indicators of head trauma. *BMC Sports Sci Med Rehabil*. 2022;14(1):39.

Chapter 11

1. Jarvis C. *Physical Examination & Health Assessment*. 8th ed. Elsevier; 2019.

2. Ball J, Dains J, Flynn J, Solomon BS, Stewart RW. *Seidel's Guide to Physical Examination, An Interprofessional Approach*. 10th ed. Elsevier; 2021.

3. Cass SP. Ocular injuries in sports. *Curr Sports Med Rep*. 2012;11(1):11-15.

4. Toldi JP, Thomas JL. Evaluation and management of sports-related eye injuries. *Curr Sports Med Rep*. 2020;19(1):29-34.

5. Meida N, Setyawati I. The influence of corneal foreign body on eye infection. In: *Proceedings of the Third International Conference on Sustainable Innovation 2019 Health Science and Nursing (IcoSIHSN 2019)*. Atlantis Press; 2019:58-60.

6. Bickley L, Szilagyi P, Hoffman R. *Bates' Guide to Physical Examination and History-Taking*. 13th ed. Wolters Kluwer; 2021.

7. Wu F, Liu Y, Zhang K. Examination of the retina. *New Engl J Med*. 2015;373(25):2484.

8. Thirunavukarasu AJ, Mullinger D, Rufus-Toye RM, Farrell S, Allen LE. Clinical validation of a novel web-application for remote assessment of distance visual acuity. *Eye.* 2022;36(10):2057-2061.

9. Rodrigues PF. Influence of pre-operative refraction in LASIK surgery success. *Revista Sociedade Portuguesa de Oftalmologia.* 2018;42(1).

10. Liu M, Chen Y, Wang D, et al. Clinical outcomes after SMILE and femtosecond laser-assisted LASIK for myopia and myopic astigmatism: A prospective randomized comparative study. *Cornea.* 2016;35(2):210-216.

11. Owen J. How to determine an ideal LASIK candidate. *Optometry Times.* 2019;11(5):10-11.

12. Ferri FF. *Ferri's Clinical Advisor 2022.* Elsevier; 2022.

13. Geissler KE, Borchers JR. More than meets the eye: A rapidly progressive skin infection in a football player. *Clin J Sport Med.* 2015;25(3):e54-e56.

14. Roat MI. Overview of conjunctival and scleral disorders. In: *Merck Manual.* Merck; 2014.

15. Ahmed F, House RJ, Feldman BH. Corneal abrasions and corneal foreign bodies. *Prim Care.* 2015;42(3):363-375.

16. Richardson B. *Pediatric Primary Care: Practice Guidelines for Nurses.* Jones & Bartlett Publishers; 2013.

17. Camodeca AJ, Anderson EP. Corneal foreign body. In: *StatPearls.* StatPearls Publishing; 2021.

18. Hassan HT. The evaluation of bandage soft contact lenses as a primary treatment for traumatic corneal abrasions. *Int J Clin Exp Ophthalmol.* 2020;4:041-048.

19. Patil B, Vanathi M, Raj N. Corneal laceration and penetrating injuries. In: *Corneal Emergencies.* Springer; 2022:107-132.

20. Zafar S, Canner JK, Mir T, et al. Epidemiology of hyphema-related emergency department visits in the United States between 2006 and 2015. *Ophthalmic Epidemiol.* 2019;26(3):208-215.

21. Andreoli CM, Gardiner MF, Trobe J, Moreira ME. Traumatic hyphema: Clinical features and diagnosis. UpToDate; 2020.

22. Acar U, Sobaci G. Guidelines of return to play. In: *Sports-Related Eye Injuries.* Springer; 2020:121-128.

23. Chang H-YP, Huynh N, Borboli-Gerogiannis S. Eye injuries associated with orbital or periorbital trauma. *Invest Ophthalmol Vis Sci.* 2012;53(14):4962.

24. Kholaki O, Hammer DA, Schlieve T. Management of orbital fractures. *Atlas Oral Maxillofac Surg Clin North Am.* 2019;27(2):157-165.

25. Homer N, Huggins A, Durairaj VD. Contemporary management of orbital blowout fractures. *Curr Opin Otolaryngol Head Neck Surg.* 2019;27(4):310-316.

26. Kriz PK, Zurakowski RD, Almquist JL, et al. Eye protection and risk of eye injuries in high school field hockey. *Pediatrics.* 2015;136(3):521-527.

27. Thomas JR, Kriet JD, Humphrey CD, Eng J, Sivam S. Modern approaches to facial and athletic injuries. *Facial Plast Surg Clin North Am.* 2022;30(1):xi.

28. Vinger PF. *The Mechanisms and Prevention of Sports Eye Injuries.* Protective Eyewear Certification Council; 2012.

29. Nagpal M, Chaudhary P, Wachasundar S, Eltayib A, Raihan A. Management of recurrent rhegmatogenous retinal detachment. *Indian J Ophthalmol.* 2018;66(12):1763-1771.

30. Lazarus R. 5 tips for hard contact lenses. Optometrists Network. Accessed November 4, 2022. www.optometrists.org/general-practice-optometry/optical/guide-to-contact-lenses/guide-to-hard-contact-lenses/5-tips-for-hard-contact-lenses/#:~:text=Hard%20contact%20lenses%20are%20often,plastic%20material%20(typically%20silicone)

31. Hou A, Jin ML, Goldman D. The protective effects of soft contact lenses for contact sports: A novel porcine model for corneal abrasion biomechanics. *Eye Contact Lens.* 2022;48(5):228-230.

32. Mittal V, Jain R, Mittal R, Vashist U, Narang P. Successful management of severe unilateral chemical burns in children using simple limbal epithelial transplantation (SLET). *Br J Ophthalmol.* 2016;100(8):1102-1108.

33. Coronica R, Murty C. Ocular emergencies: Screening tool and alert protocol. *Insight.* 2015;40(4):5-13.

34. Borrione P, Quaranta F, De Luca V, et al. Ophthalmologic findings in contact sport disciplines. *Sports Med Phys Fitness.* 2016;56(12):1598-1601.

35. Akhtar N, Haneef M, Saeed M, Niaz A, Rehman MA-u-R, Khan MW. Proptosis in ENT department: Presentation and management. *Ann Punjab Med Coll.* 2018;12(4).

36. Turbert D, Shelton B. Sports eye safety. American Academy of Ophthalmology. November 7, 2022. www.aao.org/eye-health/tips-prevention/injuries-sports

37. Farrington T, Onambele-Pearson G, Taylor RL, Earl P, Winwood K. A review of facial protective equipment use in sport and the impact on injury incidence. *Br J Oral Maxillofac Surg.* 2012;50(3):233-238.

38. Prevent Blindness. Preventing eye injuries. Accessed October 9, 2022. https://preventblindness.org/recommended-sports-eye-protectors

39. Gilaberte Y, Trullàs C, Granger C, de Troya- Martín M. Photoprotection in outdoor sports: A review of the literature and recommendations to reduce risk among athletes. *Dermatol Ther (Heidelb).* 2022;12(2):329-343.

40. Shiels A, Hejtmancik JF. Biology of cataracts and opportunities for treatment. *Annu Rev Vis Sci.* 2019;5:123-149.

Chapter 12

1. Ball J, Dains J, Flynn J, Solomon BS, Stewart RW. *Seidel's Guide to Physical Examination: An Interprofessional Approach.* 10th ed. Elsevier; 2022.

2. Bickley L, Szilagyi P, Hoffman R. *Bates' Guide to Physical Examination and History-Taking.* 13th ed. Wolters Kluwer; 2021.

3. Jarvis C. *Physical Examination & Health Assessment.* 8th ed. Elsevier; 2019.

4. Domino F, Barry K, Baldor RA, Golding J, Stephens MB. *The 5-Minute Clinical Consult Premium 2022.* Wolters Kluwer; 2021.

5. Walling AD, Dickson G. Hearing loss in older adults. *Am Fam Physician.* 2012;85(12):1150-1156.

6. McDaid D, Park A-L, Chadha S. Estimating the global costs of hearing loss. *Int J Audiol.* 2021;60(3):162-170.

7. Lieu JE, Kenna M, Anne S, Davidson L. Hearing loss in children: A review. *JAMA.* 2020;324(21):2195-2205.

8. Perez-Carpena P, Lopez-Escamez JA. Current understanding and clinical management of Ménière's disease: A systematic review. *Semin Neurol.* 2020;40(1):138-150.

9. Ferri FF. *Ferri's Clinical Advisor 2022.* Elsevier; 2022.

10. Rosenfeld RM, Schwartz SR, Cannon CR, et al. Clinical practice guideline: Acute otitis externa. *Otolaryngol Head Neck Surg.* 2014;150(1 suppl):S1-S24.

11. Chhetri SS. Acute otitis media: A simple diagnosis, a simple treatment. *Nepal Med Coll J.* 2014;16(1):33-36.

12. Dinc AE, Damar M, Ugur MB, et al. Do the angle and length of the eustachian tube influence the development of chronic otitis media? *Laryngoscope.* 2015;125(9):2187-2192.

13. Esposito S, Bianchini S, Argentiero A, Gobbi R, Vicini C, Principi N. New approaches and technologies to improve accuracy of acute otitis media diagnosis. *Diagnostics (Basel).* 2021;11(12):2392.

14. Sangha K, Steinberg I, McCombs J. The impact of antibiotic treatment time and class of antibiotic for acute otitis media infections on the risk of revisits. *Value in Health.* 2019;22:S163.

15. Dolhi N, Weimer AD. Tympanic membrane perforations. In: *StatPearls.* StatPearls Publishing; 2021.

16. Zakaria M, Othman N, Lih AC. Is the degree of hearing loss truly dependent on the site of tympanic membrane perforation? *Oman Med J.* 2016;31(1):83-84.

17. Sur D, Plesa M. Treatment of allergic rhinitis. *Am Fam Physician.* 2015;92(11):985-992.

18. Settipane R, Kaliner M. Nonallergic rhinitis. *Am J Rhinol Allergy.* 2013; 27(suppl 1):S48-S51.

19. Agnihotri NT, McGrath KG. Allergic and nonallergic rhinitis. *Allergy Asthma Proc.* 2019;40(6):376-379.

20. Hansen MJ, Carson PJ, Leedahl DD, Leedahl ND. Failure of a best practice alert to reduce antibiotic prescribing rates for acute sinusitis across an integrated health system in the Midwest. *J Manag Care Spec Pharm.* 2018;24(2):154-159.

21. DeMuri GP, Gern JE, Moyer SC, Lindstrom MJ, Lynch SV, Wald ER. Clinical features, virus identification, and sinusitis as a complication of upper respiratory tract illness in children ages 4-7 years. *J Pediatr.* 2016;171:133-139.

22. Wang J, Dou X, Liu D, et al. Assessment of the effect of deviated nasal septum on the structure of nasal cavity. *Eur Arch Otorhinolaryngol.* 2016;273(6):1477-1480.

23. Andreeff R. Epistaxis. *JAAPA.* 2016;29(1):46-47.

24. Fox R, Nash R, Liu ZW, Singh A. Epistaxis management: Current understanding amongst junior doctors. *J Laryngol Otol.* 2016;130(3):252-255.

25. Boyali E, Patlar S, Ergin M, et al. The types of injury, regions and frequency in athletes participating universities taekwondo championship. *Turk J Sport Exerc.* 2019;21(1):52-57.

26. Hogrefe C. Facial trauma. In: *Sports-Related Fractures, Dislocations and Trauma.* Springer; 2020:753-802.

27. Liu J, Yan Z, Zhang M. [Clinical diagnosis and treatment of allergic pharyngitis]. *Lin Chung Er Bi Yan Hou Tou Jing Wai Ke Za Zhi.* 2015;29(15):1401-1405.

28. Sykes EA, Wu V, Beyea MM, Simpson MT, Beyea JA. Pharyngitis: Approach to diagnosis and treatment. *Can Fam Physician.* 2020;66(4):251-257.

29. Luo R, Sickler J, Vahidnia F, Lee Y-C, Frogner B, Thompson M. Diagnosis and management of group A streptococcal pharyngitis in the United States, 2011-2015. *BMC Infect Dis.* 2019;19(1):193.

30. Abati S, Bramati C, Bondi S, Lissoni A, Trimarchi M. Oral cancer and precancer: A narrative review on the relevance of early diagnosis. *Int J Environ Res Public Health.* 2020;17(24):9160.

31. American Cancer Society. Oral cavity and oropharyngeal cancer. 2016. Updated January 12, 2022. Accessed December 20, 2022. www.cancer.org/cancer/oralcavityandoropharyngealcancer/detailedguide/oral-cavity-and-oropharyngeal-cancer-key-statistics

32. Stoopler ET, Sollecito TP. Recurrent gingival and oral mucosal lesions. *JAMA.* 2014;312(17):1794-1795.

33. Kumar S. Evidence-based update on diagnosis and management of gingivitis and periodontitis. *Dent Clin North Am.* 2019;63(1):69-81.

34. Merle CL, Richter L, Challakh N, et al. Orofacial conditions and oral health behavior of young athletes: A comparison of amateur and competitive sports. *Scand J Med Sci Sports.* 2022;32(5):903-912.

35. Martonffy AI. Oral health: Prevention of dental disease. *FP Essent.* 2015;428:11-15.

Chapter 13

1. Centers for Disease Control and Prevention. Leading causes of death. Updated September 6, 2022. Accessed November 5, 2022. www.cdc.gov/nchs/fastats/leading-causes-of-death.htm

2. Centers for Disease Control and Prevention. United States Cancer Statistics. Updated May 29, 2018. Accessed November 2022. https://gis.cdc.gov/Cancer/USCS/#/Demographics/

3. Vinjamaram S. Non-Hodgkin lymphoma (NHL). Medscape. Updated August 3, 2021. Accessed December 8, 2022. http://emedicine.medscape.com/article/203399-overview

4. Papadakis MA, McPhee SJ, Rabow MW, McQuaid KR. *Current Diagnosis & Treatment.* 62nd ed. McGraw Hill; 2023.

5. Ferri FF. *Ferri's Clinical Advisor 2023*. Elsevier; 2023.

6. American Cancer Society. Cancer facts and statistics. 2022. Accessed November 10, 2022.www.cancer.org/research/cancerfactsstatistics/cancerfactsfigures

7. Lash BW. Hodgkin lymphoma. Medscape. Updated November 9, 2021. Accessed December 8, 2022. http://emedicine.medscape.com/article/201886-overview

8. Porter RE. *The Merck Manual of Diagnosis and Therapy*. 20th ed. Merck, Sharp & Dohme Corp; 2018.

9. American Cancer Society. Late and long-term side effects of Hodgkin lymphoma treatment. Updated May 1, 2018. Accessed December 9, 2022. www.cancer.org/cancer/hodgkin-lymphoma/after-treatment/lifestyle-changes.html

10. Seiter K. Acute lymphoblastic leukemia (ALL). Medscape. Updated July 2, 2021. Accessed December 10, 2022. https://emedicine.medscape.com/article/207631-overview

11. Seiter K. Acute myeloid leukemia (AML). Medscape. Updated December 6, 2022. Accessed December 10, 2022. https://emedicine.medscape.com/article/197802-overview

12. Christi MM. Chronic lymphocytic leukemia (CLL). Medscape. Updated November 10, 2022. Accessed December 10, 2022. https://emedicine.medscape.com/article/199313-overview

13. DuPrey KM. Lyme disease in athletes. *Curr Sports Med Rep*. 2015;14(1):51-55.

14. Kullberg BJ, Vrijmoeth HD, van de Schoor F, et al. Lyme borreliosis: Diagnosis and management. *BMJ*. 2020;369:m1041.

15. Wormser GP, Dattwyler RJ, Shapiro ED, et al. The clinical assessment, treatment, and prevention of Lyme disease, human granulocytic anaplasmosis, and babesiosis: Clinical practice guidelines by the Infectious Diseases Society of America. *Clin Infect Dis*. 2006;43(9):1089-1134.

16. Centers for Disease Control and Prevention. Division of Vector-Borne Diseases (DVBD). Updated February 11, 2022. Accessed Oct 20, 2022. www.cdc.gov/ncezid/dvbd/

17. Marques AR, Strle F, Wormser GP. Comparison of Lyme disease in the United States and Europe. *Emerg Infect Dis*. 2021;27(8):2017-2024.

18. Meyerhoff JO. Lyme disease. Medscape. Updated September 12, 2022. Accessed December 11, 2022.http://emedicine.medscape.com/article/330178-overview

19. Centers for Disease Control and Prevention. Lyme disease. Updated January 19, 2022. www.cdc.gov/lyme/index.html Accessed December 10, 2022.

20. Lantos PM, Rumbaugh J, Bockenstedt LK et al. Clinical Practice Guidelines by the Infectious Diseases Society of America, American Academy of Neurology, and American College of Rheumatology: 2020 guidelines for the prevention, diagnosis, and treatment of Lyme disease. *Neurology*. 2021;96(6):262-273.

21. Hansen-Dispenza H. Raynaud phenomenon. Medscape. Updated Aug 4, 2022. Accessed December 11. 2022. http://emedicine.medscape.com/article/331197-overview.

22. Centers for Disease Control and Prevention. Lupus. Updated July 1, 2020. Accessed December 11, 2022. www.cdc.gov/lupus/.

23. American College of Rheumatology. Lupus. Updated December 2021. Accessed December 11, 2022. www.rheumatology.org/I-Am-A/Patient-Caregiver/Diseases-Conditions/Lupus

24. Vleugels RA. Discoid lupus erythematosus. Medscape. Updated June 11, 2020. Accessed December 12, 2022. https://emedicine.medscape.com/article/1065529-overview

25. Kauffman CL. Drug-induced lupus erythematosus. Medscape. Updated June 22, 2020. Accessed December 12, 2022. https://emedicine.medscape.com/article/1065086-overview

26. Femia A. Neonatal and pediatric lupus erythematosus. Medscape. Updated May 17, 2021. Accessed December 12, 2022. https://emedicine.medscape.com/article/1006582-overview

27. Raghunath S, Guymer EK, Glikmann-Johnston Y, et al. Fibromyalgia, mood disorders, cognitive test results, cognitive symptoms and quality of life in systemic lupus erythematosus. *Rheumatology (Oxford)*. 2022;62(1):190-199.

28. Staud R. Are patients with systemic lupus erythematosus at increased risk for fibromyalgia? *Curr Rheumatol Rep*. 2006;8(6):430-435.

29. American College of Rheumatology. Fibromyalgia. Updated December 2021. Accessed December 27, 2022. www.rheumatology.org/I-Am-A/Patient-Caregiver/Diseases-Conditions/Fibromyalgia

30. Aringer M, Costenbader K, Daikh D, et al. 2019 European League Against Rheumatism/American College of Rheumatology classification criteria for systemic lupus erythematosus. *Arthritis Rheumatol*. 2019;71(9):1400-1412.

31. Bartels CM. Systemic lupus erythematosus (SLE), Medscape. Updated November 11, 2022. Accessed December 11, 2022.https://emedicine.medscape.com/article/332244-overview

32. Balsamo S, dos Santos-Neto L. Fatigue in systemic lupus erythematosus: An association with reduced physical fitness. *Autoimmun Rev*. 2011;10(9):514-518.

33. Mertz P, Schlencker A, Schneider M, et al. Towards a practical management of fatigue in systemic lupus erythematosus. *Lupus Sci Med*. 2020;7(1):e000441.

34. Boomershine CS. Fibromyalgia. Medscape. Updated September 14, 2021. Accessed December 12, 2022.https://emedicine.medscape.com/article/329838-overview

35. Jiao J, Vincent A, Cha SS, et al. Physical trauma and infection as precipitating factors in patients with fibromyalgia. Am J Phys Med Rehabil. 2015;94(12):1075-1082.

36. Bair MJ, Krebs EE. Fibromyalgia. *Ann Intern Med*. 2020;172(5):ITC33-ITC48.

37. Sumpton JE, Moulin DE. Fibromyalgia. *Handb Clin Neurol*. 2014;119:513-27.

38. Wolfe F, Clauw DJ, Fitzcharles MA, et al. The American College of Rheumatology preliminary diagnostic criteria for fibromyalgia and measurement of symptom severity. *Arthritis Care Res.* 2010;62(5):600-610.

39. Segura-Jiménez V, Álvarez -Gallardo IC, Estévez- López F, et al. Differences in sedentary time and physical activity between female patients with fibromyalgia and healthy controls: The Al-Ándalus Project. *Arthritis Rheumatol.* 2015;67(11):3047-3057.

40. Gavilán-Carrera B, Acosta-Manzano P, Soriano-Maldonado A, et al. Sedentary time, physical activity, and sleep duration: Associations with body composition in fibromyalgia. The Al-Ándalus Project. *J Clin Med.* 2019;8(8):1260.

41. Santos E, Campos MA, Párraga-Montilla JA, et al. Effects of a functional training program in patients with fibromyalgia: A 9-year prospective longitudinal cohort study. *Scand J Med Sci Sports.* 2020;30(5):904-913.

42. Roberts JR. Chronic fatigue syndrome (myalgic encephalomyelitis). Medscape. Updated September 6, 2020. Accessed December 27, 2022. https://emedicine.medscape.com/article/235980-overview

43. Centers for Disease Control and Prevention. Myalgic encephalomyelitis/chronic fatigue syndrome. Updated November 25, 2022. Accessed December 27, 2022.www.cdc.gov/me-cfs/

44. Institute of Medicine. Myalgic encephalomyelitis/chronic fatigue syndrome. Updated August 12, 2022. Accessed December 27, 2022. www.nih.gov/mecfs/about-mecfs

45. Centers for Disease Control and Prevention. Symptoms of ME/CFS. Updated January 27, 2021. Accessed January 27, 2022. www.cdc.gov/me-cfs/symptoms-diagnosis/symptoms.html

46. Leray E, Moreau T, Fromont A, et al. Epidemiology of multiple sclerosis. *Rev Neurol (Paris).* 2016;172(1):3-13.

47. Magyari M, Sorensen PS. The changing course of multiple sclerosis: Rising incidence, change in geographic distribution, disease course, and prognosis. *Curr Opin Neurol.* 2019;32(3):320-326.

48. National Multiple Sclerosis Society. Multiple sclerosis. 2020. Accessed December 28, 2022. www.nationalmssociety.org

49. Peterson S, Jalil A, Beard K, et al. Updates on efficacy and safety outcomes of new and emerging disease modifying therapies and stem cell therapy for multiple sclerosis: A review. *Mult Scler Relat Disord.* 2022;68:104125.

50. Luzzio C. Multiple sclerosis. Medscape. Updated January 3, 2022. Accessed December 28, 2022.https://emedicine.medscape.com/article/1146199-overview

51. Thompson AJ, Banwell BL, Barkhof F, et al. Diagnosis of multiple sclerosis: 2017 revisions of the McDonald criteria. *Lancet Neurol.* 2018; 17(2):162-173.

52. Andary MT. Guillain-Barré syndrome. Medscape. Updated January 14, 2022. Accessed December 28, 2022. https://emedicine.medscape.com/article/315632-overview

53. National Institute of Neurological Disorders and Stroke. Guillain-Barré syndrome. Updated July 25, 2022. Accessed December 28, 2022. www.ninds.nih.gov/health-information/disorders/guillain-barre-syndrome?search-term=Guillain

54. Bentley SA, Ahmad S, Kobeissy FH, Toklu HZ. Concomitant Guillain-Barré syndrome and COVID-19: A meta-analysis of cases. *Medicina (Kaunas).* 2022;58(12):1835.

55. Andary MT, Robert HM. Guillain Barre syndrome treatment and management. *Update Mayo.* 2018:1-9.

56. Rothschild BM. Gout and pseudogout. Medscape. Updated July 12, 2022. Accessed December 28, 2022. https://emedicine.medscape.com/article/329958-overview

57. McCormick N, Rai SK, Lu N, et al. Estimation of primary prevention of gout in men through modification of obesity and other key lifestyle factors. *JAMA Netw Open.* 2020;3(11):e2027421.

58. Smith HR. Rheumatoid arthritis (RA). Medscape. Updated January 31, 2022. Accessed December 29, 2022. https://emedicine.medscape.com/article/331715-overview

59. Firestein GS, Budd RC, Gabriel SE, Koretzky GA, McInnes IB, O'Dell JR. *Firestein & Kelly's Textbook of Rheumatology.* 11th ed. Elsevier; 2021.

60. Lozada CJ. Osteoarthritis. Medscape. Updated November 30, 2022. Accessed December 28, 2022. https://emedicine.medscape.com/article/330487-overview

61. Llewellyn A, Jones-Diette J, Kraft J, et al. Imaging tests for the detection of osteomyelitis: A systematic review. *Health Technol Assess.* 2019;23(61):1-128.

62. Gandhi J. Osteomyelitis. Medscape. Updated July 11, 2022. Accessed December 29, 2022. https://emedicine.medscape.com/article/1348767-overview#a1

63. Femia A. Dermatomysotis. Medscape. Updated July 21, 2022. Accessed December 29, 2022. https://emedicine.medscape.com/article/332783-overview

64. Seetharaman M. Polymyositis. Medscape. Updated December 21, 2022. Accessed December 29, 2022. https://emedicine.medscape.com/article/335925-overview

65. Chohan S, Chohan A. Recurrence of a rare subtype of Guillain-Barré syndrome following a second dose of the shingles vaccine. *Cureus.* 2022;14(10):e30717.

66. Principi N, Esposito S. Do vaccines have a role as a cause of autoimmune neurological syndromes? *Front Public Health.* 2020;8:361.

67. Toussirot É, Bereau M. Vaccination and induction of autoimmune diseases. *Inflamm Allergy Drug Targets.* 2015;14(2):94-98.

68. Schwartz AM, Kugeler KJ, Nelson CA, Marx GE, Hinckley AF. Use of commercial claims data for evaluating trends in Lyme disease diagnoses, United States, 2010-2018. *Emerg Infect Dis.* 2021;27(2):499-507.

69. Lister TA, Crowther D, Sutcliffe SB, et al. Report of a committee convened to discuss the evaluation and staging of patients with Hodgkin's disease: Cotswolds meeting. *J Clin Oncol.* 1989;7:1630.

70. Cheson BD, Fisher RI, Barrington SF, et al. Recommendations for initial evaluation, staging, and response assessment of Hodgkin and non-Hodgkin lymphoma: the Lugano classification. *J Clin Oncol.* 2014;32:3059.

Chapter 14

1. Parsons JT. *2014-15 NCAA Sports Medicine Handbook.* 25th ed. National Collegiate Athletics Association; 2014.

2. U.S. Department of Labor. Regulations Standard 29 CFR: Bloodborne pathogens. Updated May 14, 2019. Accessed October 21, 2022. www.osha.gov/laws-regs/regulations/standardnumber/1910/1910.1030

3. U.S. Department of Labor. A-Z Index. 2022. Accessed October 31, 2022. www.osha.gov/a-z

4. National Federation of State High School Associations. General guidelines for sport hygiene, skin infections and communicable diseases. Updated January 2022. Accessed October 31, 2022. www.nfhs.org/media/5546438/2022-nfhs-general-guidelines-for-sports-hygiene-skin-infections-and-communicable-diseases-final-3-8-22.pdf

5. U.S. Environmental Protection Agency. Selected EPA-registered disinfectants. Updated October 17, 2022. Accessed October 31, 2022. www.epa.gov/pesticide-registration/selected-epa-registered-disinfectants

6. U.S. Department of Labor. Bloodborne pathogen and needlestick prevention. 2022. Accessed October 31, 2022. www.osha.gov/SLTC/bloodbornepathogens/bloodborne_quickref.html

7. Porter RE, ed. *The Merck Manual of Diagnosis and Therapy.* 20th ed. Merck, Sharp & Dohme Corp; 2018.

8. Centers for Disease Control and Prevention. Adult immunization schedule. Updated February 17, 2022. Accessed October 21, 2022. www.cdc.gov/vaccines/schedules/hcp/imz/adult.html

9. Centers for Disease Control and Prevention. Child and Adolescent Immunization Schedule. Updated February 17, 2022. Accessed October 21, 2022. www.cdc.gov/vaccines/schedules/hcp/imz/child-adolescent.html

10. Chen RT, Clark TA, Halperin SA. The yin and yang of paracetamol and paediatric immunizations. *Lancet* 2009;374(9698):1305-1306.

11. Office of Disease Prevention and Health Promotion. Healthy People 2030. Updated October 17, 2022. Accessed October 21, 2022. https://health.gov/healthypeople

12. Huang AS, Cortese MM, Curns AT, et al. Risk factors for mumps at a university with a large mumps outbreak. *Public Health Rep.* 2009;124(3):416-426.

13. Commission on Accreditation of Athletic Training Programs. 2020 Standards. Pages 15-74. Updated June 2022. Accessed October 21, 2022. https://caate.net/Portals/0/Documents/Standards%20and%20Procedures%20for%20Accreditation%20of%20Professional%20Programs%20Updated%209.6.2022.pdf?ver=IHxl9QQJspd34B-DTRbF_mQ%3d%3d

14. Shafer A, Atkinson W, Friedman C, et al. Advisory Committee on Immunization Practices; Centers for Disease Control and Prevention (CDC). Immunization of health care personnel: Recommendations of the Advisory Committee on Immunization Practices (ACIP). *MMWR Recomm Rep.* 2011;60(RR-7):1-45.

15. Aaron D, Nagu TJ, Rwegasha J, Komba E. Hepatitis B vaccination coverage among healthcare workers in Tanzania: How much, who and why? *BMC Infect Dis.* 2017;17(1):786.

16. Malik S, Das RS, Khan T, Anto AG, Rajagopal L, Das Bhattacharya S. Building the evidence for hepatitis B vaccination programs for students and researchers working with biological samples in Indian institutes of higher education. *Hum Vaccin Immunother.* 2021;17(12):5595-5602.

17. Centers for Disease Control and Prevention. Influenza (flu). Updated October 13, 2022. Accessed October 21, 2022. www.cdc.gov/flu/index.htm

18. Grohskopf LA, Blanton LH, Ferdinands JM, et al. Prevention and control of seasonal influenza with vaccines: Recommendations of the Advisory Committee on Immunization Practices—United States, 2022-2023. *MMWR Recomm Rep.* 2022;71(1):1-28.

19. Howe W. Preventing infectious disease in sports. *Phys Sportsmed.* 2003;31(2):23-29.

20. Lam W, Dawson A, Fowler C. Health promotion intervention to prevent early childhood human influenza at the household level: A realist review to identify implications for programmes in Hong Kong. *J Clin Nurs.* 2015;24(7-8):891-905.

21. U.S. National Library of Medicine. Reportable diseases. 2022. Accessed June 8, 2022. https://medlineplus.gov/ency/article/001929.htm

22. Centers for Disease Control and Prevention. National Notifiable Diseases Surveillance System (NNSAA). Updated September 12, 2022. Accessed October 22, 2022. www.cdc.gov/nndss/index.html

23. Kelly H. The classical definition of a pandemic is not elusive. *Bull World Health Org.* 2011;89:540-541.

24. Johns Hopkins Medicine. Severe acute respiratory syndrome (SARS). 2022. Accessed October 23, 2022. www.hopkinsmedicine.org/health/conditions-and-diseases/severe-acute-respiratory-syndrome-sars

25. Liu C. Research and development on therapeutic agents and vaccines for COVID-19 and related human coronavirus disease. *ACS Cent Sci.* 2020;6(3):315-331.

26. Samavati L, Uhal BD. ACE2, much more than just a receptor for SARS-COV-2. *Front Cell Infect Microbiol.* 2020;10:317.

27. Johns Hopkins Medicine. Coronavirus Resource Center. Updated 2022. Accessed October 22, 2022. https://coronavirus.jhu.edu/map.html

28. Cutler J, Schleihauf E, Hatchette TF, et al. Investigation of the first cases of human-to-human infection with the new swine-origin influenza A (H1N1) virus in Canada. *CMAJ.* 2009;4(181):159-163.

29. Shetty K. Epstein-Barr virus (EBV) infectious mono-nucleosis (mono). Medscape. Updated April 21, 2021. Accessed October 22, 2022. https://emedicine.medscape.com/article/222040-overview

30. Omari MS. Infectious mononucleosis (IM) in emergency medicine. Medscape. Updated May 24, 2019. Accessed October 20, 2022. https://emedicine.medscape.com/article/784513-workup#c7

31. Ferri FF. *Ferri's Clinical Advisor 2023*. Elsevier; 2023.

32. Becker JA, Smith JA. Return to play after infectious mononucleosis. *Sports Health*. 2014;6(3):232-238.

33. O'Connor TE, Skinner LJ, Kiely P, Fenton JE. Return to contact sports following infectious mononucleosis: The role of serial ultrasonography. *Ear Nose Throat J*. 2011;8:E21-E24.

34. Camacho C. Acute mumps. Updated April 29, 2019. Accessed October 20, 2022. http://emedicine.medscape.com/article/784603-overview

35. Centers for Disease Control and Prevention. Measles history. Updated November 5, 2020. Accessed October 23, 2022. www.cdc.gov/measles/about/history.html

36. Chen S. Measles. Medscape. Updated June 6, 2019. Accessed October 21, 2022. http://emedicine.medscape.com/article/966220-overview

37. World Health Organization. Rubella. Updated October 4, 2019. Accessed October 25, 2022. www.who.int/media-centre/factsheets/fs367/en/

38. Centers for Disease Control and Prevention. Measles, mumps, rubella, varicella vaccines. Updated September 9, 2020. Accessed September 9, 2022. www.cdc.gov/vaccinesafety/vaccines/mmrv-vaccine.html

39. Ezike E. Pediatric rubella. Medscape. Updated April 18, 2022. Accessed October 25, 2022.http://emedicine.medscape.com/article/968523-overview

40. Mayo Clinic. Rubella. Updated 2021. Accessed October 23, 2022. www.mayoclinic.org/diseases-conditions/rubella/basics/definition/con-20020067

41. Anderson WE. Varicella-zoster virus (VZV). Medscape. Updated September 20, 2022. Accessed October 25, 2022. http://emedicine.medscape.com/article/231927-overview

42. Agel J, Ransone J, Dick R, Oppliger R, Marshall SW. Descriptive epidemiology of collegiate men's wrestling injuries: National Collegiate Athletics Association injury surveillance system, 1988-1989 through 2003-2004. *J Athl Train*. 2007;42(2):303-310.

43. National Federation of State High School Associations. NFHS Medical Release Form for Wrestlers to Participate with Skin Lesion(s): State Medical Advisory Committee (SMAC). Updated April 2022. Accessed October 25, 2022. www.nfhs.org/media/882323/2022-23-nfhs-wrestling-skin-lesion-form-final-april-2022.pdf

44. Khan ZZ. Varicella-zoster virus (VZV) medication. Medscape. Updated September 30, 2022. Accessed October 25, 2022. https://emedicine.medscape.com/article/231927-medication#3

45. Bonanni P, Breuer J, Gershon A, et al. Varicella vaccination in Europe—Taking the practical approach. *BMC Med*. 2009;28(7):26.

46. Centers for Disease Control and Prevention. 2020 Viral Hepatitis Surveillance Report. Updated August 18, 2022. Accessed October 25, 2022. www.cdc.gov/hepatitis/statistics/2020surveillance/index.htm

47. Samji NS. Viral hepatitis. Medscape. Updated June 12, 2017. Accessed October 26, 2022. http://emedicine.medscape.com/article/775507-overview

48. Anish EJ. Viral hepatitis: Sports-related risk. *Curr Sports Med Rep*. 2004;3(2):100-106.

49. Buxton BP, Daniell JE, Buxton BH, Okasaki EM, Ho KW. Prevention of hepatitis B virus in athletic training. *J Athl Train*. 1994;29(2):107-112.

50. Gilroy RA. Hepatitis A. Medscape. Updated May 8, 2019. Accessed October 26, 2022. http://emedicine.medscape.com/article/177484-overview

51. Pyrsopoulos NT. Hepatitis B. Medscape. Updated October 5, 2022. Accessed October 25, 2022. http://emedicine.medscape.com/article/177632-overview

52. Tobe K, Matsuura K, Ogura T, et al. Horizontal transmission of hepatitis B virus among players of an American football team. *Arch Intern Med*. 2000;160:2541-2545.

53. Kashiwagi S, Hayashi J, Ikematsu H, Nishigori S, Ishihara K, Kaji M. An outbreak of hepatitis B in members of a high school sumo wrestling club. *JAMA*. 1982;9(248):3213-3214.

54. Dhawan VK. Hepatis C. Medscape. Updated October 7, 2019. Accessed October 25, 2022. https://emedicine.medscape.com/article/177792-overview

55. Roy PK. Hepatitis D. Medscape. Updated October 20, 2021. Accessed October 21, 2022. http://emedicine.medscape.com/article/178038-overview

56. Khan ZZ. Group A streptococcal infections. Medscape. Updated April 8, 2021. Accessed October 21, 2022. http://emedicine.medscape.com/article/228936-overview

57. Venkataraman R. Toxic shock syndrome. Medscape. Updated October 8, 2020. Accessed October 25, 2022. http://emedicine.medscape.com/article/169177-overview

58. Schulz SA. Necrotizing fasciitis. Medscape. Updated October 12, 2022. Accessed October 22, 2022. https://emedicine.medscape.com/article/2051157-overview

59. Woods CJ. Group B streptococcus (GBS) infections. Medscape. Updated April 21, 2021. Accessed October 25, 2022. http://emedicine.medscape.com/article/229091-overview

60. Mazumder SA. Group D streptococcus (GDS) infections (Streptococcus bovis/Streptococcus gallolyticus). Medscape. Updated March 2, 2021. Accessed October 25, 2022. http://emedicine.medscape.com/article/229209-overview

61. Herchline TE. Staphylococcal infections. Medscape. Updated March 9, 2022. Accessed October 22, 2022. http://emedicine.medscape.com/article/228816-overview

62. Perloff SA. MRSA skin infection in athletes. Medscape. Updated June 23, 2022. Accessed October 23, 2022. http://emedicine.medscape.com/article/108972-overview

63. Kourtis AP, Hatfield K, Baggs J, et al. Vital signs: Epidemiology and recent trends in methicillin-resistant and in methicillin-susceptible Staphylococcus aureus bloodstream infections—United States. *MMWR Morb Mortal Wkly Rep*. 2019;68(9):214-219.

64. Baorto EP. Staphylococcus aureus infection. Medscape. Updated July 27, 2021. Accessed November 2, 2022. https://emedicine.medscape.com/article/971358-overview

65. Rogers S. A practical approach to preventing CA-MRSA infections in the athletic training setting. *Athl Ther Today*. 2008;13(4):35-38.

66. Centers for Disease Control and Prevention. Methicillin-resistant Staphylococcus aureus (MRSA) infections. Updated June 26, 2019. Accessed October 25, 2022. www.cdc.gov/mrsa/community/index.html#anchor_1548173148

67. Howes DS. Encephalitis. Medscape. Updated August 7, 2018. Accessed October 25, 2022. http://emedicine.medscape.com/article/791896-overview

68. Soto RA, Hughes ML, Staples E, Lindsey NP. West Nile virus and other domestic notifiable arboviral diseases—United States May 6, 2022. *MMWR Morb Mortal Wkly Rep*. 2022;71(18):628-632.

69. Anderson A. Arthropod pests and the diseases they carry: Prevention in the community and athletic setting. *Athl Ther Today*. 2004;9(3):16-21.

70. Salinas JD. West Nile virus. Medscape. Updated March 31, 2021. Accessed October 21, 2022. http://emedicine.medscape.com/article/312210-overview

71. Centers for Disease Control and Prevention. Division of Vector-Borne Diseases (DVBD). Updated February 11, 2022. Accessed October 20, 2022. www.cdc.gov/ncezid/dvbd/

72. U.S. Environmental Protection Agency. Tips to prevent mosquito bites. Updated July 18, 2022. Accessed October 23, 2022. www.epa.gov/insect-repellents/tips-prevent-mosquito-bites

73. Navalkele BD. Zika virus. Medscape. Updated June 20, 2021. Accessed October 27, 2022. http://emedicine.medscape.com/article/2500035-overview

74. Centers for Disease Control and Prevention. Zika and pregnancy. Updated March 17, 2022. Accessed October 27, 2022. www.cdc.gov/pregnancy/zika/data/index.html

75. Centers for Disease Control and Prevention. Zika virus. Updated December 22, 2021. Accessed October 27, 2022. www.cdc.gov/zika/reporting/index.html

76. Hennessey M, Fischer M, Staples JE. 2016. Zika virus spreads to new areas—region of the Americas May 2015–January 2016. *MMWR Morb Mortal Wkly Rep*. 2016;65(3):55-58.

77. Splete H. Vaccine candidate shows promise in phase 1 trial. Medscape. Updated February 19, 2021. Accessed October 27, 2022. www.medscape.com/viewarticle/946141

78. Croker C, Civen R, Keough K, Ngo V, Narutani A, Schwartz B. Notes from the field: Aseptic meningitis outbreak associated with echovirus 30 among high school football players — Los Angeles County, California, 2014. *MMWR Morb Mortal Wkly Rep*. 2015;63(51):1228.

79. Alexander JP Jr, Chapman LE, Pallansch MA, Stephenson WT, Torok TJ, Anderson LT. Coxsackievirus B2 infection and aseptic meningitis: A focal outbreak among members of a high school football team. *J Infect Dis*. 1993;167(5):1201-1205.

80. Begier EM, Oberste MS, Landry ML, et al. An outbreak of concurrent echovirus 30 and coxsackievirus A1 infections associated with sea swimming among a group of travelers to Mexico. *Clin Infect Dis*. 2008;47(5):616-623.

81. Wan C. Viral meningitis. Medscape.. Updated July 17, 2018. Accessed October 27, 2022. http://emedicine.medscape.com/article/1168529-overview

82. Vasudeva SS. Meningitis. Medscape.. Updated July 11, 2022. Accessed November 3, 2022. https://emedicine.medscape.com/article/232915-overview

83. World Health Organization. Meningococcal meningitis. Updated September 2021. Accessed October 23, 2022. www.who.int/mediacentre/factsheets/fs141/en/

84. Gondim F. Meningococcal meningitis. Medscape. Updated July 16, 2018. Accessed October 27, 2022. http://emedicine.medscape.com/article/1165557-overview

85. Centers for Disease Control and Prevention. Bacterial meningitis. Updated July 15, 2021. Accessed October 27, 2022. www.cdc.gov/meningitis/bacterial.html

86. Davies HD, Jackson MA, Rice SG; Committee on Infectious Diseases; Council on Sports Medicine and Fitness. Infectious diseases associated with organized sports and outbreak control. *Pediatrics*. 2017;140(4):e20172477.

87. Centers for Disease Control and Prevention. Influenza (flu): 2022-2023 preliminary in-season burden estimate. Accessed May 25, 2022. www.cdc.gov/flu/about/burden/preliminary-in-season-estimates.htm

88. Centers for Disease Control and Prevention. Influenza (flu): 2021-22 flu burden prevented by vaccination. Accessed May 28, 2022. www.cdc.gov/flu/about/burden-averted/2021-2022.htm

89. Clark DP, Pazdernik NJ. Biological warfare: Infectious disease and bioterrorism. *Biotechnology*. 2016:687-719.

90. Mak LY, Beasley I, Kennedy PTF. Chronic viral hepatitis in athletes: An overlooked population? *Br J Sports Med*. 2023;57(2):72-74.

Chapter 15

1. Lee PJ, Papachristou GI. New insights into acute pancreatitis. *Nat Rev Gastroenterol Heptaol*. 2019;16(8):479-496.

2. Sekimoto M, Takada T, Kawarada Y, et al. JPN Guidelines for the management of acute pancreatitis: Epidemiology, etiology, natural history, and outcome predictors in acute pancreatitis. *J Hepatobiliary Pancreat Surg*. 2006;13(1):10-24.

3. Ferri FF. *Ferri's Clinical Advisor 2023*. Elsevier; 2023.

4. Tang JC. Acute pancreatitis. Medscape. 2021. Accessed November 30, 2022. http://emedicine.medscape.com/article/181364-overview

5. Safizadeh Shabestari SA, Ho SB, Chaudhary P, et al. Drug-induced acute pancreatitis in a bodybuilder: A case report. *J Med Case Rep*. 2022;16(1):114.

6. Kumar V, Issa D, Smallfield G, et al. Acute pancreatitis secondary to the use of the anabolic steroid trenbolone acetate. *Clin Toxicol.* 2019;57(1):60-62.

7. Liane B-J, Magee C. Guerilla warfare on the pancreas? A case of acute pancreatitis from a supplement known to contain anabolic-androgenic steroids. *Mil Med.* 2016;181(10):e1395-e1397.

8. Binet Q, Dufour I, Agneessens E, et al. The second case of a young man with L-arginine-induced acute pancreatitis. *Clin J Gastroenterol.* 2018;11(5):424-427.

9. Papadakis MA, McPhee SJ, Rabow MW, McQuaid KR. *Current Diagnosis & Treatment.* 62nd ed. McGraw Hill; 2023.

10. Noel RA, Braun DK, Patterson RE, et al. Increased risk of acute pancreatitis and biliary disease observed in patients with type 2 diabetes: A retrospective cohort study. *Diabetes Care.* 2009;32(5):834-38.

11. Centers for Disease Control and Prevention. *National Diabetes Statistics Report.* Updated June 29, 2022. Accessed November 30, 2022. www.cdc.gov/diabetes/data/statistics-report/index.html 2022.

12. Centers for Disease Control and Prevention. Leading causes of death. Updated September 6, 2022. Accessed November 5, 2022. www.cdc.gov/nchs/fastats/leading-causes-of-death.htm

13. Porter RE. *The Merck Manual of Diagnosis and Therapy.* 20th ed. Merck, Sharp & Dohme Corp; 2018.

14. Khardori R. Type 1 diabetes mellitus. Medscape. Updated November 21, 2022. Accessed November 30, 2022. http://emedicine.medscape.com/article/117739-overview

15. Smeeks FC. Acute hypoglycemia. Medscape. Updated September 9, 2020. Accessed November 30, 2022. https://emedicine.medscape.com/article/767359-overview

16. Hamby O. Diabetic ketoacidosis (DKA). Medscape. 2021. Accessed December 1, 2022. https://emedicine.medscape.com/article/118361-overview

17. American Diabetes Association Professional Practice Committee. Diabetes technology: Standards of medical care in diabetes—2020. *Diabetes Care.* 2020;45:S77-S88.

18. American Diabetes Association. Understanding A1c diagnosis. 2022. Accessed November 30, 2022. https://diabetes.org/diabetes/a1c/diagnosis?loc=db-slabnav

19. Goyal A, Gupta Y, Singla R, et al. American Diabetes Association "Standards of Medical Care—2020 for Gestational Diabetes Mellitus": A critical appraisal. *Diabetes Ther.* 2020;11(8):1639-44.

20. Colberg SR, Sigal RJ, Yardley JE, et al. Physical activity/exercise and diabetes: A position statement of the American Diabetes Association. *Diabetes Care.* 2016;39(11):2065-2079.

21. Hamby O. Hypoglycemia. Medscape. Updated August 23, 2021. Accessed November 30, 2022. https://emedicine.medscape.com/article/122122-overview

22. Wolfson TS, Hamula MJ, Jazrawi LM. Impact of diabetes mellitus on surgical outcomes in sports medicine. *Phys Sportsmed.* 2013;41(4):64-77.

23. Yardley JE, Colberg SR. Update on management of type 1 diabetes and type 2 diabetes in athletes. *Curr Sports Med Rep.* 2017;16(1):38-44.

24. Harris GD, White RD. Diabetes in the competitive athlete. *Curr Sports Med Rep.* 2012;11(6):309-315.

25. Cheadle C. Supporting student-athletes with type 1 diabetes. National Collegiate Athletics Association. 2022. Accessed December 1, 2022. www.ncaa.org/sports/2015/3/17/supporting-student-athletes-with-type-1-diabetes.aspx

26. Arima H, Cheetham T, Christ-Crain M, et al. Changing the name of diabetes insipidus: A position statement of the working group to consider renaming diabetes insipidus. *Arch Endocrinol Metab.* 2022;66:868-870.

27. Kim SM. Insulin pumps. Medscape. Updated January 31, 2018. Accessed December 1, 2022. https://emedicine.medscape.com/article/2139073-overview

28. Palermi S, Serio A, Vecchiato M, et al. Potential role of an athlete-focused echocardiogram in sports eligibility. *World J Cardiol,* 2021;13(8):271-297.

29. Khardori R. Type 2 diabetes mellitus. Medscape. Updated May 31, 2022. Accessed November 30, 2022. https://emedicine.medscape.com/article/117853-overview

30. Lee SL. Hyperthyroidism and thyrotoxicosis. Medscape. Updated February 8, 2022. Accessed December 1, 2022. http://emedicine.medscape.com/article/121865-overview

31. Kitahara CM, Sosa JA. Understanding the ever-changing incidence of thyroid cancer. *Nat Rev Endocrinol.* 2020;16(11):617-618.

32. Sharma PK. Thyroid cancer. Medscape. Updated August 17, 2022. Accessed December 1, 2022. https://emedicine.medscape.com/article/851968-overview#a2 2022

33. Orlander PR. Hypothyroidism. Medscape. Updated May 25, 2022. Accessed December 1, 2022. http://emedicine.medscape.com/article/122393-overview

Chapter 16

1. Ashack KA, Burton KA, Johnson TR, et al. Skin infections among US high school athletes: A national survey. *J Am Acad Dermatol.* 2016;74(4):679-684.

2. Wong HK. Acute urticaria. Medscape. Updated March 21, 2018. Accessed November 10, 2022. http://emedicine.medscape.com/article/137362-overview

3. Ferri FF. *Ferri's Clinical Advisor 2023.* Elsevier; 2023.

4. Laube S. Dermographism urticaria. Medscape. Updated June 11, 2018. Accessed November 12, 2022. http://emedicine.medscape.com/article/1050294-overview.

5. Schwartz RA. Cholinergic urticaria. Medscape. Updated June 6, 2022. Accessed November 11, 2022. http://emedicine.medscape.com/article/1049978-overview

6. Porter RE. *The Merck Manual of Diagnosis and Therapy.* 20th ed. Merck, Sharp & Dohme Corp; 2018.

7. Maltseva N, Borzova E, Fomina D, et al. Cold urticaria—What we know and what we do not know. *Allergy.* 2021;76(4):1077-1094.

8. Handler MZ. Solar urticaria. Medscape. Updated April 11, 2022. Accessed November 9, 2022. http://emedicine.medscape.com/article/1050485-overview

9. American Academy of Dermatology. Types of skin cancer. 2022. Accessed November 11, 2022. www.aad.org/public/spot-skin-cancer/learn-about-skin-cancer/types-of-skin-cancer

10. Fromm LJ. Epidermal inclusion cyst. Medscape. Updated September 17, 2020. Accessed November 9, 2022. http://emedicine.medscape.com/article/1061582-overview

11. Koyfman A. Pilonidal cyst and sinus. Medscape. Updated August 9, 2022. Accessed November 12, 2022. https://emedicine.medscape.com/article/788127-overview

12. Stevens DL, Bisno AL, Chambers HF, et al. Practice guidelines for the diagnosis and management of skin and soft tissue infections: 2014 update by the Infectious Diseases Society of America. *Clin Infect Dis.* 2014;59(2):e10-e52.

13. Sartelli M, Guirao X, Hardcastle TC, et al. 2018 WSES/SIS-E consensus conference: Recommendations for the management of skin and soft-tissue infections. *World J Emerg Surg.* 2018;13(1):1-24.

14. Bradby C. Atopic dermatitis in emergency medicine. Medscape. Updated April 26, 2021. Accessed November 10, 2022. http://emedicine.medscape.com/article/762045-overview

15. Anderson CK. Asteatotic eczema. Medscape. Updated November 6, 2020. Accessed November 12, 2022. https://emedicine.medscape.com/article/1124528-overview

16. Habashy J. Psoriasis. Medscape. Updated September 14, 2022. Accessed November 11, 2022. http://emedicine.medscape.com/article/1943419-overview

17. Hammadi AA. Psoriatic arthritis. Medscape. Updated January 24, 2022. Accessed November 11, 2022. http://emedicine.medscape.com/article/2196539-overview

18. Menter A, Gelfand JM, Connor C, et al. Joint American Academy of Dermatology–National Psoriasis Foundation guidelines of care for the management of psoriasis with systemic nonbiologic therapies. *J Am Acad Dermatol.* 2020;82(6):1445-1486.

19. American Academy of Dermatology. Skin cancer incidence rates. Updated April 4, 2022. Accessed November 11, 2022. www.aad.org/media/stats/conditions/skin-cancer

20. American Cancer Society. Cancer Facts and Statistics. Updated 2022. Accessed November 10, 2022. www.cancer.org/research/cancerfactsstatistics/cancerfactsfigures

21. Wysong A, Gladstone H, Kim D, et al. Sunscreen use in NCAA collegiate athletes: Identifying targets for intervention and barriers to use. *Prev Med.* 2012;55(5):493-496.

22. Parsons JT. *2014-15 NCAA Sports Medicine Handbook.* 25th ed. National Collegiate Athletics Association; 2014.

23. John SM, Trakatelli M, Gehring R, et al. Consensus Report: Recognizing non-melanoma skin cancer, including actinic keratosis, as an occupational disease—a call to action. *J Eur Acad Dermatol Venereol.* 2016;30:38-45.

24. Bader RS. Basal cell carcinoma. Medscape. Updated February 14, 2022. Accessed November 10, 2022. http://emedicine.medscape.com/article/276624-overview

25. American Cancer Society. Key statistics for basal and squamous cell skin cancers. Updated January 12, 2022. Accessed November 11, 2022. www.cancer.org/cancer/skincancer-basalandsquamouscell/detailedguide/skin-cancer-basal-and-squamous-cell-key-statistics

26. Wells JW. Cutaneous squamous cell carcinoma. Medscape. Updated September 24, 2021. Accessed November 12, 2022. http://emedicine.medscape.com/article/1965430-overview.

27. Skin Cancer Foundation. Mohs surgery. 2022. Accessed November 10, 2022. www.skincancer.org/treatment-resources/mohs-surgery

28. American Cancer Society. Key statistics for melanoma skin cancer. Updated January 11, 2022. Accessed November 11, 2022. www.cancer.org/cancer/skincancer-melanoma/detailedguide/melanoma-skin-cancer-key-statistics

29. De La Garza H, Maymone MB, Vashi NA. Impact of social media on skin cancer prevention. *Int J Environ Res Public Health.* 2021;18(9):5002.

30. Najmi M, Brown AE, Harrington SR, et al. A systematic review and synthesis of qualitative and quantitative studies evaluating provider, patient, and health care system-related barriers to diagnostic skin cancer examinations. *Arch Dermatol Res.* 2022;314(4):329-340.

31. Culp MB, Benard V, Dowling NF, et al. Ocular melanoma incidence rates and trends in the United States, 2001-2016. *Eye.* 2021;35(2):687-689.

32. American Academy of Dermatology. What to look for: ABCDEs of melanoma. 2022. Accessed May 25, 2022. www.aad.org/public/diseases/skin-cancer/find/at-risk/abcdes

33. Tan WW. Malignant melanoma. Medscape. Updated June 10, 2022. Accessed November 11, 2022. http://emedicine.medscape.com/article/280245-overview

34. Tan WW. Malignant melanoma staging. Medscape. Updated March 23, 2022. Accessed November 12, 2022. http://emedicine.medscape.com/article/2007147-overview.

35. Papadakis MA, McPhee SJ, Rabow MW, McQuaid KR. *Current Diagnosis & Treatment.* 62nd ed. McGraw Hill; 2023.

36. Castellani JW, Young AJ, Ducharme MB, et al. American College of Sports Medicine position stand: Prevention of cold injuries during exercise. *Med Sci Sports Exerc.* 2006;38(11):2012-2029.

37. Hulme S. Emergent management of frostbite. Medscape. Updated June 22, 2021. Accessed November 11, 2022. http://emedicine.medscape.com/article/770296-overview

38. Zonnoor B. Frostbite. Medscape. Updated October 13, 2020. Accessed November 12, 2022. http://emedicine.medscape.com/article/926249-overview

39. Cappaert TA, Stone JA, Castellani JW, et al. National Athletic Trainers' Association position statement: Environmental cold injuries. *J Athl Train*. 2008;43(6):640-658.

40. National Collegiate Athletics Association. Wrestling Skin Evaluation and Participation Status Form. 2022. Accessed November 12, 2022. https://ncaaorg.s3.amazonaws.com/championships/sports/wrestling/rules/RulesMWR_SkinEvalPartStatForm.pdf

41. National Federation of State High School Associations. General guidelines for sport hygiene, skin infections and communicable diseases. Updated January 2022. Accessed October 31, 2022. www.nfhs.org/media/5546438/2022-nfhs-general-guidelines-for-sports-hygiene-skin-infections-and-communicable-diseases-final-3-8-22.pdf

42. National Federation of State High School Associations. NFHS Medical Release Form for Wrestlers to Participate with Skin Lesion(s): State Medical Advisory Committee (SMAC). Updated April 2022. Accessed October 25, 2022. www.nfhs.org/media/882323/2022-23-nfhs-wrestling-skin-lesion-form-final-april-2022.pdf

43. Powell JR, Boltz AJ, Robison HJ, et al. Epidemiology of injuries in National Collegiate Athletic Association men's wrestling: 2014-2015 through 2018-2019. *J Athl Train*. 2021;56(7):727-733.

44. Lewis LS. Impetigo. Medscape. Updated September 24, 2019. Accessed November 9, 2022. http://emedicine.medscape.com/article/965254-overview

45. Williams C, Wells J, Klein R, Sylvester T, Sunenshine R; Centers for Disease Control and Prevention (CDC). Notes from the field: Outbreak of skin lesions among high school wrestlers—Arizona, 2014. *MMWR Morb Mortal Wkly Rep*. 2015;64(20):559-560.

46. Zinder SM, Basler RS, Foley J, et al. National Athletic Trainers' Association position statement: Skin diseases. *J Athl Train*. 2010;45(4):411-428.

47. Peterson AR, Nash E, Anderson B. Infectious disease in contact sports. *Sports Health*. 2019;11(1):47-58.

48. Satter EK. Folliculitis. Medscape. 2020 Updated October 8, 2020. Accessed November 12, 2022. https://emedicine.medscape.com/article/1070456-overview

49. National Athletic Trainers Association. Official statement from the National Athletic Trainers' Association on communicable and infectious diseases in secondary school sports. 2007. Accessed November 12, 2022. www.nata.org/sites/default/files/CommunicableInfectiousDiseases-SecondarySchoolSports.pdf

50. Perloff SA. MRSA skin infections in athletes. Medscape. Updated June 23, 2022. Accessed November 12, 2022. http://emedicine.medscape.com/article/108972-overview

51. Rogers S. A practical approach to preventing CA-MRSA infections in the athletic training setting. *Athl Ther Today*. 2008;13(4):35-38.

52. National Athletic Trainers Association. Official Statement from the National Athletic Trainers' Association on Community-Acquired MRSA Infections (CA-MRSA). 2005. Accessed November 13, 2022. www.nata.org/sites/default/files/mrsa.pdf

53. National Collegiate Athletics Association. Appendix C - Skin Infections in Wrestling. In: Follis A, ed. *21-22 and 22-23 Wrestling Rules Book*. National Collegiate Athletics Association; 2019:99-102.

54. National Federation of State High School Associations. Sports-Related Skin Infections Position Statement and Guideline. Updated January 2022. Accessed November 12, 2022. www.nfhs.org/media/5546437/2022-nfhs-sports-related-skin-infections-position-statement-and-guidelines-final-3-8-22.pdf

55. Rao J. Acne vulgaris. Medscape. 2020 Updated August 27, 2020. Accessed November 12, 2022. http://emedicine.medscape.com/article/1069804-overview

56. Ayoade FO. Herpes simplex. Medscape. 2021 Updated May 24, 2021. Accessed November 11, 2022. http://emedicine.medscape.com/article/218580-overview

57. Landry GL, Chang CJ, Harmon KG, et al. Herpes and tinea in wrestling: Managing outbreaks, knowing when to disqualify. *Phys Sportsmed*. 2004;32(10):34-42.

58. Landry GL, Chang CJ, D. Mees P, et al. Treating and avoiding herpes and tinea infections in contact sports. *Phys Sportsmed*. 2004;32(10):43-44.

59. Cyr PR, Dexter W. Viral skin infection: Preventing outbreaks in sports settings. *Phys Sportsmed*. 2004;32(7):33-38.

60. Awasthi S, Friedman HM. An mRNA vaccine to prevent genital herpes. *Transl Res*. 2022;242:56-65.

61. Janniger CK. Herpes zoster. Medscape. 2021. Accessed June 2, 2022. http://emedicine.medscape.com/article/1132465-overview

62. Khan ZZ. Varicella-zoster virus (VZV). Medscape. Updated September 30, 2022. Accessed November 11, 2022. http://emedicine.medscape.com/article/231927-overview

63. Khan ZZ. Varicella-zoster virus (VZV) medication. Medscape. Updated September 30, 2022. Accessed October 25, 2022. https://emedicine.medscape.com/article/231927-medication#3

64. Bhatia AC. Molluscum contagiosum. Medscape. Updated September 21, 2020. Accessed November 10, 2022. http://emedicine.medscape.com/article/910570-overview

65. Gearhart PA. Human papillomavirus (HPV). Medscape. Updated February 20, 2020. Accessed November 9, 2022. http://emedicine.medscape.com/article/219110-overview

66. Handler MZ. Tinea capitis. Medscape. Updated February 21, 2020. Accessed November 12, 2022. http://emedicine.medscape.com/article/1091351-overview

67. Nowicka D, Bagłaj-Oleszczuk M, Maj J. Infectious diseases of the skin in contact sports. *Adv Clin Exp Med*. 2020;29(12):1491-1495.

68. Paradise SL, Hu Y-WE. Infectious dermatoses in sport: A review of diagnosis, management, and return-to-play recommendations. *Curr Sports Med Rep*. 2021;20(2):92-103.

69. Shukla S. Tinea corporis. Medscape. Updated September 17, 2020. Accessed November 9, 2022. http://emedicine.medscape.com/article/1091473-overview

70. Winderkehr M. Tinea curis. Medscape. Updated September 11, 2020. Accessed November 9, 2022. http://emedicine.medscape.com/article/1091806-overview

71. Robbins CM. Tinea pedis. Medscape. Updated September 11, 2020. Accessed November 11, 2022. http://emedicine.medscape.com/article/1091684-overvie

72. Sayed C. Tinea versicolor clinical presentation. Medscape. Updated June 9, 2020. Accessed November 10, 2022. http://emedicine.medscape.com/article/1091575-clinical

73. Barry ME. Scabies. Medscape. Updated October 12, 2020. Accessed November 10, 2022. http://emedicine.medscape.com/article/1109204-overview

74. Guenther LCC. Pediculosis and pthiriasis (lice infestation). Medscape. 2019. Accessed November 29, 2022. https://emedicine.medscape.com/article/225013-overview

75. Centers for Disease Control and Prevention. Scabies—Treatment. Updated October 31, 2018. Accessed November 12, 2022. www.cdc.gov/parasites/scabies/treatment.html

76. Centers for Disease Control and Prevention. Head lice—Treatment. Updated October 15, 2019. Accessed November 12, 2022. www.cdc.gov/parasites/lice/head/treatment.html

77. Centers for Disease Control and Prevention. Sexually Transmitted Disease Surveillance 2020. Updated April 12, 2022. Accessed November 18, 2022. www.cdc.gov/std/statistics/2020/overview.htm#Syphilis

78. U.S. National Library of Medicine. Reportable diseases. 2022. Accessed March 17, 2022. https://medlineplus.gov/ency/article/001929.htm

79. Centers for Disease Control and Prevention. Division of Vector-Borne Diseases (DVBD). Updated February 11, 2022. Accessed October 20, 2022. www.cdc.gov/ncezid/dvbd

80. Arnold TC. Brown recluse spider envenomation. Medscape. Updated October 14, 2021. Accessed November 11, 2022. http://emedicine.medscape.com/article/772295-overview

81. Patti L, Bryczkowski C, Landgraf B. Brown recluse spider bite. *J Edu Teach Emerg Med*. 2019;4(3):V30-V32.

82. Burns BD. Insect bites. Medscape. 2021. Accessed November 30, 2022. https://emedicine.medscape.com/article/769067-overview

83. Diehl K, Lindwedel KS, Mathes S, Görig T, Gefeller O. Tanning bed legislation for minors: A comprehensive international comparison. *Children (Basel)*. 2022;9(6):768.

Chapter 17

1. World Health Organization. Fact sheets: Mental disorders. Accessed August 2, 2022. www.who.int/news-room/fact-sheets/detail/mental-disorders

2. World Health Organization. The World Health Report 2020: Mental Health. Accessed March 2022. www.who.int/health-topics/mental-health#tab=tab_2

3. American Psychiatric Association. *Diagnostic and Statistical Manual of Mental Disorders*. 5th ed. American Psychiatric Association; 2013.

4. Knudsen-Martin C, Huenergardt D. A socio-emotional approach to couple therapy: Linking social context and couple interaction. *Fam Process*. 2010;49:369-384.

5. Gouttebarge V, Castaldelli-Maia JM, Gorczynski P, et al. Occurrence of mental health symptoms and disorders in current and former elite athletes: A systematic review and meta-analysis. *Br J Sports Med*. s2019;53(11):700-706.

6. National Collegiate Athletics Association. 2022-23 NCAA banned drugs. Updated 2022. Accessed July 20, 2022. www.ncaa.org/2015-16-ncaa-banned-drugs

7. Anxiety and Depression Association of America. Anxiety disorders. Accessed April 20, 2022. https://adaa.org

8. Bhatia MS, Goyal A. Anxiety disorders in children and adolescents: Need for early detection. *J Postgrad Med*. 2018;64(2):75-76.

9. Spitzer RL, Kroenke K, Williams JBW, Lowe B. A brief measure for assessing generalized anxiety disorder: The GAD-7. *Arch Intern Med*. 2006;166(10):1092-1097.

10. Junge A, Feddermann-Demont N. Prevalence of depression and anxiety in top-level male and female football players. *BMJ Open Sport Exerc Med*. 2016;2(1):e000087.

11. Good BJ, Kleinman AM. Culture and anxiety: Cross-cultural evidence for the patterning of anxiety disorders. In: *Anxiety and the Anxiety Disorders*. Routledge; 2019:297-324.

12. Jefferies P, Ungar M. Social anxiety in young people: A prevalence study in seven countries. *PLoS One*. 2020;15(9):e0239133.

13. Mangolini VI, Andrade LH, Lotufo-Neto F, Wang Y-P. Treatment of anxiety disorders in clinical practice: A critical overview of recent systematic evidence. *Clinics (Sao Paulo)*. 2019;74:e1316.

14. Valdes B, Salani D, King B, De Oliveira GC. Recognition and treatment of psychiatric emergencies for health care providers in the emergency department: Panic attack, panic disorder, and adverse drug reactions. *J Emerg Nur*. 2021;47(3):459-468.

15. Karthikeyan V, Nalinashini G, Raja EA. A study of panic attack disorder in human beings and different treatment methods. *J Crit Rev*. 2020;7:1166-1169.

16. Macauley K, Plummer L, Bemis C, Brock G, Larson C, Spangler J. Prevalence and predictors of anxiety in healthcare professions students. *Health Prof Educ*. 2018;4(3):176-185.

17. Asnaani A, Richey JA, Dimaite R, Hinton DE, Hofmann SG. A cross-ethnic comparison of lifetime prevalence rates of anxiety disorders. *J Nerv Ment Dis*. 2010;198(8):551-555.

18. Bonfils KA, Lysaker PH, Yanos PT, et al. Self-stigma in PTSD: Prevalence and correlates. *Psychiatry Res*. 2018;265:7-12.

19. Hoppen TH, Morina N. The prevalence of PTSD and major depression in the global population of adult war survivors: A meta-analytically informed estimate in absolute numbers. *Eur J Psychotraumatol.* 2019;10(1):1578637.

20. Lateef T, Witonsky K, He J, Ries Merikangas K. Headaches and sleep problems in US adolescents: Findings from the National Comorbidity Survey–Adolescent Supplement (NCS-A). *Cephalalgia.* 2019;39(10):1226-1235.

21. Ferentinos P, Preti A, Veroniki AA, et al. Comorbidity of obsessive-compulsive disorder in bipolar spectrum disorders: Systematic review and meta-analysis of its prevalence. *J Affect Disord.* 2020;263:193-208.

22. Anxiety and Depression Association of America. Generalized anxiety disorder (GAD). August 2, 2022. https://adaa.org/understanding-anxiety/generalized-anxiety-disorder-gad

23. Reardon CL, Factor RM. Considerations in the use of stimulants in sport. *Sports Med.* 2016;46(5):611-617.

24. Reardon CL. The sports psychiatrist and psychiatric medication. *Int Rev Psychiatry.* 2016;28(6):606-613.

25. Roy-Byrne P, Russo J, Dugdale DC, Lessler D, Cowley D, Katon W. Undertreatment of panic disorder in primary care: Role of patient and physician characteristics. *J Am Board Fam Pract.* 2002;15(6):443-450.

26. Fleming L. *Anxiety: Specific Phobias Management (Behavioral Health).* Elsevier; 2020.

27. Hedden S, Kennet J, Lipari R. *Behavior Health Trends in the United States: Results From the 2014 National Survey on Drug Use and Health.* Substance Abuse and Mental Health Services Administration; 2014.

28. World Health Organization. *World Health Statistics 2022.* World Health Organization; 2022.

29. Deng J, Zhou F, Hou W, et al. The prevalence of depressive symptoms, anxiety symptoms and sleep disturbance in higher education students during the COVID-19 pandemic: A systematic review and meta-analysis. *Psychiatry Res.* 2021;301:113863.

30. Gorczynski PF, Coyle M, Gibson K. Depressive symptoms in high-performance athletes and non-athletes: A comparative meta-analysis. *Br J Sports Med.* 2017;51(18):1348-1354.

31. Coyle M, Gorczynski P, Gibson K. "You have to be mental to jump off a board any way": Elite divers' conceptualizations and perceptions of mental health. *Psychol Sport Exerc.* 2017;29:10-18.

32. Choi KW, Kim YK, Jeon HJ. Comorbid anxiety and depression: Clinical and conceptual consideration and transdiagnostic treatment. *Adv Exp Med Biol.* 2020;1191:219-235.

33. de Haan S. Bio-psycho-social interaction: An enactive perspective. *Int Rev Psychiatry.* 2021;33(5):471-477.

34. Drew M, Vlahovich N, Hughes D, et al. Prevalence of illness, poor mental health and sleep quality and low energy availability prior to the 2016 Summer Olympic Games. *Br J Sports Med.* 2018;52(1):47-53.

35. Grandner MA, Hall C, Jaszewski A, et al. Mental health in student athletes: Associations with sleep duration, sleep quality, insomnia, fatigue, and sleep apnea symptoms. *Athl Train Sports Health Care.* 2021;13(4):e159-e167.

36. Kroenke K, Spitzer RL, Williams JB. The PHQ-9: Validity of a brief depression severity measure. *J Gen Intern Med.* 2001;16(9):606-613.

37. Beard C, Hsu K, Rifkin L, Busch A, Björgvinsson T. Validation of the PHQ-9 in a psychiatric sample. *J Affect Disord.* 2016;193:267-273.

38. Baron DA, Baron SH, Tompkins J, Polat A. Assessing and treating depression in athletes. In: Baron D, Reardon C, Baron S, eds. *Clinical Sports Psychiatry: An International Perspective.* Wiley-Blackwell; 2013.

39. Larzelere MM, James E III, Arcuri M. Treating depression: What works besides meds? *J Fam Practice.* 2015;64(8):454-459A.

40. Park LT, Zarate CA Jr. Depression in the primary care setting. *New Engl J Med.* 2019;380(6):559-568.

41. van Eeden AE, van Hoeken D, Hoek HW. Incidence, prevalence and mortality of anorexia nervosa and bulimia nervosa. *Curr Opin Psychiatry.* 2021;34(6):515-524.

42. Smink F, van Hoeken D, Hoek H. Epidemiology of eating disorders: Incidence, prevalence and mortality rates. *Curr Psychiatry Rep.* 2012;14(4):406-414.

43. Mancine RP, Gusfa DW, Moshrefi A, Kennedy SF. Prevalence of disordered eating in athletes categorized by emphasis on leanness and activity type—A systematic review. *J Eat Disord.* 2020;8:47.

44. Bratland-Sanda S, Sundgot-Borgen J. Eating disorders in athletes: Overview of prevalence, risk factors and recommendations for prevention and treatment. *Eur J Sport Sci.* 2013;13(5):499-508.

45. Joy E, Kussman A, Nattiv A. 2016 update on eating disorders in athletes: A comprehensive narrative review with a focus on clinical assessment and management. *Br J Sports Med.* 2016;50(3):154-162.

46. van Eeden AE, van Hoeken D, Hoek HW. Incidence, prevalence and mortality of anorexia nervosa and bulimia nervosa. *Curr Opin Psychiatry.* 2021;34(6):515-524.

47. Dobrescu SR, Dinkler L, Gillberg C, Råstam M, Gillberg C, Wentz E. Anorexia nervosa: 30-year outcome. *Br J Psychiatry.* 2020;216(2):97-104.

48. Hilbert A. Binge-eating disorder. *Psychiatr Clin North Am.* 2019;42(1):33-43.

49. Kaye WH, Bulik CM. Treatment of patients with anorexia nervosa in the US—A crisis in care. *JAMA Psychiatry.* 2021;78(6):591-592.

50. Raevuori A, Keski-Rahkonen A, Hoek HW. A review of eating disorders in males. *Curr Opin Psychiatry.* 2014;27(6):426-430.

51. Currie A, Blauwet C, Bindra A, et al. Athlete mental health: Future directions. *Br J Sports Med.* 2021;55(22):1243-1244.

52. McCance-Katz EF. The Substance Abuse and Mental Health Services Administration (SAMHSA): New directions. *Psychiatr Services*. 2018;69(10):1046-1048.

53. Centers for Disease Control and Prevention. Adolescent Behaviors and Experiences Survey (ABES). Accessed August 18, 2022. www.cdc.gov/healthyyouth/data/abes.htm?s_cid=tw-zaza-2022-abes

54. Jones CM, Clayton HB, Deputy NP, et al. Prescription opioid misuse and use of alcohol and other substances among high school students—Youth Risk Behavior Survey, United States, 2019. *MMWR Suppl*. 2020;69(1):38-46.

55. Centers for Disease Control and Prevention. Binge drinking. www.cdc.gov/alcohol/fact-sheets/binge-drinking.htm

56. National Institute on Drug Abuse. Overdose death rates. Accessed August 18, 2022. https://nida.nih.gov/research-topics/trends-statistics/overdose-death-rates

57. National Institutes of Health. *Misuse of Prescription Drugs Research Report*. 2022. Accessed August 2022. www.nlm.nih.gov/medlineplus/prescriptiondrugabuse.html

58. Tolliver BK, Anton RF. Assessment and treatment of mood disorders in the context of substance abuse. *Dialogues Clin Neurosci*. 2015;17(2):181-190.

59. Bahji A, Mazhar MN, Hudson CC, Nadkarni P, MacNeil BA, Hawken E. Prevalence of substance use disorder comorbidity among individuals with eating disorders: A systematic review and meta-analysis. *Psychiatry Res*. 2019;273:58-66.

60. Mowlem FD, Rosenqvist MA, Martin J, Lichtenstein P, Asherson P, Larsson H. Sex differences in predicting ADHD clinical diagnosis and pharmacological treatment. *Eur Child Adolesc Psychiatry*. 2019;28(4):481-489.

61. Faraone SV, Banaschewski T, Coghill D, et al. The World Federation of ADHD International Consensus Statement: 208 evidence-based conclusions about the disorder. *Neurosci Biobehav Rev*. 2021;128:789-818.

62. Han DH, McDuff D, Thompson D, Hitchcock ME, Reardon CL, Hainline B. Attention-deficit/hyperactivity disorder in elite athletes: A narrative review. *Br J Sports Med*. 2019;53(12):741-745.

63. Katzman MA, Bilkey TS, Chokka PR, Fallu A, Klassen LJ. Adult ADHD and comorbid disorders: Clinical implications of a dimensional approach. *BMC Psychiatry*. 2017;17(1):302.

64. World Anti-Doping Agency. Therapeutic use exemptions. Accessed April 20, 2022. www.wada-ama.org/en/athletes-support-personnel/therapeutic-use-exemptions-tues

65. Kuriala GK. Covid-19 and its impact on global mental health. *Sens Int*. 2021;2:100108.

66. Prochaska JO, DiClemente CC. Stages and processes of self-change of smoking: Toward an integrative model of change. *J Consult Clin Psychol*. 1983;51(3):390-395.

67. Littell JH, Girvin H. Stages of change: A critique. *Behavi Modif*. 2002;26(2):223-273.

68. Prochaska JO, Norcross JC, DiClemente CC. Applying the stages of change. *Psychother Australia*. 2013;19(2):10-15.

69. Parsons JT. *2014-15 NCAA Sports Medicine Handbook*. 25th ed. National Collegiate Athletics Association; 2014.

70. American Association for Marriage and Family Therapy. Code of Ethics. 2015. Accessed October 5, 2023. www.aamft.org/Legal_Ethics/Code_of_Ethics.aspx

Chapter 18

1. Molina M. Meet the 21 military veterans representing Team USA at the Paralympic Games. US Department of Veterans Affairs. Updated August 27, 2021. Accessed October 17, 2022. https://news.va.gov/93655/meet-the-21-military-veterans-representing-team-usa-at-the-paralympic-games

2. Vergun D. Military athletes represent US at Tokyo Olympics. U.S. Department of Defense. 2021. Accessed October 17, 2022. www.defense.gov/News/News-Stories/Article/Article/2690855/19-military-athletes-to-represent-us-at-tokyo-olympics

3. Invictus Games Foundation. Invictus Games. 2022. Accessed September 11, 2022. https://invictusgamesfoundation.org/foundation/story

4. National Center for Education Statistics. Number and percentage of children served under Individuals with Disabilities Act: Institute of Educational Sciences; 2020-2021. Accessed September 11, 2022. https://nces.ed.gov/programs/digest/d21/tables/dt21_204.70.asp

5. Fagher K, Dahlstrom O, Jacobsson J, et al. Injuries and illnesses in Swedish Paralympic athletes: A 52-week prospective study of incidence and risk factors. *Scand J Med Sci Sports*. 2020;30(8):1457-1470.

6. Ferrara MS, Buckley WE. Athletes with disabilities injury registry. *Adapt Phys Activ Q*. 1996;13(1):50-60.

7. DePauw KP, Gavron SJ. *Disability Sport*. Human Kinetics; 2005.

8. Boyajian-O'Neill L, Cardone D, Dexter W, et al. The preparticipation examination for the athlete with special needs: Working Group of the Preparticipation Physical Evaluation. *Phys Sportsmed*. 2004;32(9):13-42.

9. Patel DR, Greydanus DE. The pediatric athlete with disabilities. *Pediatr Clin North Am*. 2002;49(4):803-827.

10. Ramirez M, Yang J, Bourque L, et al. Sports injuries to high school athletes with disabilities. *Pediatrics*. 2009;123(2):690-696.

11. Gawroński W, Sobiecka J. The development of medical care in Polish Paralympic sport. *Rehabilitacja Medyczna*. 2018;22(4):39-48.

12. Hawkeswood JP, O'Connor R, Anton H, et al. The preparticipation evaluation for athletes with disability. *Int J Sports Phys Ther*. 2014;9(1):103.

13. Siow HM, Cameron DB, Ganley TJ. Preparticipation sports evaluation: Issues for healthy children and athletes with disabilities. *J Pediatr Orthop*. 2010;30:S10-S20.

14. Jacob T, Hutzler Y. Sports-medical assessment for athletes with a disability. *Disabil Rehabil*. 1998;20(3):116-119.

15. Roberts TT, Leonard GR, Cepela DJ. Classifications in brief: American Spinal Injury Association (ASIA) Impairment Scale. *Clin Orthop Relat Res.* 2017;475(5):1499-1504.

16. Kirshblum S, Snider B, Rupp R, et al. Updates of the international standards for neurologic classification of spinal cord injury: 2015 and 2019. *Phys Med Rehabil Clin N Am.* 2020;31(3):319-330.

17. Dec KL, Sparrow KJ, McKeag DB. The physically-challenged athlete. *Sports Med.* 2000;29(4):245-258.

18. Patel DR, Greydanus DE. Sport participation by physically and cognitively challenged young athletes. *Pediatr Clin North Am.* 2010;57(3):795-817.

19. Black SA. Triathlon participation for the physically challenged athlete: Medical considerations. *Curr Sports Med Rep.* 2007;6(3):195-199.

20. Allen KJ, Leslie SW. Autonomic Dysreflexia. In: *StatPearls.* Treasure Island (FL): StatPearls Publishing; May 30, 2023.

21. Wan D, Krassioukov AV. Life-threatening outcomes associated with autonomic dysreflexia: A clinical review. *J Spinal Cord Med.* 2014;37(1):2-10.

22. Krassioukov A. Autonomic dysreflexia: Current evidence related to unstable arterial blood pressure control among athletes with spinal cord injury. *Clin J Sport Med.* 2012;22(1):39-45.

23. Sparkes AC, Brighton J. Autonomic dysreflexia and boosting in disability sport: Exploring the subjective meanings, management strategies, moral justifications, and perceptions of risk among male, spinal cord injured, wheelchair athletes. *Qual Res Sport Exerc Health.* 2020;12(3):414-430.

24. Sherrill C. A*dapted Physical Activity, Recreation, and Sport: Crossdisciplinary and Lifespan.* 6th ed. McGraw-Hill; 2004.

25. Bhambhani Y, Mactavish J, Warren S, et al. Boosting in athletes with high-level spinal cord injury: Knowledge, incidence and attitudes of athletes in Paralympic sport. *Disabil Rehabil.* 2010;32(26):2172-2190.

26. Mazzeo F, Santamaria S, Iavarone A. "Boosting" in Paralympic athletes with spinal cord injury: Doping without drugs. *Funct Neurol.* 2015;30(2):91-98.

27. Griggs KE, Price MJ, Goosey-Tolfrey VL. Cooling athletes with a spinal cord injury. *Sports Med.* 2015;45(1):9-21.

28. Grossman F, Flueck JL, Perret C, Meeusen R, Roelands B. The thermoregulatory and thermal responses of individuals with a spinal cord injury during exercise, acclimation and by using cooling strategies-a systematic review. *Front Physiol.* 2021;12:636997.

29. Goosey-Tolfrey V, Paulson T, Graham-Paulson T. Practical considerations for fluid replacement for athletes with a spinal cord injury. In: Meyer F, Szygula Z, Wilk B, eds. *Fluid Balance, Hydration, and Athletic Performance.* CRC Press; 2016:333-355.

30. Casa DJ, DeMartini JK, Bergeron MF, et al. National Athletic Trainers' Association position statement: Exertional heat illnesses. *J Athl Train.* 2015;50(9):986-1000.

31. Hosokawa Y, Adami PE, Stephenson BT, et al. Prehospital management of exertional heat stroke at sports competitions for Paralympic athletes. *Br J Sports Med.* 2022;56(11):599-604.

32. Anderson M, Barnum M. *Foundations of Athletic Training: Prevention, Assessment, and Management.* Lippincott Williams & Wilkins; 2021.

33. Kasitinon D, Royston A, Wernet L, et al. Health-related incidents among intercollegiate wheelchair basketball players. *PM R.* 2021;13(7):746-755.

34. Zarkou A F-FE. The influence of physiologic and atmospheric variables on spasticity after spinal cord injury. *NeuroRehabilitation.* 2021;48(3):353-363.

35. Walter M, Ruiz I, Squair JW, et al. Prevalence of self-reported complications associated with intermittent catheterization in wheelchair athletes with spinal cord injury. *Spinal Cord.* 2021;59(9):1018-1025.

36. Poirier C, Dinh A, Salomon J, et al. Prevention of urinary tract infections by antibiotic cycling in spinal cord injury patients and low emergence of multidrug resistant bacteria. *Med Mal Infect.* 2016;46(6):294-299.

37. Copp AJ, Adzick NS, Chitty LS, et al. Spina bifida. *Nat Rev Dis Primers.* 2015;1(1):15007.

38. Umphred DA, Lazaro RT. *Neurological Rehabilitation.* Elsevier Health Sciences; 2012.

39. Soler GJ, Bao M, Jaiswal D, et al. Focus: Medical technology: A review of cerebral shunts, current technologies, and future endeavors. *Yale J Biol Med.* 2018;91(3):313-321.

40. Nath A, Smith BR, Thakur KT. Major advances in neuroinfectious diseases in the past two decades. *Lancet Neurol.* 2022;21(4):308-310.

41. National Library of Medicine. Polio and Post-Polio Syndrome. 2022. Accessed March 17, 2022. https://medlineplus.gov/polioandpostpoliosyndrome.html

42. Lai AM, Stanish WD, Stanish HI. The young athlete with physical challenges. *Clin Sports Med.* 2000;19(4):793-819.

43. National Federation of State High School Associations. NFHS rules changes affecting risk (1982-2021). 2021. Accessed September 19, 2022. www.nfhs.org/media/4860165/1982-2021-nfhs-risk-minimization-rules-final-9-8-21.pdf

44. Parsons J. NCAA Guideline 3a: Protective Equipment. In: Parsons JT. *2014-15 NCAA Sports Medicine Handbook.* 25th ed. National Collegiate Athletics Association; 2014:104-108.

45. Anderson TM, McKirgan KL, Hastings JD. Seated pressures in daily wheelchair and sports equipment: Investigating the protective effects of cushioned shorts. *Spinal Cord Ser Cases.* 2018;4(47):47-53.

46. Moore G, Durstine JL, Painter P, et al. *ACSM's Exercise Management for Persons With Chronic Diseases and Disabilities*. 4th ed. Human Kinetics; 2016.

47. Meier NF, Lee DC, Sui X, Blair SN. Physical activity, cardiorespiratory fitness, and incident glaucoma. *Med Sci Sports Exerc*. 2018;50(11):2253-2258.

48. Winnick JP, Porretta DL. *Adapted Physical Education and Sport*. Human Kinetics; 2016.

49. Buchman CA, Gifford RH, Haynes DS, et al. Unilateral cochlear implants for severe, profound, or moderate sloping to profound bilateral sensorineural hearing loss: A systematic review and consensus statements. *JAMA Otolaryngol Head Neck Surg*. 2020;146(10):942-953.

50. American Psychiatric Association. *Diagnostic and Statistical Manual of Mental Disorders*. 5th ed Text Revision. American Psychiatric Association; 2022.

51. Zeldin AS. Intellectual disability. Medscape. Updated November 16, 2021. Accessed September 19, 2022. https://emedicine.medscape.com/article/1180709-overview#a8

52. Klenck C, Gebke K. Practical management: Common medical problems in disabled athletes. *Clin J Sport Med*. 2007;17(1):55-60.

53. Bottos S, Chambers C, Oberlander T, et al. *Pain in Children and Adults with Developmental Disabilities*. Brookes; 2006.

54. Birrer RB. The Special Olympics athlete: Evaluation and clearance for participation. *Clin Pediatr*. 2004;43(9):777-782.

55. ASIA and ISCoS International Standards Committee. The 2019 revision of the International Standards for Neurological Classification of Spinal Cord Injury (ISNCSCI)—What's new? *Spinal Cord*. 2019;57:815-817.

56. Maloney PL, Pumpa KL, Miller J, Thompson KG, Jay O. Extended post-exercise hyperthermia in athletes with a spinal cord injury. *J Sci Med Sport*. 2021;24(8):831-836.

57. Forsyth P, Miller J, Pumpa K, Thompson KG, Jay O. Independent influence of spinal cord injury level on thermoregulation during exercise. *Med Sci Sports Exerc*. 2019;51(8):1710-1719.

58. Sherrill C. *Adapted Physical Activity, Recreation and Sport: Cross Disciplinary and Lifespan*. 6th ed. McGraw Hill; 2004.

59. Crutchfield KE. Managing patients with neurological disorders who participate in sports. *Sports Neurol*. 2014;20(6):1657-1666.

60. Sparks AC & Brighton, J. Autonomic dysreflexia and boosting in disability sport: Exploring the subjective meanings, management strategies, moral justifications, and perceptions of risk among male, spinal cord injured, wheelchair athletes. *Qualitative Research in Sport, Exercise and Health*. 2020;12(3):414-430.

INDEX

ABOUT THE AUTHORS

Katie Walsh Flanagan, EdD, ATC, LAT, is a professor in the department of health education and promotion at East Carolina University (ECU), where she has worked for over two and a half decades, and is a certified athletic trainer by the Board of Certification (BOC). She was hired in 1995 as director of the sports medicine and athletic training program at East Carolina University; served as a lecturer and assistant athletic trainer at California State University, Fresno; and served as the head athletic trainer for the Chicago Power, a men's professional soccer team. She has also assisted as an athletic trainer for various sports in international competitions, including the 1996 Summer Olympic Games and the 1987 Pan American Games. Flanagan is a practicing athletic trainer and has volunteered in ECU Athletics for the past 28 years. In 2012, Flanagan was elected to the North Carolina Athletic Trainers' Association Hall of Fame. The organization named her the College/University Athletic Trainer of the Year in 2000 and 2006. In 2023 she was elected to the Mid-Atlantic Athletic Trainers' Association Hall of Fame. She received the National Athletic Trainers' Association (NATA) Most Distinguished Athletic Trainer Award in 2010 and NATA's Service Award in 2006. In 2017, she was named a NATA board member as the director of District Three, where she served until 2022. Flanagan is an author of three medical textbooks and a prolific speaker on athletic emergencies and on weather and safety policies.

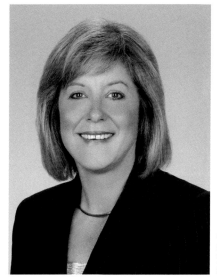
© Katie Walsh Flanagan

Micki Cuppett, EdD, LAT, ATC, FNAP, has more than 30 years of experience as an athletic trainer, medical educator, and administrator. She has directed athletic training programs at two universities, both at the undergraduate and graduate levels. In addition to educating athletic training students, Micki also taught medical, nursing, physical therapy, and pharmacology students in the University of South Florida College of Medicine and helped initiate the interprofessional education program. She is now a consultant in the areas of strategic planning, interprofessional education, leadership, accreditation, AT education, medical simulation, and innovation.

Prior to starting her own consulting business, Cuppett was the executive director for the Commission on Accreditation of Athletic Training Education (CAATE). During her tenure in the position, she oversaw the successful recognition of CAATE by the Council for Higher Education Accreditation, converted all accreditation documentation and processes to an electronic platform, and implemented an entirely virtual office. She is a fellow of the National Academies of Practice and the USF Health Leadership Institute. Cuppett has received numerous professional awards and hall of fame inductions throughout her professional career.

© Micki Cuppett

CONTRIBUTORS

Tamara C. Valovich McLeod, PhD, ATC, FNATA
  Professor
  Director of Athletic Training Programs
  A.T. Still University
  Mesa, Arizona

Layne A. Prest, PhD, LIMHP, LMFT
  Couple and Family Therapist at PeaceHealth Southwest
  Washington
  Behavioral Scientist at Family Medicine Residency
  Clinical Assistant Professor at University of Washington
  Vancouver, Washington

A special thank-you to these contributors for their work on the previous editions:

Joseph Armen, DO

Helen E. Bateman, MD

Larry Collins, PA-C, DFAAPA, ATC

Christine Curran, MD

David Eichenbaum, MD

Richard Figler, MD

Joseph Garry, MD, CAQ, FACSM

Todd L. Kanzenbach, MD, CAQ

Lawrence J. Kusior, MD, FAAOS

Mary H. Lien, MD

Sara McDade, MD

Monique Mokha, PhD, ATC

Tiffany O'Connor, MS, ATC/L, OTC

Sally A. Perkins, MS, ATC, CAATE

Arnold M. Ramirez, MD

Dorraine Reynolds, PharmD

Patrick Sexton, EdD, ATC, CSCS

Charles B. Slonim, MD, FACS

Laurie Small, MD

Bryan W. Smith, MD, PhD

Kevin B. Sneed, PharmD, CRPh

Daniel J. Van Durme, MD, FAAFP

M. Craig Whaley, MD

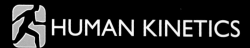
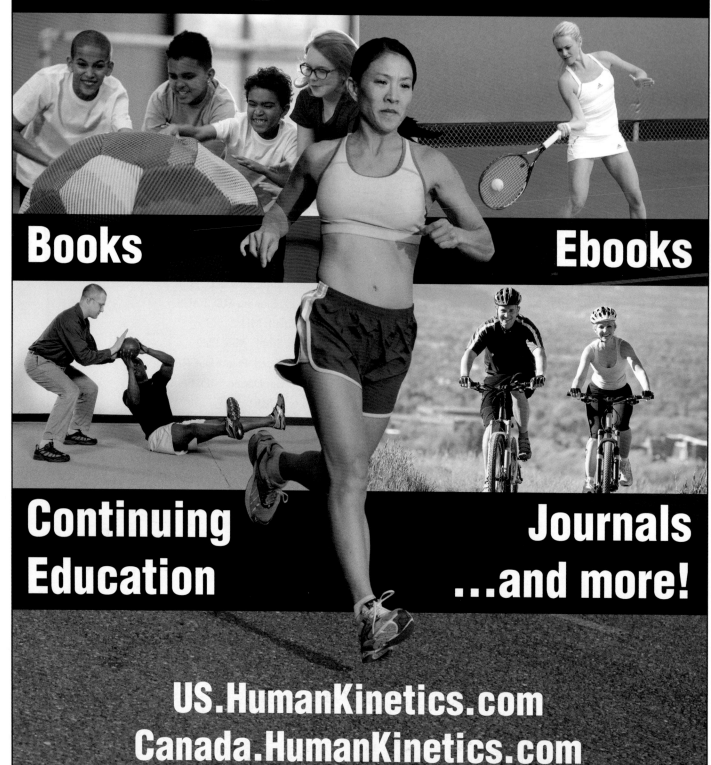